PAIN MANAGEMENT

ANESTHESIOLOGY: A PROBLEM-BASED LEARNING APPROACH SERIES

Pain Management
Edited by Magdalena Anitescu

PAIN MANAGEMENT

A PROBLEM-BASED LEARNING APPROACH

EDITED BY

Magdalena Anitescu, MD, PhD

ASSOCIATE PROFESSOR
DIRECTOR, PAIN MEDICINE FELLOWSHIP PROGRAM SECTION CHIEF
DIVISION OF PAIN MANAGEMENT DEPARTMENT OF ANESTHESIA AND CRITICAL CARE
UNIVERSITY OF CHICAGO MEDICAL CENTER

OXFORD
UNIVERSITY PRESS

OXFORD
UNIVERSITY PRESS

Oxford University Press is a department of the University of Oxford. It furthers the University's objective of excellence in research, scholarship, and education by publishing worldwide. Oxford is a registered trade mark of Oxford University Press in the UK and certain other countries.

Published in the United States of America by Oxford University Press
198 Madison Avenue, New York, NY 10016, United States of America.

Library of Congress Cataloging-in-Publication Data
Names: Anitescu, Magdalena, editor.
Title: Pain management: a problem-based learning approach /
edited by Magdalena Anitescu.
Other titles: Pain management (Anitescu)
Description: New York, NY: Oxford University Press, [2018] |
Includes bibliographical references.
Identifiers: LCCN 2018011687 | ISBN 9780190271787 (hardcover)
Subjects: | MESH: Pain Management | Problem-Based Learning
Classification: LCC RB127 | NLM WL 704.6 | DDC 616/.0472—dc23
LC record available at https://lccn.loc.gov/2018011687

1 3 5 7 9 8 6 4 2

Printed by Sheridan Books, Inc., United States of America

CONTENTS

CONTRIBUTORS

Hassan Aboumerhi, MD
Department of Anesthesia and Critical Care
University of Chicago Medicine
Chicago, IL

Deepti Agarwal, MD
Assistant Professor
Department of Anesthesiology and Pain Management
Advocate Illinois Masonic Medical Center
Chicago, IL

Jumana T. Alshaikh, MD
Department of Neurology
University of Chicago Medicine
Chicago, IL

Magdalena Anitescu, MD, PhD
Associate Professor
Director, Pain Medicine Fellowship Program
Section Chief, Division of Pain Management
Department of Anesthesia and Critical Care
University of Chicago Medical Center
Chicago, IL

Ajay Antony, MD
Fellow, Division of Multidisciplinary Pain Medicine
Department of Anesthesiology
University of Florida College of Medicine
Gainesville, FL

Melinda Aquino, MD
Assistant Professor of Anesthesiology
Pain Management, and Regional Anesthesiology
Albert Einstein College of Medicine
Montefiore Medical Center
Bronx, NY

David Arnolds, MD
Department of Anesthesiology and Critical Care
The University of Chicago
Chicago, IL

Juan Francisco Asenjo, MD, FRCPC
Professor
Department of Anesthesia and Alan Edwards McGill Pain Treatment Unit
McGill Center Pain Clinic
McGill University Health Centre
Montreal, QC, Canada

Ignacio Badiola, MD
Instructor of Anesthesiology
Department of Anesthesiology and Critical Care
Perelman School of Medicine
University of Pennsylvania
Philadelphia, PA

Nancy J. Beckman, PhD
Assistant Professor
Department of Psychiatry and Behavioral Neuroscience
University of Chicago
Chicago, IL

Alan Berkman, MD
Physician Lead
Complex Pain Program
St. Paul's Hospital
Vancouver, BC, Canada

Esther Caballero-Manrique, MD, PhD
Center for Pain Medicine
Department of Anesthesiology
University of Vermont Medical Center
Burlington, VT

Randy L. Calisoff, MD
Department of Physical Medicine and Rehabilitation
Northwestern University Feinberg School of Medicine
Chicago, IL

Kenneth D. Candido, MD
Advocate Illinois Masonic Medical Center
Chicago, IL

Benjamin Cantu, MD
Advocate Illinois Masonic Medical Center
Chicago, IL

Sarah Choxi, MD
Clinical Associate
Anesthesia & Critical Care
The University of Chicago
Chicago, IL

Andrea Dellaria, MD
Musculoskeletal Fellow
Department of Neurology
University of Chicago
Chicago, IL

David Dickerson, MD
Department of Anesthesia and Critical Care
Division of Pain Management
University of Chicago Medicine
Chicago, IL

Bora Dinc, MD
Advocate Illinois Masonic Medical Center
Chicago, IL

Dan Dirzu, MD
Anesthesia and Intensive Care Consultant
Emergency County Hospital Cluj-Napoca
University of Medicine and Pharmacy "Iuliu Hatieganu" Cluj
Cluj-Napoca, Romania

Ali Ebrahimi, MD
Interventional Pain Medicine Fellow
Northwestern University
Feinberg School of Medicine
Department of Anesthesiology
Evanston, IL

Nabil Elkassabany, MD, MSCE
Department of Anesthesiology and Critical Care
Perelman School of Medicine
University of Pennsylvania
Philadelphia, PA

Dalia H. Elmofty, MD
Assistant Professor
Department of Anesthesia and Critical Care
Division of Pain Management
University of Chicago Medicine
Chicago, IL

David Frim, MD
Department of Surgery
Division of Neurosurgical Surgery
University of Chicago Medicine
Chicago, IL

Shuchita Garg, MD
Clinical Assistant Professor of Anesthesiology
University of Cincinnati Medical Center
Cincinnati, OH

Alexandra Dubikovsky Golden, MD
Department of Anesthesia and Critical Care
University of Chicago Medicine
Chicago, IL

David Gordon, MD
Department of Anesthesia
Division of Pain Management
University of California at San Francisco
San Francisco, CA

Radhika P. Grandhe, MD
Assistant Professor
Department of Anesthesiology
University of New Mexico
Albuquerque, NM

John Henry Harrison, MD
Department of Anesthesia and Critical Care
University of Chicago Medicine
Chicago, IL

Julia K. Hunter, MD, MPH
Addiction Medicine Physician
UHS Binghamton General Hospital
Binghamton, NY

Ifeyinwa C. Ifeanyi, MD
Assistant Professor
Department of Anesthesiology and Perioperative Medicine
MD Anderson Cancer Center
Houston, TX

Afzaal Iqbal, MD
Pain Management Physician
Hoag Memorial Hospital Presbyterian
Newport Beach, CA

Reem Jan, MBBS
Assistant Professor
Section of Rheumatology
Department of Medicine
University of Chicago
Chicago, IL

Saima Kamal, MD
Assistant Professor
Department of Anesthesiology and Pain Medicine
University of Oklahoma Health Sciences Center
Oklahoma City, OK

Joel Kent, MD
Professor of Anesthesiology
Physical Medicine and Rehabilitation Director
Division of Pain Medicine University of Rochester
School of Medicine and Dentistry
Rochester, NY

Ahmad Khattab, DO
Department of Anesthesia & Critical Care
The University of Chicago Medicine
Chicago, IL

Faraz Khursheed, MD
Fellow
Division of Multidisciplinary Pain Medicine
Department of Anesthesiology
University of Florida College of Medicine
Gainesville, FL

Ivana Knezevic, MD
Clinical Research Coordinator
Advocate Illinois Masonic Medical Center
Chicago, IL

Nebojsa Nick Knezevic, MD, PhD
Advocate Illinois Masonic Medical Center
Chicago, IL

Lynn Kohan, MD
University of Virginia
Charlottesville, VA

Teresa M. Kusper, DO
Advocate Illinois Masonic Medical Center
Chicago, IL

Alina Lazar, MD
Assistant Professor
Department of Anesthesia and Critical Care
University of Chicago Medicine
Chicago, IL

James Liadis, MD
Georgetown University Hospital
Washington, DC

Alexei Lissounov, MD
Advocate Illinois Masonic Medical Center
Chicago, IL

Jiabin Liu, MD, PhD
Assistant Professor
Department of Anesthesiology and Critical Care
Perelman School of Medicine
University of Pennsylvania
Philadelphia, PA

Tariq M. Malik, MD
Assistant Professor
Department of Anesthesia and Critical Care
Division of Pain Mangement
University of Chicago Medicine
Chicago, IL

Issam A. Mardini, MD, PhD
Department of Anesthesiology and Critical Care
Perelman School of Medicine
University of Pennsylvania
Philadelphia, PA

Marc O. Maybauer, MD, PhD, EDIC, FCCP, FASE
Professor and Consultant
Department of Anaesthesia
Manchester Royal Infirmary
Central Manchester University Hospitals NHS Foundation Trust
Manchester Academic Health Science Centre and University of Manchester
Manchester, UK

Andrew J. McNeil, DO
Fellow
Division of Multidisciplinary Pain Medicine
Department of Anesthesiology
University of Florida College of Medicine
Gainesville, FL

Giuliano Michelagnoli, MD
Fellow of Spine Anesthesia
Montreal General Hospital
McGill University Health Centre
Montreal, QC, Canada

Geeta Nagpal, MD
Northwestern University
Feinberg School of Medicine
Department of Anesthesiology
Evanston, IL

Christine Oryhan, MD
Anesthesiologist and Pain Medicine Physician
Associate Pain Medicine Fellowship Director
Virginia Mason Medical Center
Seattle, WA

Ovidiu Palea, MD
Anesthesiologist
Washington Metro Pain Institute
Greenbelt, MD
MedStar Washington Hospital Center
Washington, DC

Carlos A. Pino, MD
Associate Professor
Center for Pain Medicine
Department of Anesthesiology
University of Vermont Medical Center
Burlington, VT

Heena Pranav, MD
Department of Anesthesia and Critical Care
University of Chicago Medicine
Chicago, IL

Edit Racz, MD, FIPP
Péterfy Sándor Hospital and Trauma Center
Department of Anesthesia
Critical Care and Pain Medicine
Budapest, Hungary

Rahul Rastogi, MD
Clinical Associate Professor
Director of Pain Medicine
Department of Anesthesia
University of Iowa Carver College of Medicine
Iowa City, IA

Ashley Reed, MD
Department of Anesthesia and Critical Care
University of Chicago Medicine
Chicago, IL

Helene Rubeiz, MD
Associate Professor
Department of Neurology
University of Chicago Medicine
Chicago, IL

Chirag Shah, MD
Department of Anesthesia and Critical Care
University of Chicago Medicine
Chicago, IL

Nirav N. Shah, MD
Multidisciplinary Interventional Pain Fellow
Department of Anesthesiology and Critical Care
University of Chicago
Chicago, IL

Tulsi Singh, MD
Resident in Physical Medicine and Rehabilitation
Department of Physical Medicine and Rehabilitation
Perelman School of Medicine
University of Pennsylvania
Philadelphia, PA

Vinita Singh, MD
Assistant Professor of Anesthesiology
Emory University School of Medicine
Atlanta, GA

Virtaj Singh, MD
Seattle Spine and Sport
Seattle, WA

Denis Snegovskikh, MD
Adjunct Clinical Professor
Department of Anesthesiology
Yale New Haven Hospital
New Haven, CT

Dmitri Souza, MD, PhD
Clinical Professor of Anesthesiology
Ohio University
Center for Pain Medicine
Western Reserve Hospital
Cuyahoga Falls, OH

Agnes Stogicza, MD, FIPP, CIPS
University of Washington
Department of Anesthesia and Pain Medicine
Seattle, WA

Shaan Sudhakaran, MD
Department of Anesthesia and Critical Care
Division of Pain Management
University of Chicago Medicine
Chicago, IL

Marie B. Tobin, MD
Professor
Director of Consult-Liaison and Emergency Psychiatry
Department of Psychiatry and Behavioral Neuroscience
University of Chicago
Chicago, IL

Bartha Peter Tohotom, MD, FIPP
Péterfy Sándor Hospital and Trauma Center
Department of Anesthesia
Critical Care and Pain Medicine
Budapest, Hungary

Andrea Trescot, MD, FIPP
Pain and Headache Center
Wasilla, AK

Tatiana Tverdohleb, MD
Advocate Illinois Masonic Medical Center
Chicago, IL

Mercy A. Udoji, MD
Assistant Professor
Department of Anesthesiology and Perioperative Medicine
University of Alabama
Birmingham, AL

Matthew Valeriano, MD
Department of Anesthesiology and Critical Care Medicine
University of New Mexico School of Medicine
Albuquerque, NM

Kevin Vorenkamp, MD
Anesthesiologist and Pain Medicine Physician
Virginia Mason Medical Center
Seattle, WA

David R. Walega, MD
Division of Pain Medicine
Department of Anesthesiology
Northwestern University Feinberg School of Medicine
Chicago, IL

Roger Wang, DO
Schwab Rehabilitation Hospital
Chicago, IL

Daniel Warren, MD
Anesthesiologist and Pain Medicine Physician
Virginia Mason Medical Center
Seattle, WA

James Wolf, MD
Clinical Instructor
Department of Anesthesiology
Center for Pain Medicine
University of Vermont College of Medicine
Burlington, VT

Anna Woodbury, MD, CAc
Assistant Professor of Anesthesiology
Associate Program Director
Emory Multidisciplinary Pain Fellowship
Emory University School of Medicine
Division Chief for Pain Management
Veterans Affairs Medical Center
Atlanta, GA

Andrew Wuenstel, MD
Department of Anesthesiology and Critical Care
The University of Chicago School of Medicine
Chicago, IL

Sarah T. Yang, MD
Schwab Rehabilitation Hospital
Chicago, IL

Fardin Yousefshahi, MD
Associate Professor
Department of Anesthesia
Tehran University of Medical Sciences & Fellow of Regional Anesthesia and Pain Medicine
Montreal General Hospital
McGill University Health Centre
Montreal, QC, Canada

Dawen Zhang, MD
Department of Medicine
University of Chicago
Chicago, IL

DIGITAL MEDIA ACCOMPANYING THE BOOK

Individual purchasers of this book are entitled to free personal access to accompanying digital media in the online edition. Please refer to the access token card for instructions on token redemption and access.

These online ancillary materials, where available, are noted with iconography throughout the book.

✔ Test

The corresponding media can be found on *Oxford Medicine Online* at: http://oxfordmedicine.com/painmanagementreview

If you are interested in access to the complete online edition, please consult with your librarian.

1.

OCCIPITAL NEURALGIA

Andrea Dellaria, Nirav N. Shah, and Helene Rubeiz

STEM CASE AND KEY QUESTIONS

A 48-year-old female with no past medical history presents in the clinic with 3 weeks of right-sided posterior scalp pain that radiates to the top of her head. She describes the pain as "piercing" and "shooting." Her neurologic exam is normal and her pain is reproduced upon palpation of the posterior scalp in the distribution of the greater occipital nerve (GON). On the basis of the history and examination, the clinician considers the diagnosis of occipital neuralgia (ON).

WHAT IS ON? WHAT IS THE DIFFERENTIAL DIAGNOSIS?

The patient reports that she has brief episodes of sharp, shooting pain, but also has a dull ache in the same distribution that seems to be always present. She also reports skin sensitivity over the involved area that can be triggered by brushing her hair. Although the suspicion is high for ON, the clinician also takes into consideration that the patient can suffer from migraines, tension-type headache, or cervicogenic headache. In order to establish a positive diagnosis, the clinician performs an ultrasound-guided GON block that provides temporary relief.

WHAT IS THE ANATOMIC BASIS FOR ON?

Although the patient had significant relief, her pain returns quickly despite the use of a combination of local anesthetic and steroids. This prompts the clinician to conduct additional diagnostic tests, including an MRI of the cervical spine to rule out cervical disk herniation at a high spinal segment.

WHAT TYPES OF STRUCTURAL LESIONS SHOULD BE RULED OUT WHEN MAKING THE DIAGNOSIS OF ON?

In examining the newly performed MRI, the clinician looks for possible fracture, Chiari malformation, or cervical nerve compression; fortunately, no structural abnormality is noted on the patient's cervical spine MRI. She asks what could be causing her pain.

WHAT IS THE PROPOSED PATHOPHYSIOLOGIC MECHANISM FOR IDIOPATHIC ON?

In explaining to the patient why she has unrelenting pain, the clinician describes the trajectory of the GON and the fact that it may become stretched as it passes between the inferior oblique muscle of the head and the semispinalis muscle. Because the patient continues to have pain, the clinician recommends a trial of physical therapy and gabapentin.

WHAT OPTIONS FOR CONSERVATIVE MANAGEMENT ARE AVAILABLE?

The patients enrolls in physical therapy for 2 months and her pain stabilizes; however, she feels that it is still nagging, and the clinician escalates the analgesic regimen to include, in addition to 1800 mg gabapentin, baclofen 10 mg every 8 hours and amitriptyline 25 mg at bedtime. Several months later, her pain is still significant. Furthermore, she reports that her symptoms are interfering with her ability to work. She wants to know if there is anything else that can be done.

WHAT INTERVENTIONAL PROCEDURES ARE AVAILABLE?

Because an occipital nerve block (ONB) provides the patient with temporary relief for several weeks, the clinician decides to perform a radiofrequency ablation of the GON; the procedure is successful and provides the patient with excellent control of her pain to values of 1/10 to 2/10 for 6 months; however, her pain returns. The clinician discusses an occipital nerve stimulator placement with the patient. She quickly agrees to the procedure. She is once more pain-free, with excellent return of function and quality of life.

DISCUSSION

DEFINITION OF ON

The International Classification of Headache Disorders (ICHD-3) describes ON as a paroxysmal, shooting pain typically located in the area of the posterior scalp. The pain is localized to the distribution of the occipital nerve and its branches. In the ICHD-3 classification scheme, ON is grouped under the "painful cranial neuropathies and other facial pains," along with other cranial neuralgias.[1] ON can be differentiated from trigeminal and glossopharyngeal neuralgia based on the anatomic location of symptoms. Other primary headaches considered in the differential diagnosis include migraine, tension-type headache, primary stabbing headache (PSH), and cervicogenic headache. These headaches can be differentiated from ON by a thorough headache history and an exam with attention to key features. A local anesthetic nerve block administered to the occipital nerve with resultant pain relief will make the diagnosis certain.

ANATOMIC BASIS OF ON

The GON arises from the dorsal ramus of the C2 spinal nerve. It courses underneath the splenius capitis, longissimus, and semispinalis muscles. It enters the scalp, where it then runs through the aponeurosis of the trapezius muscle just inferior to the superior nuchal ridge. At this point, it becomes subcutaneous and lies in close proximity to the occipital artery.[2]

ON can involve any of the three occipital nerves. As the GON arises from the second cervical spinal nerve and runs through the semispinalis capitis and trapezius muscles, it supplies skin sensation from the external occipital protuberance up to the vertex (Figure 1.1).

The lesser occipital nerve is formed by divisions of the second and third cervical spinal nerves, and runs upward along the posterior border of the sternocleidomastoid muscle. The lesser occipital nerve supplies sensory fibers to the scalp lateral to the area supplied by the GON. The third occipital nerve arises from the third cervical nerve and gives sensation to the upper posterior neck and lower occipital scalp.[3]

ETIOLOGY

ON was first described as a distinct clinical entity in 1821. The GON is involved in up to 90% of patients. The lesser and third occipital nerves are less frequently involved, with involvement of the third nerve considered to be infrequent. Involvement of the greater and lesser occipital nerves together occurs in approximately 9% of cases.[2] Most cases of ON are idiopathic and ON is considered to be a primary cranial neuralgia. The GON has a variable anatomic course and can encounter entrapment or irritation caused by nearby structures. Structural lesions requiring intervention must be ruled out.

DIAGNOSIS AND INVESTIGATIONS

Given the abundance of potential mechanisms, serious pathology should be investigated by undertaking a full neurologic examination. In palpating the GON, a useful landmark is the external occipital protuberance. To find the nerve, one should palpate approximately 2 cm lateral and 2 cm inferior to the bony structure.[4] Following examination, patients should be referred for imaging of the cervical spine. Appropriate serum evaluation should be undertaken dependent upon suspected etiology.

DIFFERENTIAL DIAGNOSIS OF ON

In most cases, no obvious structural or systemic etiology can be found and the neuralgia is termed idiopathic. However, imaging and diagnostic studies should be undertaken to rule out an underlying etiology. There are many case reports in the literature pointing to diverse causes. These include a craniocervical junction meningioma presenting only as ON, as well as reports of osteochondroma and schwannoma of the

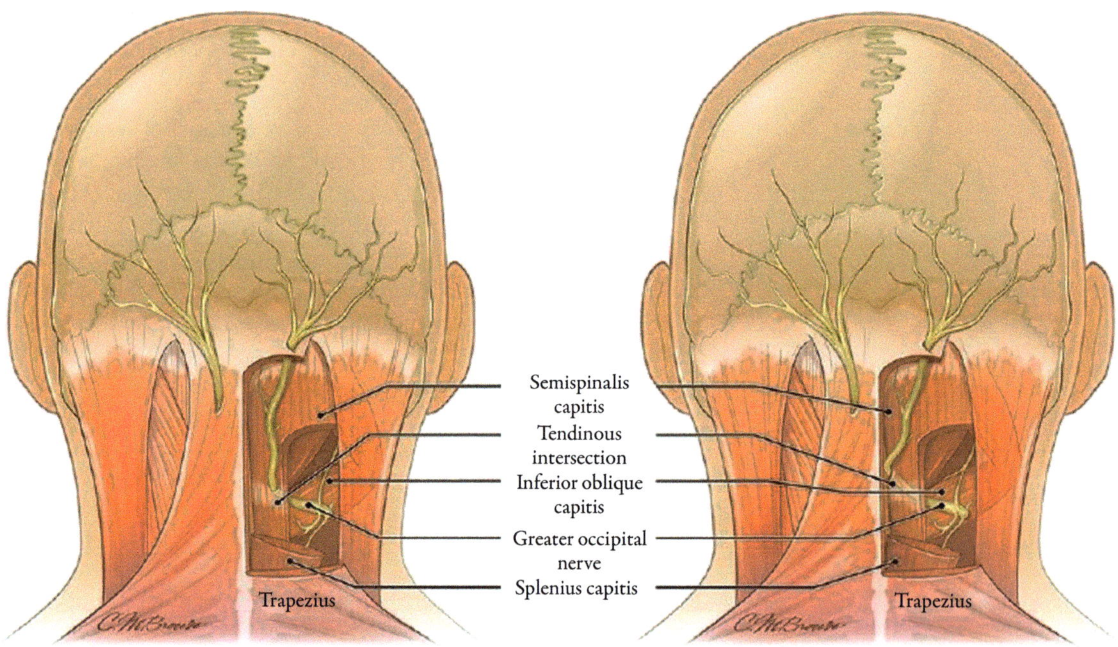

Figure 1.1. Trajectory of the occipital nerves. Tubbs RS, Watanabe K, Loukas M, Cohen-Gadol AA. The Intramuscular Course of the Greater Occipital Nerve: Novel Findings with Potential Implications for Operative Interventions and Occipital Neuralgia. Surg Neurol Int 31-Oct-2014;5:155.

upper cervical spine with similar presentations.[5–7] Other structural etiologies that have been identified in patients include cervicomedullary dural arteriovenous malformations that became symptomatic after hemorrhage.[8] ON has also been identified as the presenting feature in traumatic fracture and nerve compression, Chiari malformation, neurosyphilis, and hypertrophic cervical pachymeningitis.[9]

PATHOPHYSIOLOGY OF IDIOPATHIC ON

The GON can become irritated by nearby anatomic structures anywhere along its course through the posterior head and neck. At its origin from the C2 dorsal ramus, it is vulnerable to compression at the atlanto-axial joint, especially if the nerve has a variant anatomic course. Additionally, the GON is vulnerable to stretch injury as it passes between the inferior oblique muscle of the head and the semispinalis muscle. One proposed mechanism has been compression by the nearby occipital artery.[9]

SYMPTOMS AND CLINICAL MANIFESTATIONS

Patients will typically describe a paroxysmal pain that is shooting, stabbing, or "electric." The pain can be severe, and duration may range from several seconds to minutes. Some patients may also have a milder continuous pain in the same anatomic region, with paroxysmal episodes superimposed. Patients may describe associated dysesthesia, allodynia, or hypesthesia. The sensory disturbances are typically located in the dermatome supplied by the relevant affected cervical spinal nerve. On examination, pain can often be reproduced upon nerve palpation, either at the root or along its course more peripherally. ON is typically unilateral but it may present bilaterally. A patient may report pain in the frontal or retro-orbital areas. This is theorized to be secondary to neural interconnections with the trigeminal spinal nuclei in the upper cervical cord.[3]

TREATMENT

A typical approach to treating a patient with ON is to start with the least invasive and most conservative management. Escalation to interventional techniques can occur if the patient has persistent and/or severe symptoms or symptoms that interfere with daily routines.

CONSERVATIVE MANAGEMENT OF ON

Patients are often referred for physical therapy. Sometimes short-term immobilization of the neck with a brace may be tried. Pharmacologic treatments can include anti-inflammatory agents, acetaminophen, muscle relaxants, selective serotonin reuptake inhibitors (SSRIs), anticonvulsants, and tricyclic antidepressants. There is no evidence in the literature to support any one medication, and the prescription often depends upon the side-effect profile.

INTERVENTIONAL PROCEDURE FOR ON

The literature on ON often includes mention of similar and related headache syndromes (cervicogenic headache, cluster headache, migraine), many of which have shared clinical manifestations and overlapping diagnostic criteria with ON, such as tenderness to palpation (TTP) or reproduction of headache pain with occipital nerve pressure (RHPONP). While it is not consistent among the syndromes, diagnostic and therapeutic ONB with local anesthetic plus or minus steroids may have some efficacy in treatment of multiple headache syndromes.[10] This efficacy may speak to a shared or overlapping etiology for the syndromes.

Once conservative therapy has failed for a patient diagnosed with ON per the diagnostic criteria published by the International Headache Society, several interventional treatments are available; however, it is important to note that currently no standard of care exists and that the studies that have been performed are limited factors like sample size, variability between protocols, and the limited nature of the studies themselves.[11,12] The interventional options include local anesthetic injections with or without corticosteroids, botulinum neurotoxin (BoNT) injection, occipital nerve stimulation (ONS), occipital pulsed radiofrequency (PRF), and cryoablation. For intractable cases resistant to all conservative and interventional therapies, surgical rhizotomy is considered.[11,13]

While local anesthetic nerve blocks with and without steroid are both diagnostic and therapeutic, short duration of action limits their use in prolonged relief of ON.[11,14] Some studies seem to indicate that repetitive series of ON blocks may be more effective for a longer duration than single diagnostic and therapeutic blocks; however, more and better-controlled studies are warranted before this can be concluded. Similarly, adding steroids to local anesthetic in blocks appears to benefit transformed migraine headaches, but the evidence for benefit with other types of headache syndromes is insufficient or contradictory; more and better-controlled studies are warranted.[15] For ON specifically, there are no studies supporting the addition of steroids for increased efficacy or duration of response; a host of steroid side effects, ranging from cutaneous atrophy and alopecia to Cushing's syndrome, have been documented.[3]

PRF Ablation

PRF ablation has recently emerged as a safe, noninvasive, and potentially long-term treatment for refractory ON.[16] While the exact mechanism of action of PRF is uncertain, PRF is thought to be a temperature-independent, nondestructive neuromodulatory process that involves alteration of synaptic transmission via the emission of electrical fields and that avoids deafferentation pain, a much-feared and difficult-to-treat complication of conventional continuous radiofrequency ablation.[16] To date there have been two promising prospective studies and one retrospective study on the benefits of PRF for the treatment of ON; however, results from a more recent double-blind randomized controlled comparative-effectiveness study were more tempered. Cohen et al. found that, while PRF resulted in a statistically significant improvement in average occipital pain in comparison to steroid injection through the 6-month follow-up period, worst occipital pain was significantly improved only through the 3-month follow-up and average overall headache pain only through 6 weeks. Further, they found that, while PRF may have a superior analgesic effect, secondary outcome measures, such as decrease in pain medication taken or improvement in sleep quality, were not seen.[10]

Cryoablation

Cryoablation is an interventional technique that involves placement of a cryoprobe into tissues and inducing a drastic temperature decrease, which has been shown to create a conduction block in the targeted nerve. Ice-crystal formation around the nerve in question damages the vasa nervorum, leading to endoneural edema and wallerian degeneration of the nerve axon; concomitant preservation of the myelin sheath and endoneurium allows eventual regeneration of the nerve and potentially avoids the development of deafferentation pain. This technique has been shown to achieve reliable pain relief with lasting effect in chronic neuropathic pain conditions by blocking nerve conduction in afferent and efferent pain pathways. The extent and duration of pain relief are proportional to the temperature decrement and length of exposure to the decreased temperature.[17] While the literature for cryoablation utilized in the treatment of ON is scant, one recent study has shown promising results in terms of efficacy and safety. In a retrospective study of 38 patients, Kim et al. demonstrated a nearly 60% improvement in pain for an average duration of 6.1 months, with a complication rate of 7.5%. Three patients suffered minor adverse events that resolved fully with no lasting sequelae.[11]

ONS

ONS is touted as having a relatively high rate of success with a long duration of action; however, there are relatively few studies available. The 2015 Congress of Neurological Surgeons provided evidence-based guidelines for the treatment of patients with medically refractory ON.[18] After reviewing the available evidence, the panel concluded that ONS recommendations in refractory ON were Level III evidence, with multiple publications reviewed having only single-digit sample sizes. The ONS technique, which is surgical and thus requires an advanced skill set, appears to be limited by a high rate of complications, such as lead migration, hardware failure/fracture/erosion, or infection, which may necessitate a return to the operating room for revision.[13,16] However, recent developments in less-invasive implantation techniques and advances in hardware technology have led to a resurgence of interest in ONS.[19]

BoNT Nerve Block Injections

Since the 1970s and the first use of BoNT to treat strabismus, its use has evolved into treatment of numerous pain conditions. BoNT inhibits the release of acetylcholine at nerve terminals by inhibiting the soluble *N*-ethylmaleimide-sensitive factor attachment protein receptor (SNARE) complex; therefore, BoNT has been used effectively to treat spasticity and dystonia along with their accompanying pain. However, the fortuitous clinical observation of improvement in pain symptoms independent of muscle hyperactivity improvement in the setting of BoNT injection has led to further research into the underlying mechanisms of this effect in both animal studies and clinical settings.[20] Animal studies seem to indicate that BoNT may inhibit the release of various pain-modulating neurotransmitters, such as glutamate, substance P, and calcitonin gene-related peptide, as well as inhibit pain-sensing transmembrane receptors, via its interference with the SNARE complex.[21] Further, there is also evidence from animal studies that the analgesic mechanism of BoNT may also involve retrograde axonal transport to the spinal cord from the site of injection, which implies that there is both a peripheral and central nervous system component to BoNT's antinociceptive properties.[21] It is important to note that evidence from human studies suggests that complete denervation or nerve transection may be a predictor of poor pain response to BoNT.[20] Should this be borne out in more robust studies, it could suggest that BoNT should be trialed prior to neurodestructive interventions. To date, two small studies have evaluated BoNT as a treatment for ON. Kapural et al. demonstrated a median 4-month decrease in scores on the VAS (Visual Analog Scale) from 8 ± 1.8 to 2 ± 2.7, and an improvement in the PDI (Pain Disability Index) from 51.5 ± 7.6 to 19.5 ± 21 in a retrospective series of six patients who received BoNT nerve blockade versus 0.5% bupivacaine diagnostic/therapeutic blocks, which improved pain for only 1.9 ± 0.5 weeks.[22] A prospective pilot study of six patients by Taylor et al. demonstrated a 3-month improvement in headache-specific quality of life measures, with an improvement in lancinating pain but no significant change in dull/aching or pins/needles pain; furthermore, there was no significant reduction in pain medication usage.[22]

OCCIPITAL NEURALGIA OVERVIEW

ON is categorized as a painful cranial neuralgia, like trigeminal neuralgia, and they share some common characteristics and features. As with other neuralgias, the symptoms are brief, paroxysmal, and lancinating. The course can be monophasic, relapsing-remitting, or chronic.[24] Often, the affected nerve can be directly palpated and may reproduce symptoms. According to the ICHD-3 criteria, the diagnosis is certain if symptoms are improved after a local anesthetic nerve block. There are no epidemiologic studies of ON, and the incidence in the population is uncertain. There have been studies suggesting a slight female predominance.[25]

ONBs are routinely performed under ultrasound guidance, which provides excellent visualization of needle placement and deposit of medication around the nerves while avoiding complications, such as intravascular injections.[26] In some cases, the occipital nerve may be entrapped close to the occipital artery; in those rare cases, surgical decompression of the nerve may provide benefit.[27]

CONCLUSIONS

- ON is classified as a primary cranial neuralgia and is characterized by paroxysmal episodes of sharp pain in the distribution of the occipital nerve.
- ON is often idiopathic and is thought to arise from compression or irritation of the occipital nerves by nearby anatomic structures along their course through the posterior neck and head.
- Secondary structural causes should be investigated before diagnosis of idiopathic ON is made.

REFERENCES

1. Occipital neuralgia—ICHD-3 Beta, The International Classification of Headache Disorders. 3rd ed. (Beta version). 2017. Available at: https://www.ichd-3.org/13-painful-cranial-neuropathies-and-other-facial-pains/13-4-occipital-neuralgia/. Accessed June 26, 2017.
2. Choi I, Jeon S. Neuralgias of the head: occipital neuralgia. *J Korean Med Sci*. 2016;31(4):479–488. doi:10.3346/jkms.2016.31.4.479.
3. Dougherty C. Occipital neuralgia. *Curr Pain Headache Rep*. 2014;18(5):411. doi:10.1007/s11916-014-0411-x.
4. Loukas M, El-Sedfy A, Tubbs RS, et al. Identification of greater occipital nerve landmarks for the treatment of occipital neuralgia. *Folia Morphol*. 2006;65(4):337–342.
5. Kim N, Yang S, Koo J, Jeong S. Occipital neuralgia as the only presenting symptom of foramen magnum meningioma. *J Clin Neurol*. 2009;5(4):198–200. doi:10.3988/jcn.2009.5.4.198.
6. Arasil E, Erdem A, Yüceer N. Osteochondroma of the upper cervical spine. *Spine*. 1996;21(4):516–518. doi:10.1097/00007632-199602150-00021.
7. Garza I. Craniocervical junction schwannoma mimicking occipital neuralgia. *Headache*. 2007; 47(8): 1204–1205. doi:10.1111/j.1526-4610.2007.00887.x
8. Hashiguchi A, Mimata C, Ichimura H, Kuratsu J. Occipital neuralgia as a presenting symptom of cervicomedullary dural arteriovenous fistula. *Headache*. 2007;47(7):1095–1097. doi:10.1111/j.1526-4610.2007.00865.x.
9. Cesmebasi A, Muhleman M, Hulsberg P, et al. Occipital neuralgia: anatomic considerations. *Clin Anat*. 2014;28(1):101–108. doi:10.1002/ca.22468.
10. Cohen SP, Peterlin BL, Fulton L, et al. Randomized, double-blind, comparative-effectiveness study comparing pulsed radiofrequency to steroid injections for occipital neuralgia or migraine with occipital nerve tenderness. *Pain*. 2015;156(12):2585–2594.
11. Kim CH, Hu W, Gao J, Dragan K, Whealton T, Julian C. Cryoablation for the treatment of occipital neuralgia. *Pain Physician*. 2015;18(3):E363–E368.
12. Nadler SF, Weingand K, Cruse RJ. The physiologic basis and clinical applications of cryotherapy and thermotherapy for the pain practitioner. *Pain Physician*. 2004;7(3):395–399.
13. Ducic I, Felder JM III, Fantus SA. A systematic review of peripheral nerve interventional treatments for chronic headaches. *Ann Plast Surg*. 2014;72(4):439–445.
13. Mathew NT. The prophylactic treatment of chronic daily headache. *Headache*. 2006;40(10):1552–1564.
14. Tobin J, Flitman S. Occipital nerve blocks: when and what to inject? *Headache*. 2009;49(10):1521–1533.
15. Manolitsis N, Elahi F. Pulsed radiofrequency for occipital neuralgia. *Pain Physician*. 2014;17:E709–E717.
16. Myers R, Heckman H, Powell H. Axonal viability and the persistence of thermal hyperalgesia after partial freeze lesions of nerve. *J Neurol Sci*. 1996;139(1):28–38.
17. Sweet JA, Mitchell LS, Narouze S, et al. Occipital nerve stimulation for the treatment of patients with medically refractory occipital neuralgia: Congress of Neurological Surgeons systematic review and evidence-based guideline. *Neurosurgery*. 2015;77(3):332–341.
18. Slavin K. Peripheral nerve stimulation for neuropathic pain. *Neurotherapeutics*. 2008;5(1):100–106.
19. Sandrini G, De Icco R, Tassorelli C, Smania N, Tamburin S. Botulinum neurotoxin type A for the treatment of pain: not just in migraine and trigeminal neuralgia. *J Headache Pain*. 2017;18(1):38.
20. Kim DW, Lee SK, Ahnn J. Botulinum toxin as a pain killer: players and actions in antinociception. *Toxins*. 2015;7(7):2435–2453.
21. Kapural L, Stillman M, Kapural M, McIntyre P, Guirguis M, Mekhail N. Botulinum toxin occipital nerve block for the treatment of severe occipital neuralgia: a case series. *Pain Pract*. 2007;7(4):337–340.
22. Taylor M, Silva S, Cottrell C. Botulinum toxin type-A (Botox®) in the treatment of occipital neuralgia: a pilot study. *Headache*. 2008;48(10):1476–1481.
23. Gadient P, Smith J. The neuralgias: diagnosis and management. *Curr Neurol Neurosci Rep*. 2014;14(7):459. doi:10.1007/s11910-014-0459-3.
24. Koopman J, Dieleman J, Huygen F, de Mos M, Martin C, Sturkenboom M. Incidence of facial pain in the general population. *Pain*. 2009;147(1):122–127. doi:10.1016/j.pain.2009.08.023.
25. Narouze S. Occipital neuralgia diagnosis and treatment: the role of ultrasound. *Headache*. 2016;56(4):801–807. doi:10.1111/head.12790.
26. Cornely C, Fischer M, Ingianni G, Isenmann S. Greater occipital nerve neuralgia caused by pathological arterial contact: treatment by surgical decompression. *Headache*. 2010;51(4):609–612. doi:10.1111/j.1526-4610.2010.01802.x.

REVIEW QUESTIONS

1. A 56-year-old male comes to clinic for evaluation of subacute, sharp, shooting pain located over the left posterior neck and scalp. He has no pain with neck flexion and no pain located in the distribution of the trigeminal nerve. He is otherwise healthy, with no significant past medical history. His neurologic exam is normal. What would confirm your suspected diagnosis?

   A. CT neck
   B. MRI cervical spine
   C. Pain relief following local anesthetic nerve block
   D. A trial of nonsteroidal anti-inflammatory drugs (NSAIDs)

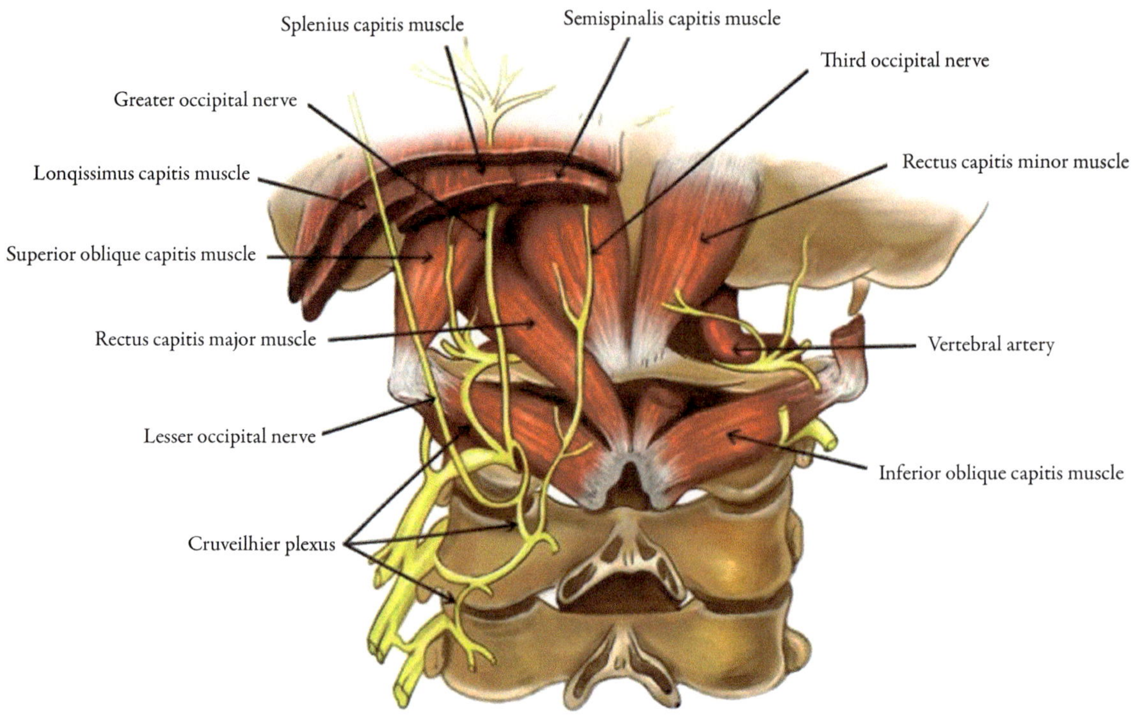

Figure 1.2. Interneural connections allow occipital irritation to manifest as trigeminal neuralgia. Choi I, Jeon S. Neuralgias of the head: occipital neuralgia. *J Korean Med Sci*. 2016; 31(4): 479. doi:10.3346/jkms.2016.31.4.479.

2. A patient with previously diagnosed ON, managed well with conservative therapy, develops sharp pain in her forehead and dull, aching pain behind her eyes. What is the anatomic basis for this?

   A. Trigeminocervical interneuronal connections
   B. Involvement of the GON
   C. Cruveilhier plexus
   D. Referred pain to the facial nerve

3. Which nerve is involved most commonly in ON?

   A. Third occipital nerve
   B. Lesser occipital nerve
   C. GON
   D. Dorsal ramus of C2

ANSWERS

1. C. When considering the diagnosis of ON, the first step should be to see if the pain responds to a local nerve block. If the pain is relieved, the diagnosis of ON is certain. Further diagnostic studies can then be undertaken depending upon the clinician's suspicion about the underlying cause.

2. A. In this case, the patient is reporting pain that can be referred to the distribution of the trigeminal nerve. Some patients may also experience pain in the frontal and orbital regions due to trigeminocervical connections in the trigeminal spinal nuclei. The Cruveilhier plexus is a connection among the C1, C2, and C3 sensory branches. These neural interconnections can be a cause for resistant pain and therapy failure. It is theorized that anatomic variants in the plexus can result in refractory pain even after intervention (Figure 1.2).

3. C. The GON is the most frequently involved.

QUESTIONS AND ANSWERS

This chapter has accompanying questions and answers that are available to subscribers as part of the Oxford eLearning platform. To access the questions, follow the link below, or go to http://oxfordmedicine.com/painmanagementreview

2.

TRIGEMINAL NEURALGIA

Jumana T. Alshaikh, Shaan Sudhakaran, and Helene Rubeiz

STEM CASE AND KEY QUESTIONS

A 51-year-old woman presents with a 2-week history of episodic, brief, sharp, shocklike pain in her face involving the left upper teeth and left cheek, radiating to the left pre-auricular region. She has been having several attacks of pain daily, each lasting approximately 10 seconds. The attacks are triggered by touching the left side of her upper lip, eating, drinking, brushing her teeth, smiling, or exposure to a breeze of cold air. She has tried over-the-counter analgesics, including acetaminophen and ibuprofen, without relief. She has visited two dentists, who did not find a dental cause for her symptoms. She is crying in the clinic because the pain was unbearable. Her neurologic exam is normal. She is diagnosed with trigeminal neuralgia (TN), based on the description of her pain.

WHAT IS TN?

TN is a condition characterized by recurrent, unilateral, brief episodes of severe stabbing facial pain of sudden onset and termination, involving a branch of the trigeminal nerve. This patient's pain involves the maxillary division (V2) of the left trigeminal nerve.

WHAT CAUSES TN?

The most common cause of TN is vascular compression due to a tortuous vascular loop (most frequently the superior cerebellar artery). Compression of the trigeminal nerve by other structural lesions, such as a vestibular schwannoma, meningioma, cyst, aneurysm, or arteriovenous malformation (AVM), can also cause TN. It can also be seen with demyelinating lesions in the brainstem caused by multiple sclerosis (MS). This patient has not had any imaging at this point; therefore, the cause of her TN is not yet determined.

WHAT WORKUP IS NEEDED TO ESTABLISH THE DIAGNOSIS?

The diagnosis of TN is made based on the clinical history and unremarkable neurologic examination. Contrast-enhanced MRI of the brain with fine cuts through the trigeminal nerves, along with brain MRA, is useful for evaluation of neurovascular compression and secondary causes of TN. This patient meets the International Classification of Headache Disorders, 3rd edition (ICHD-3), criteria for classical TN (detailed below).

WHAT MEDICATIONS ARE USED FOR PAIN RELIEF IN TN?

First-line treatment is carbamazepine or oxcarbazepine. Other medications that may be effective include lamotrigine, baclofen, gabapentin, or phenytoin. The patient is started on 300 mg gabapentin three times per day to be titrated to a total dose of 1800 mg over the next 2 to 3 weeks.

IS THERE A SURGICAL OPTION FOR PATIENTS?

The patient returns in 4 weeks and reports that the gabapentin has been controlling the pain partially, with scores decreasing from 8/10 to 6/10; she still complains, though, of episodes of lancinating pain, but they are a little more tolerable. However, she is not satisfied with the treatment and is inquiring what other options are available, and specifically if she can benefit from surgical intervention. You explain to the patient that, since medical therapy has failed, you can refer her to a neurosurgeon for consultation about possible microvascular decompression (MVD). This surgery requires a craniotomy under general anesthesia, and MVD can be associated with many complications, although complications are rare.

ARE THERE NONSURGICAL OPTIONS FOR PATIENTS?

After the neurosurgeon explains the surgical procedure, the patient decides that the risks may be too great for her to take and she inquires about alternatives to surgical interventions. You explain that there are percutaneous options available. Radiofrequency (RF) ablation is emerging as an effective and relatively safe technique. It can be pulsed or continuous. It is performed under light sedation and is well tolerated in the elderly and high-risk patients with multiple comorbidities.

CAN PATIENTS ACHIEVE REMISSION?

The patient also inquires about her prognosis. She is particularly concerned about constant pain and if she will ever be pain-free, especially since gabapentin makes her overly sedated. In describing the disease prognosis, you tell her that many patients with classical TN experience periods of remission during which they can be weaned off medications. However, pain may recur months or years later. For most patients, the duration and severity of pain progressively increase over time.

Discussion

TN, also known as tic douloureux, is a disorder characterized by recurrent paroxysms of brief unilateral facial pain limited to one or more branches of the trigeminal nerve. The maxillary (V2) and mandibular (V3) branches are most often affected at equal frequency.[1] The pain is described as stabbing, shooting, lancinating, or electric shocklike. The episodes of pain are brief, lasting a few seconds to a minute. Pain is triggered by innocuous sensory stimuli on the same side of the face, produced by activities such as touching, chewing/eating, brushing the teeth, smiling, speaking, or exposure to wind.[1] Patients' avoidance of potential pain triggers can affect their daily activities. For example, patients may adjust their diet to liquefied food.[2] Some patients may lose weight from reduced food intake. Many patients present to a dentist initially, and some receive unnecessary invasive dental procedures, such as extractions or root canal treatments, for management of their pain.[2–3] The incidence of TN is 4 to 13 per 100,000 per year, with a higher prevalence among females.[4–8] Average age of onset is around age 50 or later, but TN can affect any age group.[4–5]

Diagnostic criteria for classical TN, according to the beta version of ICHD-3 (ICHD-3 Beta), include:[9]

A. At least three attacks of unilateral facial pain fulfilling criteria B and C

B. Occurring in one or more divisions of the trigeminal nerve, with no radiation beyond the trigeminal distribution

C. Pain has at least three of the following four characteristics:

   1. Recurring in paroxysmal attacks lasting from a fraction of a second to 2 minutes
   2. Severe intensity
   3. Electric shocklike, shooting, stabbing, or sharp in quality
   4. Precipitated by innocuous stimuli to the affected side of the face*

D. No clinically evident neurologic deficit**

E. Not better accounted for by another ICHD-3 diagnosis.

Notes

* Some attacks may be, or may appear to be, spontaneous, but there must be at least three that are precipitated in this way to meet this criterion.

** Hypesthesia or hypalgesia in the affected trigeminal region always indicates axonal damage. When either is present, there is trigeminal neuropathy and extensive diagnostic workup is necessary to exclude symptomatic cases. Some patients have hyperalgesia in the painful region, which should not necessarily lead to a diagnosis of trigeminal neuropathy because it may reflect the patient's increased attention to the painful side.

In most patients with TN, there is no pain between attacks; however, in a minority of cases, a continuous dull or burning background pain may precede, or linger after, the more severe paroxysms. (ICHD-3 Beta subform: classical TN with concomitant persistent facial pain.)

According to ICHD-3 Beta, TN is divided into either classical TN (without apparent cause other than neurovascular compression) or secondary TN caused by MS or a space-occupying lesion, such as a tumor, cerebral aneurysm, or AVM.[9] The International Association for the Study of Pain (IASP) has produced a different classification system that includes three categories: idiopathic TN (no apparent cause), classical TN (caused by neurovascular compression), and secondary TN (caused by major neurologic disease, e.g., cerebellopontine angle tumor or MS).[10]

ETIOLOGY

TN is most commonly caused by neurovascular compression, usually arterial compression from a redundant or tortuous arterial loop impinging on the trigeminal nerve root adjacent to its entry zone into the pons, causing focal demyelination (Figure 2.1).[11]

The superior cerebellar artery is the vessel frequently implicated.[12] In patients with TN, neurovascular contact is prevalent on both the symptomatic and the asymptomatic side, but tends to be more severe on the symptomatic side, causing displacement or atrophy of the trigeminal nerve. In

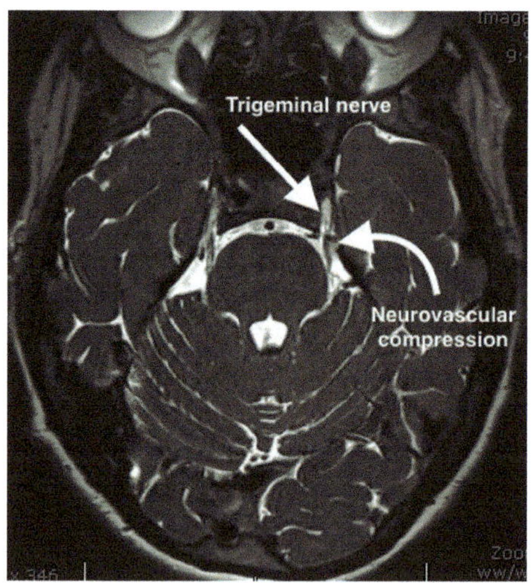

Figure 2.1. Brain MRI, axial view, FIESTA sequence, showing compression of the left trigeminal nerve root entry zone by a vascular loop, crossing and distorting the nerve.

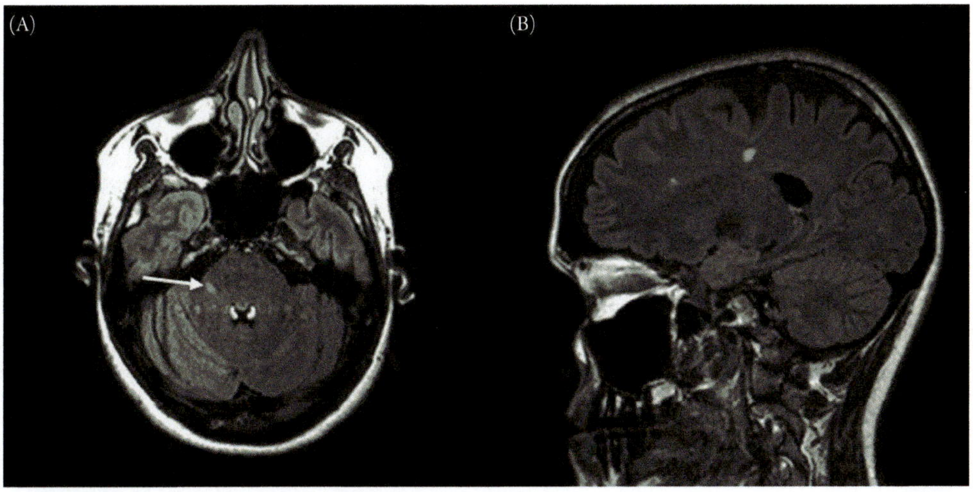

Figure 2.2. Brain MRI, FLAIR sequences, of a 53-year-old female with right-sided facial pain due to MS-related trigeminal neuralgia (TN). (A) Axial view showing right pontine demyelinating lesion (white arrow), which is likely the cause of her TN. (B) Sagittal view showing periventricular demyelinating lesions consistent with MS.

one study, neurovascular compression was present on the symptomatic side in 89% of patients, compared to 78% on the asymptomatic side. However, severe neurovascular compression was present on the symptomatic side in 53% and on the asymptomatic side in only 13% of cases.[4]

Occasionally, TN can be secondary to MS, with a demyelinating lesion in the brainstem (Figure 2.2).[13] Patients with MS have a 20-fold increased risk of developing TN and it can be bilateral in up to 30% of patients.[1] Therefore, a young patient with bilateral TN and other neurologic signs and symptoms should be evaluated for MS.

Cerebellopontine angle tumors, such as epidermoid cysts, vestibular schwannoma, meningioma, and lipoma, can also cause TN (Figure 2.3).[14]

Other causes of TN include compression by a venous loop, pontine cavernous malformation, or aneurysm.[15–16] TN without neurovascular compression presents at an earlier age than TN with neurovascular compression. In one study, the mean age of onset in patients with neurovascular compression was 51 years, compared to 42 years in patients without neurovascular compression.[17]

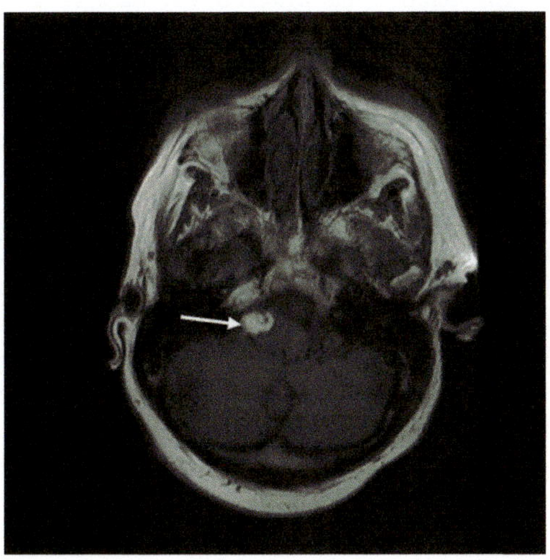

Figure 2.3. T1-weighted brain MRI without contrast showing a 13 x 11 mm lipoma (white arrow) in the right cerebellopontine angle of a 69-year-old female causing secondary trigeminal neuralgia (TN) in the right maxillary and mandibular areas of her face.

DIAGNOSTIC TOOLS

TN is a clinical diagnosis based on patient history. Neuroimaging using high-resolution brain MRI with gadolinium in conjunction with brain MRA is helpful for determining the anatomy of the trigeminal nerve and adjacent vessels and identifying patients with neurovascular compression.[18–21] MRI is also useful for the evaluation of secondary causes of TN, such as MS and cerebellopontine angle lesions.

TREATMENT

Initial treatment of TN is pain control by pharmacologic agents. Surgery is reserved for patients who are refractory to medical therapy. In secondary TN, the underlying medical condition should be treated as well. Antiepileptic agents are the mainstay of medical therapy. The best studied and most effective first-line treatment is carbamazepine, followed by oxcarbazepine.[22] Carbamazepine is generally used at the lowest effective dose, with a gradual dose escalation (up to 100 to 200 mg three times a day). In a number of patients, larger doses are often required. In one study of patients with classical TN, carbamazepine was effective in 98% of patients and oxcarbazepine was effective in 94% of patients. Withdrawal of therapy in the study was mostly due to intolerable side effects, rather than failure of treatment.[23] In another study, the most common adverse effects of carbamazepine were fatigue, memory impairment, and somnolence.[24]

Other medications that have been used, but with limited available evidence on their efficacy, are lamotrigine, baclofen, pregabalin, pimozide, tizanidine, clonazepam, gabapentin, and phenytoin.[25–33] Over-the-counter analgesics, such as acetaminophen and NSAIDs, are ineffective in TN. Patients with classical TN with concomitant persistent facial pain are poorly responsive to conservative treatment and neurosurgical interventions.

There is minimal high-grade (level I) evidence regarding therapy after first-line medications fail. One must take into account the patient's comorbidities with regard to surgical intervention versus less invasive therapies. MRI should be obtained in order to rule out other conditions and to assist with procedural intervention. If there is a mass or malformation, it may be amenable to resection. It is prudent to refer the patient for initial surgical evaluation to ensure adequate informed consent.

Vascular compression plays a prominent role in TN. MVD has become increasingly common over the past 30 years. The target area is at the trigeminal nerve–pontine junction. The surgical approach is through the posterior fossa via a suboccipital craniotomy. Pain is generated from compression of the trigeminal nerve by the superior cerebellar artery. Once the artery is isolated, a piece of padded Teflon felt is placed between the nerve and artery to minimize compression. Brainstem evoked potentials are monitored to minimize the risk of intraoperative cranial nerve damage. Pain relief outcomes seem to be similar in patients < 50 years old and patients > 70 years old. Initial pain relief rates are from 87% to 98%, and pain relief at 1 to 2 years is 75% to 80%, and at 8 to 10 years it is 58% to 64%.[34] MVD has the lowest pain recurrence rate but has some significant risk. Cranial nerve palsies in CN VII and CN VIII can occur as a complication of surgery. Other rare but serious complications include cerebellar injury, hearing loss, and CSF leakage.[35] Further details regarding the anatomic approach and long-term outcomes for decompression are beyond the scope of this book.

One of the most studied interventions is RF ablation of the gasserian ganglion or its branches. RF ablation works by running current through nervous tissue, creating heat around the nerve. An electric field is created around the tip of the electrode. This field oscillates with alternating current, causing friction between molecules in the tissue. The RF system is able to monitor frequency, temperature, and voltage. RF current tends to be high frequency and low energy. The threshold for cell damage is 42°C. Theoretically, the cellular damage is thought to affect thinly myelinated or nonmyelinated fibers first, therefore affecting primarily pain fibers. In practice, there is often concomitant change in all sensory function.

In order to approach the gasserian ganglion for RF ablation, a submental view is obtained with the C-arm in the AP view. In order to visualize the foramen ovale, a small tilt toward the ipsilateral side may be required. Needle entry should be placed a few centimeters lateral from the corner of the mouth. Needle trajectory should avoid entering the oral cavity. To ensure sterile conditions, the procedure should be repeated with a new needle if the oral cavity is entered. Once the needle has entered the foramen ovale, the C-arm should be rotated laterally to assess depth. The tip of the needle should be at the angle of the petroclival junction (Figure 2.4).

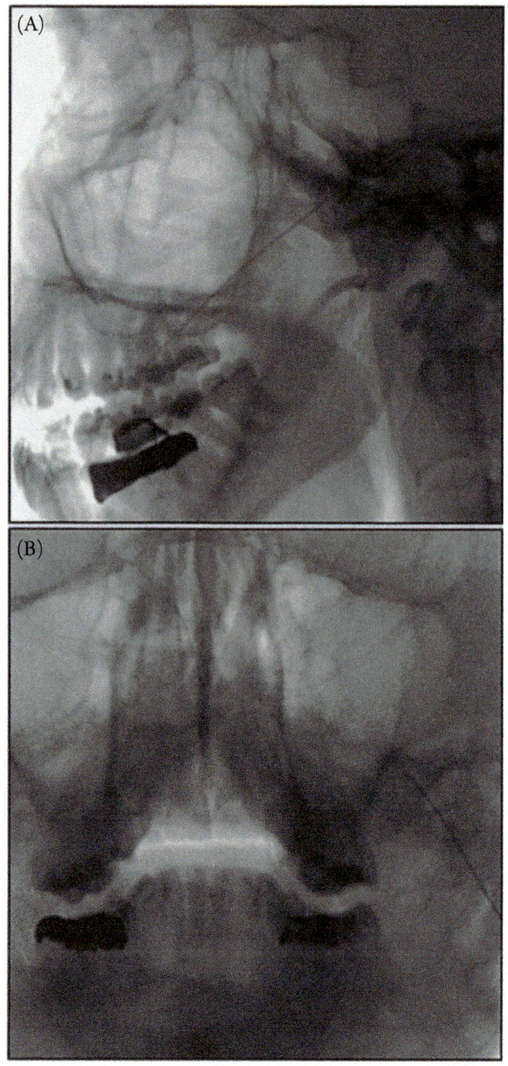

Figure 2.4. Fluoroscopic needle entry for radiofrequency procedures. (A) Lateral image to determine depth of needle. Needle entry is through the foramen ovale. (B) Trajectory to guide needle into foramen ovale.

Once the needle has entered Meckel's cave, aspiration will usually yield CSF. Nerve localization is confirmed with sensory stimulation at 0.2 to 1 V, with a frequency of 50 Hz. Small movements and rotation of the needle will change which branch of the trigeminal nerve is affected. In general, straight electrodes are preferred for V3 symptoms and curved electrodes for V1 or V2 involvement, given the angle made from the needle entry point. A temperature of 60°C to 90°C immediately leads to protein coagulation and cell death. RF ablation is often performed in cycles of ~1 minute. Cycles can be repeated until hypalgesia is appreciated at the target site.[36] According to a large review by Kanpolat et al., with continuous RF ablation, immediate pain relief occurred in 97.6% of patients. Pain recurred in 7.7% of patients by 6 months, 42.3% by 5 years, and 59% by 20 years.[37]

Pulsed RF ablation involves minimal to no tissue damage in the target nerve; rather, it is thought to affect signal transduction pathways, and thus it is thought to incur less sensory deficit than continuous RF ablation. At about 1 year after intervention, 55.9% of patients had at least 80% pain relief.[38] Classically, a 50-kHz current is delivered in 20-msec pulses at a frequency of about 2 Hz for 120 seconds. Pauses between pulses allow for dissipation of heat. The temperature of the tip is limited to 42°C, which is inadequate for neuronal tissue destruction. The greatest current is distal to the tip of the electrode, which enables perpendicular placement. IV sedation should be held temporarily, with sensory stimulation to ensure correct placement of the needle. The area with the pulsed lesion should have reduced sensation to pinprick (hypalgesia).[39]

Mild dysesthesias can occur in up to one out of four patients. The most common adverse side effects include loss of, or decreased, corneal reflex (5.7%), masseter paresis (3.0%), and masseter paralysis (1.1%). Less common (< 1%) but significant complications include oculomotor nerve palsy, corneal keratitis, abducens nerve palsy, and anesthesia dolorosa. Anesthesia dolorosa is a feared complication in which the patient has decreased sensation but pain that can sometimes be more severe than the initial neuralgia.

Chemical neurolysis typically provides pain relief for a few months. It causes destruction of nerve fibers and Wallerian degeneration of Schwann cells and axons. Neurons take about 3 to 6 months for regeneration. The most common agent used for TN is 100% glycerol. The needle takes an approach similar to that used for RF ablation (the needle is inserted into the trigeminal cistern through the foramen ovale). Once the final needle position is confirmed with fluoroscopy, the patient is placed in a sitting position and small doses of glycerol are injected (up to 0.5 mL). The patient should remain seated for 2 hours after the injection.[34] Pain relief may not occur for 7 days. There is significant variation in reported rates of pain recurrence, and recurrence rate is likely to vary with practitioner experience. (Alcohol neurolysis has also been used but is associated with severe pain on injection and a high recurrence rate.) Chemical neurolysis has remained a prominent treatment in Third World countries but has recently fallen out of favor in the United States due to sometimes unpredictable chemical spread.

Local anesthetic and steroid combination blocks have been shown to temporarily alleviate pain but should not be used as sole treatment. In 1975, Adler[40] demonstrated an injection with high-concentration bupivacaine into the gasserian ganglion. Although the study included only five patients, length of the paroxysm-free period after the procedure ranged from 7 months to 4 years. The injection approach involved needle advancement into Meckel's space and injection of 1.5 mL of 0.5% bupivacaine through a catheter without epinephrine. Confirmation was established with anesthesia and hypalgesia to the appropriate dermatomes. Corneal reflex returned in all patients after 24 to 72 hours.[40] Goto et al. used a combination of bupivacaine and tetracaine. They observed that the addition of tetracaine prolongs the analgesic effect when compared to bupivacaine only. They proposed that peripheral nerve injection is an acceptable alternative to more invasive procedures and has fewer side effects.[41]

An emerging technology for peripheral neuropathy is neuromodulation. It is based on the gate theory, which posits that small nerve fiber transmissions can be overridden by stimulation of larger nerve fibers. Leads are threaded in close proximity to the affected nerves and send stimulatory signals to the large fibers. This causes constant paresthesias that override pain fiber transmission. Neuromodulation is a newer technology and studies of its use for peripheral nerve stimulation are still in the early stages. A retrospective case series by Amin et al. described supraorbital peripheral nerve stimulator insertion in ten patients with chronic headaches. Patients underwent a 5- to 7-day trial and those with at least 50% improvement went on to the implant phase. VAS scores were reduced from 7.5 to 3.5 30 weeks after implantation.[42] Data for TN are lacking at this time, but neuromodulation will likely prove to have utility as a treatment modality.

If the above interventions fail, other procedures that may be considered include gamma knife radiation, Botox injections, balloon microcompression, cryoablation, and peripheral neurectomy. Data for these interventions are not as robust, and long-term pain relief is not as adequate as that with surgical intervention.

PROGNOSIS

There are no studies about the natural history of TN, perhaps because the excruciating nature of TN pain requires early treatment.[43] Remission periods are common in patients with TN, but symptoms are likely to recur. In patients who remain pain-free for a prolonged period, a medication weaning trial should be attempted. In one study, 65% of patients had recurrence of their pain within 5 years. In 23% of patients, the pain recurred after a remission period of more than 10 years.[8]

CONCLUSIONS

- TN is characterized by severe, unilateral, paroxysmal facial pain in the distribution of one of the divisions of the trigeminal nerve and is triggered by innocuous physical stimuli.
- The most common cause of TN is neurovascular compression by an aberrant arterial loop. Other causes include MS and cerebellopontine angle lesions. TN can also be idiopathic.
- The diagnosis is made clinically based on patient history. MRI of the brain is a useful tool to evaluate for neurovascular compression and secondary causes of TN.
- First-line pharmacologic treatment is carbamazepine or oxcarbazepine.
- Failure of medical therapy should lead to surgical consultation and risk stratification.
- RF ablation is an excellent choice for patients with significant comorbidities or who prefer to avoid craniotomy.
- Many patients achieve spontaneous remission, but the recurrence rate for TN is high.

REFERENCES

1. Cheshire WP. Cranial neuralgias. *Continuum*. 2015;21(4):1072–1085.
2. Allsop MJ, Twiddy M, Grant H, et al. Diagnosis, medication, and surgical management for patients with trigeminal neuralgia: a qualitative study. *Acta Neurochir (Wien)*. 2015;157(11):1925–1933.
3. Von Eckardstein KL, Keil M, Rohde V. Unnecessary dental procedures as a consequence of trigeminal neuralgia. *Neurosurg Rev*. 2015;38(2):355–360.
4. Maarbjerg S, Wolfram F, Gozalov A, Olesen J, Bendtsen L. Significance of neurovascular contact in classical trigeminal neuralgia. *Brain*. 2015;138(Pt 2):311–319.
5. Maarbjerg S, Gozalov A, Olesen J, Bendtsen L. Trigeminal neuralgia—a prospective systematic study of clinical characteristics in 158 patients. *Headache*. 2014;54(10):1574–1582.
6. Katusic S, Williams DB, Beard CM, Bergstralh EJ, Kurland LT. Epidemiology and clinical features of idiopathic trigeminal neuralgia and glossopharyngeal neuralgia: similarities and differences, Rochester, Minnesota, 1945–1984. *Neuroepidemiology*. 1991;10(5-6):276–281.
7. Macdonald BK, Cockerell OC, Sander JW, Shorvon SD. The incidence and lifetime prevalence of neurological disorders in a prospective community-based study in the UK. *Brain*. 2000;123(Pt 4):665–676.
8. Katusic S, Beard CM, Bergstralh E, Kurland LT. Incidence and clinical features of trigeminal neuralgia, Rochester, Minnesota, 1945–1984. *Ann Neurol*. 1990;27(1):89–95.
9. The International Classification of Headache Disorders, 3rd ed. (Beta version). *Cephalalgia*. 2013;33(9):629–808.
10. Cruccu G, Finnerup NB, Jensen TS, et al. Trigeminal neuralgia: new classification and diagnostic grading for practice and research. *Neurology*. 2016;87(2):220–228.
11. Chen GQ, Wang XS, Wang L, Zheng JP. Arterial compression of nerve is the primary cause of trigeminal neuralgia. *Neurol Sci*. 2014;35(1):61–66.
12. Lorenzoni J, David P, Levivier M. Patterns of neurovascular compression in patients with classic trigeminal neuralgia: a high-resolution MRI-based study. *Eur J Radiol*. 2012;81(8):1851–1857.
13. Cruccu G, Biasiotta A, Di Rezze S, et al. Trigeminal neuralgia and pain related to multiple sclerosis. *Pain*. 2009;143(3):186–191.
14. Khan Afridi EA, Khan SA, Qureshi WU, et al. Frequency of cerebellopontine angle tumours in patients with trigeminal neuralgia. *J Ayub Med Coll Abbottabad*. 2014;26(3):331–333.
15. Adachi K, Hasegawa M, Hayashi T, Nagahisa S, Hirose Y. A review of cavernous malformations with trigeminal neuralgia. *Clin Neurol Neurosurg*. 2014;125:151–154.
16. Hong W, Zheng X, Wu Z, et al. Clinical features and surgical treatment of trigeminal neuralgia caused solely by venous compression. *Acta Neurochir (Wien)*. 2011;153(5):1037–1042.
17. Ko AL, Lee A, Raslan AM, Ozpinar A, Mccartney S, Burchiel KJ. Trigeminal neuralgia without neurovascular compression presents earlier than trigeminal neuralgia with neurovascular compression. *J Neurosurg*. 2015;123(6):1519–1527.
18. Hughes MA, Frederickson AM, Branstetter BF, Zhu X, Sekula RF. MRI of the trigeminal nerve in patients with trigeminal neuralgia secondary to vascular compression. *AJR Am J Roentgenol*. 2016;206(3):595–600.
19. Lee A, Mccartney S, Burbidge C, Raslan AM, Burchiel KJ. Trigeminal neuralgia occurs and recurs in the absence of neurovascular compression. *J Neurosurg*. 2014;120(5):1048–1054.
20. Cai J, Xin ZX, Zhang YQ, Sun J, Lu JL, Xie F. Diagnostic value of 3D time-of-flight MRA in trigeminal neuralgia. *J Clin Neurosci*. 2015;22(8):1343–1348.
21. Leal PR, Hermier M, Souza MA, Cristino-Filho G, Froment JC, Sindou M. Visualization of vascular compression of the trigeminal nerve with high-resolution 3T MRI: a prospective study comparing preoperative imaging analysis to surgical findings in 40 consecutive patients who underwent microvascular decompression for trigeminal neuralgia. *Neurosurgery*. 2011;69(1):15–25.
22. Gomez-Arguelles JM, Dorado R, Sepulveda JM, et al. Oxcarbazepine monotherapy in carbamazepine-unresponsive trigeminal neuralgia. *J Clin Neurosci*. 2008;15(5):516–519.
23. Di Stefano G, La Cesa S, Truini A, Cruccu G. Natural history and outcome of 200 outpatients with classical trigeminal neuralgia treated with carbamazepine or oxcarbazepine in a tertiary centre for neuropathic pain. *J Headache Pain*. 2014;15:34. https://doi.org/10.1186/1129-2377-15-34
24. Besi E, Boniface DR, Cregg R, Zakrzewska JM. Comparison of tolerability and adverse symptoms in oxcarbazepine and carbamazepine in the treatment of trigeminal neuralgia and neuralgiform headaches using the Liverpool Adverse Events Profile (AEP). *J Headache Pain*. 2015;16(1):81. https://doi.org/10.1186/s10194-015-0563-z
25. Shaikh S, Yaacob HB, Abd Rahman RB. Lamotrigine for trigeminal neuralgia: efficacy and safety in comparison with carbamazepine. *J Chin Med Assoc*. 2011;74(6):243–249.
26. Pérez C, Navarro A, Saldaña MT, Martínez S, Rejas J. Patient-reported outcomes in subjects with painful trigeminal neuralgia receiving pregabalin: evidence from medical practice in primary care settings. *Cephalalgia*. 2009;29(7):781–790.
27. Zakrzewska JM, Chaudhry Z, Nurmikko TJ, Patton DW, Mullens EL. Lamotrigine (Lamictal) in refractory trigeminal neuralgia: results from a double-blind placebo controlled crossover trial. *Pain*. 1997;73(2):223–230.
28. Lechin F, Van Der Dijs B, Lechin ME, et al. Pimozide therapy for trigeminal neuralgia. *Arch Neurol*. 1989;46(9):960–963.
29. Pandey CK, Singh N, Singh PK. Gabapentin for refractory idiopathic trigeminal neuralgia. *J Indian Med Assoc*. 2008;106(2):124–125.
30. Steardo L, Leo A, Marano E. Efficacy of baclofen in trigeminal neuralgia and some other painful conditions. A clinical trial. *Eur Neurol*. 1984;23(1):51–55.
31. Fromm GH, Aumentado D, Terrence CF. A clinical and experimental investigation of the effects of tizanidine in trigeminal neuralgia. *Pain*. 1993;53(3):265–271.
32. Caccia MR. Clonazepam in facial neuralgia and cluster headache. Clinical and electrophysiological study. *Eur Neurol*. 1975;13(6):560–563.
33. Tate R, Rubin LM, Krajewski KC. Treatment of refractory trigeminal neuralgia with intravenous phenytoin. *Am J Health Syst Pharm*. 2011;68(21):2059–2061.
34. Nurmikko TJ, Eldridge PR. Trigeminal neuralgia—pathophysiology, diagnosis and current treatment. *Br J Anaesth*. 2001;87(1):117–132.
35. Zakrzewska JM, Mcmillan R. Trigeminal neuralgia: the diagnosis and management of this excruciating and poorly understood facial pain. *Postgrad Med J*. 2011;87(1028):410–416.
36. Emril DR, Ho KY. Treatment of trigeminal neuralgia: role of radiofrequency ablation. *J Pain Res*. 2010;3:249–254.
37. Kanpolat Y, Savas A, Bekar A, Berk C. Percutaneous controlled radiofrequency trigeminal rhizotomy for the treatment of idiopathic trigeminal neuralgia: 25-year experience with 1,600 patients. *Neurosurgery*. 2001;48(3):524–532.
38. Chua NH, Halim W, Beems T, Vissers KC. Pulsed radiofrequency treatment for trigeminal neuralgia. *Anesth Pain Med*. 2012;1(4):257–261.
39. Van Zundert J, Brabant S, Van De Kelft E, Vercruyssen A, Van Buyten JP. Pulsed radiofrequency treatment of the gasserian ganglion in patients with idiopathic trigeminal neuralgia. *Pain*. 2003;104(3):449–452.
40. Adler P. The use of bupivacaine for blocking the gasserian ganglion in major trigeminal neuralgia. *Int J Oral Surg*. 1975;4(6):251–257.
41. Goto F, Ishizaki K, Yoshikawa D, Obata H, Arii H, Terada M. The long lasting effects of peripheral nerve blocks for trigeminal neuralgia using high concentration of tetracaine dissolved in bupivacaine. *Pain*. 1999;79(1):101–103.

42. Amin S, Buvanendran A, Park KS, Kroin JS, Moric M. Peripheral nerve stimulator for the treatment of supraorbital neuralgia: a retrospective case series. *Cephalalgia.* 2008;28(4):355–359.
43. Bennetto L, Patel NK, Fuller G. Trigeminal neuralgia and its management. *BMJ.* 2007;334(7586):201–205.
44. Al-Ubaidy SS, Nally FF. Adverse reactions to carbamazepine (Tegretol). *Br J Oral Surg.* 1976;13(3):289–293.
45. Sedky K, Lippmann S. Psychotropic medications and leukopenia. *Curr Drug Targets.* 2006;7(9):1191–1194.

REVIEW QUESTIONS

1. A 59-year-old female presents to clinic with right upper lip and cheek pain for 2 weeks. She is diagnosed with TN. Which of the following is true regarding pain in TN?

   A. Often bilateral
   B. Constant
   C. Shooting quality
   D. Most common location is the forehead.

2. The onset of classical TN typically occurs in which of the following age groups?

   A. 50s
   B. Teens
   C. 20s
   D. 30s

3. A 45-year-old female presents to clinic with episodes of severe shooting pain in her left upper teeth and lip that last for 30 seconds and are triggered by chewing, talking, and drinking cold or hot beverages. Between these episodes, she has constant moderate-intensity pain affecting the same area. She has no neurologic deficits on exam. Brain MRI is normal. Per ICHD-3, how would you classify her pain?

   A. Secondary TN
   B. Classical TN with concomitant persistent facial pain
   C. Classical migraine
   D. Classical TN, purely paroxysmal

ANSWERS

1. C. TN pain is described as shooting, stabbing, lancinating, or electric shocklike. In most patients, it is unilateral. Answer B is incorrect because it is episodic, occurring in brief attacks of severe pain that last from a fraction of a second to 1 minute (although patients with classical TN with concomitant persistent facial pain have constant pain of mild to moderate intensity between the episodes).[9] The most common locations for the pain are the areas innervated by either the maxillary or mandibular divisions of the trigeminal nerve.[1] The ophthalmic division of the trigeminal nerve, which supplies the forehead, is the least likely of the other divisions to be involved in TN.

2. A. Mean age of onset of TN is the 50s.[4–5] It is less common in younger adults and is rare in children.

3. B. Per ICHD-3, patients with TN are said to have classical TN when it is idiopathic or due to neurovascular compression. Secondary TN is diagnosed when a secondary cause is found, such as MS or cerebellopontine angle tumor. Since her brain MRI was normal and she has no neurologic deficits, she has classical TN. Because she has constant moderate-intensity pain between the attacks of severe pain, she has classical TN with concomitant persistent facial pain. Her pain does not meet the criteria for migraine.[9]

QUESTIONS AND ANSWERS

This chapter has accompanying questions and answers that are available to subscribers as part of the Oxford eLearning platform. To access the questions, follow the link below, or go to http://oxfordmedicine.com/painmanagementreview

3.

MECHANICAL CHRONIC JAW PAIN

Radhika P. Grandhe, Matthew Valeriano, and Dmitri Souza

STEM CASE AND KEY QUESTIONS

A 25-year-old female presents to her primary care provider with a chief complaint of mechanical jaw pain. The pain has been occurring for the past 12 months and is described as a constant, dull ache that is localized over the temporalis and masseter muscles bilaterally. She notes that the pain is at its worst when she first wakes up and is exacerbated by activities requiring mandibular function, such as eating. The patient also describes associated bitemporal headaches. She denies any prior history of migraines but does note that she has been under a tremendous amount of stress (she was fired from her job a little over a year ago and has been out of work ever since). She admits to nail biting and teeth clenching during times of emotional stress. The patient is started on a course of nonsteroidal anti-inflammatory drugs (NSAIDs) with instructions to consume a soft diet over the following weeks.

At her follow-up appointment, the patient describes ongoing jaw pain. She is referred to the pain medicine clinic for further evaluation.

HOW ARE TEMPOROMANDIBULAR DISORDERS (TMDS) DIAGNOSED? WHAT FURTHER DETAILS SHOULD BE GATHERED FROM THE PHYSICAL EXAM?

On physical examination, the patient is a well-nourished female who appears anxious. A thorough oral exam does not reveal any lesions, plaques, or ulcers. Anterior neck and cervical spine exam are also unremarkable. The diagnostic criteria for TMDs (DC/TMD) are used to further characterize the patient's overall symptoms. No abnormal mandibular movements are noted. The patient has a maximal incisal opening of 32 mm. Maximum assisted opening is 40 mm, with an audible click at 36 mm. The patient's pain symptoms are reproduced with assisted opening. Left and right lateral excursions of the mandible are 8 mm and 9 mm, respectively. Further examination reveals diffuse tenderness to palpation along the temporalis and masseter muscles bilaterally. Only minimal tenderness is found with palpation of the temporomandibular joint (TMJ). Examination of the oral cavity and dentition shows moderate signs of tooth wear. Psychosocial assessment is performed with the Patient Health Questionnaire (PHQ-9) and shows moderate depression. With the history and physical exam findings, a working diagnosis of TMD secondary to myofascial pain and dysfunction is made.

WHAT OTHER DIAGNOSTIC STUDIES SHOULD BE PERFORMED? WHAT OTHER DIAGNOSES SHOULD BE CONSIDERED IN THE DIFFERENTIAL?

As an initial screening tool, a panoramic radiograph is ordered to give an overview of the patient's teeth and bony structures. The radiograph reveals no odontogenic or osseous pathology. Given the low suspicion for TMJ arthritis, no further imaging studies are indicated.

Although the patient's headaches are likely secondary to ongoing jaw pain, there is concern for the possibility of temporal arteritis. An erythrocyte sedimentation rate (ESR) and C-reactive protein (CRP) level are ordered and are found to be within normal limits.

WHAT SHOULD BE DONE NEXT? WHAT TREATMENT SHOULD BE INITIATED?

The patient is educated about her diagnosis and is given self-care techniques to employ over the following weeks. These include use of cold/hot packs, massage, jaw exercises to strengthen the muscles of mastication, and general relaxation techniques. She is educated about parafunctional oral behaviors that could be contributing to her overall symptoms. In addition to receiving self-care techniques, the patient is referred to a dentist for an occlusal splint fitting, given the high likelihood of bruxism.

WHAT ELSE SHOULD BE CONSIDERED WHEN DEALING WITH TMDS?

The patient returns to clinic with moderate improvement in her overall pain symptoms. She states that her pain has decreased by approximately 50%. The patient inquires whether there are any other options to help alleviate her symptoms. Given the patient's coexisting depression, the decision is made to initiate a low dose of amitriptyline. In addition, the patient is referred to a psychotherapist for cognitive-behavioral therapy (CBT), biofeedback, and relaxation techniques. She is also referred to a physical therapist and receives soft tissue mobilization, trigger-point dry needling, and electrical stimulation. With better relaxation and pain coping strategies, the patient continues to improve over the following weeks.

DISCUSSION

Temporomandibular disorder is a general term that refers to structural and functional disorders associated with the TMJ and/or muscles of mastication. In many patients, mechanical chronic jaw pain is related to TMDs. TMDs are the most common cause of nondental orofacial pain, affecting approximately 4% to 12% of the general adult population.[1] The etiology is often complex and multifactorial, varying from patient to patient. Factors that appear to put an individual at risk for TMD include: genetic predisposition, parafunctional oral habits (gum chewing, bruxism, jaw clenching), comorbid chronic pain conditions (fibromyalgia), widespread nonspecific symptoms, and concurrent psychiatric diagnoses.[2–3] There is a female predominance, with TMD symptoms occurring approximately twice as often in women as in men.[4]

REVIEW OF ANATOMY

The TMJ (Figure 3.1) is an atypical synovial joint that serves as the articulation between the condylar process of the mandible and the glenoid fossa of the temporal bone. The mandibular condyle changes significantly throughout childhood and, in some cases, can lead to facial deformities, predisposing those individuals to TMDs. The joint capsule contains an intra-articular disk that separates the joint into superior and inferior joint spaces. Unlike in other synovial joints, in the TMJ the articular surfaces of the bones involved are covered by fibrocartilage, rather than hyaline cartilage. Degenerative changes are more common in the inferior joint space. Although extensive erosion of the joint may be seen on radiographic images, a clinically significant relation between radiographic changes and TMD symptoms does not always exist.[5]

Muscles of the head, face, and cervical spine are also involved in mandibular movements required for common tasks like talking or eating. The act of mouth opening involves two sequential motions in the TMJ: posterior spin of the mandibular condyle first, followed by anteroinferior gliding motion of the intra-articular disk and condyle. Mandibular opening is largely controlled by the lateral pterygoid muscle, with assistance from the medial pterygoid for protrusion, while closing is controlled by the temporalis, masseter, and medial pterygoid, with the geniohyoid and digastric muscles assisting in retraction. Parafunctional habits, such as bruxism, can predispose individuals to myalgias in these muscle groups.[6]

DEFINITION

TMD is a collective term used for musculoskeletal disorders that affect the muscles of mastication and/or the TMJ. TMDs are often subdivided into four categories: myofascial disorders, disk displacement, intra-articular disorders, and headache attributable to TMDs.

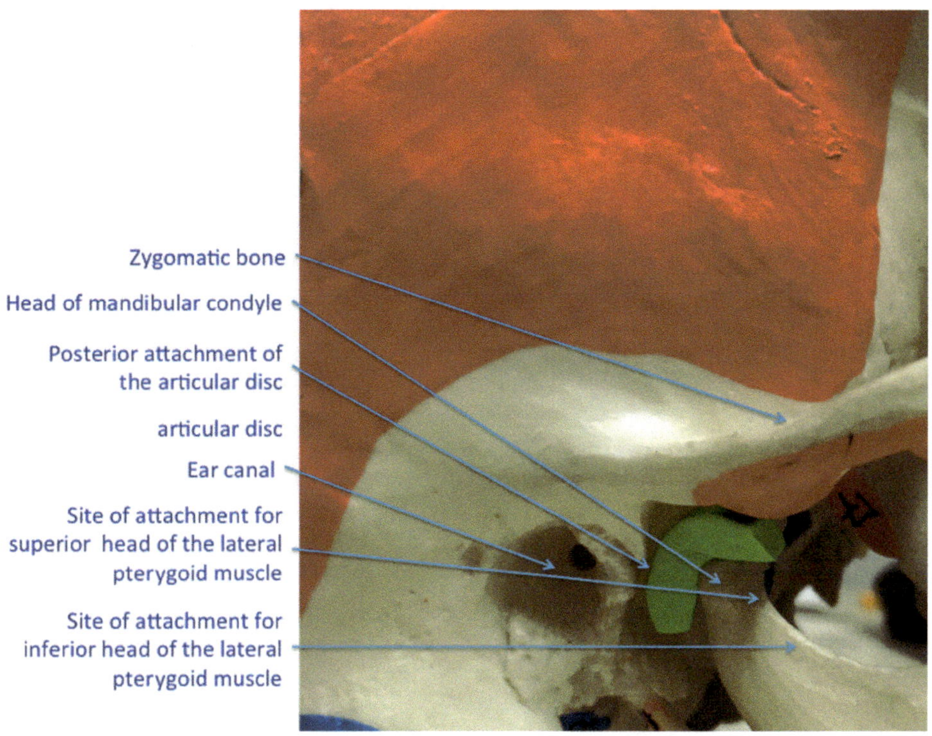

Figure 3.1. Anatomy of temporomandibular joint.

DC/TMD AND TYPES OF TMD

Diagnosis of TMD involves careful history-taking and a thorough physical examination of the TMJ and its surrounding structures. Secondary causes, such as cancer, CNS dysfunction, cerebrovascular insufficiency, cervical spine instability, infection, coronary artery disease, vasculitis, and inflammatory arthritides, which may masquerade as jaw pain, must be ruled out. Juvenile idiopathic arthritis (JIA) and temporal arteritis can frequently present with jaw pain.[7]

Patients with TMD can present with pain in the jaw area, auricular area, pre-auricular area, or temporal area, headache, toothache, orbital pain, or cervical pain.[6] Historically, the process of diagnosing TMD was not standardized until 1992, when the Research Diagnostic Criteria for TMD (RDC/TMD) were introduced. The RDC/TMD served as a well-validated and evidence-based tool to reliably diagnose TMD. In 2014, the RDC/TMD diagnostic algorithms were revised and new DC/TMD were released that included diagnostic tools for both Axis I and II disorders. The new criteria serve as a dual axis assessment not only for physical assessment of TMD pain, but also for screening for psychosocial comorbidities,[8] because many psychosomatic conditions, such as fibromyalgia, chronic widespread pain, headaches, and interstitial cystitis, have been linked with TMD. The biopsychosocial model forms the basis for the DC/TMD.[9]

The DC/TMD define many different types of TMDs and the diagnostic criteria for each (Table 3.1). The full diagnostic algorithms are beyond the scope of this chapter and interested readers may refer to the article by Schiffman and colleagues[8] for further details. The differential diagnoses to be considered while managaing a patient with mechanical jaw pain is presented in Table 3.2.

INVESTIGATIONS

The diagnosis of TMD begins with the patient's history and is subsequently confirmed through physical findings. In general, laboratory studies are not indicated. Uncertainties may emerge when details from the history and physical examination do not give a clear etiology for an individual's symptoms, and then laboratory studies may be necessary to rule out other diagnoses. Studies that may be considered include: complete blood count (infection), calcium/ phosphate levels (bone disease), creatine phosphokinase levels (muscle disease), ESR (temporal arteritis), and rheumatoid factor or autoimune workup (rheumatoid arthritis, JIA).

Imaging studies are not generally indicated for the diagnosis of TMD. However, a panoramic radiograph is commonly ordered because it gives important information about both tooth and bone pathology. It also provides a gross assessment of the sinuses and TMJs. Patients who have anatomic abnormalities (i.e., osteoarthritis, disk derangements) may benefit from further imaging studies. Maxillofacial cone-beam CT and MRI of the TMJ can provide additional data about disk pathologies.[10] However, imaging abnormalities have to be interpreted in the clinical context. A comparative study of patients with and without TMD showed no significant differences in the prevalence of osteoarthritic changes on CT scans between the two groups.[11]

TREATMENT

Management, rather than cure, is central to the treatment of TMD. The primary goal of TMD management is to alleviate jaw pain and to restore normal function. In acute cases, pain management should be initiated promptly in order to prevent peripheral or central sensitization.

Unfortunately, quality randomized controlled trials that address treatment of TMDs are scarce. A recent international consensus stated that reversible, conservative treatment should be the first-line intervention for TMDs.[12] Most patients benefit from a multimodal approach with the incorporation of education, self-care techniques, pharmacotherapy, and behavioral therapy. Overall, treatment should be individualized to the patient's symptoms, and treatment responses should be monitored every 4 to 6 weeks.[13]

Nonpharmacologic Therapies

Initially, the diagnosis should be carefully explained to the patient, along with comprehensive education about symptom management and self-care techniques. Instruction on good sleep hygiene, avoidance of parafunctional activities, relaxation and stress-management training, use of cold/hot packs, and simple home exercises can be helpful in providing a structured self-care regimen.[14]

In patients with comorbid depression or anxiety, behavioral interventions should be considered. CBT is ideal for patients with chronic pain or coexisting psychiatric conditions.[15] CBT helps to build on the self-care plan by addressing treatment adherence, providing further relaxation skills, dealing with pain cognitions and self-defeating behaviors, and creating a plan for managing flare-ups. There is evidence to support CBT and its efficacy in reducing TMD pain.[16] Biofeedback is another form of psychotherapy that is most effective for headaches. Patients are provided real-time feedback about physiologic changes through the measurement of EMG, EEG, skin conductance, and pulse volume and this process is used to teach voluntary strategies for regulating the emotions that lead to the changes.[17]

Oral appliances are other treatment adjuncts that have been used for both myogenous and arthrogenous TMD. They are particularly well suited for patients who have a history of bruxism or clenching because they not only protect the teeth, but also provide biofeedback. Evidence shows modest therapeutic benefits from splint therapy.[18]

Physical therapy is an integral component of multidisciplinary TMD management. Techniques that are used include joint mobilization, friction massage, soft tissue release, dry needling of trigger points, therapeutic exercise, TENS, iontophoresis, and low-level laser therapy. Kraus recommended a series of exercises intended to inhibit masticatory muscle strain, to improve neuromuscular control of mandibular activity, and to address aberrant joint noises or movements.[19] The efficacy of manual therapy for pain and dysfunction improvement in TMD patients is supported by varying levels of evidence.[20]

Table 3.1. SUMMARY OF DIAGNOSTIC CRITERIA FOR TEMPOROMANDIBULAR DISORDERS

CATEGORY	HISTORY AND PHYSICAL FINDINGS	SUBCATEGORY
Myalgia	History—positive for both of the following: 1. Pain in jaw, temple, ear, or front of ear 2. Pain modified with jaw movement, function, or parafunction Examination—positive for both of the following: 1. Confirmed pain in temporalis or masseter 2. Reproduction of customary pain with one of following provocation tests: — Palpation of temporalis/masseter — Maximum unassisted or assisted opening movements	Local myalgia—Pain localized to site of palpation Myofascial pain—Pain spreading beyond site of palpation but within muscle boundary Myofascial pain with referral—Pain spreading beyond boundary of muscle being palpated
Arthralgia	History—same as myalgia (above) Examination—positive for both of the following: 1. Confirmed pain in TMJ 2. Reproduction of customary pain at TMJ with at least one of the following provocation tests: — Palpation of the lateral pole or around the lateral pole — Maximum unassisted or assisted opening, right or left lateral movements, or protrusive movements	
Intra-articular disorders	History—positive for one of the following: 1. Any TMJ noise with jaw movement or function (last 30 days) 2. Report of any noise present during exam Examination—positive for one of the following: 1. Click, pop, and/or snap on both opening/closing movements with palpation of jaw opening/closing (≥ 1 out of 3 repetitions); OR 2a. Click, pop, and/or snap detected with palpation of opening/closing movements (≥ 1 out of 3 repetitions) AND 2b. Click, pop, and/or snap detected with palpation of right or left lateral movement, or protrusive movements (≥ 1 out of 3 repetitions)	Disk displacement with reduction—Jaw does not lock Disk displacement with intermittent locking—Jaw locks with limited mouth opening and then unlocks Degenerative joint disease — No click, pop, snap — Crepitus with any movement
	History—positive for both of the following: 1. Jaw locked so that the mouth would not open all the way 2. Limitation in jaw opening; interferes with ability to eat	Disk displacement without reduction with limited opening —Maximum assisted opening < 40 mm Disk displacement without reduction without limited opening—Maximum assisted opening > 40 mm
	History—positive for both of the following: 1. Jaw locking/catching in wide-open mouth position (last 30 days) 2. Inability to close mouth from wide-open position without a self-maneuver	Subluxation—No exam required
Headache attributed to TMD	History—positive for both of the following: 1. Headache of any type in the temple 2. Headache modified with jaw movement, function, or parafunction Examination—positive for both of the following: 3. Confirmation of headache location in the area of the temporalis muscle 4. Reproduction of customary headache with one of following provocation tests: — Palpation of temporalis muscle — Maximum unassisted or assisted opening, right or left lateral movements, or protrusive movements	

Table 3.2. **DIFFERENTIAL DIAGNOSIS OF MECHANICAL JAW PAIN**

I. Temporomandibular joint disorder	III. Headache disorders
1. Osseous pathology	1. Migraine headache
a. Degenerative arthritis	2. Cluster headache
b. Systemic arthritides	3. Tension headache
c. Fracture	4. Temporal arteritis
d. Neoplasm	
e. Congenital/ developmemtal disorders	IV. Associated structures
2. Nonosseous pathology	1. Dental infection
a. Disk disorders	2. Nondental oral lesions
b. Hypomobility	3. Sinusitis
c. Hypermobility (dislocation/ subluxation)	4. Salivary gland pathology
d. Neoplasm	5. Otitis media
e. Congenital/ developmental disorders	6. Trigeminal neuralgia
	7. Glossopharyngeal neuralgia
II. Disorders of Muscles of Mastication	8. Postherpetic neuralgia
1. Muscle pain	9. Cervical spine disorders
a. Myalgia, tendonitis, myositis, muscle spasm	
2. Contracture	
3. Hypertrophy	
4. Neoplasm	
5. Movement disorders	
6. Central pain disorders	

Complementary therapies, such as auricular acupuncture and tai chi, provide analgesia and help improve TM joint mobility. They can be used as adjuvant therapy with conventional therapies for management of chronic jaw pain.

Pharmacologic Therapies

Pharmacotherapy is very helpful in the treatment of acute TMJ and is often the first step. Initially, a short 10- to 14-day course of NSAIDs can be prescribed. For patients with masticatory muscle pain, a centrally acting muscle relaxant, such as cyclobenzaprine or tizanidine, may be beneficial. Other pharmacologic therapies that have been shown to be effective for myogenous or neuropathic pain are gabapentin, benzodiazepines, and amitriptyline.[21–22] Amitriptyline is particularly useful in patients suffering from chronic symptoms or in patients who have comorbid psychiatric conditions, such as depression. Its analgesic action is mediated by inhibition of serotonin and norepinephrine (NE) reuptake in adrenergic and serotoninergic neurons, which potentiates the descending inhibitory pain pathways.[23]

Interventional Therapies

For patients who are not responsive to the therapies described, more invasive treatment may be required. Interventional therapies include intra-articular corticosteroid injections, trigger-point muscle injections, Botox injections, and surgery. Botulinum toxin (Botox) injections of the masticatory muscles, namely temporalis, masseter, or other muscles, is one of the treatment modalities used in masticatory muscle myofascial pain. Botox acts by inhibiting presynaptic release of acetylcholine (Ach) and relieving muscle tension. A recent systematic review showed lack of consensus about the effects of botulinum toxin, although most studies showed a beneficial effect.[24]

For patients with osteoarthritis who are suffering from acute TMJ pain, intra-articular corticosteroid injections can be used. Repeated injections are not recommended due to risk of damage to the capsule or disk and formation of fibrous tissue. TMJ injections can be done blind or utilizing fluoroscopic or ultrasound guidance. A recently published systematic review suggests that autologous blood injections for TMJ disorders may provide significant pain relief. However, there are concerns about fibrotic changes in the TMJ after whole-blood injections.[25] There are animal studies and clinical reports that indicate that platelet-rich plasma (PRP) injections can effectively complement conventional management strategies without provocation of fibrotic changes in the TMJ, as well as provide superior pain relief and improved function compared to traditional treatments.[25–30]

Minimally invasive surgeries, such as arthrocentesis or arthroscopy, may be useful for some patients with internal derangement of the TMJ that has been refractory to conservative treatment. Accurate diagnosis through detailed imaging studies will dictate what type of surgery is indicated (i.e., arthroscopy, arthrotomy, reconstruction). An open surgical approach is pursued for ankylosis, TMJ tumors, and growth abnormalities.[31] Supplementation with vitamin D may also be used in chronic benign cases of TMD.[32]

CONCLUSIONS

- TMDs are a common hindrance to many patients.
- TMDs are often subdivided into four categories: myofascial (most common), arthralgia, intra-articular disorders, and headache attributable to TMDs.
- Diagnosis is largely based on history and physical exam findings. The DC/TMD provide a reliable, evidence-based set of criteria for accurate diagnosis of TMD.
- The differential diagnosis for jaw pain is broad, and non TMJ causes must be ruled out initially.
- Initial treatment should be aimed at education and self-care. Short courses of pharmacologic management may be considered on an individual basis, depending on the patient's symptoms.
- Adjunctive biobehavioral therapy is of utmost importance for individuals with chronic pain or comorbid psychiatric disorders.
- Interventional procedures, such as intra-articular injections of steroid or PRP or Botox injections of masticatory muscles, can be useful in some patients.

- Surgery is considered only when an accurate diagnosis has been made of specific structural pathology that has been refractory to conservative treatment.

REFERENCES

1. National Institute of Dental and Craniofacial Research. Facial pain. http://www.nidcr.nih.gov/DataStatistics/FindDataByTopic/FacialPain/
2. Hoffmann RG, Kotchen JM, Kotchen TA, Cowley T, Dasgupta M, Cowley AW. Temporomandibular disorders and associated clinical comorbidities. *Clin J Pain*. 2011;27(3):268–274. doi:10.1097/AJP.0b013e31820215f5.
3. Plesh O, Adams SH, Gansky SA. Temporomandibular joint and muscle disorder-type pain and comorbid pains in a national US sample. *J Orofac Pain*. 2011;25(3):190–198.
4. Slade GD, Bair E, Greenspan JD, et al. Signs and symptoms of first-onset TMD and sociodemographic predictors of its development: the OPPERA prospective cohort study. *J Pain*. 2013;14(12)(suppl):T20-32-3. doi:10.1016/j.jpain.2013.07.014.
5. Nordahl S, Alstergren P, Appelgren A, Appelgren B, Eliasson S, Kopp S. Pain, tenderness, mandibular mobility, and anterior open bite in relation to radiographic erosions in temporomandibular joint disease. *Acta Odontol Scand*. 1997;55(1):18–22.
6. Shaffer SM, Brismée J-M, Sizer PS, Courtney CA. Temporomandibular disorders. Part 1: anatomy and examination/diagnosis. *J Manual Manipulative Ther*. 2014;22(1):2–12.
7. Frei R. Study finds high rates of temporomandibular joint pain in juvenile idiopathic arthritis. *Pain Medicine News*. April 15, 2016.
8. Schiffman E, Ohrbach R, Truelove E, et al. Diagnostic criteria for temporomandibular disorders (DC/TMD) for clinical and research applications: recommendations of the International RDC/TMD Consortium Network and Orofacial Pain Special Interest Group. *J Oral Facial Pain H*. 2014;28(1):6–27.
9. Shephard MK, MacGregor EA, Zakrzewska JM. Orofacial pain: a guide for the headache physician. *Headache*. 2013;54(1):22–39. doi:10.1111/head.12272.
10. Petscavage-Thomas JM, Walker EA. Unlocking the jaw: advanced imaging of the temporomandibular joint. *AJR Am J Roentgenol*. 2014;203(5):1047–1058. doi:10.2214/AJR.13.12177.
11. Al-Ekrish AA, Al-Juhani HO, Alhaidari RI, Alfaleh WM. Comparative study of the prevalence of temporomandibular joint osteoarthritic changes in cone beam computed tomograms of patients with or without temporomandibular disorder. *Oral Surg Oral Med Oral Pathol*. 2015;120(1):78–85. doi:10.1016/j.oooo.2015.04.008.
12. Greene CS. Managing the care of patients with temporomandibular disorders: a new guideline for care. *J Am Dent Assoc*. 2010;141(9):1086–1088.
13. Mehta NR, Scrivani SJ, Spierings ELH. Dental and facial pain. In: Benzon HT, Rathmell JP, Wu CL, eds. *Practical Management of Pain*. 5th ed. Philadelphia, PA: Elsevier/Saunders; 2013:424–440.
14. Dworkin SF, Huggins KH, Wilson L, et al. A randomized clinical trial using research diagnostic criteria for temporomandibular disorders-axis II to target clinic cases for a tailored self-care TMD treatment program. *J Orofac Pain*. 2002;16(1):48–63.
15. Aggarwal VR, Lovell K, Peters S, Javidi H, Joughin A, Goldthorpe J. Psychosocial interventions for the management of chronic orofacial pain. *Cochrane Database Syst Rev*. 2011;11 CD008456. doi:10.1002/14651858.CD008456.pub2.
16. List T, Axelsson S. Management of TMD: evidence from systematic reviews and meta-analyses. *J Oral Rehabil*. 2010;37(6):430–451.
17. Kerns RD, Sellinger J, Goodin BR. Psychological treatment of chronic pain. *Annu Rev Clin Psychol*. 2011;7:411–344. doi:10.1146/annurev-clinpsy-090310-120430.
18. Ebrahim S, Montoya L, Busse JW, Carrasco-Labra A, Guyatt GH, Medically Unexplained Syndromes Research Group. The effectiveness of splint therapy in patients with temporomandibular disorders: a systematic review and meta-analysis. *J Am Dent Assoc*. 2012;143(8):847–857.
19. Shaffer SM, Brismée J-M, Sizer PS, Courtney CA. Temporomandibular disorders. Part 2: Conservative management. *J Manual Manipulative Ther*. 2014;22(1):13–23. doi:10.1179/2042618613y.0000000061.
20. Calixtre LB, Moreira RFC, Franchini GH, Alburquerque-Sendín F, Oliveira AB. Manual therapy for the management of pain and limited range of motion in subjects with signs and symptoms of temporomandibular disorder: a systematic review of randomised controlled trials. *J Oral Rehab*. 2015;42(11):847–861. doi:10.1111/joor.12321.
21. Kimos P, Biggs C, Mah J, et al. Analgesic action of gabapentin on chronic pain in the masticatory muscles: a randomized controlled trial. *Pain*. 2007;127(1-2):151–160. doi:10.1016/j.pain.2006.08.028.
22. Rizzatti-Barbosa CM, Nogueira MTP, de Andrade ED, Ambrosano GMB, de Barbosa JRA. Clinical evaluation of amitriptyline for the control of chronic pain caused by temporomandibular joint disorders. *Cranio*. 2003;21(3):221–225.
23. Smith HS, Argoff CE, McCleane G. Antidepressants as analgesics. In: Benzon HT, Rathmell JP, Wu CL, eds. *Practical Management of Pain*. 5th ed. Philadelphia, PA: Elsevier/Saunders; 2013:530–542.
24. Chen Y-W, Chiu Y-W, Chen C-Y, Chuang S-K. Botulinum toxin therapy for temporomandibular joint disorders: a systematic review of randomized controlled trials. *Int J Oral Maxillofac Surg*. 2015;44(8):1018–1026. doi:10.1016/j.ijom.2015.04.003.
25. Coser R, da Silveira H, Medeiros P, Ritto FG. Autologous blood injection for the treatment of recurrent mandibular dislocation. *Int J Oral Maxillofac Surg*. 2015;44(8):1034–1037.
26. Comert Kilic S, Gungormus M, Sumbullu MA. Is arthrocentesis plus platelet-rich plasma superior to arthrocentesis alone in the treatment of temporomandibular joint osteoarthritis? A randomized clinical trial. *J Oral Maxillofac Surg*. 2015;73(8):1473–1483.
27. Hegab AF, Ali HE, Elmasry M, Khallaf MG. Platelet-rich plasma injection as an effective treatment for temporomandibular joint osteoarthritis. *J Oral Maxillofac Surg*. 2015;73(9):1706–1713.
28. Hanci M, Karamese M, Tosun Z, Aktan TM, Duman S, Savaci N. Intra-articular platelet-rich plasma injection for the treatment of temporomandibular disorders and a comparison with arthrocentesis. *J Cranio Maxill Surg*. 2015;43(1):162–166.
29. Pihut M, Szuta M, Ferendiuk E, Zenczak-Wieckiewicz D. Evaluation of pain regression in patients with temporomandibular dysfunction treated by intra-articular platelet-rich plasma injections: a preliminary report. *Biomed Res Int*. 2014;2014:132369.
30. Kutuk N, Bas B, Soylu E, et al. Effect of platelet-rich plasma on fibrocartilage, cartilage, and bone repair in temporomandibular joint. *J Oral Maxillofac Surg*. 2014;72(2):277–284.
31. González-García, R. The current role and the future of minimally invasive temporomandibular joint surgery. *Oral Maxillofac Surg Clin North Am*. 2015;27(1):69–84.
32. Shipton EA, Shipton EE. Vitamin D and pain: vitamin D and its role in the aetiology and maintenance of chronic pain states and associated comorbidities. *Pain Res Treat*. 2015:2015;904967.

REVIEW QUESTIONS

1. All of the following therapies for mechanical jaw pain are currently used in common clinical practice and might be effective except:

   A. Ear acupuncture
   B. Occlusive oral splint
   C. Reducing oral intake
   D. Musculoskeletal manual therapy

2. Which of the following conditions has a high degree of association with TMJ dysfunction?

A. Fibromyalgia
B. Pelvic inflammatory disease
C. Myocardial infarction
D. Spinal stenosis

3. With TMDs, osseous changes seen on CT are:

A. Related to severity of pain
B. Related to degree of incisal opening
C. Related to palpable tenderness of TMJ
D. Not significantly different between patients with and without chronic TMJ pain

ANSWERS

1. C. Various types of manual therapy for masticatory muscles, exercises, and acupuncture have been used for treatment of mechanical jaw/TMJ pain, based on individual presentation. Dentists use a variety of oral splints to reduce sleep bruxism and muscle tension. Intake of soft foods might be considered for some patients, but decreasing oral food intake is not a recommended approach.[19]

2. A. TMJ dysfunction is multifactorial and is best explained using the biopsychosocial model. It has been demonstrated to have high association with psychosomatic conditions, such as fibromyalgia, back pain, headaches, hypermobility, and interstitial cystitis. Pelvic inflammatory disease, myocardial infarction, and spinal stenosis are not generally included in psychosomatic conditions.[9]

3. D. The severity of degenerative changes seen on CT has not demonstrated any correlation with clinical symptoms of TMD, such as pain scores, degree of TMJ tenderness, or the extent of mouth opening. Also, osseous abnormalities on imaging were not found to be significantly different in patients with and without TMJ pain. This lends further credence to the biopsychosocial model of TMD.[6,11]

QUESTIONS AND ANSWERS

This chapter has accompanying questions and answers that are available to subscribers as part of the Oxford eLearning platform. To access the questions, follow the link below, or go to ✔ http://oxfordmedicine.com/painmanagementreview

4.

POSTCRANIOTOMY PAIN AND CHIARI MALFORMATION PAIN

Andrew Wuenstel, David Frim, and Magdalena Anitescu

STEM CASE AND KEY QUESTIONS

A 16-year-old female has had severe, intermittent headaches for a few years, but they are worsening. The headaches are triggered by coughing, with severe occipital pain for 2 minutes followed by dull pain for 10 minutes. Her primary care physician recommends acetaminophen and naproxen, but there is no improvement in her symptoms over the next 2 weeks. A brain MRI shows cerebellar tonsillar herniation 6 mm below the foramen magnum, consistent with Chiari malformation type 1 (CM1). Her primary care physician consults neurosurgery for further evaluation.

WHAT IS CM1? WHAT OTHER SYMPTOMS MIGHT BE PRESENT ON DIAGNOSIS?

The patient is evaluated by a neurosurgeon. A detailed neurologic examination reveals only the absence of a gag reflex. An MRI of the spine to assess for a syrinx is negative. The neurosurgeon determines that there are no neurologic deficits requiring surgical intervention and recommends conservative medical management for the patient's headache. The patient is referred to neurology for ongoing observation and medical treatment.

WHAT ARE THE GENERAL INDICATIONS FOR SURGERY FOR CM1?

The neurologist gradually introduces topiramate, amitriptyline, and gabapentin, which improve the patient's symptoms. The headaches are less severe and of shorter duration. Some of the medications are tapered off over a period of years, and the headaches resolve.

WHAT CAUSES THE PAIN WITH CM1? WHAT MEDICAL THERAPIES ARE AVAILABLE FOR PAIN MANAGEMENT?

With the resolution of her headaches, the patient stops seeing the neurologist. The neurosurgeon evaluates the patient annually for neurologic deficits, but eventually informs her that she no longer needs follow-up unless new symptoms arise.

At the age of 26, a few weeks after having her first child, the patient hits her head on a car door. Severe headaches, similar to the headaches she experienced when she was 16 years old, return. She sees her neurologist, who restarts her previous medications. After 8 weeks of acetaminophen, ibuprofen, sumatriptan, amitriptyline, gabapentin, and topiramate, the patient notes little improvement in her headaches. The patient meets with her neurosurgeon and insists that, given her young age, limited response to medical management, and inability to care for her young child, she needs a surgical intervention.

WHAT SURGICAL INTERVENTIONS ARE AVAILABLE FOR CM1? HOW OFTEN DOES SURGERY IMPROVE CHIARI PAIN?

The patient is evaluated in the anesthesia preoperative assessment clinic before a posterior fossa decompression surgery. The anesthesiologist plans to continue all medications on the morning of surgery and to use opioids for postoperative pain management, tapering to ketorolac and acetaminophen by postoperative day (POD) 2. He also recommends a low-dose ketamine infusion during surgery.

IS THERE ANY EVIDENCE TO GUIDE PERIOPERATIVE MANAGEMENT OF CHIARI PAIN?

The patient undergoes a posterior fossa decompression without complications and is given hydromorphone for pain control and diazepam for muscle spasms postoperatively. On POD 1, the patient transitions from hydromorphone to ketorolac and is discharged with hydrocodone/acetaminophen on POD 3. Within the first week, the patient's headache improves and the pain physician slowly tapers her medications. Over the next 2 months, however, the headaches return and are similar in intensity, although different in character, to those she experienced before surgery.

WHAT INTERVENTIONAL PROCEDURES OR INFUSIONS ARE AVAILABLE TO HELP TREAT PAIN FROM CM1? HOW OFTEN DO THESE THERAPIES PROVIDE PAIN RELIEF?

The patient is evaluated in the pain clinic and is given a ketamine infusion. The intensity of headaches lessens, but they are still debilitating. On physical examination, she has muscle tenderness on her posterior neck superficial to the surgical site, concerning for myofascial trigger points. Trigger-point injections improve her neck pain, but not the occipital headaches. Occipital neuralgia is one possible etiology and the anesthesiologist attempts a bilateral greater occipital nerve block with local anesthetic. The headaches improve, but do not entirely resolve. The patient returns to the pain clinic after 1 month because her headaches have returned. A second bilateral greater occipital nerve block is performed, with similar successful results. After she returns with recurrent pain treated with repeat blocks, the anesthesiologist recommends an occipital nerve radiofrequency ablation. The patient undergoes bilateral greater occipital nerve ablation, with lasting improvement of symptoms. She continues to take gabapentin and amitriptyline.

DISCUSSION

CM1 is a congenital anomaly at the craniocervical junction characterized by inferior displacement of the cerebellar structures through the foramen magnum.[1] There are four subtypes of CM (Table 4.1). Symptoms of CM1 have been noticed in children as young as 1 year old, but they usually develop in adults from 25 to 45 years old.[1] The diagnosis is established with MRI. How many cases of CM1 are symptomatic is not known, but in one series, only 32% of cases detected on MRI were symptomatic.[2] The majority of patients with CM1 are asymptomatic, but the prevalence in the general population is estimated to be 0.24% to 3.6%[3] (Figure 4.1).

Table 4.1. **TYPES AND CHARACTERISTICS OF CHIARI MALFORMATION**

TYPE	CHARACTERISTICS
CM1 (common)	• Cerebellar tonsils displaced > 5–6 mm (adolescents and adults) below foramen magnum • Cerebellar tonsillar displacement of 3–5 mm may also be diagnostic with other symptoms[a] • May/may not have syringomyelia (syrinx)
CM2 (or Arnold-Chiari malformation)	• Cerebellar vermis and tonsils displaced below foramen magnum • Beaked tectum on MRI • Myelomeningocele, most serious form of spina bifida • Other possible anomalies: hydrocephalus, inferior displacement of fourth ventricle, elongation and thinning of lower pons and medulla, stenosis or atresia of cerebral aqueduct, upward displacement of upper cerebellum into middle fossa, cerebellar dysplasia, colpocephaly of posterior lateral ventricles, elongation of lower pons and medulla
CM3 (rare)	• "Cerebellar" encephalocele • Small posterior fossa, often with displaced structures into encephalocele and inferior displacement of brainstem into spinal canal • High mortality rate in infants • Severe neurologic deficits
CM4 (obsolete term)	• Complete cerebellar agenesis

Adapted from References 1 and 4.

Abbreviations: CM, Chiari malformation.

[a] In most cases, the anatomic finding confirms the diagnosis when CM is suspected based on clinical signs.

ETIOLOGY AND PATHOGENESIS

Two main theories for the development of CM predominate. The first theory is that cerebrospinal fluid (CSF) does not flow through the foramen magnum because of crowding by herniated cerebellar tonsils.[4] In this case, the goal of surgery is to restore CSF flow via a suboccipital craniectomy with removal of the laminar arch at C1 and possibly opening the dura with a duraplasty.[4] Another theory is that the inadequate size of the posterior fossa causes the symptoms. In that case, the goal of surgery is to remove a large portion of the suboccipital region to expand the posterior fossa.[4] The first surgical method is more popular, but there is still extensive debate about the pathogenesis of CM1.[4]

Regardless of the cause of the condition, CM1 is associated with many signs and symptoms, with each patient having a different response to pain treatment before and after surgical decompression. There are some cases of acquired CM from noncommunicating hydrocephalus causing intracranial hypertension and descent of the cerebellar structures into the foramen magnum.[5] Some examples are CM caused by multiple lumbar punctures, brain tumors, and malfunction of lumboperitoneal shunts.

PRESENTING SYMPTOMS

CM1 produces an array of symptoms. The common pathophysiology underlying the symptoms is brainstem compression and obstruction.[4,6–8] The most common symptom is a tussive headache lasting from a few seconds to a few minutes, which may be associated with posterior neck pain running down the shoulders.[4] There may be a frontal headache or pain/paresthesia in the upper extremity.[4] One study found that headaches triggered by Valsalva maneuvers were occipital 80% of the time and frontal 60% of the time.[9] The most common inciting factors were coughing and sexual activity, but sneezing, bowel movements, crying, laughing, playing a wind instrument, or any exertion were other possible triggers.[1,9] A tussive headache is caused by a sudden increase in intrathecal pressure from obstructed CSF flow at the foramen magnum.[6] Some of

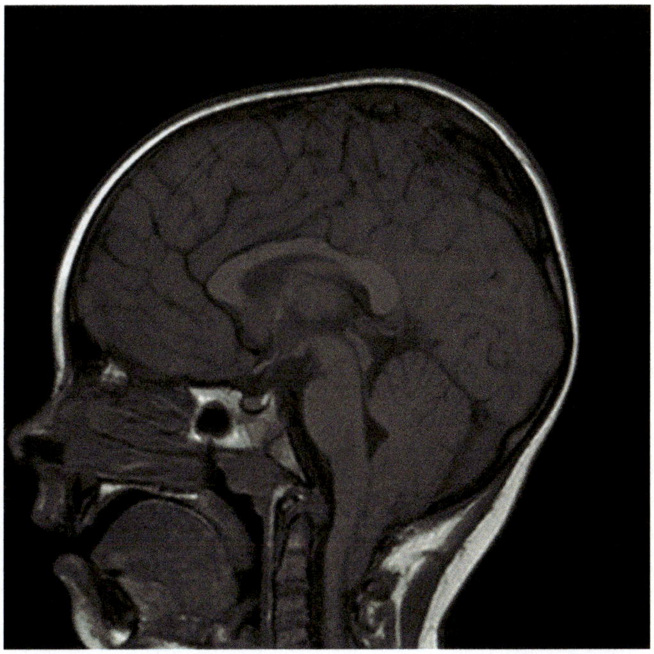

Figure 4.1. Chiari 1 malformation in a 5-year-old patient. The left cerebellar tonsil extends up to 2.8 cm below the level of the foramen magnum to the upper C3 level.

Table 4.2. **PRIMARY AND SECONDARY SIGNS AND SYMPTOMS OF CHIARI MALFORMATION TYPE 1**

PRIMARY	SECONDARY
Tussive headache	Papilledema
Visual changes	Absent gag reflex (CN IX involvement)
Syncope ("drop attacks")	Hoarseness (CN X involvement)
Muscle weakness	Tinnitus
Sensory deficits	Hyporeflexia
Dysphagia	Hyperreflexia
Dysarthria	Babinski's sign
Ataxia	Positive Romberg sign
Sleep apnea	Nystagmus (vertical and downbeating)
	Speech delay
	Seizures
	Tremor

Adapted with permission from Yassari & Frim.[4]

the more severe symptoms are apneic episodes or drop attacks, which are syncopal episodes lasting a few seconds that are usually triggered by physical activity.[4]

Compression of the brainstem in CM1 may cause apnea via three mechanisms: direct depression of the respiratory center, dysfunction of the ascending reticular activating system, or paralysis of movement in the upper respiratory wall or vocal cords.[7] Drop attacks are hypothesized to be due to dysautonomia caused by hindbrain compression.[8] There have also been case reports of CM diagnosed after aspiration pneumonia, likely from to dysphagia or vocal cord dysfunction.[10] Secondary symptoms of CM that are caused by nerve compression appear in Table 4.2.

SYRINGOMYELIA

The most common anatomic anomaly associated with CM1, occurring in 40% to 75% of patients, is syringomyelia.[1] A syrinx, a fluid-filled cyst within the spinal cord, represents a dilation of the central canal of the spinal cord and is also called a syringohydromyelia. It can be found in any portion of the spinal cord, but in CM1 it is generally located in the cervical spinal cord[1] (Figure 4.2).

A syrinx tends to be diagnosed at an early age and can produce neurologic deficits that become severely debilitating if it progresses.[1] A syrinx may cause pain, numbness, and weakness in the distribution of the spinal nerve roots affected.[11] Most patients with a syrinx (fluid-filled cavity) have little or no pain. The pathogenesis of syringomyelia is debated, but a leading theory is that blockage of CSF flow at the foramen magnum creates pressure back-up in the spine and venous engorgement of the Virchow-Robin spaces that dilates the central canal.[11] Most surgeons agree that the presence of syringomyelia with CM is an indication for surgery to restore normal CSF flow at the foramen magnum and to halt potential enlargement of the syrinx and worsening of symptoms.[4]

ASSOCIATED DISORDERS

Patients with CM1 and syringomyelia may suffer from scoliosis if the spinal cord grows toward the paraspinal muscles; unequal growth of the vertebral column leads to asymmetry of the spine.[1,12] Depending on its severity, scoliosis can contribute to poor posture and musculoskeletal pain. Arachnoiditis, which may mimic an occipital headache, is caused by rubbing of the herniated cerebellar tonsils against the spinal meninges.[1] The incidence of hydrocephalus in CM1 is 10%, but it is almost ubiquitous in CM2.[1,13] Tethered cord syndrome, associated with CM1, can cause severe back pain radiating into the legs and groin, along with nerve damage if it is not corrected.[14] The association between hereditary disorders of connective tissue (HDCT), most commonly Ehlers-Danlos and Marfan syndromes, and CM1 is 12.7%. In one study of 1,262 patients whose condition did not improve after surgery, 125 (9.9%) had HDCT.[15] The occipital headache in these patients may have been caused by atlanto-occipital or atlanto-axial joint instability.[15] Other disorders, such as Klippel-Feil syndrome and achondroplasia, have also been associated with CM.[16]

DIAGNOSIS

The diagnosis of CM is made with MRI. Historically, CM has been defined as the herniation of cerebellar tonsils ≥ 5 mm below the foramen magnum.[4] With the increased sensitivity of MRI, some patients present with classic Chiari symptoms

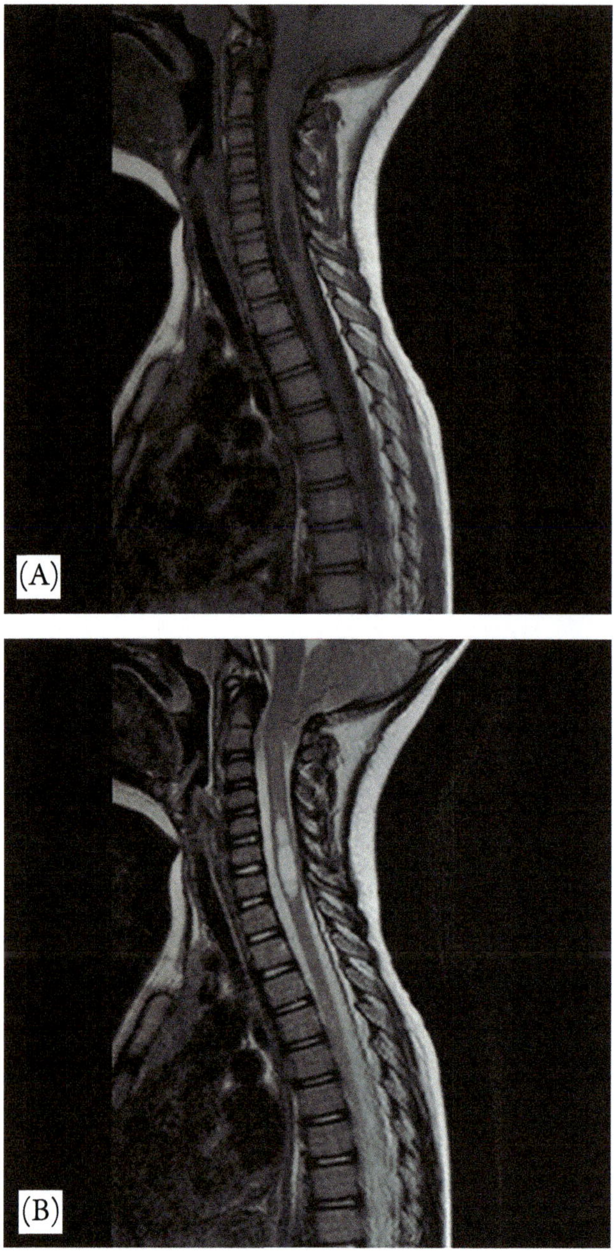

Figure 4.2. Syrinx is present in a 5-year-old patient with worsening headaches. There is a multiloculated lower cervical syrinx craniocaudally extending from the C4-C5 level to C7-T1 (image A). Faint T2 hyperintensity within the upper cervical cord at C2-C3 represents pre-soft syrinx (image B).

and herniation < 5 mm, while others are asymptomatic with herniation > 5 mm, making this definition questionable.[4,17] A full-spine MRI is required to evaluate for a syrinx and a CT is used to evaluate for bony abnormalities.

Given the incidence of asymptomatic CM1, even if a patient meets the anatomic criteria, the CM may not be the cause of the patient's occipital headache. Other causes of headaches, such as migraine, tension headache, sinus headache, posttraumatic headache, cluster headache, medication-overuse headache, meningitis, subarachnoid hemorrhage, hydrocephalus, and hypertension, need to be considered.[4] In one study, the incidence of migraines in patients with CM1 was 15%, and 11% had chronic migraine.[18] Although the incidence of migraines was similar in patients with CM1 and the general population, the frequency of chronic migraine was threefold higher in patients with CM1.[18] The high correlation between the disorders may lead a clinician to mistreat an occipital migraine headache.

PATHOPHYSIOLOGY OF PAIN IN CM

The pathophysiology of pain in CM1 is not completely understood. Most of the pain comes from the compression of the brainstem and cerebellum, producing sensory dysfunction and central pain sensitization, but the pain is multifactorial.[19] The pain associated with a syrinx is a central neuropathic pain, and the symptoms depend on the location of the syrinx.[20] Valsalva maneuvers, such as coughing, temporarily elevate intrathecal pressure (and likely intracranial pressure) and cause cerebellar tonsillar movement toward the cervical spine, producing a headache.[6] There is no effective medical treatment for intermittent intracranial pressure elevations; the only definitive treatment is surgical decompression.[6]

Central sensitization can develop after repeated exposure to noxious stimuli, causing a lower threshold for nociceptive activation; responses to nociceptive input are amplified.[21] Central sensitization may convert nociceptive-specific neurons to wide-dynamic neurons that respond to innocuous and less noxious stimuli, resulting in allodynia, which is the triggering of a pain response from a normally nonpainful stimulus.[21] Central sensitization requires activation of NMDA receptors, which is why ketamine (an NMDA receptor antagonist) is frequently used in treatment.[21] There is no single defining molecular interaction at fault, but rather a collection of transmitters (glutamate, substance P, kinin, bradykinin, nitric oxide, brain-derived neurotrophic factor) and receptors (AMPA, NMDA, metabotropic glutamate receptor subtypes or mGlu) that promote pain.[21] Central sensitization is common and may be triggered by central pain from a syrinx, peripheral nerve compression of the greater occipital nerve, brainstem compression causing central nerve inflammation, or any other chronic pain. This predisposes patients with CM to other central pain sensitization syndromes, such as complex regional pain syndrome, fibromyalgia, and temporomandibular joint disorder.[19]

Occipital neuralgia is pain isolated to the sensory distribution of the greater or lesser occipital nerves and may be a cause of peripheral neuropathic pain in CM1. It is typically a constant deep or burning pain, with intermittent intense shooting pain.[22] Intermittent subclinical cerebellar herniation may contribute to irritation of cervical nerves, especially C2 and C3, which presents as occipital neuralgia. After decompressive surgery, dissection of the surgical field may trigger myofascial pain or occipital neuralgia. The nerve roots of the greater and lesser occipital nerves emerging at C2 and C3 are one site for peripheral nerve blockade, either at that level or in the suboccipital region.

TREATMENTS

Medical Management

Unfortunately, only a few studies have investigated the efficacy of medication to treat CM pain. Many medications have become standard treatments based on their efficacy in treating other neuropathic and central pain syndromes. Some medications are used to exclude other disorders from the differential diagnosis. Triptans (serotonin receptor agonists), for example, are used to exclude migraines; however, the side effects can be misleading because they include mild headache, neck pain, and numbness. Other medications have been studied in other species, but have not been studied in humans. In canines, for example, many veterinarians have reduced CSF production with acetazolamide, cimetidine, omeprazole, and furosemide, to control syrinx symptoms, but there have been no trials in humans.[23]

Acetaminophen

Many patients will have taken acetaminophen for pain, with mixed results. Acetaminophen is a first-line management of headaches; however, because of the often extreme and complex pain in many patients with CM, it has limited utility. In one evaluation of acetaminophen for postoperative pain after a suboccipital craniectomy in children, acetaminophen alternating with ibuprofen every 2 hours significantly decreased postoperative pain scores, length of hospital stay, narcotic requirement, and antiemetic requirement.[24] The investigators postulated that this protocol would be helpful in adults, but they did not study an adult population.[24]

Nonsteroidal Anti-Inflammatory Drugs (NSAIDs)

Many patients will take NSAIDs for pain relief. The only support for the use of NSAIDs with CM is the acetaminophen/ibuprofen protocol mentioned for children.[24] The main concern with perioperative NSAID use is possible postoperative bleeding. One study found no significant postoperative hemorrhage with an acetaminophen/ibuprofen protocol used in pediatric patients after a craniotomy for brain tumor resection.[25] Although ibuprofen has minimal effects on platelet function and ketorolac has only a moderate effect, there is no prospective trial evaluating the safety of NSAIDs in craniotomy.[26] Currently, the routine administration of NSAIDs perioperatively cannot be recommended and should be addressed with the neurosurgeon for each case.

Muscle Relaxants

Baclofen, cyclobenzaprine, diazepam, tizanidine, or orphenadrine (anticholinergic, antihistamine) may be used to control muscle spasms, especially in the postoperative period.

Anticonvulsants

In neuropathic pain, there is a shift in the composition and distribution of sodium and calcium channels that may result in spontaneous and high-frequency firing from ectopic sites. Most anticonvulsants inhibit these signals by blocking sodium and calcium channels in a use-dependent fashion.[27] Other anticonvulsants potentiate GABA in the central nervous system to modulate pain.[27] There are no data available on use of phenytoin, carbamazepine, oxcarbazepine, valproate, lamotrigine, or levetiracetam for CM. One trial evaluated CM1 pain management with topiramate. The study had 28 patients, only some had CM1, but they did show some improvement in headache and sleep normalization.[28] One prospective crossover study of dogs compared quality of life with the addition of gabapentin or topiramate to carprofen (a NSAID commonly used in dogs). The results showed no improvement in quality of life with the addition of topiramate.[29]

Gabapentin

Gabapentin is a common first-line therapy in neuropathic pain. The mechanism of action may be gabapentin's inhibition of voltage-gated calcium channels via antagonism of the $\alpha_{2\delta}$ subunit, which is upregulated in pain, and it may disrupt NMDA events responsible for central sensitization.[30] Despite its common use, the only trial evaluating the efficacy of gabapentin in CM was in dogs, which showed that adding gabapentin to an existing NSAID therapy improved the quality of life of the dog, while adding topiramate did not have any impact.[29]

Tricyclic Antidepressants (TCAs)

TCAs, such as amitriptyline, nortriptyline, desipramine, and imipramine, have been studied in the treatment of neuropathic pain[31] and have been shown to improve pain in two-thirds of patients with peripheral neuropathic pain.[32] TCAs may block reuptake of serotonin and norepinephrine and thereby enhance descending inhibitory signals.[30] TCAs have minor effects at NMDA, H_1-histaminergic, and μ opioid receptors.[30] Side effects of TCAs are sedation, anticholinergic effects, constipation, urinary retention, and possible slowing of atrioventricular or intraventricular conduction.[30]

Selective Serotonin Reuptake Inhibitors (SSRIs) and Serotonin-Norepinephrine Reuptake Inhibitors (SNRIs)

SSRIs and SNRIs are effective in treating neuropathic pain.[32] Their action may be similar to that of TCAs.[30] In patients with neuropathic pain, SNRIs have been found to be effective in one of every four or five patients, and SSRIs in one out of every seven patients.[32] There are no published data to support the use of SSRIs (paroxetine, fluoxetine, citalopram) or SNRIs (venlafaxine, duloxetine, milnacipran) in CM pain, but they are used in treating CM pain before and after surgery.

Pain Interventions

After medical therapies fail, patients may try interventional therapies. Most neurosurgeons will not recommend surgery unless there is a specific indication for it. It is not uncommon for patients treated in a pain clinic to have a craniotomy and still suffer chronic, debilitating pain after surgery.

Ketamine Infusion

Ketamine is an NMDA antagonist utilized in treating chronic pain patients. Ketamine has been shown to reduce postoperative pain and opioid consumption even in opiate-dependent patients with chronic pain after various surgeries.[33] In chronic pain patients, ketamine was superior to placebo in treating central and peripheral neuropathic pain. Administration of

0.3 to 0.7 mg/kg of ketamine over 30 minutes was associated with a 31% to 51% chance of improving chronic pain in patients suffering from central sensitization.[34] In our clinic, a retrospective study of 42 patients who had pain after posterior fossa decompression revealed that 11 of 15 patients (73%) who received a lidocaine or ketamine infusion had improvement in symptoms (unpublished data, research presented at the American Society of Regional Anesthesia and Pain Medicine [ASRA] Fall Meeting, 2014). The dose and rate of infusion differ in various studies, making a specific regimen difficult to recommend.[35]

Current literature suggests ketamine infusions perioperatively or in the pain clinic may benefit CM patients with chronic pain. One possible side effect of ketamine may be increased intracranial pressure (ICP). Case reports published in the 1970s showed an increase in ICP in patients with obstructed ventricular systems.[36] More recent evidence suggests that ketamine may decrease ICP.[37–38] Until the effects of ketamine on ICP have been thoroughly studied, the safety of ketamine use in CM patients is controversial.

Lidocaine Infusion

There are no published trials evaluating the efficacy of lidocaine infusions on CM pain, but there are multiple studies evaluating lidocaine infusions perioperatively and in the pain clinic to treat acute, subacute, and chronic pain. In one meta-analysis, perioperative lidocaine infusions to treat pain after breast surgery showed no improvement in pain scores up to POD 3. The infusions, however, decreased cumulative analgesic use at 72 hours postoperatively and decreased the risk of developing chronic pain.[39] But in another study, perioperative lidocaine infusions did not decrease opioid consumption before hospital discharge.[40]

Lidocaine infusions have been shown to improve central neuropathic pain, peripheral neuropathic pain, and persistent postoperative pain.[35] Each study used different infusion doses and durations, making it difficult to recommend a single protocol. In our pain clinic, infusion therapies (lidocaine, ketamine) administered every 4 to 6 weeks decreased persistent pain from posterior fossa decompression in up to 70% of the patients (unpublished data, research presented at ASRA Fall Meeting, 2014).

Trigger-Point Injection

Trigger points are focal, irritable spots located within skeletal muscles that are palpated as taut bands. They are hypothesized to be caused by leakage of acetylcholine at the neuromuscular junction, resulting in a persistent contracture.[41] Trigger points arise from acute trauma or surgery and can cause an occipital headache in postsurgical craniotomy patients. They are treated conservatively with physical therapy or more aggressively with steroid or local anesthetic injections. There is currently no good evidence to support trigger-point injections for the treatment of headache disorders, although they have been used with peripheral nerve blocks for headache treatment.[42]

Botulinum Neurotoxin Injections

Botulinum toxin A (Botox) injected into skin, muscle, and joints can treat peripheral inflammatory and neuropathic pain.[43] Some studies have shown pain improvement in acute/chronic migraines, chronic joint pain, mono/polyneuropathy, chronic low back pain (with injection into paraspinal muscles), and myofascial pain.[43] The exact mechanism of analgesia of Botox is unknown, but it blocks pain to a greater extent than muscle paralysis alone.[43] Botox may block SNARE (soluble NSF-N-ethylmaleimide sensitive fusion-receptor) proteins in inflammatory cells, preventing cytokine release, or it may travel retrograde (spinopetal transport) into the dorsal root ganglion and inhibit neurotransmitter release and activation of satellite cells or neighboring neurons.[43] It may even undergo transcytosis to travel into the brainstem.[43]

Occipital Nerve Block

Multiple peripheral nerve branches innervate the posterior scalp, extending up toward the vertex and laterally behind the ears. After surgical decompression, as a result of the division of muscle and distortion of anatomy superficial to the posterior fossa, many patients can have occipital nerve entrapment that causes occipital neuralgia and cervicogenic headache. A peripheral nerve block is both diagnostic and therapeutic for occipital neuralgia. Nerve blocks have been efficacious in the treatment of cervicogenic headaches.[42] When methylprednisolone was injected into the greater and lesser occipital nerve in 180 patients, 94% experienced complete pain relief for 10 to 77 days.[44] In a double-blind, randomized controlled trial, an anesthetic block of both occipital nerves (greater and lesser) with a mixture of lidocaine, bupivacaine, epinephrine, clonidine, and fentanyl resulted in a 50% decrease in the pain of cervicogenic headache.[45] Headache duration, frequency, and limitations in functional activity after the intervention were less than in the control group. In a smaller case series of the same patients, 47 patients were given occipital nerve injections with the goal of being pain-free for 6 months; 41 patients (87%) required repeat blocks.[46] Interestingly, the investigators found that, for every 3 years of headache history, the patient required one additional block beyond the original injection to maintain adequate pain control. In our clinic, in a retrospective study of 21 patients with CM1 who had persistent pain after posterior fossa decompression and who underwent various interventional procedures, 13 patients (62%) reported improvement in symptoms (unpublished data, research presented at ASRA Fall Meeting, 2014).

Occipital Nerve Radiofrequency Ablation

If pain after an occipital nerve block recurs, ablation or implantation of a peripheral nerve stimulator may be considered. Surgical decompression of the greater occipital nerve from the scar tissue engulfing it after posterior fossa decompression surgery has also been successfully performed.[22]

Table 4.3. CHICAGO CHIARI OUTCOME SCALE

PAIN	NONPAIN	FUNCTIONALITY	COMPLICATIONS	TOTAL SCORE
1 = Worse	1 = Worse	1 = Unable to attend	1 = Persistent complication, poorly controlled	4 = Incapacitated
2 = Unchanged and refractory to medication	2 = Unchanged or improved but impaired	2 = Moderate impairment (< 50% attendance)	2 = Persistent complication, well controlled	8 = Impaired outcome
3 = Improved or controlled with medication	3 = Improved and unimpaired	3 = Mild impairment (> 50% attendance)	3 = Transient complication	12 = Functional outcome
4 = Resolved	4 = Resolved	4 = Fully functional	4 = Uncomplicated course	16 = Excellent outcome

Reproduced with permission and modified from Aliaga et al.[50]

Occipital Nerve Stimulators

Occipital nerve stimulation is a form of neuromodulation that is a reversible, nondestructive therapy. Typical candidates include patients with occipital neuralgia.[47] In one retrospective study of 22 patients who underwent an occipital neurostimulator trial, 15 (68%) patients had a successful neurostimulator trial and permanent implantation; 13 of 15 (87%) had persistent pain relief at a mean follow-up of 18.9 months (range 6 to 51 months).[48] Six (40%) patients with a permanent implant required additional surgeries for complications. Although this approach is promising, the high rate of complications requiring a second surgery and poor pain relief in two (13%) patients requires caution when recommending this option to patients with chronic pain.

Surgical Interventions

Good surgical outcomes are not guaranteed for patients with CM. Some neurosurgeons recommend that the only absolute indications for surgery are the presence of a syrinx, a syncopal episode triggered by exertion or a Valsalva maneuver, central apnea, or dysphagia causing aspiration pneumonia.[4] After medical management and interventional management have failed, the surgical options available for a posterior fossa decompression are suboccipital craniectomy, C1 arch laminectomy, and expansile duraplasty.[4] Debate is ongoing about which surgical procedure provides the best outcome.[4] Although surgery helps the majority of patients, it may not cure all. Among children less than 16 years old who undergo surgery, 90% to 95% have complete or near-complete resolution of symptoms by 1 year postoperatively.[4] The resolution of symptoms in adults ranges from 60% to 100% after surgery.[4,49]

There are many tools available to assess the overall level of patient improvement after medical/surgical intervention. One tool that we commonly use is the Chicago Chiari Outcome Scale (CCOS; see Table 4.3), which assigns higher scores to patients with better outcomes, including less pain, fewer nonpain symptoms, improved functionality, and fewer complications.[50]

CONCLUSIONS

- CMs are characterized by inferior movement of the cerebellar structures through the foramen magnum. CM1, the most common, is often asymptomatic.
- Symptoms are a tussive headache or headache triggered by a Valsalva maneuver. Other possible signs include neurologic deficits from a syrinx, central apnea, sleep apnea, or a syncopal episode with a Valsalva maneuver.
- CM1 is diagnosed with MRI.
- In adults, the success of surgical interventions ranges from 60% to 100%. Medical and interventional therapies are preferred before pursuing a posterior fossa decompression.
- Medical therapies include traditional neuropathic pain medications (with limited to no studies available in patients with CM). Interventional pain therapies are lidocaine infusion, ketamine infusion, and occipital nerve block. Radiofrequency ablation and nerve stimulators have not been studied in patients with CM, but offer promising results in pain control.

REFERENCES

1. Fernández AA, Guerrero AI, Martínez MI, et al. Malformations of the craniocervical junction (Chiari type I and syringomyelia: classification, diagnosis and treatment). *BMC Musculoskelet Dis.* 2009;10(suppl 1):S1.
2. Strahle J, Muraszko KM, Kapurch J, Bapuraj JR, Garton HJ, Maher CO. Chiari malformation type I and syrinx in children undergoing magnetic resonance imaging. *Neurosurg Pediatr.* 2011;8(2):205–213.
3. Kahn EN, Muraszko KM, Maher CO. Prevalence of Chiari I malformation and syringomyelia. *Neurosurg Clin North Am.* 2015;26(4):501–507.
4. Yassari R, Frim D. Evaluation and management of the Chiari malformation type 1 for the primary care pediatrician. *Pediatr Clin North Am.* 2004;51(2):477–490.
5. Payner T, Prenger E, Berger T, Crone K. Acquired Chiari malformations. *Neurosurgery.* 1994;34(3):429–434.

6. Sansur C, Heiss J, DeVroom H, Eskioglu E, Ennis R, Oldfield E. Pathophysiology of headache associated with cough in patients with Chiari I malformation. *Neurosurgery.* 2003;98(3):453–458.
7. Shiihara T, Shimizu Y, Mitsui T, Saitoh E, Sato S. Isolated sleep apnea due to Chiari type I malformation and syringomyelia. *Pediatr Neurol.* 1995;13(3):266–267.
8. Straus D, Foster K, Zimmerman F, Frim D. Chiari drop attacks: surgical decompression and the role of tilt table testing. *Pediatr Neurosurg.* 2009;45(5):384–389.
9. Martins HA, Ribas VR, Lima MD, et al. Headache precipitated by Valsalva maneuvers in patients with congenital Chiari I malformation. *Arq Neuropsiquiatr.* 2010;68(3):406–409.
10. Tsao TC, Juang YC, Chiang YC, Tsai YH, Lan RS, Lee CH. Pneumonia preceding respiratory failure. *Chest.* 1991;99(5):1294–1295.
11. Schijman E. History, anatomic forms, and pathogenesis of Chiari I malformations. *Childs Nerv Syst.* 2004;20(5):323–328.
12. Caldarelli M, Di Rocco C. Diagnosis of Chiari I malformation and related syringomyelia: radiological and neurophysiological studies. *Childs Nerv Syst.* 2004;20(5):332–335.
13. Nohria V, Oakes J. Chiari I malformation: a review of 43 patients. *Pediatr Neurosurg.* 1991;16(4-5):222–227.
14. Milhorat T, Bolognese P, Nishikawa M, et al. Association of Chiari malformation type I and tethered cord syndrome: preliminary results of sectioning filum terminale. *Surg Neurol.* 2009;72(1):20–35.
15. Milhorat TH, Bolognese PA, Nishikawa M, McDonnell NB, Francomano CA. Syndrome of occipitoatlantoaxial hypermobility, cranial settling, and Chiari malformation type I in patients with hereditary disorders of connective tissue. *J Neurosurg-Spine.* 2007;7(6):601–609.
16. Loukas M, Shayota BJ, Oelhafen K, et al. Associated disorders of Chiari type I malformations: a review. *Neurosurg Focus.* 2011;31(3):E3.
17. Barkovich A, Wippold F, Sherman J, Citrin C. Significance of cerebellar tonsillar position on MR. *Am J Neuroradiol.* 1986;7(5):795–799.
18. Kaplan Y, Oksuz E. Chronic migraine associated with the Chiari type 1 malformation. *Clin Neurol Neurosurg.* 2008;110(8):818–822.
19. Thimineur M, Kitaj M, Kravitz E, Kalizewski T, Sood P. Functional abnormalities of the cervical cord and lower medulla and their effect on pain: observations in chronic pain patients with incidental mild Chiari I malformation and moderate to severe cervical cord compression. *Clin J Pain.* 2002;18(3):171–179.
20. Ducreux D. Mechanisms of central neuropathic pain: a combined psychophysical and fMRI study in syringomyelia. *Brain.* 2006;129(4):963–976.
21. Latremoliere A, Woolf C. Central sensitization: a generator of pain hypersensitivity by central neural plasticity. *J Pain.* 2009;10(9):895–926.
22. Li F, Ma Y, Zou J, et al. Micro-surgical decompression for greater occipital neuralgia. *Turk Neurosurg.* 2012;22(4):427–429.
23. Rusbridge C. Chiari-like malformation and syringomyelia. *Eur J Companion Anim Pract.* 2013;23(3):70–89.
24. Smyth MD, Banks JT, Tubbs RS, Wellons JC III, Oakes WJ. Efficacy of scheduled nonnarcotic analgesic medications in children after suboccipital craniectomy. *J Neurosurg-Pediatr.* 2004;100(suppl 2):183–186.
25. Bauer DF, Waters AM, Tubbs RS, et al. Safety and utility of scheduled nonnarcotic analgesic medications in children undergoing craniotomy for brain tumor. *Neurosurgery.* 2010;67(2):353–356.
26. Bozzo J, Escolar G, Hernández MR, Galán AM, Ordinas A. Prohemorrhagic potential of dipyrone, ibuprofen, ketorolac, and aspirin: mechanisms associated with blood flow and erythrocyte deformability. *J Cardiovasc Pharmacol.* 2001;38(2):183–190.
27. Rogawski MA, Löscher W. The neurobiology of antiepileptic drugs for the treatment of nonepileptic conditions. *Nat Med.* 2004;10(7):685–692.
28. Klocheva EG, Komiakhov AV, Zhukova MV. The use of topiramate in patients with combined craniovertebral anomaly [In Russian]. *Zh Nevrol Psikhiatr.* 2009;109(9):49–51.
29. Plessas I, Volk HA, Rusbridge C, Vanhaesebrouck AE, Jeffery ND. Comparison of gabapentin versus topiramate on clinically affected dogs with Chiari-like malformation and syringomyelia. *Vet Rec.* 2015;177(11):288–288. doi:10.1136/vr.103234.
30. Ryder SA, Stannard CF. Treatment of chronic pain: antidepressant, antiepileptic and antiarrhythmic drugs. *Contin Educ Anaesth Crit Care Pain.* 2005;5(1):18–21.
31. O'Connor AB, Dworkin RH. Treatment of neuropathic pain: an overview of recent guidelines. *Am J Med.* 2009;122(suppl): S22–S32.
32. Sindrup SH, Otto M, Finnerup NB, Jensen TS. Antidepressants in the treatment of neuropathic pain. *Basic Clin Pharmacol Toxicol.* 2005;96(6):399–409.
33. Loftus RW, Yeager MP, Clark JA, et al. Intraoperative ketamine reduces perioperative opiate consumption in opiate-dependent patients with chronic back pain undergoing back surgery. *Anesthesiology.* 2010;113(3):639–646.
34. Patil S, Anitescu M. Efficacy of outpatient ketamine infusions in refractory chronic pain syndromes: a 5-year retrospective analysis. *Pain Med.* 2012;13(2):263–269.
35. Kosharskyy B, Almonte W, Shaparin N, Pappagallo M, Smith H. Intravenous infusions in chronic pain management. *Pain Physician.* 2013;16(3):231–249.
36. Bar-Joseph G, Guilburd Y, Tamir A, Guilburd JN. Effectiveness of ketamine in decreasing intracranial pressure in children with intracranial hypertension. *J Neurosurg- Pediatr.* 2009;4(1):40–46.
37. Zeiler FA, Teitelbaum J, West M, Gillman LM. The ketamine effect on ICP in traumatic brain injury. *Neurocrit Care.* 2014;21(1):163–173.
38. Zeiler FA, Teitelbaum J, West M, Gillman LM. The ketamine effect on intracranial pressure in nontraumatic neurological illness. *J Crit Care.* 2014;29(6):1096–1106.
39. Chang YC, Liu CL, Liu TP, Yang PS, Chen MJ, Cheng SP. Effect of perioperative intravenous lidocaine infusion on acute and chronic pain after breast surgery: a meta-analysis of randomized controlled trials. *Pain Pract.* 2017;17(3):336–343.
40. Wuethrich PY, Romero J, Burkhard FC, Curatolo M. No benefit from perioperative intravenous lidocaine in laparoscopic renal surgery: a randomised, placebo-controlled study. *Eur J Anaesthesiol.* 2012;29(11):537–543.
41. Zhuang X, Tan S, Huang Q. Understanding of myofascial trigger points. *Chin Med J.* 2014;127(24):4271–4277.
42. Ashkenazi A, Blumenfeld A, Napchan U, et al. Peripheral nerve blocks and trigger point injections in headache management—a systematic review and suggestions for future research. *Headache.* 2010;50(6):943–952.
43. Pellett S, Yaksh TL, Ramachandran R. Current status and future directions of botulinum neurotoxins for targeting pain processing. *Toxins.* 2015;7(11):4519–4563.
44. Anthony M. Cervicogenic headache: prevalence and response to local steroid therapy. *Clin Exp Rheumatol.* 2000;18(2)(suppl 19):S59–S64.
45. Naja ZM, El-Rajab M, Al-Tannir MA, Ziade FM, Tawfik OM. Occipital nerve blockade for cervicogenic headache: a double-blind randomized controlled clinical trial. *Pain Pract.* 2006;6(2):89–95.
46. Naja ZM, El-Rajab M, Al-Tannir MA, Ziade FM, Tawfik OM. Repetitive occipital nerve blockade for cervicogenic headache: expanded case report of 47 adults. *Pain Pract.* 2006;6(4):278–284.
47. Mammis A, Agarwal N, Mogilner AY. Occipital nerve stimulation. *Adv Tech Stand Neurosurg.* 2015;42:23–32.
48. Vadivelu S, Bolognese P, Milhorat TH, Mogilner AY. Occipital nerve stimulation for refractory headache in the Chiari malformation population. *Neurosurgery.* 2012;70(6):1430–1437.
49. Tisell M, Wallskog J, Linde M. Long-term outcome after surgery for Chiari I malformation. *Acta Neurol Scand.* 2009;120(5):295–299.
50. Aliaga L, Hekman KF, Yassari R, et al. A novel scoring system for assessing Chiari malformation type I treatment outcomes. *Neurosurgery.* 2012;70(3):656–665.

REVIEW QUESTIONS

1. A 32-year-old male presents to your office after MRI for a chronic headache reveals that he has CM. What are the most likely presenting characteristics for a CM headache?

A. Persistent frontal headache worse light and sounds
B. Persistent occipital headache worse with movement of the shoulders
C. Intermittent headache triggered by coughing
D. Intermittent headache present when the patient stands up for any period of time

2. A patient who has been diagnosed with CM1 by MRI ask his physician why his headache is so severe only when he coughs. What is the best answer for this patient?

A. Coughing causes an increase in intra-abdominal pressure, which causes a spinal pressure wave that presses on the CM.
B. Coughing increases the pressure in his head.
C. Coughing causes his ears to "pop," which is painful with a CM.
D. It is unknown why coughing causes pain with CM.

3. A 26-year-old female presents to your clinic with a history of CM1, diabetes, obesity, and hypertension. She has been reading online and found a list of severe symptoms of CM that indicate she might need surgery. Which of the following is not a severe symptom caused by CM?

A. Mild bilateral arm pain
B. A fainting episode that lasts a few seconds when having a bowel movement
C. Central apnea noted on a sleep study
D. Community-acquired pneumonia

ANSWERS

1. C. The classic presentation of CM is a tussive headache or any headache triggered by a Valsalva maneuver.[4] Answer A may describe a migraine; the persistent nature and triggering by light and sound are not classic for CM headache. In patients with CM, 60% of headaches are frontal and 80% are occipital.[9] Answer B seems like a tension headache with myofascial pain in the back of his neck. Answer D seems to describe a post-dural-puncture headache, given the positional trigger.

2. B. Coughing causes a sudden increase in intrathecal pressure due to the obstructed CSF flow at the foramen magnum.[6] Answer A is not true, the pressure originates in the skull. Answer C is false, as "popping" of the patient's ears would not cause a headache.

3. D. The concerning symptoms that some neurosurgeons consider absolute indications for posterior fossa decompression are the presence of a syrinx, a syncopal episode triggered by exertion or a Valsalva maneuver, central apnea, or dysphagia causing aspiration or aspiration pneumonia.[4] Answer A is concerning for a syrinx. Community-acquired pneumonia is not related to CM; therefore, answer D is correct.

QUESTIONS AND ANSWERS

This chapter has accompanying questions and answers that are available to subscribers as part of the Oxford eLearning platform. To access the questions, follow the link below, or go to ✔ http://oxfordmedicine.com/painmanagementreview

5.

SPONTANEOUS INTRACRANIAL HYPOTENSION

Magdalena Anitescu and David Arnolds

STEM CASE AND KEY QUESTIONS

A 34-year-old female presents to a hospital with severe headaches that are worse with standing and that are accompanied by nausea and vomiting. A lumbar puncture and a brain CT are normal. Because the headaches are unresponsive to ibuprofen and hydrocodone/acetaminophen as prescribed by her internist, she is referred to an academic institution for further workup. A detailed family history is obtained upon arrival in the new center and is notable for episodes of severe positional headaches in her brother and paternal uncle. Spontaneous intracranial hypotension (SIH) is suspected. A bedside lumbar puncture for evaluation of cerebrospinal fluid (CSF) pressure is unsuccessful in obtaining spinal fluid.

WHAT IS SIH? WHAT SHOULD BE CONSIDERED IN THE DIFFERENTIAL DIAGNOSIS?

Given the difficulties in obtaining CSF during a bedside procedure, the neurologist requests a fluoroscopic-guided lumbar puncture in the interventional radiology suite to determine CSF opening pressure and to obtain CSF. A cervical tap is attempted at C1-C2 because the space appeared to be readily accessible. During the procedure, the patient feels restlessness in both legs and makes involuntary movements in her left arm, which subsequently becomes weak. The procedure is abandoned without obtaining CSF. The patient's physical examination reveals left upper extremity 3/5 motor strength and decreased sensation to pinprick and temperature on the entire left side from the toes through the T4 dermatome. A STAT spine and brain MRI demonstrates high-intensity foci at the C2 level consistent with traumatic cord injury, edema, and scant CSF. The patient is admitted to the ICU and is treated with high-dose steroids. Her symptoms began to improve following steroid treatment.

IS A SPINAL TAP ALWAYS INDICATED TO DIAGNOSE SIH? ARE THERE OTHER MEANS OF IDENTIFYING THIS DISEASE?

Daily MRIs obtained during the patient's hospitalization demonstrate improvement in the spinal cord injury, with gradual disappearance of cord edema. The patient's neurologic symptoms improve with steroids, and she is able to leave the hospital after 4 days. She has residual paresthesias in the upper extremity. Although diagnostic cysternogram and myelogram are discussed with the patient, no other additional investigations for her positional headache are attempted during her hospitalization.

WILL THIS PATIENT'S PARESTHESIAS EVER SUBSIDE?

Throughout her hospitalization and after discharge, the patient continues to have a positional headache. While her spinal cord injury continues to improve, her postural headache becomes even more severe, eventually prompting an emergency department (ED) visit.

ARE THERE ANY OTHER TREATMENTS FOR HER HEADACHE? WHAT SHOULD BE CONSIDERED FOR POTENTIAL SIH? WHAT ARE THE TREATMENT MODALITIES FOR POSITIONAL HEADACHE ASSOCIATED WITH INTRACRANIAL HYPOTENSION?

The patient's headache is not controlled in the ED despite IV opioids, but she is subsequently discharged. She becomes confined to bed and is unable to provide for her three small children. The pain is unresponsive to conservative treatment (bed rest, caffeinated drinks, fluids, oxycodone/acetaminophen, and hydromorphone). During a follow-up appointment with neurology, an upper extremity paresthesia is present (although slightly improved), the postural headache is worse, and the patient can no longer maintain an upright position without pain. She is subsequently referred to the pain clinic for an epidural blood patch (EBP).

FOR THE BLOOD PATCH PROCEDURE, SHOULD WE USE FLUOROSCOPY TO IDENTIFY THE EPIDURAL SPACE? WHEN IS AN EBP INDICATED? IS IT A TREATMENT FOR ALL POSITIONAL HEADACHES? HOW DOES A BLOOD PATCH WORK?

A thorough physical examination in the pain clinic reveals a myelopathic syndrome consistent with her month-old traumatic, iatrogenic spinal cord injury. Apart from the severely debilitating headache, accompanied by nausea and vomiting, the patient experiences increased fatigue in the left upper and lower extremities. Given her history and the uncertainty about the presence of a CSF leak, the patient is not initially offered a blood patch and is advised to continue conservative treatment. The patient insists on an EBP, however, because of her increasingly debilitating symptoms. She has been confined to bed for the last 3 weeks with severe nausea and vomiting, is unable to eat and drink, and has lost 15 lbs. She is unable to maintain an erect position for more than 5 minutes due to the pain. After a thorough discussion of risks, side effects, and possible benefits of a blood patch, the attending physician agrees to perform a lumbar EBP under fluoroscopic guidance. Immediately after the procedure, the patient's symptoms improve, and her pain score decreases by 40%. She is discharged home in good condition.

WHY DID THE LUMBAR EBP FAIL TO PROVIDE COMPLETE PAIN RELIEF? IS THERE ANY VALUE IN PERFORMING ANOTHER LUMBAR EBP? HOW MANY BLOOD PATCHES CAN BE PERFORMED FOR A POSTURAL HEADACHE OR A POST-DURAL-PUNCTURE HEADACHE (PDPH)?

The patient's positional headache improves during the following week. While the pain decreased by 60%, she continues to complain of intermittent nausea. A second EBP, performed 1 week later, results in 100% pain relief. During follow-up phone calls, the patient is pain free and is discharged from the pain clinic. She continues to follow up with her neurologist for her residual neurologic deficit, which improves during the next year.

DISCUSSION

SIH, also known as spontaneous aliquorrhea, was first described in 1938 by G. Schaltenbrand. It is characterized by new-onset postural headache in the absence of known dural puncture.[1,2] SIH was once considered a very rare disease, but new evidence suggests that SIH affects a large number of young and middle-aged adults, with a prevalence of 1 per 50,000[3] and an estimated annual incidence of 5 per 100,000.[4] SIH affects women more often than men, with a female to male ratio of approximately 2:1. The peak age of onset is around age 40. Headache due to SIH is frequently misdiagnosed, most often as migraine headache, subdural hemorrhage, or meningitis, both in the ED and by specialists, which delays appropriate treatment.[4,5]

ETIOLOGY AND PATHOGENESIS

Similar to PDPH, with which it shares many characteristics, SIH is caused by CSF leaks.[5] The definitive cause of CSF leak is largely unknown in SIH, although several hypotheses have been suggested.[6] Structural weakness of the spinal meninges predisposes to the formation of dural defects that allow CSF to leak into the epidural space. Ruptured congenital subarachnoid (Tarlov) cysts or meningeal diverticula (Figure 5.1) are commonly present in patients with SIH.[3,5]

The association between connective tissue disease and spontaneous CSF leaks (Table 5.1) was first described in 1994, and subsequently was confirmed by numerous studies.[7] Growing scientific evidence links the presence of SIH to a heritable connective tissue disorder (HCTD). It is estimated that about 16% to 38% of patients with confirmed SIH also have an underlying HCTD. HCTD entities identified in SIH patients include Marfan syndrome, Ehlers-Danlos syndrome, Loys-Dietz syndrome, and benign hypermobility syndrome.[7–11]

The pathophysiologic mechanisms that predispose patients with HCTD to CSF leaks and subsequent SIH are not clear. Studies in mouse models of Marfan syndrome suggest that attenuation of dural tissue with fibroconnective disorganization and inherent structural weakness in the dura itself are responsible for the high rate of dural tears and subsequent CSF leak.

Another source of spontaneous CSF leak may be congenital osseous spurs or acquired degenerative disk disease that pierces the dura.[13,14] Extradural pathology is a rare cause of SIH, but several case reports have described CSF leaks associated with vertebral osteophytes, most often at the cervical level. SIH in these cases is most often treated conservatively.[16]

In rare cases, degenerative disk disease can result in calcified intervertebral disks that contribute to dural breech, ongoing CSF leak, thoracic subdural hematomas, and an altered level of consciousness. These severe cases require surgical interventions to seal the defect and correct the underlying cause[9] (Figure 5.2).

CLINICAL MANIFESTATIONS

Positional and Other Headache

SIH manifests as the new onset of severe headaches, partially or completely improved by lying down; the headache usually worsens within 15 minutes of assuming an upright position. The headache can be diffuse or localized, most commonly at the occipital or suboccipital areas and more rarely in the frontal or temporal zone.[17] In a majority of cases, the headache is bilateral, although it can sometimes start as a focal and unilateral discomfort that progresses to a holocephalic headache if the patient remains upright. Valsalva-type maneuvers often aggravate the headache.[17]

Although the postural component of the headache is the hallmark of SIH, some patients report exertional headaches,[3] headaches that appear at the end of the day,[17] and even paradoxical headaches that worsen when the patient lies down. Therefore, a thorough differential diagnosis needs to be considered with any new-onset daily headache (Table 5.2).

In addition to the classical postural headache, headaches attributed to spontaneous CSF leaks may also manifest as:

1. Nonorthostatic, lingering, chronic daily headaches or pressure sensations

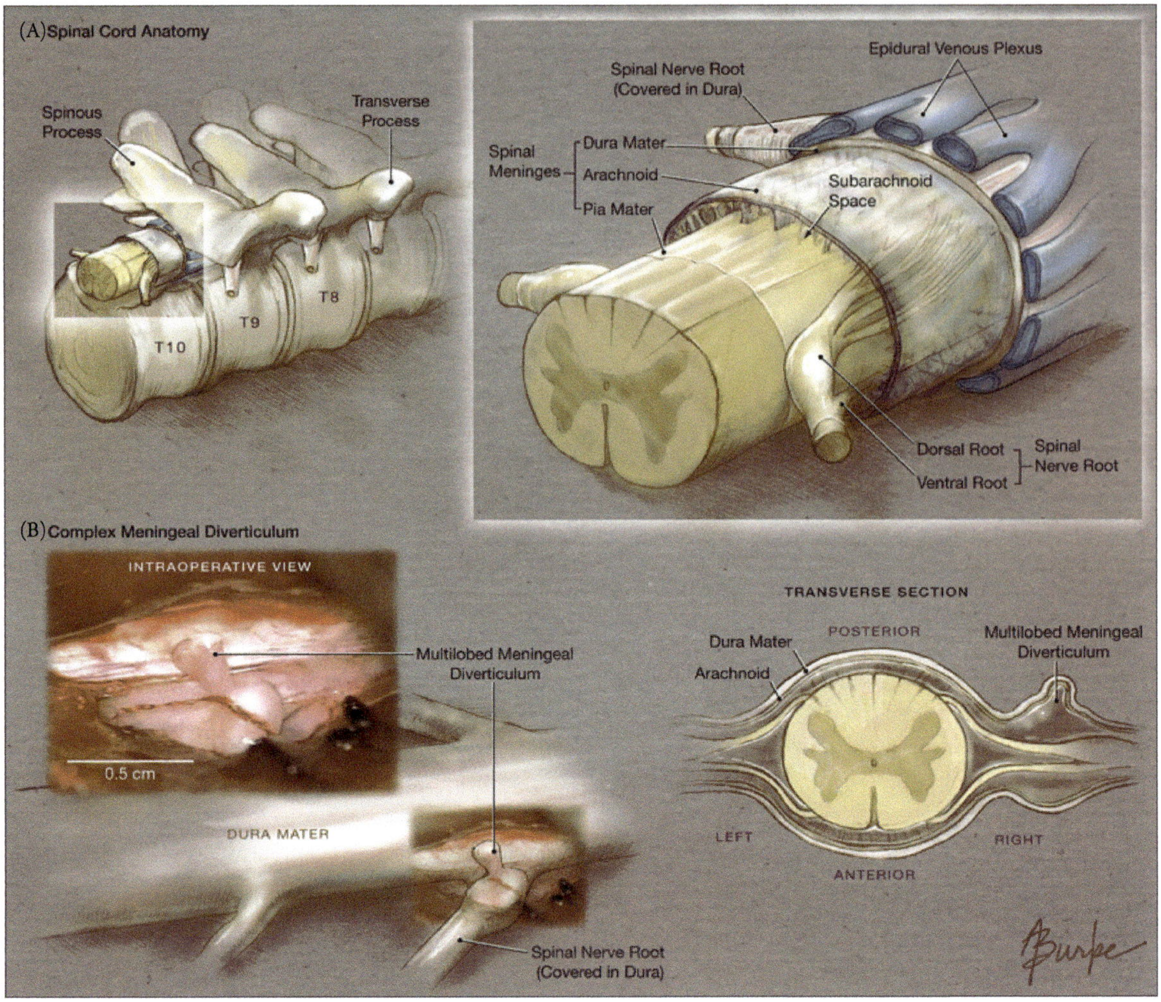

Figure 5.1. Complex meningeal diverticulum arising from a thoracic nerve root sleeve. Reproduced with permission from Schievink.[5]

2. Lingering daily headaches or cervical/interscapular pain days/weeks before the orthostatic headaches
3. "Transformed orthostatic headaches" that start as postural headaches but then progress to become a chronic daily headache

Table 5.1. **CONNECTIVE TISSUE DISORDERS ASSOCIATED WITH SPONTANEOUS INTRACRANIAL HYPOTENSION**

DEFINITE SYNDROMES	VARIOUS CONNECTIVE TISSUE TRAITS
Marfan syndrome	Isolated skeletal features of Marfan syndrome
Ehlers-Danlos syndrome	Isolated joint hypermobility
Autosomal dominant polycystic kidney disease	Joint hypermobility with fascial thinning
	Spontaneous retinal detachment

Modified from Schievink et al.[7]

4. Acute "thunderclap" onset of headache that resembles a subarachnoid hemorrhage followed by subsequent development of orthostatic headaches[16]
5. Paradoxical postural headache with pain in the recumbent position that disappears in the upright position[18]
6. Postural headaches that occur only in the second half of the day[19]
7. Exertional headaches[20]
8. Intermittent headaches or no headache (acephalgic form) if the CSF leak is very small[17,21]

Miscellaneous Symptoms

A variety of symptoms have been reported in patients with SIH. Posterior neck pain or stiffness, nausea, and vomiting are common, occurring in approximately 50% of patients, and suggest meningeal irritation.[7] Changes in hearing, tinnitus, and a disturbed sense of balance are the second most common symptoms of SIH and can be explained by stretching of CN VIII during downward displacement of the brain (Table 5.3).

(A) (B)

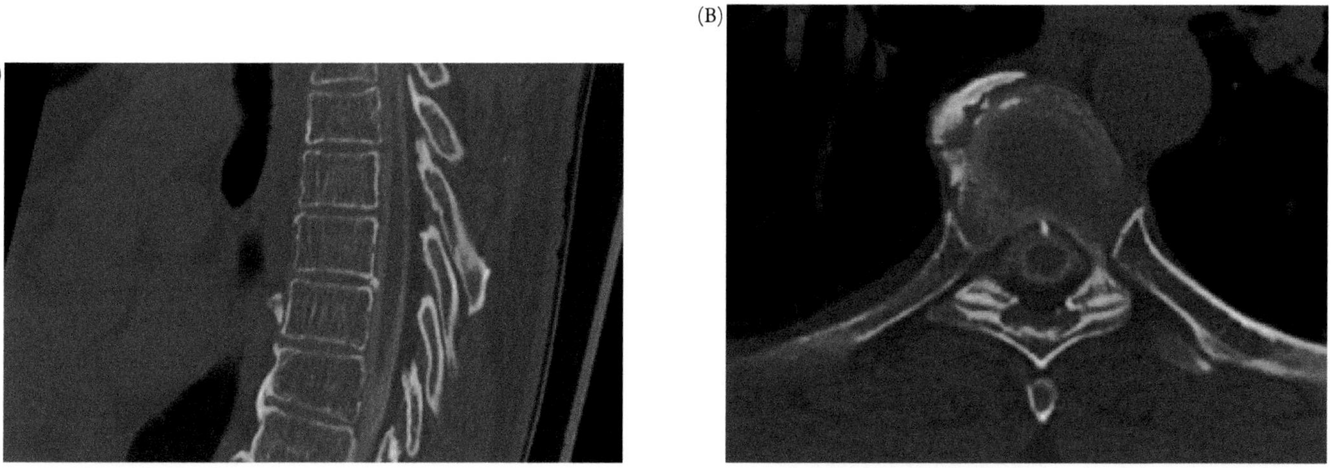

Figure 5.2. (A) CT myelogram, sagittal view, of calcified T6-T7 intervertebral disk indenting the thecal sac. (B) Axial CT myelogram showing calcified disk protrusion and accumulation of dye ventral to the thecal sac.

Rare symptoms include visual blurring or visual field defect (optic nerve involvement), diplopia (abducens or trochlear nerve involvement), facial numbness or pain (trigeminal nerve involvement), hyperprolactinemia and galactorrhea (distortion of the pituitary stalk), parkinsonism, ataxia, cerebellar hemorrhage, and coma.

Spinal manifestations include interscapular pain and, rarely, pain at the level of CSF leak. Quadriplegia and radicular symptoms have been described when cervical spinal nerve roots are stretched or epidural venous plexuses are dilated. Spinal manifestations occur in about 6% of patients with SIH, may be present at the cervical, thoracic, or lumbar levels,

Table 5.2. **DIFFERENTIAL DIAGNOSIS OF SPONTANEOUS INTRACRANIAL HYPOTENSION**

HEADACHE DISORDER	AGE OF ONSET	FEMALE: MALE RATIO	CONNECTIVE TISSUE DISORDER	HEADACHE FEATURES	ASSOCIATED FEATURES	CONFIRMATORY TESTING
New daily persistent headache	15–50 (mean 35)	2:1	No	Bilateral, migraine or tension-type	Nausea, fatigue, preceding viral illness	None
Spontaneous intracranial hypotension	20–60 (mean 40)	2:1	Yes	Bilateral, better in recumbency	Visual aura, cranial nerve dysfunction, nausea	MRI, LP, myelogram
Subarachnoid hemorrhage	> 20 (mean 50)	1.5:1	Yes	Bilateral, instantaneous	Meningismus, cranial nerve dysfunction	CT, LP
Carotid/vertebral artery dissection	20–70 (mean 45)	1:1	Yes	Unilateral, neck pain	Horner syndrome, cranial nerve dysfunction, pulsatile tinnitus	Angiography
Cerebral venous sinus thrombosis	Any age	3:1	No	Bilateral often, but unilateral if headache is the only symptom	Seizure, papilledema, visual changes, cranial nerve dysfunction	MRI/MRV, angiography
Benign intracranial hypotension	20–40 (mean 30)	8:1	No	Bilateral, worse in recumbancy	Papilledema, visual changes, abducens nerve palsy	LP
Posttraumatic headache	Any age	1.5:1	No	Bilateral, tension-type	Dizziness, neuropsychological symptoms	None
Meningitis	Any age	1:1	No	Bilateral	Fever, meningismus, systemic illness	LP

Modified from Schievink et al.[3]

ABBREVIATIONS: CT, computer tomography; LP, lumbar puncture; MRI, magnetic resonance imaging; MRV, magnetic resonance venography.

Table 5.3. **DIAGNOSTIC CRITERIA FOR SPONTANEOUS INTRACRANIAL HYPOTENSION**

A. Orthostatic headache	Diffuse and/or dull headache that worsens within 15 minutes after sitting or standing, with more than one of the following: 1. Neck stiffness 2. Tinnitus 3. Hypacusia 4. Photophobia 5. Nausea
B. At least one of the findings in the right-side column	1. Low opening pressure (< 60 mm H_2O) 2. Sustained improvement of symptoms after epidural blood patching 3. Demonstration of an active CSF leak 4. Cranial MRI changes of intracranial hypotension (brain sagging or pachymeningeal enhancement)
C. No recent history of dural puncture or other cause of CSF fistula	
D. Headache not attributable to another disorder	

Modified from Schievink et al.[26]

and consist mainly of myelopathy or radiculopathy caused by massive CSF accumulation compressing the nerve roots. Treatment of the underlying CSF leak resolves the symptoms[22] (Figure 5.3).

Given the variable presentations of SIH, new diagnostic criteria have recently been developed.[23]

DIAGNOSTIC MODALITIES

Cranial MRI

MRI is used for noninvasive diagnosis of SIH. There are five characteristic imaging features specific for SIH on the MRI.

1. Subdural fluid collection occurs in approximately 50% of patients with SIH. Fluid is localized mainly over the cerebral convexities but does not cause an appreciable mass effect. Other locations include the posterior fossa and retroclival space. An untreated CSF leak can cause a mass effect from growing subdural hematomas.
2. Enhancement of the pachymeninges is the commonly described abnormality of SIH. The enhancement is diffuse, involves both supra- and infratentorial compartments, and spares the leptomeninges[27] (Figure 5.4).
3. Engorgement of venous structures is detected when SIH affects the dural venous sinuses or large cerebral veins, and it rarely occurs in isolation.
4. Pituitary hyperemia can in some instances mimic a pituitary tumor or hyperplasia.
5. Sagging of the brain is specific for SIH and may or may not be accompanied by ventricular collapse.

Most features visible on MRI are explained by compensatory changes from loss of CSF. The Monro-Kellie theory postulates that the sum of the volumes of intracranial blood, CSF, and cerebral tissue must remain constant in an intact cranium. Therefore, loss of CSF through multiple leaks is compensated for by an increased volume of vascular components. This accounts for vessel engorgement and pachymeningeal enhancement.

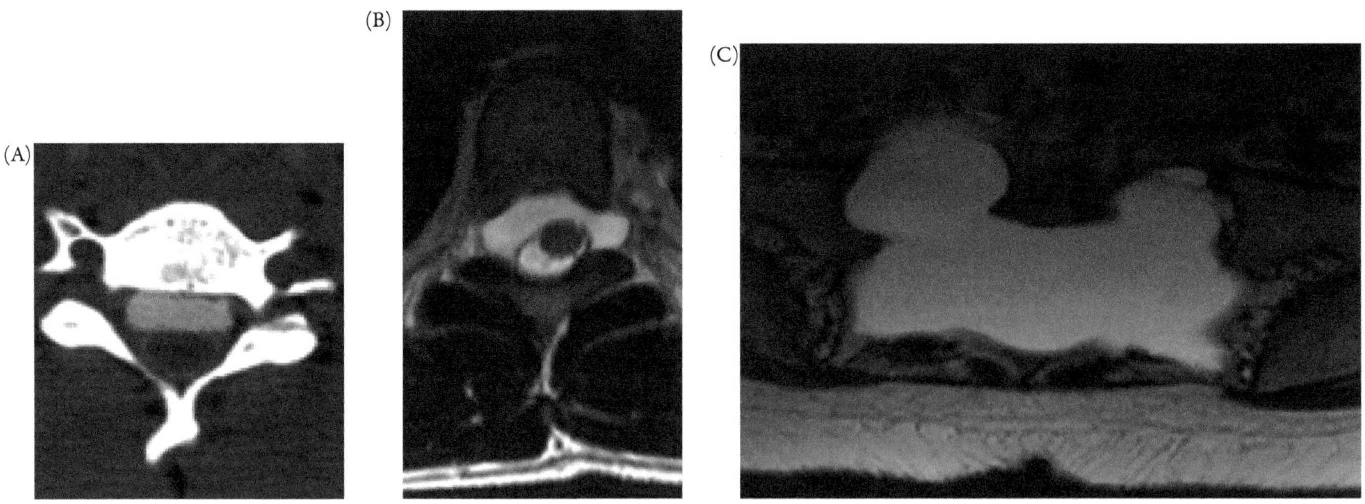

Figure 5.3. (A) Cervical myelopathy in spontaneous intracranial hypotension (SIH) demonstrating extensive CSF collections. (B) Thoracic myelopathy and radiculopathy in SIH with axial postmyelography images showing extrathecal fluid collection in the thoracic spine. (C) Lumbosacral radiculopathy in SIH with MR images revealing lumbosacral dural ectasia in patient with Marfan syndrome. Reproduced with permission from Schievink et al.[25]

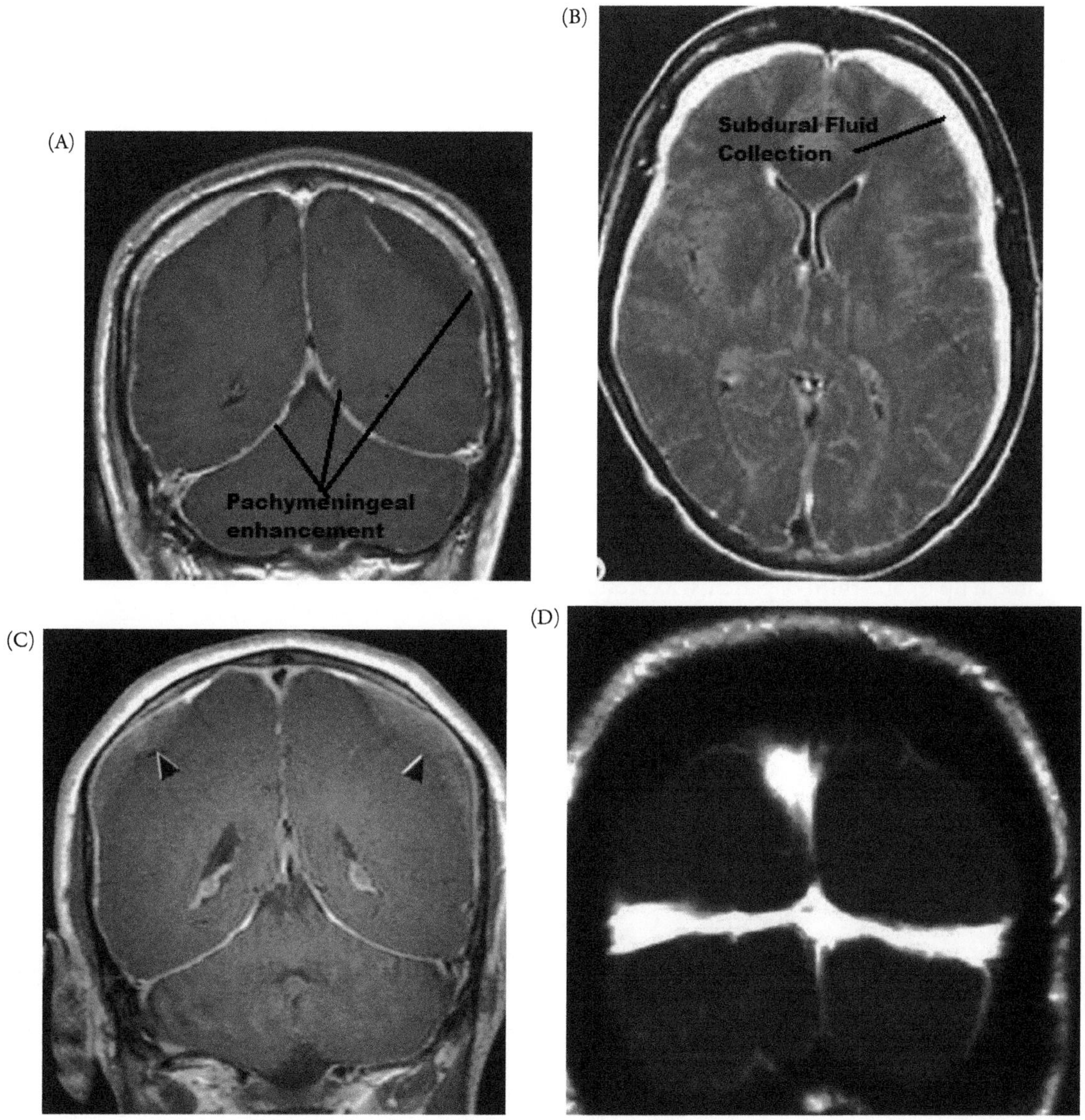

Figure 5.4. (A) MRI of pachymeningeal enhancement. (B) Gadolinium-enhanced MRI showing subdural CSF accumulation. (C) MRI showing bilateral subdural hematoma from continuous CSF leak with mass effect on underlying brain (arrowheads). (D) MRI showing engorged cerebral sinuses. (A) and (B) reproduced from Wieseman et al.[10] (C) and (D) reproduced with permission from Mokri.[18]

Spinal MRI

The main spinal MRI findings in SIH are extra-arachnoid fluid collections,[24] spinal meningeal enhancements, dilatation of anterior internal vertebral (epidural) venous plexuses, syringomyelia, and retrospinal fluid collections at C1-C2. Spinal MRI is commonly used in conjunction with radionuclide cysternography (RC) and CT myelogram to identify a CSF leak (Figure 5.5 and Figure 5.6).

Common MRI findings for both brain and spine are summarized in Table 5.4.

Cranial CT

Although less specific than MRI, CT can suggest the diagnosis of SIH based on subdural fluid accumulation or obliteration of subarachnoid cisterns and ventricular collapse.

CT Myelography

CT myelography is the diagnostic modality of choice for identifying the location and extent of CSF leak. It is performed by administering an iodinated contrast agent through a dural puncture, followed by thin-cut CT through the spine. CSF leaks are often found at the cervicothoracic or thoracolumbar junction, many times with multiple locations. Meningeal diverticula can also be identified by this technique. The sensitivity of CT myelography is unclear, and it is most appropriately performed to identify the location of CSF leak after MRI and RC suggest SIH.

RC

RC is performed by introducing a radioactive tracer into the subarachnoid space and scanning the entire neuraxis using a gamma camera. When RC is used alone, the location of CSF

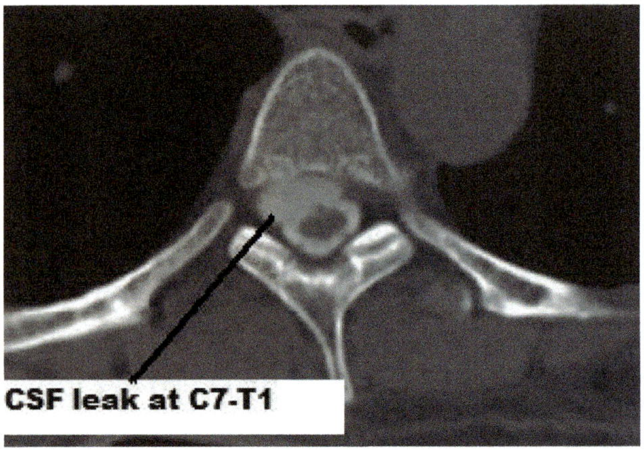

Figure 5.5. Spinal MRI showing accumulation of CSF in the ventral portions of the spine. Reproduced from Wieseman.[10]

leak remains obscure in up to one-third of patients. RC results need to be correlated with CT myelography or MRI. Typical findings include evidence of the diverticulum, early accumulation of tracer in bladder and kidney[27] (Figure 5.7), slow ascent of the tracer along the spinal axis, and decreased activity over the cerebral convexities.

Massive fluid accumulation from symptomatic CSF leak may be revealed via CT or MRI (Figure 5.5).

Lumbar Puncture

When lumbar puncture is performed in the lateral position, most patients with SIH have an opening pressure of less than 60 mm H_2O, compared to a reference range for patients without SIH of 65 to 195 mm H_2O. In some reported cases, CSF pressure was so low that CSF could be obtained only after gentle aspiration; rarely, a sucking noise with withdrawal of the stylet has been reported, signifying a subatmospheric pressure. CSF analysis can be entirely normal or have nonspecific findings, such as elevated protein concentration, lymphocytic pleocytosis, and increased erythrocyte count with or without xanthochromia.

Noninvasive diagnostic techniques, such as CT and MRI, are rarely associated with complications. However, when dural puncture is performed, arachnoiditis, nerve injury, spinal cord injury, infection, or bleeding has been reported. Additionally, the dural puncture itself can aggravate the positional headache.

TREATMENT OF SIH

Conservative Treatment

In many cases, the postural headache disappears spontaneously or is responsive to conservative treatment. As with PDPH, conservative treatment for SIH involves bed rest, oral

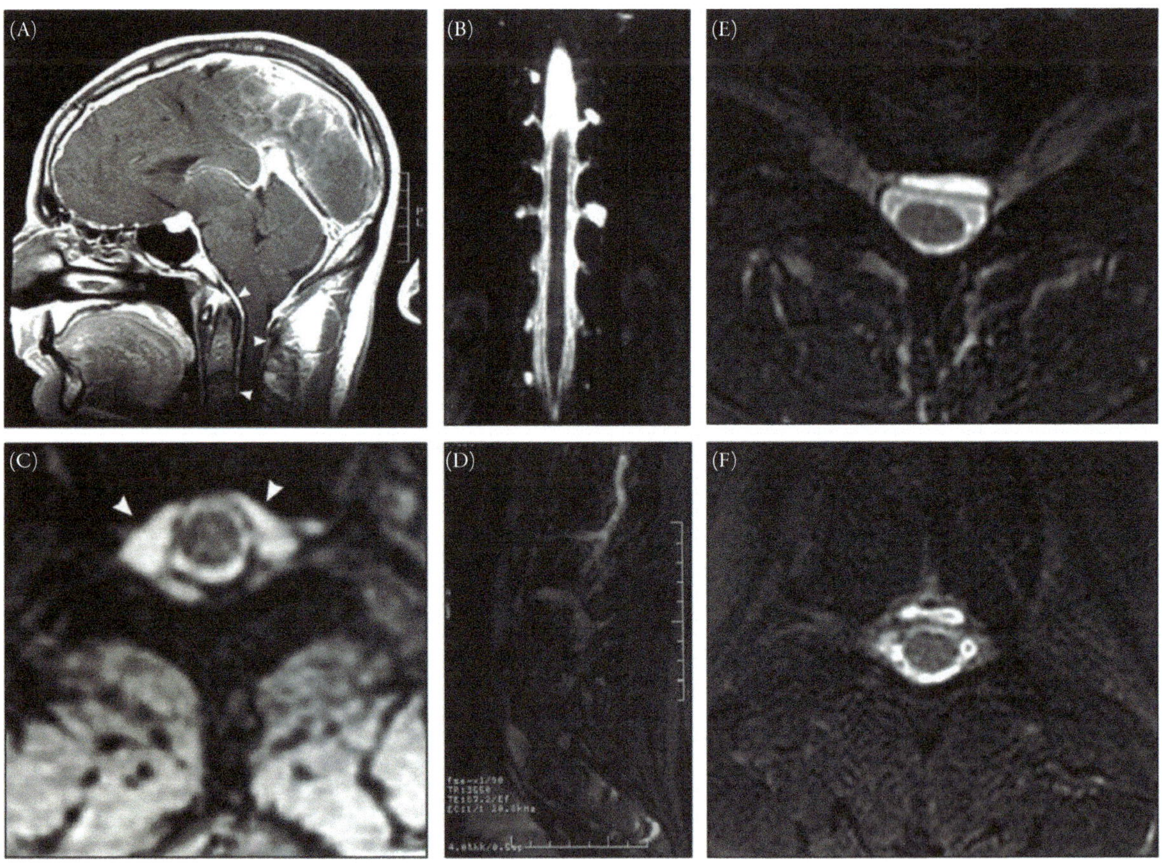

Figure 5.6. Spinal MRI showing changes in the spine. (A) CSF hypovolemia and enhancement of spinal dura (arrowheads). (B) Meningeal diverticulum and dilated nerve root sleeves. (C) Engorgement of epidural venous plexuses. (D, E, and F) Extra-arachnoid fluid collections. Reproduced with permission from Mokri.[18]

Table 5.4. **COMMON FINDINGS ON BRAIN AND SPINAL MRI IN SPONTANEOUS INTRACRANIAL HYPOTENSION**

BRAIN MRI FINDINGS	SPINAL MRI FINDINGS
Pachymeningeal enhancement	Spinal dural enhancement
Descent, sagging of the brain a. Descent of cerebellar tonsils, brainstem, and mesencephalon, with crowding of posterior fossa b. Obliteration of prepontine/perichiasmatic cisterns, with flattening of optic chiasm and anterior pons	Extra-arachnoid fluid collection
Subdural fluid collection, usually hygromas	Extradural extravasation of fluid a. May identify level of leak b. May identify the actual size of the leak
Enlargement of the pituitary	Meningeal diverticula
Engorged cerebral sinuses	Engorgement of spinous epidural venus plexus
Decreased size of the ventricles	

Modified from Mokri.[18]

hydration, generous caffeine intake, and use of an abdominal binder. These therapies are intended to decrease CSF pressure at the site of the leakage, thereby allowing for healing of the underlying meningeal defects and restoration of CSF pressure.[25] Additional conservative treatment measures include administration of intravenous caffeine or theophylline, which causes arterial vasoconstriction by blocking the adenosine receptors. As a consequence, intracranial blood flow and venous engorgement are decreased.

Invasive Techniques

When a positional headache becomes severely debilitating, does not respond to conservative treatment, or is associated with signs of cerebral nerve stretch or injury, more aggressive techniques may be indicated.

EBP is the mainstay of treatment for SIH that has failed conservative management[27] (Figure 5.8). The presumed mechanism of action is an immediate gelatinous tamponade of the dural leak, followed by fibrin deposition and fibroblastic activity. Restriction of CSF flow within the spinal epidural space may also occur, thereby interfering with CSF absorption.[26]

EBP is less effective in the treatment of a positional headache due to SIH than it is for PDPH. Two or three blood patches may be necessary for pain relief in severe cases. Blood patches are typically performed at the mid or low lumbar level, which may have less influence on the epidural venous pressure if the CSF leak is present higher in the spine. Given that most of dural diverticuli are localized at the cervicothoracic or thoracolumbar junction, placement of an EBP in the low lumbar spine is less likely to produce the desired effect. If possible, the location of the CSF leak should be identified and the EBP should be performed as close to the defect as possible.[10,27,28]

An EBP performed with 10 to 20 mL of autologus blood provides pain relief in up to 91% of patients with PDPH within 2 hours of the procedure. Only 61% have both initial and long-term relief. Sometimes a second blood patch with a

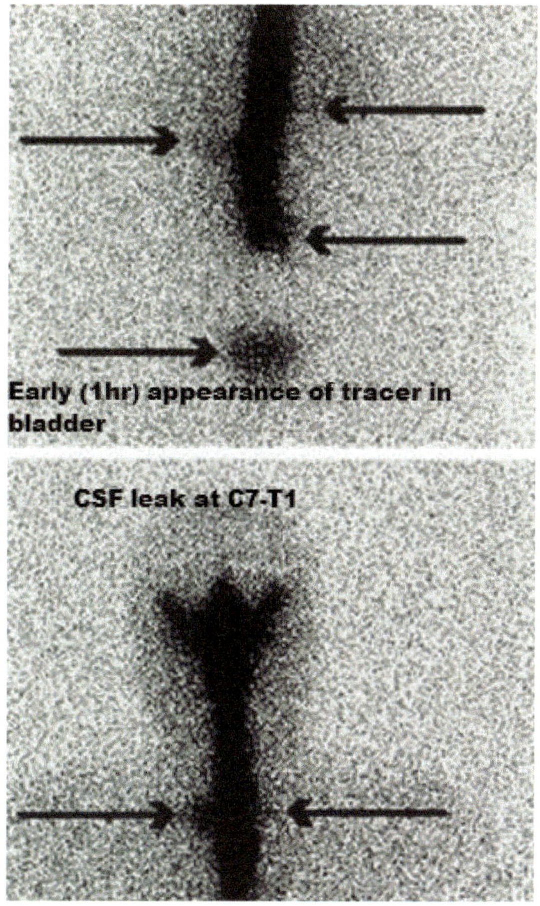

Figure 5.7. Radionuclide cysternogram showing early accumulation of tracer in bladder as well as a visible CSF leak at the C7-T1 level. Reproduced with permission from Wieseman et al.[10]

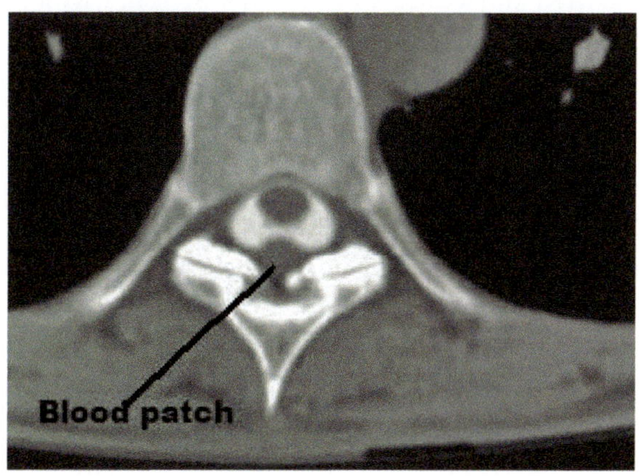

Figure 5.8. Blood deposit after completion of an epidural blood patch in a patient with positional headache. Reproduced from Wieseman et al.[10]

greater volume can be done as early as 5 days after the first procedure.[28] In one study, 87% of 80 severely debilitated patients with a refractory positional headache from SIH obtained complete symptom regression within 3 months of the first blood patch.[29] After a second EBP, 90% of the total number of patients had resolution of symptoms.[26] Repeat, high-volume (greater than 20 mL) EBPs have been associated with neurologic complications.[11] Many centers perform EBPs with patients prone and in steep Trendelenburg position to encourage cephalad spread.[12] Fluoroscopy is employed for targeted blood patches when the location of the CSF leak is known.[30] Transforaminal blood patches have been reported when the location of the leak has been identified and translaminar attempts were unsuccessful.[31]

The most common side effects of EBP are backache and back stiffness. More serious complications are very rare and consist of spinal cord and nerve root compression as a result of introduction of a blood clot, chemical meninigitis from blood leakage into the subarachnoid space via a direct meningeal defect, or arachnoiditis from accidental introduction of blood intrathecally.[29]

If the EBPs fail to provide relief after the second or third attempt, percutaneous deposit of fibrin sealant at the exact level of the CSF leak can be tried. In these situations, correct identification of the dural defect is essential for the efficacy of the treatment. Intrathecal infusion of saline or artificial CSF should not be expected to seal a CSF leak but is a good temporizing method until permanent repair of the leak can be attempted, especially in patients with decreased levels of consciousness.

Surgical treatment is reserved for patients in whom all other methods of treatment have failed. More specifically, surgery should be considered if the symptoms are debilitating and have failed appropriate management, and the site of the leak has been identified. Surgical treatment typically involves ligature of the leaking meningeal diverticulum or suture and muscle pledget in a frank dural hole, and is tailored to the specific pathology present.[25]

Data on long-term outcomes are scarce, but CSF leaks recur in approximately 10% of patients, regardless of treatment.[5] Patients with an abnormal MRI and focal spinal leak have an excellent prognosis, while those with a normal MRI and a diffuse multilevel CSF leak have a poorer prognosis.

CONCLUSIONS

- SIH typically manifests as new onset of a positional headache. Unlike in PDPH, a triggering dural puncture cannot be identified.
- SIH is becoming more frequently diagnosed, likely due to advancements in imaging and greater awareness of the condition.
- Many radiodiagnostic tools carry important risks to patients, including nerve injury and iatrogenic spinal cord injury, as occurred in our patient.
- Prompt diagnosis based on medical history, physical examination, and imaging is important to identify patients with SIH and to treat them appropriately.
- EBP, the mainstay of treatment, is less effective in SIH than in PDPH and may require multiple attempts with increasing amounts of autologous blood.

REFERENCES

1. Schaltenbrand G. Neure Anschauungen zur Pathophysiologie der Liquorzirkulation. *Zentralb Neurochir*. 1938;3:290–300.
2. Lindquist T, Moberg E. Spontaneous hypoliquorrhea. *Acta Med Scand*. 1949;132:556–561.
3. Schievink WI, Morreale VM, Atkinson JLD, et al. Surgical treatment of spontaneous spinal cerebrospinal fluid leaks. *J Neurosurg*. 1998;88:243–246.
4. Schievink WI, Roiter V. Epidemiology of cervical artery dissection. In: Baumgartner RW, Bogousslavsky J, Caso V, et al., eds. *Handbook of Cerebral Artery Dissection*. Basel, Germany: Karger; 2005:12–15.
5. Schievink WI. Spontaneous spinal cerebrospinal fluid leaks and intracranial hypotension. *JAMA*. 2006;295(19):2286–2296.
6. Diaz JH. Epidemiology and outcome of postural headache management in spontaneous intracranial hypotension. *Reg Anesth Pain Med*. 2001;26(6):582–587.
7. Mokri B, Maher CO, Sencakova D. Spontaneous CSF leaks: underlying disorder of connective tissue. *Neurology*. 2002;58:814–816.
8. Vishteh AG, Schievink WI, Baskin JJ, et al. Cervical bone spur presenting with spontaneous intracranial hypotension: case report. *J Neurosurg*. 1998;89:483–484.
9. Winter SC, Maartens NF, Anslow P, et al. Spontaneous intracranial hypotension due to thoracic disc herniation: case report. *J Neurosurg*. 2002;96:343–345.
10. Wiesemann E, Berding G, Goetz F, Windhagen A. Spontaneous intracranial hypotension: correlation of imaging findings with clinical features. *Eur Neurol*. 2006;56:204–210.
11. Benzon HT, Nemickas R, Molloy RE, Ahmad S, Melen O, Cohen B. Lumbar and thoracic epidural blood injections to treat spontaneous intracranial hypotension. *Anesthesiology*. 1996;85:920–922.
12. Paldino M, Mogilner AY, Tenner MS. Intracranial hypotension syndrome: a comprehensive review. *Neurosurg Focus*. 2003;15(6):1–8.
13. Cousins MJ, Brazier D, Cook R. Intracranial hypotension caused by cervical cerebrospinal fluid leak: treatment with epidural blood patch. *Anesth Analg*. 2004;98:1794–1797.
14. Vishteh AG, Schievink WI, Baskin JJ, et al. Cervical bone spur presenting with spontaneous intracranial hypotension: case report. *J Neurosurg*. 1998;89:483–484.
15. Wilson D, Christie J, Ferch R. Successful surgical treatment of intractable spontaneous intracranial hypotension due to a calcified thoracic disc prolapse. *J Clin Neurosci*. 2013;20(12):1773–1775.
16. Binder DK, Sarkissian V, Dillon WP, et al. Spontaneous intracranial hypotension associated with transdural thoracic osteophyte reversed by primary dural repair. *J Neurosurg Spine*. 2005;2:614–618.
17. Eross DJ, Dodick DW, Nelson KD, et al. Orthostatic headache syndrome with CSF leak secondary to bony pathology of the cervical spine. *Cephalalgia*. 2002;22:439–443.
18. Mokri B. Spontaneous low pressure, low CSF volume headaches: spontaneous CSF leaks. *Headache*. 2013;53(7):1034–1053.
19. Mokri B. Spontaneous low cerebrospinal pressure/volume headaches. *Curr Neurol Neurosci Rep*. 2004;4:117–124.
20. Schievink WI, Wijdicks EF, Meyer FB, Sonntag VK. Spontaneous intracranial hypotension mimicking aneurysmal subarachnoid hemorrhage. *Neurosurgery*. 2001;48:513–516; discussion 516–517.
21. Mokri B, Aksamit AJ, Atkinson JL. Paradoxical postural headaches in cerebrospinal fluid leaks. *Cephalalgia*. 2004;24:883–887.
22. Leep Hunderfund AN, Mokri B. Second-half-of-the day headache as a manifestation of spontaneous CSF leak. *J Neurol*. 2012;259:306–310.

23. Mokri B. Spontaneous CSF leaks mimicking benign exertional headaches. *Cephalalgia*. 2002;22:780–783.
24. Mokri B, Atkinson JL, Piepgras DG. Absent headache despite CSF volume depletion (intracranial hypotension). *Neurology*. 2000;55:1722–1724.
25. Schievink WI, Chu RM, Maya MM, Johnson JP, Cohen HC. Spinal manifestations of spontaneous intracranial hypotension. *J Neurosurg-Spine*. 2013;18(1):96–101.
26. Schievink WI, Dodick DW, Mokri B, Silberstein S, Bousser MG, Goadsby PJ. Diagnostic criteria for headache due to spontaneous intracranial hypotension: a perspective. *Headache*. 2011;51(9):1442–1444.
27. Amoozegar F, Guglielmin D, Hu W, Chan D, Becker WJ. Spontaneous intracranial hypotension: recommendations for management. *Can J Neurol Sci*. 2013;40(2):144–157.
28. Franzini A, Messina G, Chiapparini L, Bussone G. Treatment of spontaneous intracranial hypotension: evolution of the therapeutic and diagnostic modalities. *Neurol Sci*. 2013;34(1):151–155.
29. Diaz JH, Weed JT. Correlation of adverse neurological outcomes with increasing volumes and delayed administration of autologous epidural blood patches for postdural puncture headaches. *Pain Pract*. 2005;5:216–222.
30. Schievink WI. Spontaneous spinal cerebrospinal fluid leaks. *Cephalalgia*. 2008;28:1347–1356.
31. Walega D, McComb E, Rosenow J. Bilateral cervicothoracic transforaminal blood patches for persistent headache from spontaneous intracranial hypotension. *Clin J Pain*. 2011;27:357–364.

REVIEW QUESTIONS

1. A 40-year-old healthy female presents to the ED with severe headache of 2 weeks' duration; she has no complaints when she awakens in the morning or when she lies down, only with sitting and standing. What is the least invasive modality that may help with the diagnosis of her condition?

A. Brain MRI
B. Lumbar puncture with opening pressure and CSF analysis
C. Diagnostic and therapeutic EBP
D. RC

2. A 45-year-old male with Marfan syndrome is referred to the pain clinic by his neurologist due to complaints of a new, daily frontal headache that worsens when sitting up. The patient is started on conservative measures (bed rest, fluids, and caffeinated drinks) and he reports his pain is tolerable. However, when the patient is contacted to establish an appointment, despite the fact that his pain is well managed with the current conservative treatments, he demands to come urgently, directly to the procedure room, for fluoroscopically guided EBP. You:

A. Agree that the patient should be brought for immediate lumbar EBP
B. Refer the patient for head MRI to evaluate his new daily headache
C. Advise the patient that he needs a 1-month trial of bed rest, hydration, and generous consumption of caffeinated beverages before you will consider an EBP
D. Advise the patient to schedule an appointment for a new patient visit ASAP and to continue the conservative regimen with fluids, caffeinated beverages, and bed rest

3. A 52-year-old female patient presents to the ED for a severe, unilateral, pounding headache that worsens with standing and that is associated with nausea and photophobia. She reports previous episodes of this headache that responded to nasal sumatriptan that a friend gave her in the past. She also has a family history of migraines. A CT scan of the brain is unremarkable. Repeated doses of oral opioids and NSAIDs fail to control the patient's headache, and she is admitted for pain control and further diagnostic workup. MRI is obtained the next day at the recommendation of the neurology service, and is shown in Figure 5.9.

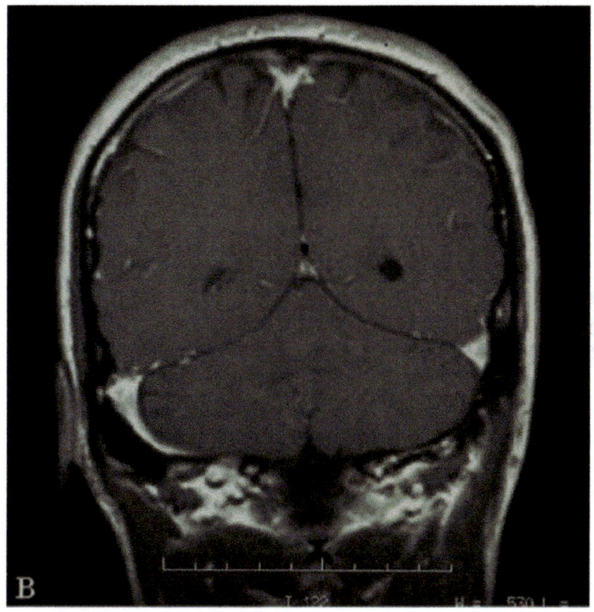

Figure 5.9. MRI. Reproduced from Paldino et al.[12]

The next step for this patient is:

A. EBP for SIH
B. RC
C. Subcutaneous sumatriptan
D. Diagnostic lumbar puncture

ANSWERS

1. A. This patient describes a positional headache, similar to PDPH. With no dural puncture reported in the history of this patient, her symptoms are most consistent with a diagnosis of SIH. Findings on brain MRI, lumbar puncture, head CT, and RC can all be used to support the diagnosis of SIH. However, given the patient's positional headache, the least invasive test should be used initially. Given its noninvasive nature, brain MRI is suggested as the initial diagnostic study of choice,[18] with the caveat that brain MRI may be

normal in up to 20% of cases of SIH.[5] While the patient may benefit from an EBP, it is not the first step in diagnosing the SIH, therefore answer C is not correct. Both lumbar puncture with opening pressure and RC are possible diagnostic tools, but they are more invasive and may further worsen the patient's refractory positional headache.

2. D. While the description of the patient's pain does suggest a diagnosis of SIH, especially in the presence of HCTD (Marfan syndrome), the differential diagnosis of new daily headache is extensive; therefore, a thorough history and physical are required prior to initiating further diagnostic and therapeutic workup. The patient already has been evaluated by a neurologist and has started on a conservative regimen with improvement of his symptoms. Answer A is incorrect because you cannot perform a procedure without evaluating the patient first. Answer B is possible, but, again, you will need to evaluate the patient before ordering tests. Waiting 1 month in bed may not be feasible for a very active patient, so answer C is not correct. Answer D is correct: you will see the patient rather urgently for evaluation while he continues the conservative regimen. The patient should be advised that if his symptoms worsen acutely, he should urgently report to the ED.[5,7]

3. C. The brain MRI shown is grossly normal, and the patient's overall symptoms are consistent with a migraine headache. While the orthostatic nature of the headache described is seen in SIH, the combined history and normal MRI suggest that treatment for migraine should be undertaken prior to further investigation of SIH. Answers A, B, and D are not correct because they list invasive modalities for diagnosis and treatment of SIH. In addition to taking a detailed history of the current and past episodes, noninvasive diagnostic modalities should be used first for confirming the diagnosis.[10,18]

QUESTIONS AND ANSWERS

This chapter has accompanying questions and answers that are available to subscribers as part of the Oxford eLearning platform. To access the questions, follow the link below, or go to http://oxfordmedicine.com/painmanagementreview

6.

CERVICOGENIC PAIN

Lynn Kohan and James Liadis

STEM CASE AND KEY QUESTIONS

A 54-year-old female presents to a pain management center with complaints of left-sided upper neck pain and headaches for the past 9 months. The pain is described as a dull ache and is rated 4/10. It is aggravated by doing work at her computer and overhead activities, such as reaching into cabinets to put away dishes. It is alleviated somewhat with rest and nonsteroidal anti-inflammatory drugs (NSAIDs), but is still present enough that she is often unable to do activities that she would like to do. She was therefore referred to a pain management center for further treatment.

A presumed diagnosis of cervicogenic headache secondary to cervical spondylosis is made and the patient undergoes cervical medial branch blocks at the third occipital nerve, C3, and C4. The patient receives greater than 75% relief after the medial branch blocks and subsequently undergoes cervical medial branch denervation.

WHAT IS CERVICOGENIC PAIN?

At the pain clinic, the patient states that her headaches are constant and started sometime after she was involved in a minor car accident, in which she was rear-ended but there was no damage to either vehicle. She had minor pain at that time but was not evaluated. Since that time, her pain has been getting worse.

WHAT SHOULD BE CONSIDERED IN THE DIFFERENTIAL DIAGNOSIS?

The patient states that her pain is left-sided and that it starts at the upper part of her neck and radiates to the back of her head. She denies photophobia, phonophobia, nausea, or vomiting. She denies any sharp or shooting pain in the back of her head. The pain is described as usually moderate in intensity but can be severe at times. She denies problems with vision or dizziness. She denies fevers or rashes. She admits to difficulty sleeping.

WHAT ARE THE DIAGNOSTIC CRITERIA?

Several diagnostic criteria proposed for cervicogenic headache are discussed in detail in this chapter. Overall, the criteria describe pain located in the neck, with some radiation pattern to the occiput, sometimes also involving pain in the frontal or temporal areas, and occasionally including shoulder pain. The symptoms are most frequently unilateral but can be bilateral. The pain is described as dull and aching, and usually nonthrobbing and nonlancinating. The pain can be increased with neck movements and specific head positions. Physical exam can reveal decreased passive range of motion with tenderness to palpation of the cervical paraspinals or upper cervical facet joints.

WHAT ARE KEY PHYSICAL EXAM FINDINGS THAT ARE CONSISTENT WITH CERVICOGENIC PAIN?

Physical examination of the patient reveals tenderness to palpation overlying the left cervical facet joints in addition to tender points within the cervical paraspinal and trapezius musculature on the left. Spurling's test is negative. Reflexes are 2+ and symmetric in her triceps, biceps, and brachioradialis. The patient has normal sensation to light touch on her bilateral upper extremities. Strength is 5/5 in all upper extremity muscle groups.

WHAT IMAGING TOOLS ARE PREDICTIVE OF CERVICOGENIC PAIN?

Cervical radiography is performed and reveals cervical spondylosis on the left greater than on the right at C2-C3 and C3-C4, as well as mild decreased disk height at C5-C6 and C6-C7. Flexion/extension films do not reveal any evidence of instability.

WHAT TREATMENT OPTIONS ARE AVAILABLE?

Interventional and medical treatment options are explained to the patient. Because she is afraid of needles, the patient prefers to take a conservative approach to treatment; therefore, a prescription for physical therapy is provided. The patient is also given a short course of diclofenac and is asked to return to the clinic in 6 weeks.

SHOULD WE PERFORM CERVICAL MEDIAL BRANCH BLOCKS OR INTRA-ARTICULAR FACET INJECTIONS UNDER FLUOROSCOPIC GUIDANCE?

Upon return to the clinic, the patient states that she is not any better. She is now open to undergoing interventional therapy.

Cervical medial branch blocks are explained in detail to the patient. After informed consent is obtained, the patient is brought to the fluoroscopy suite and cervical medial branch blocks at the third occipital nerve, C3, and C4 are performed using 0.5 mL of 0.5% bupivacaine. The patient had reported her pre-procedure pain score as 6/10. Following the procedure, she reports her pain score as 1/10. She also reports that, after the procedure, she is able to do work at her computer with significantly less pain for about 4 hours. The patient feels that her pain and function improved significantly for about 4 to 5 hours after the procedure, with subsequent gradual return to her baseline pain level.

SHOULD WE PROCEED WITH CERVICAL MEDIAL BRANCH DENERVATION UNDER FLUOROSCOPIC GUIDANCE?

Given the results of the procedure, the patient wants to proceed with cervical medial branch denervation. She is scheduled to undergo the procedure and returns to the clinic, at which time informed consent is obtained and the patient is brought to the fluoroscopy suite. Cervical medial branch denervation using thermal radiofrequency (RF) ablation at 80°C for 90 seconds is performed after sensory and motor testing are completed. The patient undergoes the procedure without complication. She notes that she has mild soreness at the site and is given an ice pack. After a brief period of observation, she is discharged home with instructions to follow up in 6 to 8 weeks.

The patient returns for her follow-up appointment 6 weeks after the denervation procedure. At this time, she states she is doing well, with a pain score of 1 to 2. She is able to perform her work-related duties without difficulty, and overall she is pleased with the outcome. She is instructed to call in the future if the pain returns. Approximately 1 year after the procedure, the patient is seen in clinic, and she notes usual pain has gradually recurred. She inquires if she can repeat the procedure.

SHOULD WE REPEAT THE CERVICAL MEDIAL BRANCH DENERVATION?

After a thorough history and examination, it is noted there are no changes from the patient's original presentation and thus it is decided to repeat her cervical medial branch denervation procedure. The patient does well, with good relief of her pain and increased function.

DISCUSSION

The term *cervicogenic headache* was introduced in 1983 by Sjaastad and colleagues, although the idea of secondary headaches from a cervical source had been referred to as early as 1853.[1] Cervicogenic headache describes head pain that is referred from bony structures or soft tissues in the neck.[2]

Cervicogenic headache is defined as a unilateral headache of varying intensity that is typically worsened with movements of the head or pressure over tender areas in the neck. The pain originates in the neck and radiates to the occipital, temporal, and/or frontal regions.[2–4] The headache is described as nonthrobbing and is of moderate to severe intensity. These clinical features, however, are similar to those of other headache disorders, such as tension-type headache, migraine without aura, or hemicrania continua, and thus cannot be used to make a definitive diagnosis.[5,6]

The prevalence of cervicogenic headache is estimated to be 0.4% to 4.1% in the general population and up to 15% to 20% in patients presenting with headache.[7,8] It is four times more common in women than in men, with a mean age of 42.9 years.[7,8] The pain is noted to have begun in the neck/occipital region in 97% of cases.[8] The condition can have a significant impact on quality of life; patients with cervicogenic headache report higher scores for bodily pain and limitation to physical functioning than patients suffering from other types of headaches.[9]

DIAGNOSTIC CRITERIA

Cervicogenic headache is a secondary headache syndrome referred from the cervical spine that is typically described as unilateral head pain that radiates from the occiput to the frontal regions. Bilateral presentations can also occur.[1] Several diagnostic criteria for cervicogenic headache have been proposed since the first use of the term by Sjaastad. Sjaastad formed the Cervicogenic Headache International Study Group in 1987, a group that published the first criteria for this diagnosis in 1990. The International Association for the Study of Pain diagnostic criteria for cervicogenic pain followed in 1994. Additional criteria were published by the Quebec Headache Study Group in 1995, and a revised version of the original criteria was proposed by Sjaastad et al. in 1998.[7] More recently, in 2004, the International Headache Society (IHS) designed a classification of headache disorders to include several diagnostic criteria for cervicogenic headache (Box 6.1).

Migraine-type symptoms, such as nausea, ipsilateral blurred vision, dizziness, and/or photophobia or phonophobia, might be present with cervicogenic headache, but usually to a lesser degree than with migraine.[7] Symptoms that might help differentiate cervicogenic headache from tension-type headache include side-locked pain, reproduction of pain by pressure on the neck muscles and by head movement, and posterior to anterior radiation of the pain.[10]

ETIOLOGY

Several anatomic pain generators have been proposed for cervicogenic headache. Some physical exam maneuvers may reproduce pain of cervicogenic headache. Similarly, painful responses to stimulation of the structures involved, as well as symptom relief upon directed interventions in structures suspected to be pain generators, may point toward positive diagnosis in this condition.[7] The upper three cervical spinal nerves can refer pain to the head.[11] Therefore, the atlanto-occipital joint, atlanto-axial joint, second and third intervertebral disks, second and third zygapophyseal facet joints, and

Box 6.1. **CERVICOGENIC HEADACHE CRITERIA ACCORDING TO THE INTERNATIONAL HEADACHE SOCIETY (INTERNATIONAL CLASSIFICATION OF HEADACHE DISORDERS, 3RD ED.; ICHD-3)**

A. Any headache fulfilling criterion C

B. Clinical, laboratory, and/or imaging evidence of a disorder or lesion within the cervical spine or soft tissues of the neck known to be able to cause headache

C. Evidence of causation demonstrated by at least two of the following:

1. Headache has developed in temporal relation to the onset of the cervical disorder or appearance of the lesion.
2. Headache has significantly improved or resolved in parallel with improvement in, or resolution of, the cervical disorder or lesion.
3. Cervical range of motion is reduced and headache is made significantly worse by provocative maneuvers.
4. Headache is abolished after diagnostic blockade of a cervical structure or its nerve supply.

D. Not better accounted for by another ICDH-3 diagnosis.

Reprinted with permission from Headache Classification Committee of the International Headache Society (IHS). The International Classification of Headache Disorders, 3rd ed. (Beta version.) *Cephalalgia.* 2013;33(9):629–808.

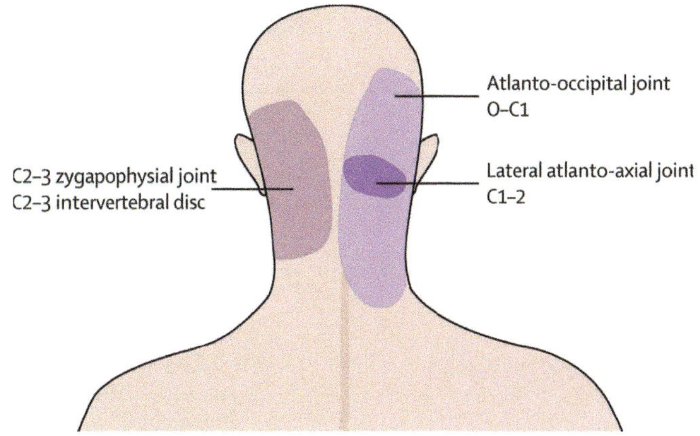

Figure 6.1. Cervicogenic headache referral patterns. Reproduced with permission from Bogduk and Govind.[11]

paravertebral muscles can all be sources of cervicogenic pain.[11] The most important clinical source of cervicogenic pain is likely cervical facet dysfunction, according to the Quebec Headache Study Group.[12]

ANATOMY

The primary pain generators in the cervical spine that can cause referred head pain include the C2-C3 facet joint, the C3-C4 facet joint, the atlanto-axial joint, the C2-C3 intervertebral disk, and the atlanto-occipital joint.[13] The innervation and referral patterns (Figure 6.1 and Table 6.1) of these common pain generators are outlined here.

Sensory nerve fibers in the descending tract of the trigeminal nerve are thought to interact with sensory fibers from the upper cervical roots in a region called the trigeminocervical nucleus.[14] The trigeminocervical nucleus (Figure 6.2), located in the upper cervical spinal cord, is thought to function as a relay station for afferent impulses from the trigeminal nerve and the upper three cervical spinal nerves. The convergence of the upper cervical and trigeminal sensory pathways enables bidirectional referral of pain sensations between the neck and areas of the head and face within the receptive fields of the trigeminal nerve.[9] This convergence of nociceptive signals from several structures has been implicated in the ability of a variety of pain generators in the cervical spine to generate cervicogenic headaches. Therefore, many have come to consider this diagnosis a pain syndrome that results from the downstream effect of numerous possible nociceptive structures in the cervical spine, as opposed to a single anatomic pain generator.[15–17]

IMAGING

While cervical radiography cannot be used to diagnose cervicogenic headache, it is helpful in identifying spondylosis and degenerative changes, which lend support to the diagnosis, in addition to ruling out other pathologies, such as fractures or neoplasms.[18] To assess for instability, flexion/extension films are warranted. There is some disagreement in the literature about the predictive value of flexion and extension views; however, there has been some evidence that hypomobility of the atlanto-occipital joint, paired with hypermobility of the C6-C7 joint, is associated with the diagnosis.[9] If "red flag" symptoms or neurologic deficits are present, an MRI is warranted, but neither CT myelogram nor MRI can be reliably used to diagnose the cause of cervicogenic headache.[18,19]

DIAGNOSTIC TESTING AND TREATMENT

A careful history, review of systems, and neurologic exam should be performed to rule out any red flags and to uncover any evidence of systemic disease.[20] During the musculoskeletal exam, one should assess for any loss of cervical range of motion. Additionally, one should assess for discomfort with palpation of the suboccipital, trapezius, and cervical paraspinal musculature and the tendinous insertions to the occiput.[21] One should also palpate for tenderness over the C1-C2 joint (corresponding to atlanto-axial pain), the C2-C3 facet joint (corresponding to pain from the third occipital nerve), and the upper facet joints. Tenderness over the occipital nerves at the level of the occiput should also be examined.

Since diagnosis cannot be confirmed by physical examination or imaging studies, anesthetic block of zygapophyseal joints, cervical nerve roots, or the medial branches is often required to confirm the diagnosis of cervicogenic headache.[11,22]

Table 6.1. **CERVICOGENIC HEADACHE PAIN AND THEIR REFERRAL PATTERNS**

PAIN GENERATOR	INNERVATION	REFERRAL PATTERN
Atlanto-occipital joint Atlanto-axial joint	Ventral ramus of Cl spinal root Medial atlanto-axial joint: recurrent meningeal branches of Cl, C2, C3 Lateral atlanto-axial joint: ventral ramus of C2 spinal nerve root	Occiput, suboccipút Occiput, suboccipút, vertex, orbit and ear
C2-C3 zygapophyseal joint	Superficial medial branch of C3 dorsal ramus (third occipital nerve)	Head, upper and lateral cervical area
C3-C4 zygapophyseal joint C2-C3 disk	Medial branch of dorsal root of C3 and C4 sinovertebral branch of superficial medial branch of C3 dorsal ramus	Head, upper and lower cervical area occiput
Greater occipital nerve (not truly a pain generator but frequently referred to as such in the literature)	Medial branch of dorsal root of C2	Occiput coincides with the distribution of the C2 dermatome

Reproduced with permission from Mehnert M, Freedman M. Update on the role of Z-joint injection and radiofrequency neurotomy for cervicogenic headache. *PM&R.* 2013;5(3):221–227.

Atlanto-Axial Joint

The atlanto-axial joint is a condylar joint allowing for flexion and extension of the head on the neck and slight lateral rotation, and it can be a common source of cervicogenic headaches.[9] The lateral portion of the joint is innervated by the C2 dorsal ramus. If tenderness over the suboccipital area or over the transverse process of C1 is appreciated, the atlanto-axial joint should be considered as a potential source of the cervicogenic headache. Unfortunately, there are no conservative treatments for lateral atlanto-axial pain. Intra-articular injection (Figure 6.3) with steroid may offer short-term relief; however, injection of this

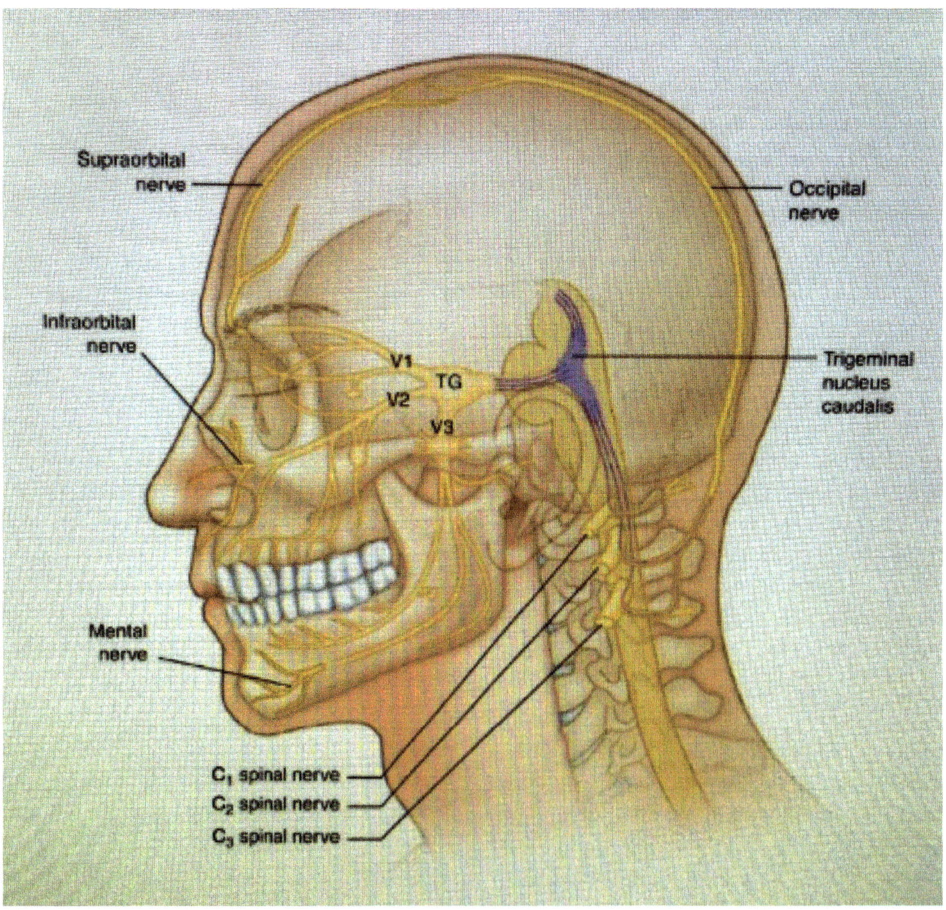

Figure 6.2. Trigeminocervical nucleus. Reproduced with permission from Narouze.[16]

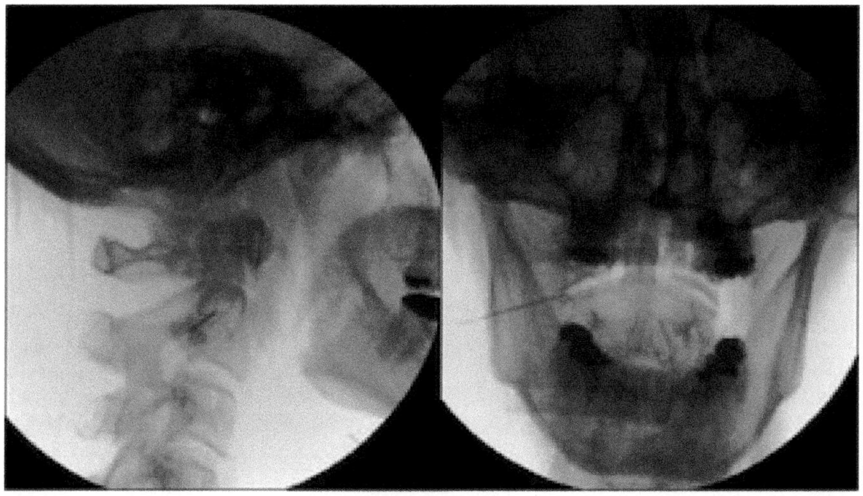

Figure 6.3. Atlanto-axial joint injection. (Left) Lateral view with a 5° oblique tilt for initial needle entry. (Right) PA view of needle entry into lateral C1-C2 joint. Reproduced with permission from Chua et al.[24]

joint has the potential for serious complications and thus is not routinely performed by most clinicians.[23] Complications from the procedure include injury to the vertebral artery and to the C2 nerve roots, which cross over the medial and posterior aspect of the joint. There have been small studies showing some utility of pulsed RF ablation to the lateral atlanto-axial joint.[9] Surgically, arthrodesis of the atlanto-axial joint is another option, with some patients noting long-term symptom relief.[14]

C2-C3 Zygapophyseal Joint

The C2-C3 zygapophyseal joint is considered to be the most common anatomic pain generator that results in cervicogenic headache, accounting for as many as 70% of the cases.[16] The C2-C3 zygapophyseal joint is supplied by the third occipital nerve. The third occipital nerve is the superficial branch of the C3 dorsal ramus. Therefore, if tenderness over the C2-C3 joint is appreciated, a diagnostic block should be performed. While this block can be performed by injecting local anesthetic intra-articularly, it is most often performed by injecting in the area of the third occipital nerve. There are varying opinions about what is considered a successful diagnostic cervical medial branch block. Clinically, most pain physicians use a reported 50% reduction in pain as an indication of a successful block.[25] This clinical benchmark is less stringent than the IHS diagnostic criteria requirement of at least a 90% decrease in pain after diagnostic blockade (discussed in Box 6.1).[10] RF ablation of the third occipital nerve has been shown to be effective in the treatment of cervicogenic headache after a successful block when performed with the proper technique.[26] Due to anatomic variance in the course of the third occipital nerve, the use of a three-needle technique, with needles placed just lateral to the joint line, above the joint, and below the joint, combined with the creation of consecutive lesions, can vastly improve the efficacy of the treatment.[26] The procedure can be performed via either a lateral or a posterior approach. The advantage of the posterior approach is that it places a conventional RF needle parallel to the nerve, thus creating a larger area of denervation.[27] In addition, with the posterior approach, bilateral procedures can be performed more easily with respect to patient positioning. Complications, which are usually self-limited, can include numbness in the cutaneous distribution of the nerve and dysesthesia and/or hypersensitivity in the areas bordering the numbness. This complication usually lasts a few days to weeks, and usually without any additional treatment requirement.[13] Temporary ataxia occurs in most patients because third occipital nerve ablation partially denervates the semispinalis capitis muscles, which results in interference with tonic neck reflexes.[28] Other possible complications include infection, hematoma, and injury to the vertebral artery or cervical nerve root if the needle is improperly positioned.[28] While RF ablation of the medial branches is more studied for neck pain, studies are emerging showing significant and sustained relief of cervicogenic headache when proper techniques are utilized[16] (Figure 6.4).

Cervical Muscles

The finding of reduced cervical range of motion, along with paraspinal tenderness, has led to the realization that cervical muscle trigger points and posterior neck attachments can also result in cervicogenic headache. Tenderness in the posterior neck muscles, especially the trapezius, sternocleidomastoid, and the splenius capitis, can cause referred pain to the occiput.[29] Since these tender areas lie above the zygapophyseal joints, it can be difficult to differentiate pain from these muscles and that from the underlying painful joints.[11]

C2-C3 Disk

Pain in the C2-C3 disk can also cause cervicogenic headache; however, cervical discography at this level is not often performed because of the potential for serious complications.

Occipital Neuralgia

Occipital nerve pain can cause cervicogenic headaches; for detailed discussion of occipital neuralgia, see Chapter 1.

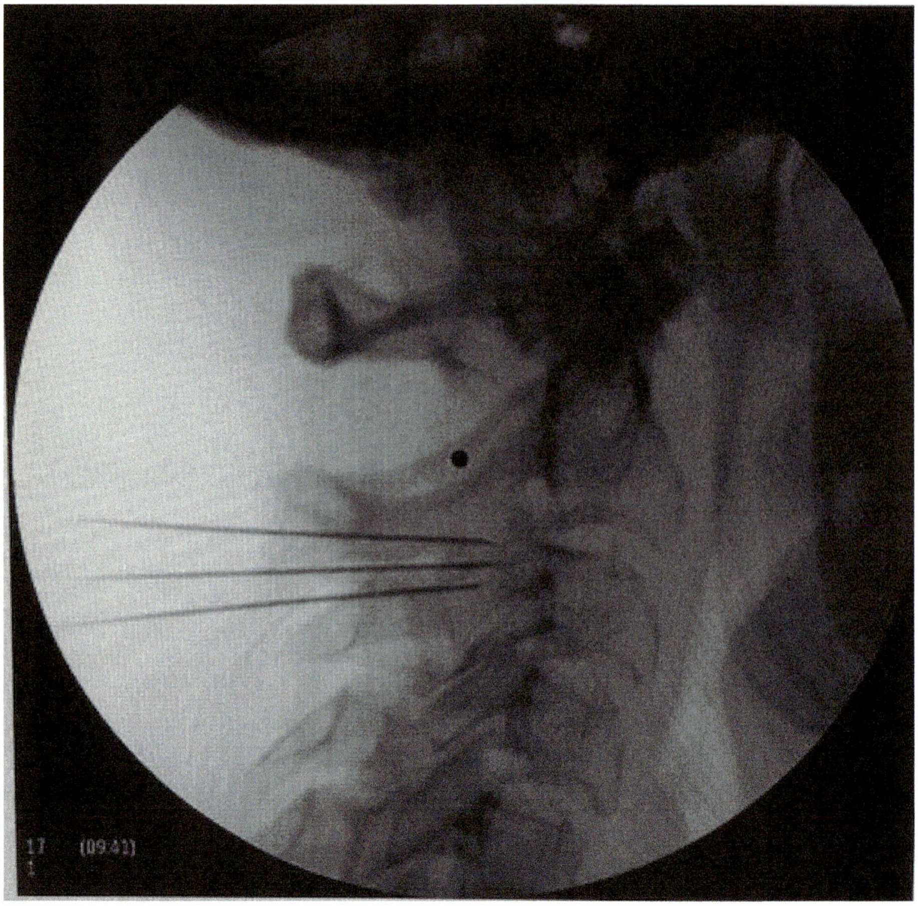

Figure 6.4. Third occipital nerve denervation. Lateral view showing three radiofrequency needles in place along the C2-C3 joint line. Reproduced with permission from Narouze.[16]

TREATMENT MODALITIES

While there is no known cure for cervicogenic headache, a number of different treatment options are available. A multimodal pain treatment plan is the best approach.

Physical therapy has been shown to have long-term efficacy for improvement of cervicogenic headaches.[30] Therapy can be initiated slowly and advanced as tolerated to include both strengthening and aerobic conditioning. Cervical mobilization and manipulation, and then progression to cervicoscapular strengthening, have been found to be beneficial techniques in therapy for patients with cervicogenic headaches.[15]

Interventional techniques can also be employed. Percutaneous RF ablation can be performed if diagnostic local anesthetic block of the cervical spinal nerve, medial branch, or zygapophyseal joint results in temporary alleviation of the pain.[27,31,32]

CONCLUSIONS

- Cervicogenic headache is referred pain from cervical structures that are innervated by the upper three cervical nerves.
- Cervicogenic headache can often be difficult to differentiate from other types of primary headaches, including tension-type headache, migraine without aura, or hemicrania continua.
- Diagnostic criteria for cervicogenic headache, according to the IHS, include: pain is referred from a source in the neck, cause of the headache is a disorder within the cervical spine or soft tissues in the neck, the headache resolves after a diagnostic block, and the pain resolves after successful treatment of the cause.
- One of the most common sites for interventional treatment is the C2-C3 zygapophyseal joint.
- RF ablation of the third occipital nerve, which supplies the C2-C3 joint, when proper technique is used, can result in successful reduction in pain.
- A multidisciplinary approach is best to improve chances of successful treatment.

REFERENCES

1. Antonaci F, Bono G, Mauri M, Drottning M, Buscone S. Concepts leading to the definition of the term cervicogenic headache: a historical overview. *J Headache Pain*. 2005;6(6):462–466.
2. Sjaastad O, Saunte C, Hovdahl H, et al. Cervicogenic headaches. A hypothesis. *Cephalalgia*. 1983;3:249–256.

3. Sjaastad O, Fredriksen TA, Pfaffenrath V. Cervicogenic headache: diagnostic criteria. The Cervicogenic Headache International Group study. *Headache*. 1998;38:442.
4. Sjaastad O, Fredriksen TA, Pfaffenrath V. Cervicogenic headache: diagnostic criteria. *Headache*. 1990;30:1975.
5. Leone M, D'Amico D, Grazzi L, et al. Cervicogenic headache: a clinical review of the current diagnostic criteria. *Pain*. 1998;78:1–5.
6. Suijlekom KA, de Vet HCW, vanden Berg SGM, Weber WEJ. Interobserver reliability of diagnostic criteria for cervicogenic headache. *Cephalalgia*. 1999;19:817–823.
7. Halderman S, Dagenais S. Cervicogenic headaches: a critical review. *Spine J*. 2001;1:31.
8. Sjaastad O, Bakketeig LS. Prevalence of cervicogenic headache: Vågå study of headache epidemiology. *Acta Neurol Scan*. 2008;117:173–180.
9. Rana MV. Managing and treating headache of cervicogenic origin. *Med Clin North Am*. 2013;97(2):267–280.
10. Headache Classification Committee of the International Headache Society (IHS). The International Classification of Headache Disorders, 3rd ed. (Beta version.) *Cephalalgia*. 2013;33(9):629–808.
11. Bogduk N. The neck and headaches. *Neurol Clin*. 2004;22(1): 151–171.
12. Meloche JP, Bergeron Y, Bellavance A, et al. Painful intervertebral dysfunction: Robert Maigne's original contribution to headache of cervical origin. The Quebec Headache Study Group. *Headache*. 1993;33:328–324.
13. Mehnert M, Freedman M. Update on the role of Z-joint injection and radiofrequency neurotomy for cervicogenic headache. *PM&R*. 2013;5(3):221–227.
14. Bogduk N. The anatomical basis for cervicogenic headache. *J Manipulative Physiol Ther*. 1992;15:67–70.
15. Pollmann W, Keidel M, Pfaffenrath V. Headache and the cervical spine: a critical review. *Cephalalgia*. 1997;17(8):801–816.
16. Bogduk N, Govind J. Cervicogenic headache: an assessment of the evidence on clinical diagnosis, invasive tests, and treatment. *Lancet Neurol*. 2009;8(10):959–968.
17. Narouze S. Practical approach to cervicogenic headache. In: Narouze S, ed. *Interventional Management of Head and Neck Pain*. New York, NY: Springer Science and Business Media; 2014:67–76.
18. Fredriksen TA, Fougner R., Tangerud A., Sjaastad O. Cervicogenic headache. Radiological investigations concerning head/neck. *Cephalalgia*. 1989;9(2):139–146.
19. Coskun O, Ulcer S, Karakurum B, et al. Magnetic resonance imaging of patients with cervicogenic headache. *Cephalalgia*. 2003;23(8):842–845.
20. Pfaffenrath V, Dandekar R, Pollmann W. Cervicogenic headache—the clinical picture, radiological finding and the hypothesis of its pathophysiology. *Headache*. 1987;27:495–499.
21. Antonaci F, Bono G, Chimento P. Diagnosing cervicogenic headache. *J Headache Pain*. 2006;7(3):145–148.
22. Van Suijlekon J, Weber WEJ, van Kleef M. Cervicogenic headache: techniques of diagnostic nerve blocks. *Clin Exp Rheumatol*. 2000;18(suppl 19):S39–S41.
23. Govind J, King W, Baily B, Bogduk N. Radiofrequency neurotomy for the treatment of third occipital headache. *J Neurol Neurosurg Psychiatry*. 2003;74:88–93.
24. Chua N, Halim W, Evers A, Vissers K. Whiplash patients with cervicogenic headache after lateral atlanto-axial joint pulsed radiofrequency treatment. *Anesth Pain Med*. 2012;1(3):162–167.
25. Narouze SN, Casanova J. The efficacy of lateral atlanto-axial intra-articular steroid injection in the management of cervicogenic headache. *Anesthesiology*. 2004;101:A1005.
26. Van Suijlekom H, Van Zundert J, Narouze S, van Kleef M, Mekhail N. Evidence-based interventional pain medicine according to clinical diagnoses: cervicogenic headache. *Pain Pract*. 2010;10(2): 124–130.
27. Lord SM, Barnsley L, Wallis BJ, et al. Percutaneous radiofrequency neurotomy for chronic cervical zygapophyseal joint pain. *N Engl J Med*. 1996;335:1721.
28. Lord S, Barnsley L, Bogduk N. Percutaneous neurotomy in the treatment of cervical zygapophyseal joint pain: a caution. *Neurosurgery*. 1995;36:732–739.
29. Freund B, Schwartz M. Post-traumatic myofascial pain of the head and neck. *Curr Pain Headache Rep*. 2002;6:361–369.
30. Jull G, Trott P, Potter H, et al: A randomized controlled trial of exercise and manipulative therapy for cervicogenic headache. *Spine*. 2002;27:1835.
31. Blume HG. Cervicogenic headaches: radiofrequency neurotomy and the cervical disk and fusion. *Clin Exp Rheumatol*. 2000;18:S53.
32. McDonald GJ, Lord SM, Bogduk N. Long-term follow-up of patients treated with cervical radiofrequency neurotomy for chronic neck pain. *Neurosurgery*. 1999;45:61.
33. Biondi D. Cervicogenic headache: a review of diagnostic and treatment strategies. *J Am Osteopath Assoc*. 2005;105(4):16S–22S.

REVIEW QUESTIONS

1. A 52-year-old male complains of pain in his neck and the back of his head. You are evaluating him for possible cervicogenic headache. Cervicogenic headache is caused by structures that innervate:

   A. The lower three cervical nerves
   B. The upper three cervical nerves
   C. The upper two thoracic nerves
   D. The lower two cervical nerves

2. The following are included in the IHS diagnostic criteria for cervicogenic headache according to the ICDH-3, except:

   A. Clinical, laboratory, and/or imaging evidence of a disorder or lesion within the cervical spine or soft tissues of the neck known to be able to cause headache
   B. The pain is referred from the first three cervical nerves
   C. The headache is not better accounted for by other ICDH-3 criteria
   D. Cervical range of motion may be reduced and the headache is made worse with provocative movements

3. While not diagnostic, typical features used to describe cervicogenic headache include all of the following except:

   A. Headache is defined as throbbing and of severe intensity
   B. Headache is worsened with movements of the head
   C. Headache can occur after whiplash injury
   D. Headache occurs in the occipital, temporal, and/or frontal region

ANSWERS

1. B. Structures innervated by the upper three cervical nerves are recognized as the cause of cervicogenic headaches.[11] These structures include the C2-C3 facet joint, the C3-C4 facet joint, the atlanto-axial joint, the C2-C3 intervertebral

disk, and the atlanto-occipital joint.[13] Answers A, C, and D are incorrect because these lower nerves do not cause referred pain to the head.[11]

2. B. The other answers are included in the IHS diagnostic criteria for cervicogenic headache. Specifically, the criteria require that there is clinical, laboratory, and/or imaging evidence of a lesion within the structures of the neck known to be able to cause headache, that the headache is not better accounted for by another diagnosis, and that the headache fulfills at least two additional criteria. These criteria include headache that develops in temporal relationship to the onset of a cervical disorder, headache that improves or resolves with improvement or resolution of a cervical disorder, reduction of cervical range of motion with headache that is exacerbated by provocative maneuvers, and headaches that are abolished by diagnostic blockade of a cervical structure or its nerve supply.[10] While answer B does correctly identify the innervation pattern of structures capable of causing cervicogenic headache, this is not part of the ICHD-3 diagnostic criteria for cervicogenic headache, and therefore B is the correct answer.[11]

3. A. Answers B, C, and D describe the typical features of cervicogenic headaches, including occurrence in the occipital, temporal, and/or frontal region of the head, worsening with head movement, and occurrence after a whiplash injury.[2] Answer A is the correct response because, while the headache can be described as moderate to severe in intensity, the pain is usually described as nonthrobbing.[5]

QUESTIONS AND ANSWERS

This chapter has accompanying questions and answers that are available to subscribers as part of the Oxford eLearning platform. To access the questions, follow the link below, or go to ✔ http://oxfordmedicine.com/painmanagementreview

7.

CERVICAL MYOFASCIAL PAIN

Roger Wang and Sarah Choxi

STEM CASE AND KEY QUESTIONS

A 36-year-old male presents to his primary care physician with an 8-month history of bilateral upper neck pain and headaches. He reports that his symptoms first began with a dull ache at the nape of his neck, which progressed to both shoulders. He is left-hand dominant and works as a video editor, spending the majority of his day sitting at a desk in front of a computer. He reports some tender spots over his neck and upper back that he feels as hard spots that he massage when pain is very severe. He self-reports poor neck posture. He denies a history of trauma, associated nausea, dizziness, or radiation into the upper extremities. The patient undergoes a 4-week trial of physical therapy and nonsteroidal anti-inflammatory drugs (NSAIDs) that briefly alleviate his pain.

WHAT IS CERVICAL MYOFASCIAL PAIN (CMP)?

The patient is concerned and he asks you to explain what he is suffering from. Because the patient is well educated and you have time before your next patient arrives, you explain the issue in detail. Neck pain is a common condition that affects two-thirds or more of the global population during their lifetimes.[1] The etiology of neck pain includes cervical disk disease (pain arising from the intervertebral disks), cervical facet-mediated pain (pain arising from the articular processes of two spinal segments also known as zygapophyseal joints), and CMP (pain arising from the muscles of the neck and upper back). In particular, CMP is often a cause of disability in the population with chronic neck pain.[2] CMP is regional pain attributed to the skeletal muscles of the shoulders and neck and their surrounding fascia. It is characterized by the presence of trigger points. A trigger point is an area of hyperirritability in a palpable, taut band of muscle fibers. On physical examination, trigger points help establish the diagnosis. Prompt treatment can prevent other muscles in the functional unit from compensating and producing more widespread and chronic pain. Patient disability is most strongly linked to the duration of pain.[2]

WHAT SHOULD BE CONSIDERED IN THE DIFFERENTIAL DIAGNOSIS?

The patient is concerned about his diagnosis and asks what else it can be, because the pain is not constant. The patient's headaches wax and wane, but the neck and shoulder pain is constant and worse with palpation. He denies photophobia or phonophobia, nausea or vomiting. He denies radiation of pain down the extremities but he does have difficulty sleeping. At this point, based on the history provided by the patient, the likely working diagnosis is myofascial pain syndrome; however, the differential diagnosis may include cervical disk disease, cervical spondylosis, cervicogenic headaches, thoracic outlet syndrome, cervical facet disease, rheumatoid arthritis, and fibromyalgia. Migraine headaches and temporomandibular joint syndrome also are found in patients with CMP.[3]

WHAT ARE THE DIAGNOSTIC CRITERIA FOR CMP? WHAT KEY PHYSICAL FINDINGS ON EXAMINATION ARE CONSISTENT WITH CMP?

The patient is referred to a pain physician for further evaluation. He reports that massage, along with superficial heat and transcutaneous electrical nerve stimulation (TENS) applied by his physical therapist, provide some relief. The pain is described as dull and aching, with occasional radiation to the back of the head, shoulders, and upper back. On physical examination, the cervical range of motion is limited due to pain. Painful bands of muscle are palpated in the trapezius and along the cervical paraspinal muscles. Strength and sensation are intact in the upper extremities. Erythrocyte sedimentation rate, C-reactive protein, a basic metabolic panel, and thyroid function tests are within normal limits. MRI reveals no significant structural or spinal canal abnormality. Electrophysiology studies, which have been contradictory and expensive in the diagnosis of CMP, are not ordered. Given the patient's clinical history and constellation of symptoms, a working diagnosis of CMP is made.

WHAT IS A TRIGGER POINT?

The patient has several areas of hypersensitive, palpable, and focal taut bands of muscle in the trapezius, rhomboid, and levator scapulae muscles bilaterally. Upon palpation, the trigger points produce radiating, referred pain into the shoulders and down the upper back, along with a muscle twitch along the scapula bilaterally.

WHAT ARE TREATMENTS FOR CMP?

Due to persistent pain after physical therapy, NSAIDs and a muscle relaxant are prescribed. Trigger-point injections in the trapezius and rhomboids are performed. The patient is encouraged to continue physical therapy for postural retraining after trigger-point injections.[4] An ergonomic evaluation at work results in installation of armrests and a keyboard at a level to maintain normal posture. The patient has good pain relief for 6 months.

SHOULD TRIGGER-POINT INJECTIONS BE PERFORMED WITH ULTRASOUND GUIDANCE?

A palpable trigger point in the trapezius is localized and marked. The musculature in the cervicothoracic spine where the palpable trigger point was detected is visualized with ultrasound. Under ultrasound guidance, a 25-G 1.5-inch needle connected to a 5-mL syringe with 0.25% bupivacaine is placed in the muscle at the exact location of the trigger point. After the clinician pinpoints and manually stabilizes the trigger point in the taut band with the fingers, the needle is quickly passed through the skin and into the trigger zone. A local twitch response or a report of referred pain indicates that the trigger zone has been entered, and 0.1 to 0.2 mL of local anesthetic is injected. The needle is pulled back to just below the skin, the angle is changed, and the needle is again inserted through the muscle to another trigger zone. In this way, a funnel-shaped volume of muscle is evaluated without withdrawing the needle through the skin. The trigger zone is explored until no further local twitch responses are obtained. By this time, the taut band is gone and the spontaneous pain of the trigger point has subsided. Ultrasound guidance helps confirm needle placement is in muscle, not in adipose tissue or other nonmuscle structures, and reduces the risk of pneumothorax.[5] Electromyography (EMG) may be beneficial for similar reasons.[6]

IS BOTULINUM TOXIN A AN OPTION FOR REFRACTORY CMP?

The patient returns for botulinum toxin A injections into the painful muscle groups, with improvement in his visual analog pain score from 6/10 to 2/10. There is notable improvement in his cervical range of motion as well as in his ability to fall asleep.[7]

DISCUSSION

Chronic nonspecific neck pain is a common complaint of patients with CMP. CMP is a painful musculoskeletal disorder characterized by the presence of a tender, taut, palpable band of muscle called a trigger point. CMP has been found in patients with headache, neck pain, low back pain, and various other musculoskeletal and systemic disorders.[9–12] The prevalence of myofascial trigger points in patients complaining of pain anywhere in the body ranges from 30% to 93%.[13] There are no objective clinical measurements for evaluating occurrence and response to treatment of CMP.

DIAGNOSTIC CRITERIA

No laboratory test or imaging has been established for the diagnosis of CMP. The diagnosis relies heavily on a detailed history and thorough physical examination, including manual manipulation of soft tissue and high clinical suspicion for CMP. Essential criteria have been proposed for the diagnosis of myofascial trigger points (Table 7.1).[14]

Trigger points are characterized by palpable, tense bands of skeletal muscle fibers that can produce local or referred pain on palpation and a local twitch response with pressure. Pressure algometry has been used to quantify the sensitivity of trigger points. A pressure meter with a 1-cm^2 rubber disk attached to a force gauge calibrated up to 10 kg is applied over a trigger point to measure the pain threshold. This method, however, is not commonly used in the clinical setting.[15]

Trigger points can be active or latent. An active trigger point is an area of tenderness at rest or on palpation. A latent trigger point produces pain on palpation but not spontaneously. A latent trigger point has some characteristics of an active trigger point, including a taut muscle band and referred pain. Autonomic dysfunction also is associated with myofascial trigger points.[14]

ETIOLOGY

Although the pathophysiology of CMP is unclear, regional pain associated with palpation of a trigger point is thought to be

Table 7.1. **DIAGNOSTIC CRITERIA FOR IDENTIFYING MYOFASCIAL TRIGGER POINTS**

CRITERIA	DESCRIPTION
Essential Criteria	Palpable taut band
	Exquisite spot of tenderness of nodule in a taut band
	Pressure on the nodule induces pain that is recognized as an experienced pain pattern
	Painful limitation to full passive range of motion for affected muscle
Confirmatory Observations	Visual or tactile identification of local twitch response
	Image of a local twitch response induced by needle penetration of a tender nodule
	Pain or altered sensation on compression of a tender nodule
	EMG demonstration of spontaneous electrical activity characteristic of active loci in a tender nodule of a taut band

Adapted from Simons et al.[14]

caused by tissue ischemia after prolonged muscle contraction. Biochemicals, such as serotonin, norepinephrine, calcitonin gene-related peptide, substance P, histamine, bradykinins, and prostaglandins, accumulate.[16] These nociceptive substances activate both peripheral receptors and dorsal horn neurons. When input persists from nociceptors of an active trigger point, central sensitization in the spinal cord may develop, and the receptive field corresponding to the original dorsal horn neuron may produce referred pain. Local infusion of phentolamine eliminated the spontaneous electrical activity during needle EMG of myofascial trigger points, suggesting that trigger points have adrenergic dependency.[17] These changes are fed into a cycle of increasing motor or sympathetic activity that can increase pain. Predisposing factors for myofascial trigger points are chronic repetitive muscle strain, poor posture, systemic diseases, and neuromusculoskeletal lesions.[18]

DIAGNOSTIC TESTING AND TREATMENT

Noninvasive therapies for trigger points are spray and stretch treatments, TENS, physical therapy, topical anesthetics, pharmacotherapy (Table 7.2), ultrasound, electrotherapy, and deep-pressure soft tissue massage.[19–24]

Invasive treatments include injections with local anesthetics and steroid, botulinum toxin A, or dry needling. Lidocaine or dry needling can completely relieve pain if local twitch responses are elicited. Only minimal relief is felt if there is no response during either injection. Inactivation of the myofascial trigger point appears to be the result of the mechanical action of the needle in the trigger point itself, because trigger points can be inactivated even when no medication is used. Using local anesthetics is more comfortable for patients and results in longer lasting pain reduction.[23] Isotonic saline injection is equally or more effective than local anesthetic injections.[25,26] Corticosteroids also have been used for treatment to prevent an inflammatory reaction, but long-acting steroids are not recommended because they may destroy muscle fibers.[27] Botulinum toxin A has a therapeutic effect in treating CMP but no more than dry needling or bupivacaine injections.[28–31]

Nociceptors are blocked during trigger-point injection if a local twitch response is elicited.[19] The mechanism of action is disruption of trigger points by the mechanical effect of the needle or chemical effect of injectate, which relaxes and lengthens the muscle fiber. The injectate causes local vasodilation, dilution, and removal of the accumulated nociceptive substrate. Other modalities include laser therapy, shockwave therapy, and hyperbaric oxygen.[32–36]

Attempts to confirm the presence of myofascial trigger points with magnetic resonance elastography have been successful. Biochemical substances associated with pain and inflammation in the CMP region have been measured. Both actions require special skills and are expensive.[37,38] Needle EMG also detected the presence of spontaneous low-voltage motor endplate activity and high-voltage activity, which is characteristic of myofascial trigger points.[39,40] Ultrasound has also been used to visualize trigger points as focal, hypoechoic, elliptical regions, with a size of 0.16 cm.[41] Even if visualization of an individual trigger point is difficult, ultrasound can be used to guide needle placement into muscle tissue instead

Table 7.2. **PHARMACOLOGIC TREATMENT OF CMP IN ADULTS**

CLASS OF MEDICATION	ROLE IN TREATMENT	EXAMPLES	ADVERSE EFFECTS
Tricyclic antidepressants (TCAs)	Commonly used for chronic pain; can help to treat associated sleep disturbances and reduce painful dysesthesia. TCAs treat nociceptive and neuropathic pain.	Amitriptyline, nortriptyline, desipramine, imipramine	Dry mouth, constipation, fluid retention, weight gain, difficulty concentrating, and cardiotoxicity
NSAIDs	The drug of choice for initial treatment of CMP.	Naproxen, ibuprofen, diclofenac, meloxicam, celecoxib	Epigastric pain, gastric ulcers, nausea, rash, bleeding, headache, edema
Skeletal muscle relaxants	Efficacious in short-term treatment of CMP.	Cyclobenzaprine, tizanidine, baclofen	Drowsiness, dry mouth, headache, dizziness
Benzodiazepines	Effectiveness in muscle spasms is moderate. The adverse effect profile, addiction potential, and inferior results when compared to muscle relaxants preclude routine use.	Diazepam, clonazepam, lorazepam, alprazolam	Drowsiness, dizziness, ataxia, headache, nausea, somnolence, sedation
Opioid analgesics	Opioids use may be counterproductive to recovery and have the potential for abuse. They may be used for short-term therapy in refractory cases.	Tramadol, Norco, Percocet	Constipation, nausea, dizziness, vertigo, headache, respiratory depression, sedation
Anticonvulsants	Gabapentin has efficacy in treating myofascial and neuropathic pain.	Gabapentin, pregabalin	Dizziness, sedation, light-headedness, somnolence, nausea, vomiting, weight gain

of adipose or other nonmuscle structures during trigger-point injections.[5] Serious complications, although rare, include pneumothorax, hematoma, intravascular injection of local anesthetic, and intrathecal injections. Direct visualization of surrounding soft tissue and structures with ultrasound reduces the risk of such complications and may improve outcomes.

CONCLUSIONS

CMP is a common cause of nonspecific regional neck pain. It is a result of repetitive strain, trauma, cervical spine pathology, or postural dysfunction. The nonspecific diagnosis and lack of objective clinical measurements for CMP make the syndrome difficult to diagnose and treat; however, the presence of trigger points is a key diagnostic criterion for CMP. Management of CMP requires a multidisciplinary approach incorporating physical therapy, pharmacotherapy, injection therapy, and behavioral modification.

REFERENCES

1. Fejer R, Kyvik KO, Hartvigsen H. The prevalence of neck pain in the world population: a systematic critical review of the literature. *Eur Spine J.* 2004;15:834–848.
2. Duyur CB, Genc H, Altuntas V, Erdem HR. Disability and related factors in patients with chronic cervical myofascial pain. *Clin Rheum.* 2009;28(6):647–654.
3. Harden RN, Cottrill J, Gagnon CM, et al. Botulinum toxin A in the treatment of chronic tension-type headache with cervical myofascial trigger points: a randomized, double-blind, placebo-controlled pilot study. *Headache.* 2009;49(5):732–743.
4. Desai M, Saini V, Saini S. Myofascial pain syndrome: a treatment review. *Pain Ther.* 2013;2(1):21–23.
5. Botwin KP, Sharma K, Saliba R, Patel BC. Ultrasound-guided trigger point injections in the cervicothoracic musculature: a new and unreported technique. *Pain Physician.* 2008;11(6):885–889.
6. Botwin KP, Patel BC. Electromyographically guided trigger point injections in the cervicothoracic musculature of obese patients: a new and unreported technique. *Pain Physician.* 2007;10(6):753–756.
7. Nicol AL, Wu II, Ferrante FM. Botulinum toxin type A injections for cervical and shoulder girdle myofascial pain using an enriched protocol design. *Anesth Analg.* 2014;118(6):1326–1335.
8. Cho IT, Cho YW, Kwak SG, Chang MC. Comparison between ultrasound-guided interfacial pulsed radio frequency and ultrasound-guided interfacial block with local anesthetic in myofascial pain syndrome of trapezius muscle. *Medicine.* 2017;96(5):e6019.
9. Han SC, Harrison P. Myofascial pain syndrome and trigger-point management. *Reg Anesth.* 1997;22(1):89–101.
10. Garvey TA, Marks MR, Wiesel SW. A prospective, randomized, double-blind evaluation of trigger-point injection therapy for low-back pain. *Spine.* 1989;14(9):962–964.
11. Ashkenazi A, Blumenfeld A, Napchan U, et al. Peripheral nerve blocks and trigger point injections in headache management—a systematic review and suggestions for future research. *Headache.* 2010;50(6):943–952.
12. Bron C, de Gast A, Dommerholt J, Stegenga B, Wensing M, Oostendorp RA. Treatment of myofascial trigger points in patients with chronic shoulder pain: a randomized, controlled trial. *BMC Med.* 2011;9.
13. Simons DG. Clinical and etiological update of myofascial pain from trigger points. *Musculoskel Pain.* 1996;4(1-2):93–121.
14. Simons D, Travell J, Simons L. *Travell & Simons' Myofascial Pain and Dysfunction: The Trigger Point Manual.* 2nd ed. Baltimore, MD: Williams & Wilkins; 1999.
15. Reeves JL, Jaeger B, Graff-Radford SB. Reliability of the pressure algometer as a measure of myofascial trigger point sensitivity. *Pain.* 1986;24(3):313–321.
16. Travell J, Rinzler SH. The myofascial genesis of pain. *Postgrad Med.* 1952;11(5):425–434.
17. Rivner MH. The neurophysiology of myofascial pain syndrome. *Curr Pain Headache Rep.* 2001;5:432–440.
18. Hong CZ, Simons DG. Pathophysiologic and electrophysiologic mechanisms of myofascial trigger points. *Arch Phys Med Rehabil.* 1998;79(7):863–872.
19. Affaitati G., Fabrizio A, Savini A, et al. A randomized, controlled study comparing a lidocaine patch, a placebo patch, and anesthetic injection for treatment of trigger points in patients with myofascial pain syndrome: evaluation of pain and somatic pain thresholds. *Clin Ther.* 2009;31:705–720.
20. Hsieh LF, Hong CZ, Chern SH, et al. Efficacy and side effects of diclofenac patch in treatment of patients with myofascial pain syndrome of the upper trapezius. *Pain Symptom Manage.* 2009;39:116–125.
21. Vernon H, Schneider M. Chiropractic management of myofascial trigger points and myofascial pain syndrome: a systematic review of the literature. *J Manipulative Physiol Ther.* 2009;32:14–24.
22. Srbely JZ, Dickey JP. Randomized controlled study of the antinociceptive effect of ultrasound on trigger point sensitivity: novel applications in myofascial therapy? *Clin Rehabil.* 2007;21:411–417.
23. Hong CZ. Lidocaine injection versus dry needling to myofascial trigger point: the importance of the local twitch response. *Am J Phys Med Rehabil.* 1994;73:256–263.
24. Yoon SH, Rah UW, Sheen SS, et al. Comparison of 3 needle sizes for trigger point injection in myofascial pain syndrome of upper and middle trapezius muscle: a randomized controlled trial. *Arch Phys Med Rehabil.* 2009;90:1332–1339.
25. Sola AE, Kuitert JH. Myofascial trigger point pain in the neck and shoulder girdle. *Northwest Med.* 1955;54:980–984.
26. Frost FA, Jessen B, Siggaard-Anderson J. A control, double-blind comparison of mepivacaine injection versus saline injection for myofascial pain. *Lancet.* 1980;1:499–501.
27. Pizzolato P, Mannheimer W. *Histopathologic Effects of Local Anesthetic Drugs and Related Substances.* Springfield, IL: Charles C Thomas; 1961:40–71.
28. Cheshire WP, Abashian SW, Mann JD. Botulinum toxin in the treatment of myofascial pain syndrome. *Pain.* 1994;59:65–69.
29. Wheeler AH, Goolkasian P, Gretz SS. A randomized, double-blind, prospective pilot study of botulinum toxin injection for refractory, unilateral, cervicothoracic, paraspinal, myofascial pain syndrome. *Spine.* 1998;23:1662–1667.
30. Kamanli A, Kaya A, Ardicoglu O, et al. Comparison of lidocaine injection, botulinum toxin injection, and dry needling to trigger points in myofascial pain syndrome. *Rheumatol Int.* 2005;25:604–611.
31. Lew HL, Lee EH, Castaneda A, et al. Therapeutic use of botulinum toxin type A in treating neck and upper-back pain of myofascial origin: a pilot study. *Arch Phys Med Rehabil.* 2008;89:75–80.
32. Carrasco TG, Guerisoli LD, Guerisoli DM, Mazzetti MO. Evaluation of low intensity laser therapy in myofascial pain syndrome. *Cranio.* 2009;27:243–247.
33. Snyder-Mackler L, Bork C, Bourbon B, et al. Effect of helium-neon laser on musculoskeletal trigger points. *Phys Ther.* 1986;66:1087–1090.
34. Chen KH, Hong CZ, Kuo FC, et al. Electrophysiologic effects of a therapeutic laser on myofascial trigger spots of rabbit skeletal muscles. *Am J Phys Med Rehabil.* 2008;87:1006–1014.
35. Bauermeister W. The diagnosis and treatment of myofascial trigger points using shockwaves (abstract). *J Musculoskelet Pain.* 2004;12(suppl 9):26.
36. Kiralp MZ, Uzun G, Dincer U, et al. A novel treatment modality for myofascial pain syndrome: hyperbaric oxygen therapy. *Natl Med Assoc.* 2009;101:77–80.

37. Shah JP, Danoff JV, Desai MJ, et al. Biochemicals associated with pain and inflammation are elevated in sites near to and remote from active myofascial trigger points. *Arch Phys Med Rehabil.* 2008;89:16–23.
38. Simons DG. New views of myofascial trigger points: etiology and diagnosis. *Arch Phys Med Rehabil.* 2008;89(1):157–159.
39. Hubbard DR, Berkoff GM. Myofascial trigger points show spontaneous needle EMG activity. *Spine.* 1993;18:1803–1807.
40. Simons DG, Hong CZ, Simons LS. Spontaneous electrical activity of trigger points (abstract). *J Musculoskelet Pain.* 1995;3(suppl 1):124.
41. Sikdar S, Shah JP, Gebreab T, et al. Novel applications of ultrasound technology to visualize and characterize myofascial trigger points and surrounding soft tissue. *Arch Phys Med Rehabil.* 2009;90(11):1829–1838.
42. Okumus M, Ceceli E, Tuncay F, Kocaoglu S, Palulu N, Yoganciogl u ZR. The relationship between serum trace elements, vitamin B_{12}, folic acid and clinical parameters in patients with myofascial pain syndrome. *Back Musculoskelet Rehabil.* 2010;23(4):187–191.
43. Gerwin R. A review of myofascial pain and fibromyalgia—factors that promote their persistence. *Acupunct Med.* 2005;23(3):121–134.
44. Bendtsen L, Jensen R. Amitriptyline reduces myofascial tenderness in patients with chronic tension-type headache. *Cephalalgia.* 2016;20(6):603–610.
45. Childers M, Feldman J, Guo H. Myofascial pain syndrome. In: Frontera W, Silver J, Rizzo T, eds. *Essentials of Physical Medicine and Rehabilitation.* 2nd ed. Philadelphia, PA: Saunders; 2008:345–354.
46. McInnis K. Repetitive strain injuries. In: Frontera W, Silver J, Rizzo T, eds. *Essentials of Physical Medicine and Rehabilitation.* 2nd ed. Philadelphia, PA: Saunders; 2008:71–76.

REVIEW QUESTIONS

1. Which of the following may potentially facilitate or perpetuate myofascial trigger points in some patients?

   A. Low creatine kinase
   B. Low aldolase
   C. Low cholesterol
   D. Low vitamin B_{12} or folate

2. After a car accident a week ago, a 42-year-old engineer reports severe neck pain that radiates down both shoulders and upper arms and mid back. The patient's car, stopped at a traffic light, was rear-ended by a pickup truck. The pain is a severe stabbing and aching sensation that is markedly exaggerated by movement of the neck. Examination reveals an otherwise intact neurologic system with 5/5 strength, intact deep tendon reflexes, and no sensory deficit. Imaging studies are essentially normal except for straightening of cervical lordosis. The patient most likely has

   A. Bilateral C5 radiculopathy
   B. Myofascial pain
   C. Fibromyalgia
   D. Thoracic outlet syndrome

3. The diagnosis of myofascial pain syndrome is confirmed when

   A. A myofascial trigger point is identified
   B. A patient has widespread muscle pain
   C. A patient is diagnosed with fibromyalgia first
   D. Regional muscle spasms are noted

ANSWERS

1. D. Low levels of vitamin B_{12} or folate may be associated with trigger points in patients who suffer from myofascial pain syndrome. Low levels of serum ferritin, thyroid- stimulating hormone, and vitamin D also are implicated in chronic CMP.[42]

2. B. Myofascial pain may result after a sudden acceleration-deceleration insult. Neck muscles may reflexively spasm, which can result in straightening of the normal cervical lordosis. Myofascial pain from cervical neck muscles may radiate between the shoulder blades and into the upper extremity. Negative imaging rules out traumatic disk herniation. Fibromyalgia is characterized by widespread musculoskeletal pain lasting at least 3 months. Thoracic outlet syndrome results from compression of nerves or blood vessels in the upper chest, which causes numbness of the fingers and pain in the shoulders, arms, and neck. It is rare to have thoracic outlet syndrome of both extremities.

3. A. Myofascial pain is dull, poorly localized, and deep, without a precise location. The diagnosis of myofascial pain syndrome is confirmed when the myofascial trigger point is identified by palpation. Myofascial pain syndrome is a regional pain syndrome; fibromyalgia is a widespread pain syndrome. There is general agreement that the two are distinct. Systemic palpation differentiates between myofascial taut bands and general muscle spasms.

QUESTIONS AND ANSWERS

This chapter has accompanying questions and answers that are available to subscribers as part of the Oxford eLearning platform. To access the questions, follow the link below, or go to ✔ http://oxfordmedicine.com/painmanagementreview

8.

NEUROGENIC THORACIC OUTLET SYNDROME

Agnes Stogicza, Virtaj Singh, and Andrea Trescot

STEM CASE AND KEY QUESTIONS

A previously healthy, high-functioning 33-year-old female was rear-ended in a low-impact motor vehicle collision (MVC). She suffered no head trauma or loss of consciousness. In the emergency department (ED), her vital signs were within normal limits, with no focal neurologic signs. A cervical spine X-ray showed loss of cervical lordosis, but no fractures. The patient was discharged from the ED with no further treatment. Immediately after the MVC, the patient complained of mild neck pain and headaches; she developed arm and hand pain within a few weeks. Three months later, she noted persistent neck pain (left side worse than right), with pain in the trapezius/periscapular region, and daily headaches. The pain also radiated down her left arm to the fourth and fifth fingers. The patient reported dropping objects occasionally. She also noticed that her left hand is often colder than the right and looks "purplish."

WHAT IS THORACIC OUTLET SYNDROME (TOS)? WHAT IS THE NEXT STEP IN THE DIAGNOSIS?

The patient saw her primary care physician, who recommended ibuprofen 400 mg three times a day, massage, and physical therapy (PT). She noted little benefit from the ibuprofen. She started massage and PT, which seemed to be beneficial for a few months. However, over time, this regimen failed to provide any lasting or significant benefit, and she returned to baseline pain or worse. She complained of worsening daily headaches that started in the left suboccipital region and constant neck pain greater on the left than on the right, and noted that her fingers would go numb and cold more and more often.

WHICH FINGERS ARE USUALLY MORE AFFECTED AND WHAT IS THE ANATOMIC BASIS FOR THIS?

Because of the ulnar sided hand numbness (fourth and fifth digits), the patient was sent for electrodiagnostic testing (EDX) to evaluate for possible cubital tunnel syndrome. EDX showed no abnormalities, to the frustration of the patient and her treating physician. Further PT, massage, and gabapentin 300 mg three times a day were prescribed. Unfortunately, gabapentin—although it helped her sleep and somewhat dulled the pain—made her forgetful, which was not acceptable at her work.

WHAT IS THE NEXT STEP IN TREATMENT?

The patient was referred to neurosurgery for evaluation, and a cervical MRI was ordered to check for radiculopathy. It showed mild degenerative changes, as well as mild C5 foraminal stenosis on the right side. Since the foraminal stenosis was on the asymptomatic side and also at a higher level than the clinical symptoms would suggest, neurosurgery did not recommended surgery.

The patient became increasingly frustrated because she had difficulty maintaining her job, since working all day at the computer significantly worsened the finger numbness and pain, and yet all the diagnostic studies to date were normal. She was referred for cognitive-behavioral therapy to learn to cope with her new condition. Nortriptyline 20 mg at night was also prescribed.

The patient found that sitting in the hot tub, running hot water on her neck and shoulder, and stretching somewhat helped temporarily, which is how she would start her mornings and finish her days, while trying to maintain family life and her job.

WHAT ARE THE NEXT STEPS IN DIAGNOSIS? WHAT SHOULD A THOROUGH PHYSICAL EXAM COVER?

Because of persistent pain, the patient was eventually referred to a pain management specialist. A thorough physical exam by this physician showed a slightly elevated left shoulder, and tenderness along the cervical facets (left greater than right). There was also tight and painful cervical musculature, with profound hypertonicity most pronounced at the left sternocleidomastoid (SCM) muscle, anterior and middle scalene muscles, upper trapezius muscle, and pectoralis minor muscle. Slight pressure in the left supraclavicular groove immediately caused pain and tingling in the fourth and fifth digits.

Cervical range of motion (ROM) was also decreased: neck extension was 40°, flexion was 40°, left lateral flexion was 35°, right lateral flexion was 25°, and left and right rotation were 70°. Upper limb tension test was positive on the left.

HOW DO YOU CONFIRM THE DIAGNOSIS OF NEUROGENIC TOS (NTOS)? WHAT IS THE ROLE OF A DIAGNOSTIC INJECTION IN THE DIAGNOSIS OF NTOS?

The pain physician performed an ultrasound-guided injection (2 mL of 1% lidocaine) into the left anterior and middle scalene muscles, as well as the left pectoralis minor muscle, which resulted in immediate resolution of both the numbness and the pain in the arm and fingers. The resident watching the procedure noted with surprise that, in spite of the local anesthetic that was injected close to the brachial plexus, the numbness decreased, whereas he had expected an increase in numbness.

WHAT ARE THE TREATMENT OPTIONS FOR THIS PATIENT?

The patient left the office rather happy, because this was the first time that her pain and numbness had resolved since her accident. However, the pain physician warned her that all of her symptoms would likely soon return, anytime between a few hours and a few weeks.

A week later, upon return of the pain, the patient returned to the pain physician, who reassessed the previous X-rays for cervical rib or aberrant first rib. Since the patient had no cervical or aberrant first rib, botulinum toxin was injected into the same muscles that had responded well previously to anterior and middle scalene and pectoralis minor injections. In a few days, the patient was mostly symptom free. She was informed that the procedure could be repeated if symptoms returned in 3 to 6 months.

DISCUSSION

TOS, also called costoclavicular syndrome, cervical rib syndrome, or scalenus anticus syndrome, refers to the compression of the neurovascular bundle on its path from the thoracic outlet above the first rib to the axilla. Depending on the compressed structures, we distinguish between nTOS, arterial TOS (aTOS), and venous TOS (vTOS).[1] In nTOS, the primary symptoms come from brachial plexus compression. nTOS represents about 90% or more of all TOS. Better known, although rarer, is the compression of the subclavian vein (vTOS), also called Paget-Shroetter disease, which occurs in about 3% of cases. Positional compression of the subclavian artery (aTOS) is potentially the most dangerous form, because of the potential for limb ischemia, but it comprises less than 1% of all TOS cases. Women are more affected with all type of TOS than men.

ETIOLOGY AND PATHOGENESIS

Compression of the exiting nerve roots at the level of the cervical spine is easily recognized, most likely because imaging techniques, such as MRI, can visualize it. Carpal and cubital tunnel syndromes are also often considered, and can generally be diagnosed with EDX. However, nerves can be compressed anywhere along their path. Just as in piriformis syndrome, which is compression of the sciatic nerve by a tight or enlarged piriformis muscle, there is a potential similar compression of the brachial plexus by the cervicothoracic musculature.

Nerves receive their blood supply by the vasa nervorum, which is highly susceptible to compression.[2] Loss of nerve function due to ischemia has been well established in studies of diabetic neuropathy. The ischemia is at least initially reversible and might account for the neurologic symptoms in nTOS.

Compression of the neurovascular bundle usually occurs at three main locations as it passes from the cervical spine to the axilla. These sites include (Figure 8.1):

- The interscalene triangle
- The costoclavicular space
- The pectoralis minor space

The most commonly observed form of nTOS is entrapment of the brachial plexus at the interscalene triangle, which is located between the first rib and the clavicle in a cephalocaudal direction and between the anterior and middle scalene muscles. The anterior, middle, and posterior scalenes originate on the C2-C7 transverse processes and attach on the first rib. Their function is to elevate the first rib, flexing the neck forward and laterally and also rotating it. The brachial plexus compression (typically the lower trunk) can occur either from tight muscles directly compressing the plexus as it passes between them, or from elevation of the first rib by the chronically tight and shortened muscles, which narrows the space for the plexus. Fibers from the C8 and T1 nerve roots—at this location already trunks of the brachial plexus—run at the most caudad part of the brachial plexus, so it is understandable that, if the

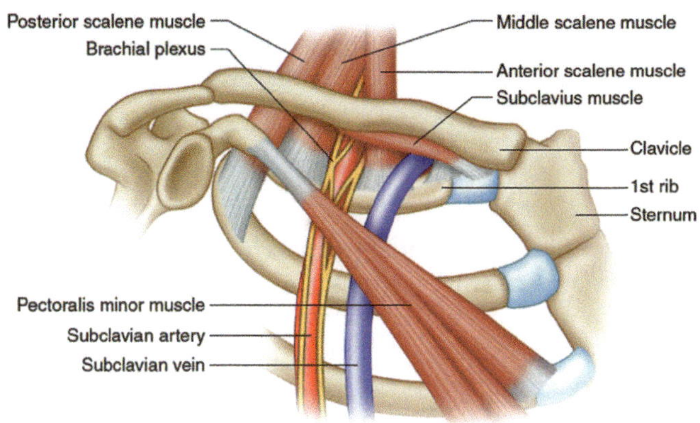

Figure 8.1. Anatomy of the brachial plexus showing the brachial plexus traveling between the scalene muscles, over the first rib, and under the pectoralis minor muscle. Reproduced with permission from Illig KA, Thompson RW, Freischlag JA, Donahue DM, Jordan SE, Edgelow PI, eds. Thoracic Outlet Syndrome. London: Springer; 2013.

plexus is pushed onto the first rib, the first symptoms will be in C8- and T1-related dermatomes. Hence, nTOS will often initially present in the hands and last two fingers. Of course, more severe cases can affect other parts of the nerve bundle, too.

This type of entrapment is often observed among MVC patients and more commonly in women than in men (by a ratio of 7:3). Patients have been shown to have tighter muscles with significantly more trigger points in the cervical musculature.[3]

One of the possible explanations for the symptom profile is that flexion-extension injuries can result in ligamentous laxity of the cervical spine, which leads to an increased muscle tone to compensate for the loss of stability. Alternatively, it may be that the actual trauma to the muscles directly results in the development of tight, shortened, and painful muscles (the scalenes themselves are subject to eccentric strain during a classic whiplash injury).[4]

The presence of an aberrant (large or higher positioned) first rib, or a cervical rib, can also contribute to the narrowing of the interscalene space and therefore compression of the neurovascular bundle. Other structural aberrations include fibrous bands, callus formations, tumor, and scalene muscle insertion variations, which can all contribute to the narrowing of the interscalene triangle.[5]

Entrapment can also happen at the costoclavicular space, which is the space between the first rib and subclavian muscle, just below the clavicle. Narrowing of the costoclavicular space can be caused by congenital anomalies (aberrant rib, clavicle, subclavian muscle, or costocoracoid ligament) or can also be acquired (postural changes, especially posteriorly and/or downwardly placed shoulder, drooping shoulder from deconditioning).[5–7]

The pectoralis minor syndrome form of entrapment occurs more distally, under the pectoralis minor tendon, just beneath its coracoid attachment. It is also called hyperabduction syndrome. This entrapment is the second most common type of nTOS. Abduction of the arm (a common technique in regional anesthesia to bring the plexus closer to the ultrasound probe when performing an infraclavicular block) pushes up the brachial plexus superficially and narrows the space under the pectoralis minor muscle. This also often results in the arm going numb when a person sleeps with arms placed above the head, even in otherwise healthy and symptom-free individuals.[8]

CLINICAL MANIFESTATIONS OF NTOS

Once the etiology and pathogenesis are understood, it is easy to understand the clinical symptoms of nTOS.

The compression of the various nerve fibers of the brachial plexus results in tingling, numbness, pain, and weakness in the upper extremity. The location and severity of the symptoms depend on the actual fibers that are compressed and the chronicity of the condition.

Having the C8 and T1 fibers compressed (at the level of the lower trunk of the brachial plexus), as explained, results in the leading symptoms of tingling and numbness in the fourth and fifth digits and pain radiating all along the arm. However, patients may also complain of symptoms in the first three digits or even the whole hand.[1,9]

Symptoms usually wax and wane initially, and then worsen with increasing muscle tightness caused by cold, stress, repetitive movements, or carrying weight. The symptoms often decrease temporarily with massage, stretching, hot tub, and acupuncture. However, without intervention, the symptoms usually gradually worsen and cause long-term suffering and frustration to the patient.

Patients often also complain of tight musculature, shoulder pain, neck pain, headaches, and limited ROM in the neck and arms.[10,11]

MODALITIES OF NTOS DIAGNOSIS

History

A good history and physical exam, as always, are key to the diagnosis. The history often reveals either trauma, such as MVC, or sports-related injury with some sort of flexion-extension injury of the neck. In a MVC, the seatbelt restrains the shoulder so that the forces can lead to nonphysiologic stretching of the upper cervicothoracic musculature. The other typical history is of a work injury with some sort of repetitive movement, such as repeated overhead activities or carrying heavy objects. Lifestyles leading to impaired posture, such as prolonged computer work or deconditioning, are also commonly seen.[12]

Physical Exam

Physical examination focuses on a very thorough neurologic and musculoskeletal exam of the cervical spine and upper extremities. We can often easily diagnose a cervical radiculopathy when presented with a typical pattern of weakness, reflex changes, and sensory loss in a specific nerve root distribution. Similarly, we can diagnose a peripheral nerve injury, such as carpal tunnel and cubital tunnel syndrome, when the neurologic changes follow the normal pattern for a given terminal branch. However, because of the very complicated anatomy of the brachial plexus as it travels through the root-trunk-division-cord-branch phases with multiple rearrangement of the actual nerve fibers, compression within the thoracic outlet can lead to a variety of presentations. These atypical neurologic complaints and findings should raise suspicion of nTOS, especially if distal hand weakness involving both median- and ulnar-innervated muscles is present. In some cases, the abductor pollicis brevis, abductor digiti minimi, and opponens pollicis muscles can be weak on exam.

The musculoskeletal exam is the other cornerstone of the diagnosis. Impaired posture, decreased cervical lordosis, and downward-sloping shoulders are typical findings. Patients almost always have decreased ROM of the neck and shoulder (or both). Palpation of the cervical and upper thoracic musculature shows painful muscles with palpable, tender, taught bands, especially in the SCM, trapezius, anterior scalene, middle scalene, and pectoralis minor muscles (Figure 8.2).[11]

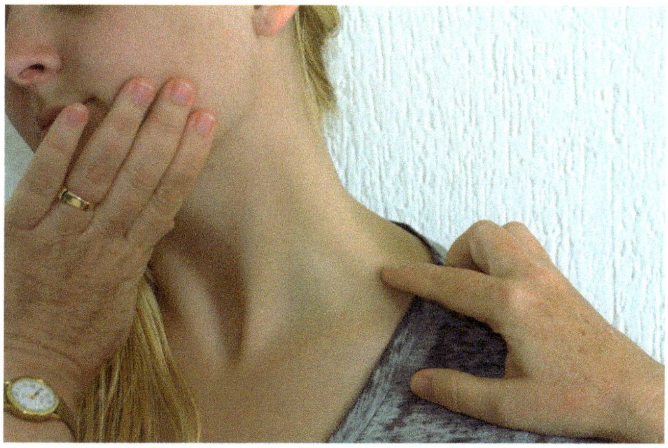

Figure 8.2. Examination of the muscles of the neck. Image courtesy of Andrea Trescot, MD.

Further examination should be done to rule out potential shoulder pathology as the primary source or contributing factor for a patient's symptoms. One should check for ROM at the shoulder to ensure the patient does not have adhesive capsulitis as well as to rule out a rotator cuff or labral tear. An injury or loss of ROM at the shoulder may contribute to compensatory cervical musculature hypertonicity or muscle-fiber shortening, which can lead to a secondary nTOS.

The upper limb tension test is a specific physical exam for nTOS (Figure 8.3). The patient abducts the arms 90°, extends the wrists 90°, and then the head is laterally flexed toward the nonsymptomatic side (ear to shoulder), while the patient observes if the symptoms worsen on the affected side. Increased numbness and tingling in the extremity and the fingers further strengthen the suspicion for nTOS.[13]

Imaging and EDX

The mainstays of the diagnosis are the history and physical exam. However, several other modalities are also used.

X-ray

Cervical ribs can be present in 0.5% of the population and are twice as common in women as in men.[14] While the presence of a cervical rib (Figure 8.4) or aberrant first thoracic rib should raise suspicion, it is not an absolute requirement for nTOS. In fact, only a minority of cases of nTOS involve a cervical rib. Instead, the majority of the cases of compression stem from spasm of the cervicothoracic musculature rather than an enlarged rib.

Decreased cervical lordosis is often observed among patients with cervical myofascial problems and nTOS; however, interpretation of this finding is difficult. It may be the root cause (due to disruption of the posterior cervical ligaments) or it may be the consequence of the increased cervical muscle tone.

MRI

MRI is not commonly used as a diagnostic tool for TOS, but it is certainly useful in ruling out other conditions, such as exiting nerve root compression (i.e., cervical radiculopathy). In some severe cases of nTOS, edema of the brachial plexus may be observed in the coronal view on MRI plexography (Figure 8.5). Some authors recommend obtaining a functional MRI scan, which can show decreased distance between the first rib and clavicle in patients with TOS.[15]

EDX

The use of EDX is controversial. While positive EDX findings can confirm the diagnosis,[16] the absence of them does not exclude nTOS. EDX is probably a relatively insensitive tool to diagnose various, often reversible, nerve compressions. Some experts, mainly neurologists and physiatrists, prefer to call only EDX-proven cases nTOS, and to call the cases without positive EDX findings nonspecific TOS. The cases where EDX test results are positive are probably advanced cases of nTOS.[12]

When EDX is positive, typical findings include low-amplitude median motor and ulnar sensory responses in the absence of evidence of cervical radiculopathy, carpal tunnel syndrome, or cubital tunnel syndrome. Another typical EDX finding (perhaps even the most sensitive finding) is diminished amplitude of the median antebrachial cutaneous sensory response.

As mentioned, nTOS is the "piriformis syndrome of the upper extremity." The diagnosis of piriformis syndrome is similarly a clinical diagnosis that only rarely has positive EDX findings. One study showed H-reflex changes in the FAIR position (hip flexion, adduction, and internal rotation); however, the technique did not establish accuracy of the H-reflex, because the study lacked symptomatic control participants (patients with sciatica, but no piriformis syndrome).[17]

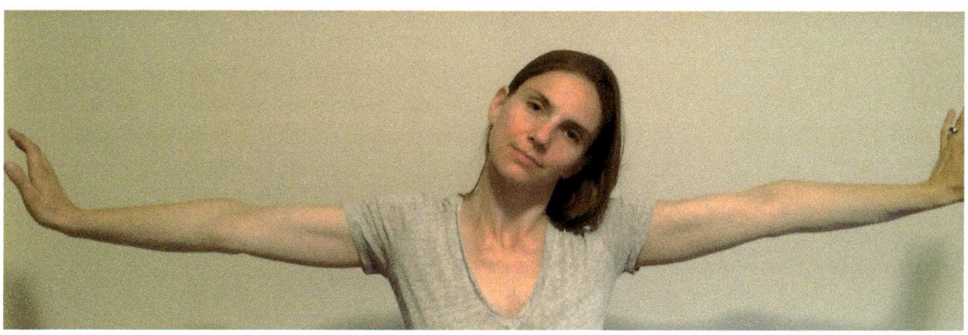

Figure 8.3. Upper limb tension test. Image courtesy of Virtaj Singh, MD.

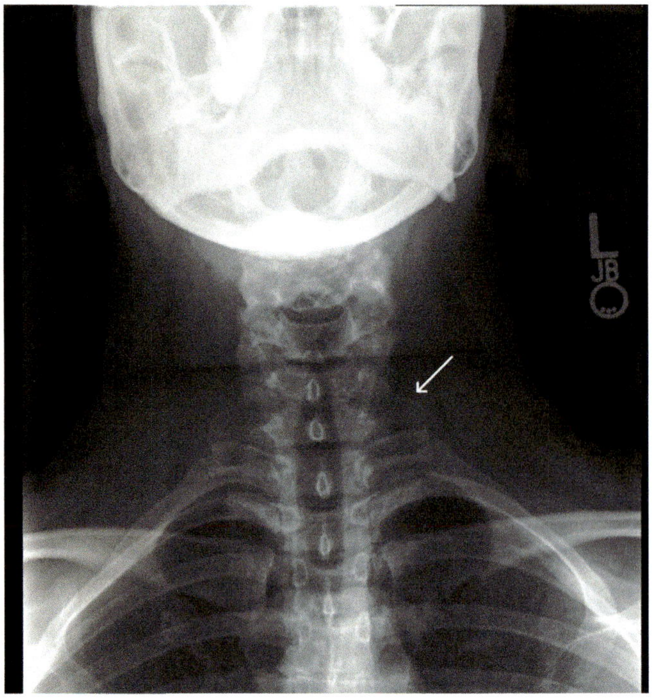

Figure 8.4. Cervical X-ray showing an enlarged C7 transverse process (arrow), also known as a cervical rib. Image courtesy of Andrea Trescot, MD.

Ultrasound Evaluation

The use of a questionnaire, combined with a thorough physical examination and ultrasound evaluation, has been proposed as a means of differentiating nTOS from other brachial plexus entrapments.[18] The ultrasound evaluation can show cervical rib impingement, vascular compromise, and fibrosis of the brachial plexus.[19]

Diagnostic Injections

Again, as in piriformis syndrome, the diagnosis of nTOS is best established by specifically relaxing the suspected compressing muscles with a small amount of local anesthetic.

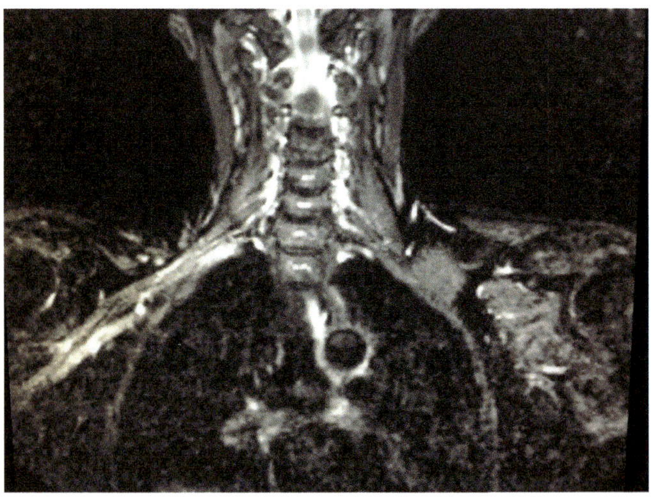

Figure 8.5. Coronal MRI showing increased signal intensity of the right brachial plexus. Stable mass also noted on the left, asymptomatic side. Image courtesy of Agnes Stogicza, MD.

If pain, numbness, and tingling resolve within a few minutes, the diagnosis of nTOS is likely.

Ultrasound-Guided Anterior Scalene Injection

When the entrapment occurs in the interscalene triangle, the anterior scalene muscles can be anesthetized. Jordan originally described electrodiagnostic-guided injections in 1998.[20] The target can also easily be localized with ultrasound, as is commonly done in interscalene nerve blocks for regional anesthesia. One can track the exiting nerve roots distally and find the trunks of the brachial plexus sandwiched between the anterior and middle scalene muscles (Figure 8.6). The other option is to find the brachial plexus at the supraclavicular location, where the divisions are organized in a bundle, superolateral to the subclavian artery. Tracking the divisions slightly cephalad again will provide an image of the scalene muscles.

After sterile prep and drape, a 25-G 4-cm needle is inserted into the muscle belly and 2 to 3 mL of local anesthetic is injected.

Care must be taken to avoid spilling local anesthetic on the brachial plexus, because that would impair the diagnostic value of the injection. After the injection, the patient should have no new numbness or weakness at the area of the brachial plexus (these symptoms signal a failed diagnostic injection).

Ultrasound-Guided Subclavian Muscle Injection

When the entrapment occurs at the costoclavicular space, in some cases it causes subclavian muscle spasm or hypertrophy. The subclavian muscle is easily visualized with ultrasound. The probe is placed on the mid-portion of the clavicle, with a slight tilt so it visualizes the subclavian muscle just beneath it (Figure 8.7). This is followed by a rather superficial injection of 1 mL of local anesthetic. The lung is in the vicinity of the target, so careful needle-tip visualization is necessary.

Ultrasound-Guided Pectoralis Minor Muscle Injection

When the entrapment occurs under the pectoralis minor muscle, the target for diagnostic injection is the pectoralis muscle, which attaches on the coracoid process and is directed medially and caudally. If the ultrasound probe is placed over the coracoid process, aimed toward the manubrium, the pectoralis minor fibers are seen longitudinally, just beneath the pectoralis major (Figure 8.8). For diagnostic purposes, 1 mL of local anesthetic is injected. The lung is in the vicinity of the target, so careful needle-tip visualization is necessary.

With all of the diagnostic injections, resolution of the symptoms can be expected within a few minutes, also with improvement in the Upper limb tension test (ULTT). The ULTT is a neurodynamic assessment by which shoulder, elbow, forearm, wrist and fingers are kept in specific position to put stress on particular nerve (nerve bias) and further modification in position of each joint is done as "sensitizer". The ULTT's are equivalent to the straight leg raise designed for the lumbar spine.

Complications of the Diagnostic Techniques

Ultrasound-guided injections of the anterior scalene, subclavian, and pectoralis minor muscles are relatively superficial, and

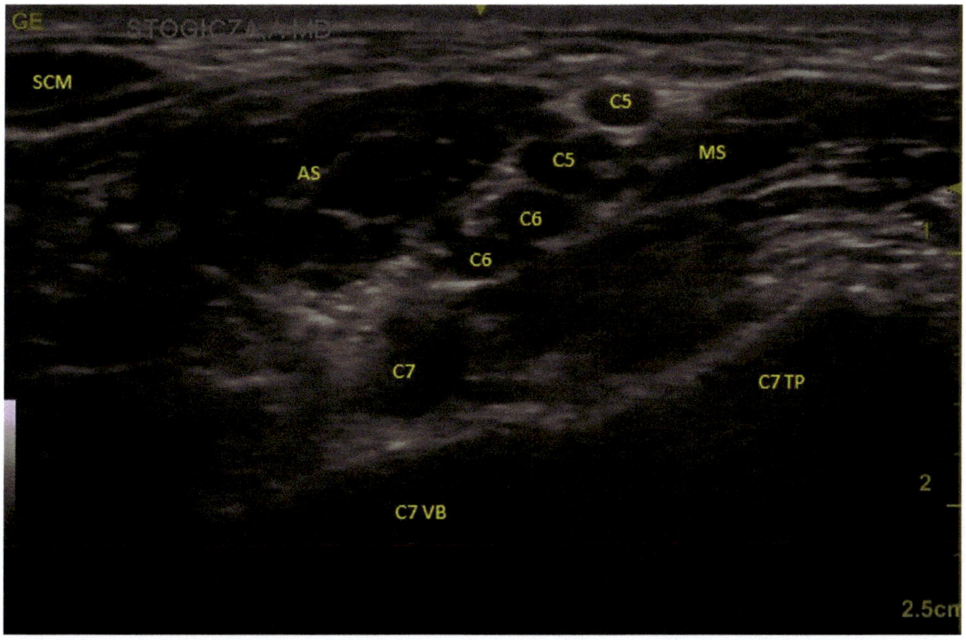

Figure 8.6. Ultrasound image of the brachial plexus at the level of the scalene muscles. Abbreviations: AS, anterior scalene muscle; C7TP, C7 transverse process; C7VB, C7 vertebral body; MS, middle scalene muscle; SCM, sternocleidomastoid muscle. Image courtesy of Agnes Stogicza, MD.

therefore are easy and safe procedures. Possible complications can be understood and avoided by considering the structures in the vicinity of the targets (Table 8.1).

TREATMENTS OF NTOS

Conservative Treatment

The mainstay of therapy is conservative, aiming to lengthen the chronically shortened cervical muscles (anterior and middle scalenes, SCM, trapezius, levator scapulae, pectoral and suboccipital muscles), thereby decreasing the entrapment. This process can be facilitated by muscle relaxants, PT, and massage. Rehabilitation should focus on improving posture, removing aggravating factors, and improving work ergonomics.[21,22]

Injection Treatment

If conservative methods fail to provide lasting improvement, minimally invasive injection techniques can offer a solution.

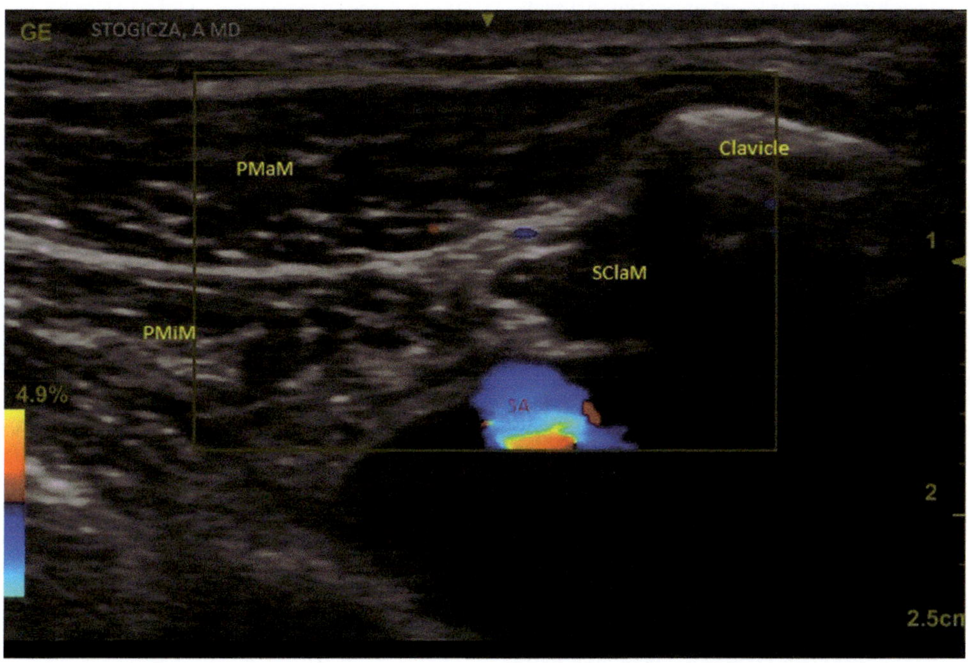

Figure 8.7. Ultrasound image of the subclavian region. Abbreviations: PMaM, pectoralis major muscle; PMiM, pectoralis minor muscle; SA, subclavian artery; SCLaM, subclavius muscle. Image courtesy of Agnes Stogicza, MD.

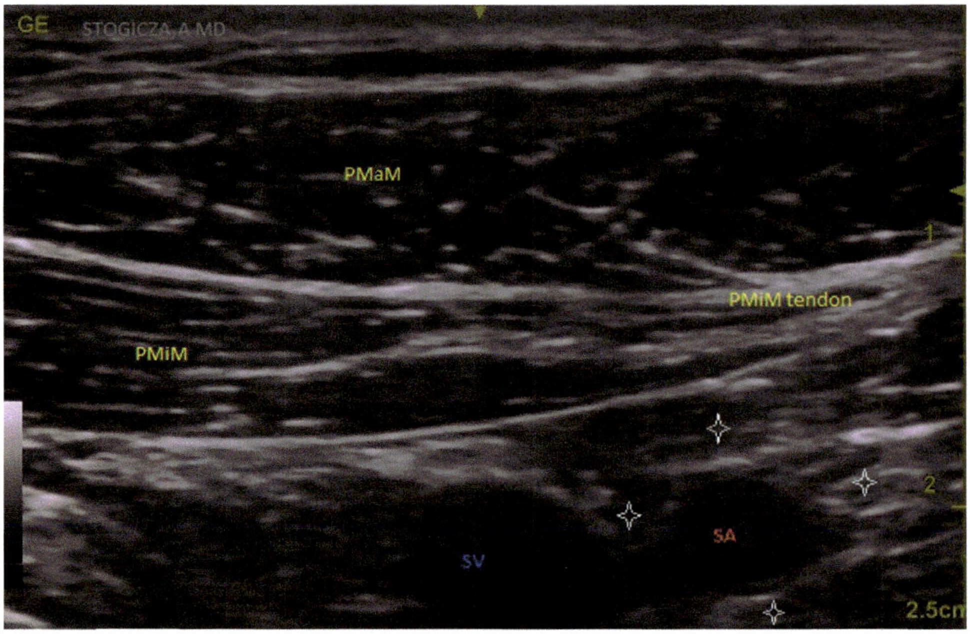

Figure 8.8. Ultrasound image of the pectoralis muscle. Abbreviations: PMaM, pectoralis major muscle; PMiM, pectoralis minor muscle; PMiM tendon, pectoralis minor muscle tendon, SA, subclavian artery; SV, subclavian vein. Image courtesy of Agnes Stogicza, MD.

Table 8.1. **STRUCTURES POTENTIALLY INJURED DURING ULTRASOUND-GUIDED INJECTIONS**

STRUCTURES AT RISK OF INJURY	POSSIBLE SIDE EFFECTS, ADVERSE EVENTS, COMPLICATIONS
Exiting nerve roots and brachial plexus	Sensory and motor block and nerve injury
Subclavian artery and vein	Intravascular injection (should cause no symptoms at this dose), possible vessel injury
Carotid and vertebral arteries	Intravascular injection, seizure, arterial dissection with brain ischemic damage
Jugular vein and thyroid venous plexus	Bleeding
Epidural injection	Minimal to no consequence with dural sleeve injected at this dose; higher doses, possible high spinal
Intrathecal injection	High spinal anesthesia
Ascending sympathetic fibers just anterior to longus colli muscle	Horner's syndrome
Vagus/recurrent laryngeal nerve	Anesthesia/damage, hoarseness
Phrenic nerve	Anesthesia/damage, unilateral diaphragmatic weakness, possible respiratory consequences with impaired lung function
Spinal cord	If needle is not visualized properly, it can cause cord injury, paralysis, and death
Lung	Pneumothorax

As myofascial pain syndrome often coexists with nTOS, or may even actually provoke nTOS, trigger-point injections can address both the myofascial pain and the neurogenic symptoms provoked by the muscle spasm. These trigger-point injections are performed in the same manner as the diagnostic injections, with slightly higher volumes of local anesthetic (3–5 mL). The duration of the benefits depends on the etiology of the nTOS and the use of other concurrently administered modalities, such as PT.

If this methods fail to provide lasting relief and the diagnosis is confirmed with diagnostic injection[23] (often under ultrasound or EMG guidance),[24] chemodenervation of the muscle with botulinum toxin is often indicated.[25,26] The injection technique is the same as the diagnostic block (with a similar risk profile, but also some risks unique to the toxin itself, such as weakness and swallowing difficulties).

Surgical Treatment

If chemodenervation provides only short-term relief, surgical treatment is a possibility. Typical surgery includes: resection of the anterior and middle scalene and pectoralis minor tenotomy,[27] and occasionally removal of the cervical or first thoracic rib.[28] Surgical interventions carry similar risks as the treatments already described, with the added risks associated with surgery.

CONCLUSIONS

- nTOS is the compression of the brachial plexus nerves as they travel from the cervical spine to the axilla.
- The symptoms initially wax and wane, and imaging and EDX may remain negative until the condition is severe.

- Diagnosis is based on a thorough history and physical examination, which can subsequently be confirmed with diagnostic injection of the spastic/dystonic muscles (most commonly the anterior scalene muscle).
- Initial treatment is conservative, but if no sustained relief is achieved, chemodenervation and surgery are possible treatment options.

REFERENCES

1. Ferrante MA. The thoracic outlet syndromes. *Muscle Nerve.* 2012;45(6):780–795.
2. Moore KL, Dailey AF, Agar AMR. *Clinically Oriented Anatomy.* 6th ed. Philadelphia, PA: Lippincott Williams & Wilkins; 2010.
3. Ettlin T, Schuster C, Stoffel R, Bruderlin A, Kischka U. A distinct pattern of myofascial findings in patients after whiplash injury. *Arch Phys Med Rehabil.* 2008;89(7):1290–1293.
4. Matsui T, Ii K, Hojo S, Sano K. Cervical neuro-muscular syndrome: discovery of a new disease group caused by abnormalities in the cervical muscles. *Neurol Med Chir.* 2012;52:75–80.
5. Atasoy E. Thoracic outlet syndrome: anatomy. *Hand Clin.* 2004;20:7–14.
6. Brantigan CO, Roos DB. Diagnosing thoracic outlet syndrome. *Hand Clin.* 2004;27:27–36.
7. Sanders RJ, Hammond SL. Etiology and pathology. *Hand Clin.* 2004;20:23–26.
8. Wilbourn AJ. Thoracic outlet syndromes. *Entrapment Neuropathies.* Philadelphia, PA: Lippincott-Raven; 1999:227–250.
9. Sunderland S. *Nerve and Nerve Injuries.* Edinburgh: Churchill Livingstone; 1978.
10. Ferrante MA. Brachial plexopathies: classification, causes, and consequences. *Muscle Nerve.* 2004;30:547–568.
11. Gujar B, Flores RH. Entrapment neuropathies and compartment syndromes. *Rheumatology.* 2014;81:671–682.
12. Trescot AM. *Peripheral Nerve Entrapment—Clinical Diagnosis and Management.* New York, NY: Springer; 2016.
13. Sanders RJ, Hammond SL, Rao NM. Diagnosis of thoracic outlet syndrome. *J Vasc Surg.* 2007;46(3):601–604.
14. Juvonen T, Satta J, Laitala P. Anomalies at the thoracic outlet are frequent in the general population. *Am J Surg.* 1995;170:33–37.
15. Smedby ORO, Klaastad F, Lilleas F, Tillung T, Fosse E. Functional imaging of the thoracic outlet syndrome in an open MR scanner. *Eur Radiol.* 2000;10:597–600.
16. Tsao BE, Ferrante MA, Wilbourn AJ, Shields RW. Electrodiagnostic features of true neurogenic thoracic outlet syndrome. *Muscle Nerve.* 2014;49(5):724–727.
17. Fishman LM, Zybert PA. Electrophysiologic evidence of piriformis syndrome. *Arch Phys Med Rehabil.* 1992;73(4):359–364.
18. Jordan SE, Ahn SS, Gelabert HA. Differentiation of thoracic outlet syndrome from treatment-resistant cervical brachial pain syndromes: development and utilization of a questionnaire, clinical examination and ultrasound evaluation. *Pain Physician.* 2007;10(3):441–452.
19. Lapegue F, Faruch-Bilfeld M, Demondion X, et al. Ultrasonography of the brachial plexus, normal appearance and practical applications. *Diagn Intervent Imaging.* 2014;95(3):259–275.
20. Jordan SE, Machleder HI. Diagnosis of thoracic outlet syndrome using electrophysiologically guided anterior scalene blocks. *Ann Vasc Surg.* 1998;12:260–264.
21. Crosby CA, Wehbe MA. Conservative treatment for thoracic outlet syndrome. *Hand Clin.* 2004;20:43–49.
22. Dobrusin R. An osteopathic approach to conservative management of thoracic outlet syndromes. *J Am Osteopath Assoc.* 1989;89:1046–1050, 1053–1057.
23. Benzon HT, Rodes ME, Chekka K, Malik K, Pearce WH. Scalene muscle injections for neurogenic thoracic outlet syndrome: case series. *Pain Pract.* 2012;12(1):66–70.
24. Torriani M, Gupta R, Donahue DM. Sonographically guided anesthetic injection of anterior scalene muscle for investigation of neurogenic thoracic outlet syndrome. *Skeletal Radiol.* 2009;38(11):1083–1087.
25. Foley JM, Finlayson H, Travlos A. A review of thoracic outlet syndrome and the possible role of botulinum toxin in the treatment of this syndrome. *Toxins.* 2012;4(11):1223–1235.
26. Jordan SE, Ahn SS, Freischlag JA, Gelabert HA, Machleder HI. Selective botulinum chemodenervation of the scalene muscles for treatment of neurogenic thoracic outlet syndrome. *Ann Vasc Surg.* 2000;14:365–369.
27. Sanders RJ. Recurrent neurogenic thoracic outlet syndrome stressing the importance of pectoralis minor syndrome. *Vasc Endovasc Surg.* 2011;45(1):33–38.
28. Franklin GM, Fulton-Kehoe D, Bradley C, Smith-Weller T. Outcome of surgery for thoracic outlet syndrome in Washington state workers' compensation. *Neurology.* 2000;54(6):1252–1257.

REVIEW QUESTIONS

1. A 20-year-old healthy female presents to the pain clinic with shoulder and arm pain and numbness and tingling in her hand that began shortly after she was involved in a rear-end MVC 2 months earlier. She had no loss of consciousness, and cervical spine X-rays were negative in the ED. What is the next step in the evaluation of this patient's complaints?

   A. Order a cervical spine MRI
   B. Perform a thorough physical examination
   C. Order EMG of the affected extremity
   D. Order repeat cervical spine X-rays

2. Physical examination shows no proximal muscle weakness or atrophy with 2+ symmetrical upper extremity reflexes. The patient also adds that the arm pain and paresthesia (tingling) are intermittent. She occasionally wakes up with a painful arm and parasthesias in her fourth and fifth digits. Increased physical activity, lifting, and carrying make her symptoms worse. Based on this, the arm pain is:

   A. Likely to be caused by C5 radiculopathy
   B. Likely to be caused by C6 radiculopathy
   C. Unlikely to be caused by C 6 radiculopathy
   D. Likely to be caused by carpal tunnel syndrome

3. What are the likely findings on physical exam of the neck?

   A. Increased ROM of the cervical spine
   B. Increased flexion, but decreased extension
   C. Tight cervical musculature and decreased ROM in all directions
   D. Positive Spurling's test

ANSWERS

1. B. In order to avoid misdiagnosis, a detailed history and physical exam are crucial in pain conditions, especially cases of

nTOS. The diagnosis of nTOS is mainly a clinical diagnosis, unless the condition is long-standing, with permanent nerve damage.[11–13] Therefore, answers A, C, and D are not correct.

2. C. Answer A is incorrect because C5 radiculopathy gives a C5 pattern, with decreased deltoid strength and/or impaired biceps reflex and decreased sensation in the upper arm at the lateral antecubital fossa down to the elbow joint. Similarly, B is incorrect because C6 root compression would present with impaired wrist extension and/or impaired biceps and brachioradialis reflex and/or decreased sensation at the lower arm/thumb. Answer D is incorrect because carpal tunnel syndrome is compression of the median nerve. It also often causes pain in the arm; however, in the hand, it affects only the thumb, index finger, middle finger, and half of the ring finger. The pinky finger is usually asymptomatic, which is not what the patient described. The correct answer is C because this picture is more likely to be associated with nTOS.[1,9]

3. C. Answer A is incorrect because most commonly after flexion-extension injury patients present with decreased ROM of the cervical spine. Extension of the neck is generally more limited and painful than flexion; however, after such an injury, both flexion and extension are decreased from baseline, so answer B is incorrect. As the patient is unlikely to have radicular compression, Spurling's test will likely be negative; therefore, D is incorrect. Patients present with tight cervical musculature and generally decreased overall ROM; therefore, answer C is correct.[12]

QUESTIONS AND ANSWERS

This chapter has accompanying questions and answers that are available to subscribers as part of the Oxford eLearning platform. To access the questions, follow the link below, or go to
✔ http://oxfordmedicine.com/painmanagementreview

9.

CHRONIC SHOULDER PAIN

Sarah T. Yang and Tariq M. Malik

STEM CASE AND KEY QUESTIONS

A 52-year-old left-hand-dominant man with no other significant past medical history presents to the clinic for right shoulder pain that has lasted for the past 6 months. A very active individual, he first noticed the pain when he could no longer do push-ups due to discomfort. His pain feels like a sharp twinge in his arm that radiates down to the elbow with certain movements in the posterior or anterior plane. Sleeping on the affected side is uncomfortable. He describes his pain as a "dull ache" that ranges from a 3 to a 6 on a 1 to 10 numerical rating scale. Tylenol temporarily alleviates the pain. He denies feeling weak and has no history of neurologic disease.

On examination, he has full range of motion for flexion, abduction, adduction, and extension. Muscle bulk is normal. Strength is 5/5 for shoulder abduction, elbow extension, elbow flexion, wrist extension, finger abduction, and grip. Pulses are 2+ and symmetric. Provocative tests (empty can, Hawkins, Yergason's, lift-off, O'Brien, cross-arm, Neer's, Spurling's) are negative. He is able to resist internal and external rotation adequately. On active range of motion, mild scapula-thoracic dyskinesia is noted in his right upper extremity, with some mild posterior capita tightness. Reflexes are symmetric and sensation is intact.

WHAT ARE THE MOST IMPORTANT ELEMENTS IN THE HISTORY OF SOMEONE WITH SHOULDER PAIN? WHAT ARE THE MOST COMMON PATHOLOGIES OF CHRONIC SHOULDER PAIN? HOW DOES THE PATIENT EXPLAIN HIS DEVELOPMENT OF THIS CONDITION SINCE HE IS SUCH AN ACTIVE PERSON?

History is most important in evaluating shoulder pain. Most painful conditions are mechanical in nature. Focused history elucidating the mechanism of injury, duration of symptoms, and movements that relieve or cause worsening of pain can help localize the pain generator in the joint. Common etiologies of chronic painful shoulder joint are tendon tears (rotator cuff or biceps tendon), subacromial impingement (leading to subacromial bursitis or tendinitis), osteoarthritis, and instability.

The patient reports that he vaguely remembers an instance during his vacation when his pain started after he was challenged by a friend to do a one-hand push-up immediately after lifting weights. He recalls that he felt a little twinge midway through the challenge but he continued with the complete set of 30 one-hand push-ups. His shoulder hurt and was mildly bruised for about 4 weeks but he did not pay much attention to it.

A CHRONIC TENDINOPATHY IS SUSPECTED. WHAT PHYSICAL EXAMINATION ELEMENTS WOULD SUPPORT THE DIAGNOSIS?

In evaluating the patient, you start by inspection of the painful shoulder in the anterior, posterior, and lateral planes, to look for asymmetry, swelling, deformity, discoloration, or scars. Palpation of the acromioclavicular (AC) joint, glenohumeral joint, bicipital groove, rotator muscles, periscapular muscles, and trigger points is then undertaken. Resisted movements with shoulder flexion, extension, and external and internal rotation suggest a rotator cuff issue. The patient has a positive Speed's test (pressure on the forearm with pain in the biceps groove) consistent with biceps tendinopathy.

WHAT IMAGING STUDIES ARE INDICATED IN THIS PATIENT?

Imaging is selected based on a working diagnosis. Shoulder radiographs do not reveal acute osseous abnormalities and the right shoulder radiograph is normal. Radiologic images of the cervical spine show normal alignment of the vertebrae, and loss of height at the C5-C6 disk with small anterior osteophytes. The remaining disks have preserved height. No focal destructive lesions are noted. An MRI of the shoulder, ordered after the X-rays, does not show convincing evidence of a labral tear but reveals low-grade tendinosis of the distal subscapularis, but otherwise intact rotator cuff musculature.

WHAT TREATMENT IS INDICATED FOR THIS PATIENT?

You advise the patient to start acetaminophen 500 mg every 6 hours as well as meloxicam 7.5 mg every day. You make a referral to physical therapy (PT) and explain to the patient that, although he is very physically active, he may benefit from directed exercises for his biceps tendinopathy to improve function and relieve pain.

A COMPLETE 6-WEEK COURSE OF PT DID NOT COMPLETELY RESOLVE HIS SYMPTOMS, BUT IT DID IMPROVE HIS RANGE OF MOTION. HE NO LONGER REQUIRES ACETAMINOPHEN REGULARLY, ALTHOUGH HE STILL ENDURES PAIN OCCASIONALLY. WHAT IS THE NEXT STEP?

At the patient's follow-up appointment, you discuss the possibility of an injection. The patient agrees, and the biceps tendon is injected with 40 mg of triamcinolone and 3 mL of bupivacaine 0.25% under direct ultrasound guidance. The patient responds favorably to the treatment and his pain is reduced significantly. With continued PT and occasional anti-inflammatory agents and acetaminophen, the patient is slowly resuming his routine exercises.

DISCUSSION

SHOULDER PAIN: INTRODUCTION

The glenohumeral joint is a ball-and-socket joint with a shallow socket. Its stability, therefore, depends on the rotator cuff and the scapular muscles. Shoulder stability is enhanced by the glenoid labrum, a ring of fibrous tissue that increases the diameter of the glenoid by over 50% both superiorly-inferiorly and anteriorly-posteriorly.

A thorough shoulder examination begins with the history. In chronic shoulder pain, the chronic nature of the pain and the details of the injury (if known) are investigated. Evaluation of chronic shoulder pain takes into account the physical structures that may be implicated in the initial injury (which can contribute to pain) and the patient's position and posture during the presumed injury.[1]

Although in certain cases pain is well localized, most shoulder pathologies are difficult to isolate.

A good shoulder examination can narrow the problem down to one of five pain- generator categories[1–3]:

1. Rotator cuff musculature-related pain
2. Shoulder instability-related pain
3. Shoulder stiffness-related pain
4. AC joint pain
5. Referred pain.

COMMON PATHOLOGIES OF CHRONIC SHOULDER PAIN

Acute injuries of the shoulder often originate from strains, tendon tears, tendinopathy, overuse, or impingement. If they are not addressed in a timely fashion, they can progress to chronic shoulder pain.

Chronic injuries of the shoulder are attributed to calcific tendinopathy, glenohumeral osteoarthritis, labral injuries with instability, AC joint pain, adhesive capsulitis, or referred pain from the cervical or thoracic spine.[3]

PHYSICAL EXAMINATION IN CHRONIC SHOULDER PAIN

A complete shoulder examination begins with thorough observation, first checking for skin discoloration, surgical scars, and muscle bulk symmetry. Inspection should be performed in the anterior, posterior, and lateral planes.

Active movements of the shoulder are evaluated. The examiner should routinely check for arm elevation, external rotation with elbows at side, external rotation at 90° of shoulder abduction, internal rotation, and horizontal flexion.

If a patient is unable to complete all planes of movement actively, movement is transitioned to passive range of motion.

Following assessment of the movements, palpation of the AC joint, glenohumeral joint, bicipital groove, rotator muscles, and periscapular muscles may elicit tenderness. Myofascial trigger points are evaluated during palpation.[2]

Additional tests to perform for the specific diagnosis of chronic shoulder pain are

1. Resisted movements—examiner should test for shoulder flexion, extension, and external and internal rotation against resistance
2. Special tests
    - Rotator cuff impingement/tear are tested by[4]:
        - Empty can test: This is a common examination that tests the supraspinatus tendon and muscle. With the patient in the sitting position, the examiner stabilizes the shoulder girdle. The patient is asked to lift the arm at 90°, with forward flexion in the scapular plane and full internal rotation and thumb down; if there is pain (less specific) and weakness (more specific) when the examiner applies pressure on the forearm of a resisting patient, the test is positive and the patient likely has a rotator cuff impingement due to supraspinatus muscle and/or tendon pathology.
        - Subscapularis lift off: With the patient standing and with the patient's hand behind, resting at the mid-back, the examiner pushes against the patient's hand. The patient tries to raise the dorsum of the hand off the back while maintaining internal rotation of the humerus and extension at the shoulder; inability to perform this maneuver is considered a positive test in subscapularis rupture or dysfunction.
        - Neer's test: With the patient in standing position, the examiner internally rotates and forcefully moves the arm through the full range of motion of forward flexion. Reports of pain are considered a positive test. The test elicits pain by impinging rotator cuff muscles between the greater tuberosity of the head of the humerus and the acromion process.
        - Hawkins test: With the shoulder flexed and the elbow bent 90°, the forearm is used to internally

rotate the shoulder to impinge the subacromial structure as in the Neer's test.

- Shoulder instability[5]
  - Load and shift test: With patient seated and the arm slightly abducted, the examiner stabilizes the scapula in one hand and grasps the humeral head in the other hand, applying anterior and posterior force. Excessive movement (more than 25%) indicates laxity of the capsule.
  - Apprehension test: This test is useful for evaluation of a torn labrum or an anterior instability problem. It is performed with the examiner grasping the patient's wrist with one hand and externally rotating the humerus to place it at 90°. The test is positive if the patient reports pain with pressure applied to the posterior aspect of the humeral head.
  - Jerk test: This test is useful for posterior instability and a torn posterior or posteroinferior labrum. It is performed with the examiner grasping the elbow of the sitting patient and elevating the arm to 90° of adduction and internal rotation. The test is positive if application of an axial compression load to the humerus through the elbow and moving the arm into horizontal adduction cause the patient to report pain.
  - Sulcus sign: This tests the glenohumeral joint capsule and ligamentous structures of the glenohumeral joint, especially the superior glenohumeral ligament and coracohumeral ligament. With the patient sitting, the examiner stabilizes the shoulder girdle and then pulls down with the hand grasping the patient's elbow; the test is positive if there is significant movement of the arm relative to the shoulder and a visible step-off deformity.
- Biceps tendinopathy is tested via the following tests.[5–7]
  - Speed's test is performed with the patient sitting and the arm in 60° of front flexion, with the forearm supinated and the elbow extended fully. The test is positive when resistance from the patient in response to the examiner's forcefully pressing down on the patient's arm at the forearm elicits pain in the bicipital groove.
  - Yergason's test evaluates the integrity of the biceps tendon, glenoid labrum, and transverse humeral ligament. It is performed with patient sitting with elbow at 90° and the forearm in neutral position. The test is positive if palpation at the bicipital groove elicits pain with downward pressure on the patient's forearm while the patient is attempting to move it in further pronation.
- Superior labral anterior posterior (SLAP) lesion evaluation
  - The anterior slide test is useful with pathology of the glenoid labrum and long biceps tendon. It is best performed with the patient in the sitting position and with the hand resting on the hip, with the thumb posteriorly. The test is positive if pain is reproduced over the anterior shoulder when the examiner, stabilizing the shoulder girdle with one hand, applies superior and anterior force along the humerus at the elbow.
  - The O'Brien test evaluates the glenoid labrum and AC joint. For this test, the patient is sitting with the arm in 90° flexion and 10° adduction. The examiner pushes downward distally on the arm while the patient resists with an upward force. The test is positive when the patient reports pain in fully internally rotated movement but not in a neutral one.
  - Crank test evaluates ligaments of the glenohumeral joint. The examiner applies gentle force on the glenohumeral joint while moving the humerus into internal and external rotation. The test is positive if pain is reproduced.[1,2,8]
- AC joint dysfunction
  - Scarf test (cross-arm adduction test) starts with elbow flexion at 90° and 90° of shoulder flexion, with the hand resting on the opposite shoulder. The test is positive if pressure applied to push the arm into further cross adduction elicits pain.[8]

The sensitivity and specificity of these tests vary. In combination, positive tests increase the probability of a correct diagnosis.

A neurologic evaluation is also performed: the examiner assesses sensation along the dermatomes and reflexes (biceps C5, brachioradialis C6, and triceps C7), and applies Spurling's compression (lateral bend with axial load on the head) for cervical spine pathology.

DIAGNOSTIC TESTS IN CHRONIC SHOULDER PAIN

The diagnostic tests should be directed and performed with the goal of not missing crucial pathology; sometimes, subacute or chronic shoulder pain may mask significant conditions, such as cancer, referred cardiac pain, or pulmonary pain.

Plain-film X-ray imaging rules out potential fractures or arthritic changes, tendon or bursal calcifications, and humeral subluxation suggesting rotator cuff injury.

Routine radiographs provide an overview of the anatomic profile; usually anteroposterior views with the arm in internal and external rotation as well as axillary views are obtained. When anterior shoulder dislocation and injury of the anterior (inferior) glenoid labrum is suspected, as is the case in Bankart lesion, special imaging may be indicated. In these cases, a Stryker notch view (palm on top of head and fingers toward the back of head, with the elbow straight up) or a West Point view (axillary view with the patient prone) may be useful in the initial phase of evaluation. Cervical spine and thoracic spine X-rays rule out bony pathology that refers pain to the shoulder.[9]

Other imaging modalities, such as ultrasound, CT, and MRI, also can be useful. CT arthrogram evaluates the capsular attachments of the labrum and assesses for small avulsion fracture of the glenoid rim or humeral head. MRI is useful in detecting soft tissue injury, but it is less specific for bone. Ultrasound can help with dynamic shoulder examination.[10]

TREATMENT OF CHRONIC SHOULDER PAIN

Treatment is directed at the etiology of the pain. In the absence of an organic cause (infection, tumor, fracture), most chronic shoulder pain is managed conservatively. The first step in conservative treatment is PT, NSAIDs, and/or acetaminophen. PT is an essential component of treatment; during initial PT evaluations, the examiner may discover biomechanical deficits and adaptations that inadvertently contribute to the persistence of pain and injury. Upon initiation of PT, the patient progresses through the phases of rehabilitation: range of motion, flexibility, strength, and, ultimately, improvement in function.[11]

Various other therapeutic modalities have been used in the treatment of shoulder injury and pain; among them are moist heat, ultrasound, cryotherapy, and transcutaneous electrical nerve stimulation (TENS). Complementary medicine, such as acupuncture, has shown benefit. However, data are too sparse for definite proof of consistent efficacy of the latter treatment modalities.

Among conservative treatments, Kinesio-Tape occupies a special role. Utilizing this treatment may help pain in shoulder impingement and may re-educate injured shoulder movement patterns, reduce pain, and decrease inflammation.[12]

In addition to conservative treatment, various procedures have been used in pain management for shoulder pain. Corticosteroid injections may prove effective in temporarily relieving pain and allowing improved function through PT sessions. Injections with hyaluronic acid preparations seem to have the same effect.[13]

If pain persists despite conservative and interventional techniques, arthroscopy may offer an advantage, because it can be both diagnostic and in some cases therapeutic. Arthroscopic inspection of the glenohumeral joint and the subacromial space may reveal bony lesions, cartilage defects, capsule and synovial lesions, bursa disorders, and ligament problems that can be effectively treated. However, surgical interventions should be considered carefully only after all conservative regimens have failed.

COMMON CONDITIONS ASSOCIATED WITH CHRONIC SHOULDER PAIN

Shoulder pain is responsible for approximately 16% of all musculoskeletal complaints. An estimated 20% of the population will suffer shoulder pain in their lifetime. In fact, shoulder pain is second only to low back pain in musculoskeletal ailments seen by primary care physicians. In 2000, the direct costs for treatment of shoulder dysfunction in the United States was estimated to have totaled $7 billion.[1,14]

Shoulder pain is chronic when it has been present for more than 6 months, regardless of whether the patient has sought treatment. Shoulder pain can be difficult to treat; only 50% of patients with new shoulder disorder episodes experience complete recovery at 6 months, and the rate increases to only 60% at 1 year.[1,2]

Chronic shoulder pain falls into six primary categories: rotator cuff disorders, glenohumeral osteoarthritis, glenohumeral instability, adhesive capsulitis, AC joint problems, and referred pain.

ROTATOR CUFF DISORDERS

The rotator cuff involves the supraspinatus, infraspinatus, teres minor, and subscapularis muscles. These muscles work together to provide dynamic range and stability in the shoulder's range of motion. Rotator cuff tendinopathy, a common cause of shoulder pain, accounts for almost 30% of shoulder pain. It arises from repetitive strain in the rotator cuff, the predominant dynamic stabilizer of the glenohumeral joint.

Pain from rotator cuff injury is exacerbated by overhead activities and night pain. Physical examination may be positive for the associated muscle fatigue and pain. Imaging is useful for ruling out osseous pathology; it can also show superior migration of the humerus, calcification in the ligaments, or a hooked acromion. MRI may be useful to diagnose and quantify the level of the tear and to evaluate muscle quality, especially if surgery is planned. Of asymptomatic patients more than 60 years old, 55% may have rotator cuff pathology.[4]

Rotator cuff tears can lead to arthropathy after a massive chronic rotator cuff injury, with glenohumeral cartilage destruction, subchondral osteoporosis, and humeral head collapse, usually in patients 70 years old and older. In these patients, external rotation lags and the hornblower's sign is positive. The hornblower's test evaluates teres minor muscle strength. The test is performed with the patient's arm elevated to 90° in the scapular plane. The examiner then flexes the elbow to 90°, and the patient is asked to externally rotate the shoulder. A positive test occurs with weakness and/or pain during this maneuver.

Treatment of the condition begins with conservative management: physical therapy, NSAIDs, and corticosteroid injections. Surgical intervention, such as arthroscopic/open rotator cuff repair or tendon transfer, may be needed. Risk factors for recurrence include age 65 or older, large tear, multiple tendons involved, and concomitant arcromioclavicular or biceps injuries at time of repair.[12]

Calcific tendinopathy is most commonly seen in the supraspinatus muscle tendon, although it may be found in any of the rotator cuff muscle tendons. History is often atraumatic, with patients describing pain most severe at rest, exacerbated by movement, and worse at night. At times, they may also describe a catching or mechanical block, with or without crepitus. Tendinopathy affects women 30 to 60 years old and is often associated with diabetes and hypothyroidism. Provocative testing for impingement will be positive. Deposits of calcium may be seen on X-ray and ultrasound, usually 1 to 1.5 cm from the supraspinatus tendon insertion. Recommended radiographic views to properly identify supraspinatus calcifications include anteroposterior, supraspinatus outlet, and axillary views. An internal rotation view will show infraspinatus and teres minor muscle calcification. An external rotation view will show subscapularis muscle calcification. MRI and CT have limited utility in diagnosis of this condition.[4,10]

Treatment of calcific tendinopathy is physical therapy, steroid injections, extracorporeal shockwave therapy, or ultrasound-guided needle lavage. When these nonoperative methods fail, surgical decompression can be performed to remove the calcium deposit.

GLENOHUMERAL OSTEOARTHRITIS

Like primary osteoarthritis, glenohumeral osteoarthritis has no known cause. It is usually monarticular. External rotation is limited because of contracture of the anterior capsule and subscapularis. Contributing factors in glenohumeral osteoarthritis are trauma, surgery, or chronic rotator cuff pathology.

Glenohumeral osteoarthritis is characterized by pain at night and with any shoulder activities. On physical examination, the anterior shoulder is flattened by muscle atrophy. Range of motion of the shoulder is decreased and the painful arc test (pain with abduction of arm in the scapular plane) is positive between 60° and 120° of abduction (pain decreases after 120° of abduction).

Radiographic images show subchondral sclerosis, osteophytes at the inferior aspect of the humeral head, and superior migration of the humeral head, indicating cuff deficiency. CT is the study of choice for bony evaluation or for preoperative evaluation should nonoperative treatment fail.[8]

GLENOHUMERAL INSTABILITY

Glenohumeral instability may be traumatic structural, atraumatic structural, or habitual nonstructural. Dislocation is usually anterior. Posterior dislocations are uncommon, but may happen after seizures or a motor vehicle accident. Most cases of glenohumeral instability are acute.

Posttraumatic instability may be recurrent, from frequent subluxations despite true relocation. Atraumatic instability may occur from ligamentous laxity, such as that found in Ehlers-Danlos or Marfan syndromes. The Beighton score determines ligamentous laxity in the chronic phase.[5] It consists of a series of five tests, the results of which can add up to a total of nine points. The score is worked out as follows:

1. One point if the patient can place his/her palms on the ground while standing with the legs straight,
2. One point for each elbow that bends backward
3. One point for each knee that bends backward
4. One point for each thumb that touches the forearm when bent

ADHESIVE CAPSULITIS

Adhesive capsulitis is characterized by pain and stiffness with decreased range of motion, especially during external rotation. The cause is not clearly identified in most cases. Adhesive capsulitis is found in 2% to 5% of the population, mostly in those around 40 to 60 years old. It is more common in females and in the nondominant extremity. Studies have shown that in 20% to 30% of those who have unilateral adhesive capsulitis, the condition may develop in the other shoulder. Adhesive capsulitis is associated with diabetes, thyroid disorders, and prolonged immobilization. The purpose of conservative treatment is to optimize function. If conservative measures fail, manipulation under anesthesia and arthroscopic surgical release may be options. The condition has been reported to self-resolve after 24 months, although such claims are not proven.[6,7]

AC JOINT INJURIES

In this condition, pain is associated with overhead activity, adduction (crossed-arm test), and palpation. X-rays may reveal osteoporosis at the distal end of the clavicle, as well as osteophytes.

The Rockwood system classifies AC joint injuries into six types.

In type I, the clavicle is not elevated and the only injury present is mild AC ligament sprain, with coracoclavicular (CC) ligament, joint capsule, deltoid, and trapezius muscle intact.

Type II shows an elevated clavicle but not above the superior border of the acromion; in addition to AC ligament rupture, the CC ligament is sprained and the joint capsule is ruptured, while the deltoid and trapezius are minimally detached.

All three ligamentous structures (AC, CC, and joint capsule) are ruptured in type III, with the deltoid and trapezius muscles detached. This elevates the clavicle above the superior border of the acromion, with a CC distance of less than 25 mm.

In type IV, the clavicle is displaced posteriorly into the trapezius because the AC, CC, and joint capsule are ruptured and the deltoid and trapezius are detached.

Type V has same characteristics as types IV and III, with the addition that the clavicle is markedly elevated, with a CC distance of more than 25 mm.

Type VI is rare; the clavicle is displaced inferiorly behind the coracobrachialis and biceps tendon.

Chronic joint pain may occur from several repeated minor injuries after a type II or type III injury. Treatment is focused on strengthening and mobilizing. A corticosteroid injection may relieve pain. Persistent cases may require distal clavicular resection.[4–6,8]

REFERRED PAIN

Pathologic processes in the cervical and thoracic spine may be accompanied by radiation of pain to the shoulder. Myofascial pain also can be referred to the shoulder. Myofascial pain is treated with myofascial release in physical therapy or with targeted trigger-point injections. Cervical and thoracic spine pathology resulting in shoulder pain requires more focused evaluation.

CONCLUSIONS

- Chronic shoulder pain is defined as persistent pain in the shoulder for more than 6 months, regardless of treatment.
- A variety of manual tests are used to optimally identify pain generators in chronic shoulder pain.
- Imaging is useful for further delineating shoulder pathology.
- Physical therapy is the first-line treatment in conservative management of chronic shoulder pain.
- In addition to physical therapy, other conservative treatments used to preserve function and decrease pain include TENS, a multimodal analgesic regimen, and corticosteroid injection.
- Surgery is reserved for cases refractory to conservative treatment.

REFERENCES

1. Brukner P, Khan K. Shoulder pain. *Clinical Sports Medicine*. 3rd ed. Sydney, Australia: Mcgraw-Hill; 2006:243–288.
2. Beach H, Gordon P. Clinical examination of the shoulder. *N Engl J Med*. 2016;375(11):e24.
3. Ma R. Shoulder impingement syndromes. In: Wyss J, Patel A, eds. *Therapeutic Programs for Musculoskeletal Disorders*. New York, NY: Demos Medical; 2013:39–48.
4. Sambandam SN, Khanna V, Gul A, Mounasamy V. Rotator cuff tears: an evidence based approach. *World J Orthop*. 2015;6(11):902–918.
5. Cadet ER. Evaluation of glenohumeral instability. *Orthop Clin North Am*. 2010;41(3):287–295.
6. Georgiannos D, Markopoulos G, Devetzi E, Bisbinas I. Adhesive capsulitis of the shoulder. Is there consensus regarding the treatment? A comprehensive review. *Open Orthop J*. 2017;28(11):65–76.
7. Le HV, Lee SJ, Nazarian A, Rodriguez EK. Adhesive capsulitis of the shoulder: review of pathophysiology and current clinical treatments. *Shoulder Elbow*. 2017;9(2):75–84.
8. Chillemi C, Franceschini V. Shoulder osteoarthritis. *Arthritis*. 2013;2013:370231.
9. Tuite MJ, Small KM. Imaging evaluation of nonacute shoulder pain. *AJR Am J Roentgenol*. 2017:24;1–9.
10. Bhatnagar A, Bhonsle S, Mehta S. Correlation between MRI and arthroscopy in diagnosis of shoulder pathology. *J Clin Diagn Res*. 2016;10(2):RC18–21.
11. Brand E. Glenohumeral osteoarthritis. In: Wyss J, Patel A, eds. *Therapeutic Programs for Musculoskeletal Disorders*. New York, NY: Demos Medical; 2013:59–66.
12. Page MJ, Green S, McBain B, et al. Manual therapy and exercise for rotator cuff disease. *Cochrane Database Syst Rev*. 2016;(6):CD012224.
13. Wilk KE, Macrina LC. Nonoperative and postoperative rehabilitation for glenohumeral instability. *Clin Sports Med*. 2013;32(4):865–914.
14. Chiaia T, Hannifin JA. Adhesive capsulitis. In: Wyss J, Patel A, eds. *Therapeutic Programs for Musculoskeletal Disorders*. New York, NY: Demos Medical; 2013:75–82.

REVIEW QUESTIONS

1. A 70-year-old construction worker reports right-sided shoulder pain that began over a year ago. His symptoms are worse at night after a full day of activity. He also suffers from stiffness in the morning. Ibuprofen and Tylenol bring him modest pain relief. What would you expect to see on X-ray?

   A. Bankart lesion
   B. Superior migration of humeral head indicating rotator cuff deficiency
   C. Cysts at distal end of clavicle
   D. Disuse osteopenia

2. What is the most common cause of adhesive capsulitis?

   A. Diabetes
   B. Age
   C. Trauma
   D. It is idiopathic.

3. A 45-year-old man has glenohumeral osteoarthritis. Which findings are most consistent with his physical examination?

   A. Increased pain with internal rotation, limited internal rotation and range of motion, and crepitus
   B. Limited range of motion with elevation, abduction, and internal rotation; pain during end range of active motion
   C. Shoulder pain with resisted shoulder movements, without restricted passive ROM
   D. Decreased range of motion, with pain at deltoid insertion

ANSWERS

1. B. In this case, the patient likely suffers unilateral chronic shoulder pain from glenohumeral osteoarthritis. Plain-film radiography of the shoulder may show subchondral sclerosis, osteophytes along the inferior aspect of the humeral head, superior migration of the humeral head indicating cuff deficiency, posterior glenoid wear, and posterior humeral head subluxation. Recommended views are AP, true anteroposterior, and axillary. The other answers are less likely.

2. D. The most common cause of adhesive capsulitis is unknown; therefore, the correct answer is D. Adhesive capsulitis is characterized by pain and stiffness with decreased range of motion, especially during external rotation, and its cause is not clearly known in most cases. Adhesive capsulitis is found in 2% to 5% of the population, mostly in those around 40 to 60 years old. It is more common in females and in the nondominant

extremity. Studies have shown that in 20% to 30% of those who have unilateral adhesive capsulitis, the condition may develop in the other shoulder.[6,7]

3. A. Glenohumeral osteoarthritis typically has increased pain and limited range of motion with internal rotation and is associated with crepitus. Answer B is consistent with subacromial bursitis and C with rotator cuff tear. Answer D describes findings usually seen with adhesive capsulitis.

QUESTIONS AND ANSWERS

This chapter has accompanying questions and answers that are available to subscribers as part of the Oxford eLearning platform. To access the questions, follow the link below, or go to ✓ http://oxfordmedicine.com/painmanagementreview

10.

CHRONIC KNEE PAIN

Randy L. Calisoff and David R. Walega

STEM CASE AND KEY QUESTIONS

A 58-year-old retired firefighter presents with bilateral knee stiffness and moderate-to-severe knee pain that is worsened with activity and weight bearing and is partially relieved by rest and ice packs on the knees. There is no history of recent trauma. Severity of symptoms has steadily progressed over the past 2 years.

WHAT IS YOUR INITIAL CLINICAL IMPRESSION AS YOU PREPARE TO EVALUATE THE PATIENT? WHAT ELEMENTS OF THE PHYSICAL EXAMINATION ARE MOST IMPORTANT TO DIAGNOSE PRIMARY KNEE OSTEOARTHRITIS (OA)?

On physical examination, there is medial joint-line tenderness bilaterally, crepitus with both passive as well as active range of motion (ROM) of the knee joints, and painful, limited knee flexion. There is mild swelling of both anterior patellar regions with associated mild warmth to palpation. Gait is slightly antalgic to the right, and manual muscle testing of the quadriceps is 4+/5 bilaterally. You plan imaging studies to confirm your suspicion of knee pain from primary knee OA. However, patellofemoral pain syndrome (PFPS) may be another possibility.

WHAT DIAGNOSTIC TESTS OR IMAGING STUDIES WILL HELP YOU DIFFERENTIATE OA FROM PFPS OR OTHER CAUSES OF KNEE PAIN? HOW WOULD THESE OPTIONS CHANGE YOUR PAIN MANAGEMENT PLAN?

AP and lateral standing radiographs are a standard diagnostic test to evaluate for OA of the knee joint and for patellofemoral arthritis. In this case, a sunrise radiograph of the knee is performed and shows no signs of PFPS. Similarly, an MRI of the knee does not show any loss of cartilage at the patellofemoral junction, but severe OA of the knee joint is seen, with full-thickness loss of cartilage in several areas of the medial and lateral compartments of the knee. You meet with the patient again and recommend surgical consultation with an orthopedic surgeon to discuss total knee arthroplasty as a treatment option. The patient wants to try all conservative nonsurgical treatments first, because she reports severe anxiety in relation to surgery of any type, and specifically she fears general anesthesia. She tells you she has a niece who suffered hypoxic brain damage following a routine appendectomy.

WHAT TREATMENT OPTIONS WOULD YOU RECOMMEND FOR THE CONSERVATIVE TREATMENT OF THIS PATIENT'S PAIN? WOULD PHYSICAL THERAPY AND KNEE JOINT IMMOBILIZATION BE SUFFICIENT? ARE THERE ANY MEDICATIONS OR INTERVENTIONS THAT YOU CAN OFFER?

The patient undergoes aggressive physical therapy, achieves moderate weight loss, and is prescribed oral nonsteroidal anti-inflammatory drugs (NSAIDs) and intra-articular steroid injections, but her pain is unrelenting. She agrees to knee replacement surgery under regional anesthesia. Upon completion of the surgery, she continues to have pain. The quality is now dull, achy, constant, and nagging and is not controlled despite many analgesic medications and physical therapy sessions. She is becoming more severely depressed and is accusing you of coercing her into have surgery.

WHAT PAIN REGIMEN CAN YOU OFFER THE PATIENT AT THIS POINT? ARE THERE ANY INTERVENTIONS THAT CAN BE ATTEMPTED IN ORDER TO CONTROL THIS PATIENT'S PAIN?

Since multiple medications, including NSAIDs and opioids, have had no mitigating effect on her pain or function, you discuss other procedural interventions to improve her pain level and quality of life. You perform image-guided diagnostic genicular nerve blocks with low-volume bupivacaine 0.5% that provide 90% reduction in pain, along with improved standing and walking tolerance for 6.5 hours. Similarly, repeat diagnostic genicular nerve blocks performed with 2% lidocaine provide 85% relief for 2 hours. A radiofrequency ablation (RFA) is ultimately performed, with profound relief of her knee pain for 10 months; when the knee pain did return, it was mild or moderate in severity, and only sometimes did it affect daily functioning and recreational activities. The patient was extremely satisfied with her treatment outcome and promised to recommend the procedure to her friends.

DISCUSSION

OA: DEFINITIONS, INCIDENCE, AND RISK FACTORS

Chronic knee pain affects 27 million people in the United States and is a leading cause of disability.[1] Seventy percent of the population more than 65 years old will have evidence of knee pain on physical examination combined with radiographic evidence of OA, and 12% will have clinical symptoms of OA.[2,3] The prevalence of chronic knee pain after total knee replacement (TKR) for OA ranges from 10% to 20%.[4]

Primary knee OA is a degenerative disorder that involves synovial inflammation, articular cartilage breakdown, subchondral bony sclerosis, and other hypertrophic changes of joints, as well as increased local concentrations of inflammatory mediators.[5] It is a common cause of knee pain. In total, these effects on the knee joint lead to a deterioration in function, with limitations of work, recreation, or sports activities due to pain and worsening joint mobility. Risk factors for primary knee OA include female sex, obesity, prior meniscal, ligamentous, or traumatic injuries of the knee, and chronic weakness of the quadriceps muscles.

PHYSICAL EXAMINATION AND DIAGNOSTIC STUDIES IN OA

A comprehensive clinical evaluation for knee pain includes joint inspection, palpation, active and passive ROM testing, and assessment of knee ligament integrity and gait. Crepitus with passive ROM, painful knee flexion, and weakness or atrophy of the quadriceps muscles with active contraction may be seen in knee OA. Weight bearing may show a valgus or varus deformity or joint malalignment. Swelling, fluid collections, or joint effusions should be noted.

Joint stiffness, loss of function, joint instability, and moderate to severe joint pain are hallmarks of OA. The American College of Rheumatology diagnostic criteria for primary knee OA include localized knee pain with joint stiffness that is particularly worse on awakening, crepitus on active ROM, and radiographs showing osteophyte formation or joint space narrowing.[6] If there is suspicion for infection based on local swelling, redness, or fluid collections, laboratory evaluation of white blood cell count, sedimentation rate, and C-reactive protein level should be considered; joint aspiration with Gram stain and cultures of synovial fluid should also be performed.

Radiography is the most common diagnostic study to assess for knee OA. Knee joint radiographs are commonly performed in the anteroposterior view with weight bearing. The intercondylar or sunrise view can identify patellofemoral arthritis or osteochondral loose bodies (Figure 10.1). The Kellgren-Lawrence scale is used to grade the severity of radiographic findings (Table 10.1). If subchondral fractures are suspected, MRI of the joint may show evidence of bone marrow edema. Figure 10.2, a T1-weighted image of the left knee, shows bone marrow edema in the medial compartment. MRI is also helpful in identifying meniscal tears and ligament injuries. Triple-phase bone scan is rarely needed but may show enhanced metabolism in regions suspicious for fracture.[7]

Table 10.2 lists the common tests used in the physical examination of an injured knee.

TREATMENT OF PRIMARY KNEE OA

Regardless of symptom severity or functional impairment, treatment goals for symptomatic knee OA include reduction of inflammation and pain, improved joint ROM, improved strength and function of the quadriceps muscles, and identification and correction of modifiable risk factors. Weight loss will decrease the load on the knee. Bracing of the knee joint can address instability. Therapeutic exercise will improve joint ROM. Passive and active physical therapy modalities can decrease local inflammation, improve ROM, and stabilize the knee through strengthening, specifically the quadriceps. Oral anti-inflammatory medications like acetaminophen, NSAIDs, and cyclooxygenase inhibitors can be used to decrease local inflammation and pain, but should be used at the lowest effective dose for the shortest period of time, especially in older patients. Topical creams, lotions, or patches that contain anti-inflammatories, capsaicin, or local anesthetics can be effective in treating pain from knee OA while limiting the risk

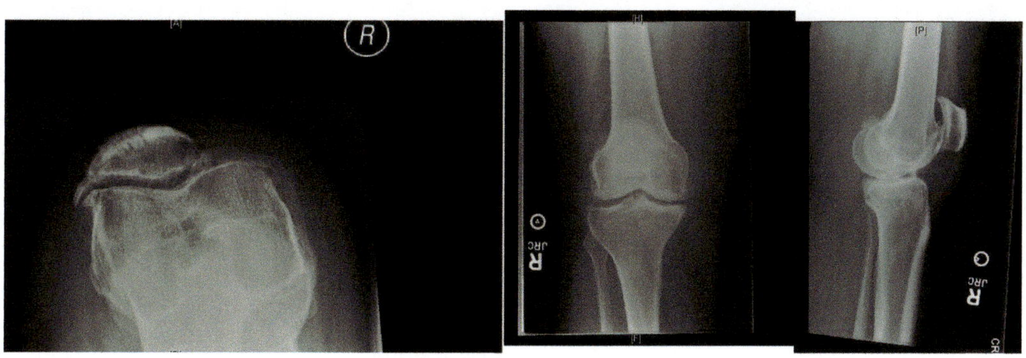

Figure 10.1. Osteochondral loose bodies, sunrise view. Image courtesy of R. Calisoff.

Table 10.1. SEVERITY OF RADIOGRAPHIC FINDINGS IN KNEE OSTEOARTHRITIS

RADIOGRAPHIC GRADE	0	I	II	III	IV
Classification	Normal	Doubtful	Mild	Moderate	Severe
Description	No features of osteoarthritis	Minute osteophytes, doubtful significance	Definite osteophytes, normal joint space	Moderate joint space reduction	Joint space greatly reduced, subchondral sclerosis
		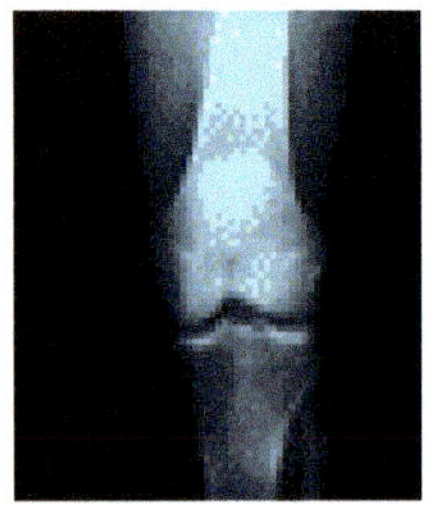	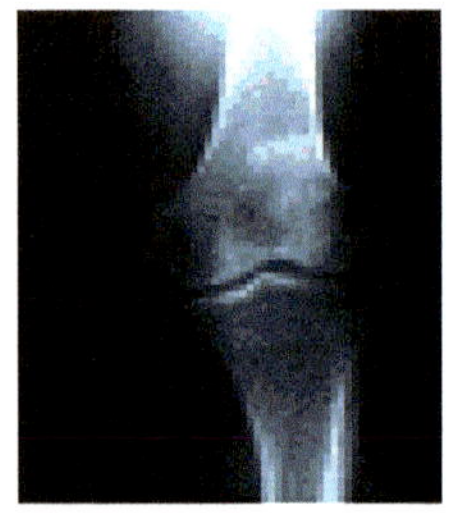	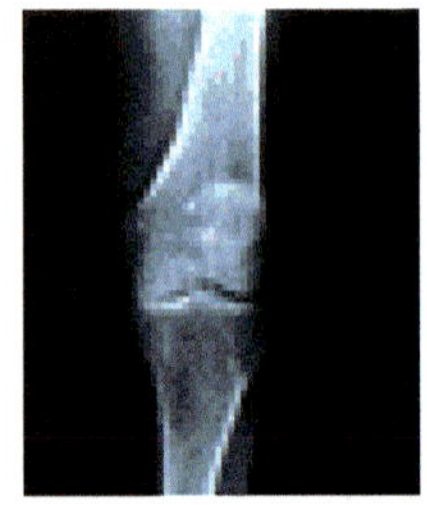	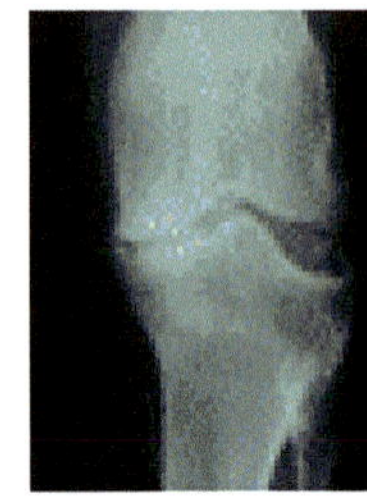

of systemic toxicity. Acupuncture has been used, but its effectiveness is questionable, with negligible effects on knee pain as reported in a large meta-analysis as well as a recent, well-designed randomized controlled trial (RCT).[8,9]

Several treatment modalities that have been reported as effective in reducing pain in OA of the knee are summarized in Table 10.3.

Intra-articular steroid injections and visco-supplementation may provide temporary benefit. Inflammatory mediators are suppressed through corticosteroid-induced blockade of prostaglandin production. Macrophage and leukocyte activity is also suppressed.

The aim of visco-supplementation with intra-articular hyaluronic acid is to restore viscoelasticity of synovial fluid in knees affected by OA and, in theory, to decrease knee pain and stiffness. Visco-supplementation is not indicated for acute knee pain flare-ups nor end-stage severe "bone-on-bone" knee OA. Visco-supplementation is controversial. A recent meta-analysis of 89 clinical trials and over 12,000 patients showed that visco-supplementation was associated with only a small and clinically irrelevant benefit.[10]

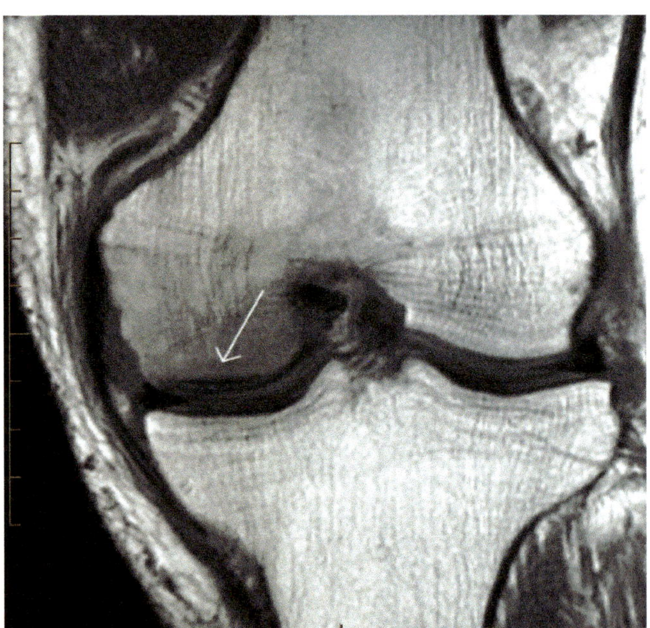

Figure 10.2. T1-weighted image of the left knee, with bone marrow edema (arrow) in the medial compartment. Image courtesy of R. Calisoff.

Regenerative therapies are an emerging treatment of primary knee OA, and aim to regenerate damaged or degenerating tissues, namely chondrocytes and intra-articular cartilage. In one type of regenerative treatment, concentrated autologous platelets (platelet-rich plasma; PRP) or mesenchymal stem cells can be harvested and sterilely injected into the knee joint; resulting local release of growth factors and potent anti-inflammatory cytokines in response to the injection can potentially induce chondrogenesis, effectively decreasing pain. A recent meta-analysis of 10 controlled trials demonstrated the superiority of PRP to placebo and to visco-supplementation in reducing knee pain and improving function, although most studies were biased in favor of PRP.[11] As early data show promise, more research is needed to confirm positive effects of regenerative therapies on knee pain related to OA.

Uncontrolled trials and case reports have shown the potential benefit of intra-articular or extra-articular pulsed radiofrequency treatment for knee pain from OA, but the quality of the data is questionable and the results have been found to be quite variable.[12,13]

Thermal RFA for chronic knee osteoarthritic pain is an emerging treatment for patients who have failed to respond to conservative therapies, who are poor surgical candidates, or who wish to avoid total knee arthroplasty. With thermal RFA, temperatures exceeding 45°C will neurolyze the targeted sensory peripheral nerve (namely, branches of the genicular nerves). Actual lesion size will depend upon RF electrode size, lesioning temperature, lesioning time, and tissue characteristics.[14] The essential sensory anatomy of the knee joint

Table 10.2. TESTS FOR PHYSICAL EXAMINATION OF THE KNEE

Inspection	Visually compare the painful knee with the asymptomatic knee and inspect the injured knee for erythema, swelling, bruising, and discoloration and symmetry of the musculature
Palpation	Check for pain, warmth, point tenderness, joint effusion, or fluid collections
Range of motion	Passive and active extension and flexion of the knee joint
Patellar apprehension test	With fingers placed at the medial aspect of the patella, attempt to subluxate the patella laterally; if this maneuver reproduces the patient's pain or a giving-way sensation, patellar subluxation is the likely cause of the patient's symptoms.
Anterior drawer test	Tests the anterior cruciate ligament. With the patient supine, the affected knee is flexed to 90° with the patient's foot fixed in slight external rotation. Place thumbs at the tibial tubercle and fingers at the posterior calf and pull anteriorly; anterior displacement is a positive sign.
Lachman test	Assesses the anterior cruciate ligament. With the patient supine and the affected knee flexed to 30°, stabilize the distal femur with one hand, grasp the proximal tibia in the other hand, and attempt to sublux the tibia anteriorly; subluxation is a positive Lachman test.
Posterior drawer test	Tests the posterior cruciate ligament. With the patient supine, the affected knee is flexed to 90° with the patient's foot in neutral rotation. Place thumbs at the tibial tubercle and fingers at the posterior calf and push posteriorly; displacement is a positive sign.
Valgus stress test	Assesses medial collateral and posterior cruciate ligaments. With the patient's leg slightly abducted, place one hand at the lateral aspect of the knee joint and the other hand at the medial aspect of the distal tibia. Apply a valgus stress to the knee in full extension (tests the posterior cruciate ligament) and at 30° of flexion (tests the medial collateral ligament).
Varus stress test	Tests lateral collateral ligament. Place one hand at the medial aspect of the knee, and the other hand at the lateral aspect of the distal fibula. Apply varus stress to the knee in full extension and then with knee flexed to 30° (tests collateral ligament).
McMurray test	Assesses meniscal injury. With the patient supine and the knee flexed to 90°, grasp the patient's heel with one hand to hold the tibia in external rotation, with the thumb at the lateral joint line and the fingers at the medial joint line. A positive McMurray test produces a thud or a click, or causes pain in a reproducible portion of the ROM.

Table 10.3. TREATMENT MODALITIES TO DECREASE PAIN AND INCREASE FUNCTION IN OSTEOARTHRITIS OF THE KNEE

TREATMENT	OBJECTIVE
Knee brace	Unload/stabilize knee joint
Cane/assistive device	Improve gait/correct antalgic patterns
Ice packs/cryotherapy	Decrease local inflammation
Heat packs	Analgesia/facilitate joint ROM
Ultrasound therapy	Deep heat penetration
Manual therapy	Improve joint ROM
TENS	Improve pain and knee stiffness
Anti-inflammatories	Decrease local or systemic inflammation and pain
Intra-articular injections	Deliver steroids for anti-inflammatory effect, or hyaluronic acid for visco-supplementation
Regenerative therapies	Enhance tissue healing or promote chondrocyte production of cartilage
Radiofrequency ablation	Block sensory afferents of the anterior knee capsule

was recently confirmed in a cadaveric study, allowing accurate neuroanatomic mapping that ensures safe and consistently successful thermal ablation can be performed.[15] The superior lateral, superior medial, and inferior medial genicular nerves, sometimes called the retinacular nerves, provide afferent pain signaling of the anterior joint capsule and have no motor component. A suprapatellar branch has also been identified but is not routinely ablated in all patients. Diagnostic blockade of these nerves with low-volume local anesthetic may predict treatment outcomes with RF ablation.

In a prospective, open-label trial, 35 patients with moderate or severe knee OA who underwent image-guided RFA of the genicular nerves had significantly decreased pain scores at 12 weeks as compared with the control group. In patients who underwent RFA, 44% reported excellent or good treatment results.[16] In a sham-controlled RCT of genicular nerve RFA, patients in the treatment group experienced, on average, a 50% reduction in pain scores at 12-week follow-up, as compared to the sham-control group.[17] Cooled RFA of the genicular nerves allows a larger lesion size and increases the likelihood of effective, complete neurolysis of the sensory target, and subsequently, predictably better clinical results.[14,18] Case series and case reports of cooled RF techniques show improved pain scores and function in patients with chronic knee pain from OA and patients with chronic knee pain following TKR, but larger, controlled trials are needed to show superior efficacy over conservative medical management. Figure 10.3 shows AP and lateral images of the knee with proper placement of RF introducer needles at the sites of the superomedial, superolateral, and inferomedial genicular nerves.

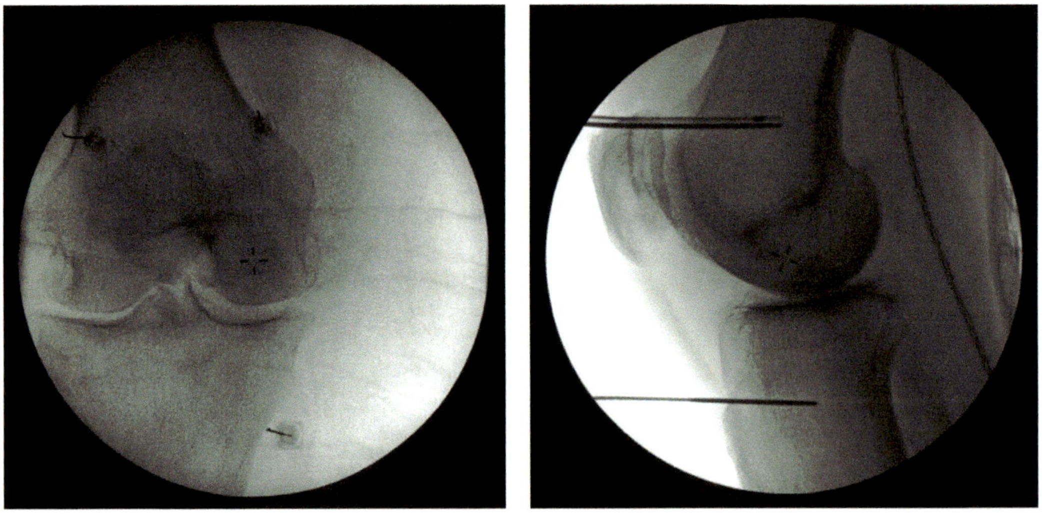

Figure 10.3. Placement of the radiofrequency ablation probes in a patient with osteoarthritic pain of the knee, lateral and PA fluoroscopic views. Image courtesy of D. Walega.

CHRONIC PAIN AFTER TOTAL KNEE ARTHROPLASTY: DEFINITION, INCIDENCE, RISK FACTORS, SIGNS, AND SYMPTOMS

The United States surpasses other developed countries on a per capita basis, with more than 600,000 TKR surgeries performed per year.[19] The rate of chronic knee pain following TKR surgery is 7% to 53% [4,20,21] and it often occurs in the absence of clinical or radiographic abnormalities. Symptoms resembling complex regional pain syndrome (CRPS) were seen in 13% of one prospective cohort of patients 6 months after TKR.[22] In another study, the presence of chronic pain was reported 3 to 4 years after surgery. Fifteen percent of TKR patients reported severe knee pain, and 7% of patients described pain as more severe than prior to surgery.[23] Risk factors for chronic knee pain following TKR include long duration of pain prior to surgery, high pain scores prior to surgery, severe pain during the first week following surgery, anxiety, depression and female sex; age appears to be inversely related to the incidence of chronic knee pain after TKR; laterality or bilaterality of surgery had no effect.[21,24]

Patients with chronic pain after TKR report worsened pain during walking, using stairs, or other weight-bearing activities. Pain was also reported to interrupt sleep. "Achiness," "tiredness," and "tenderness" in the region of the affected knee are the most common descriptors. Obvious causes of chronic knee pain following TKR include infection, hardware loosening, fracture, ligamentous laxity, or muscle atrophy, and all are required to be evaluated with a comprehensive clinical evaluation as causes of persistent postsurgical pain.

TREATMENT OF CHRONIC KNEE PAIN AFTER TOTAL KNEE ARTHROPLASTY

Physical therapy, with emphasis on knee ROM exercises and strengthening of the quadriceps and hamstring musculature, including the gastro-soleus complex, is encouraged. Modalities like ultrasound and heat should be avoided because they can cause component breakdown. Ice may be used after exercise in order to reduce swelling or edema of the knee. In addition, closed kinetic chain exercises like leg presses help reduce shear forces on the affected postsurgical knee. Maintenance and independent demonstration of a home exercise program will also help ensure optimal outcomes.

Topical analgesics may be helpful and include capsaicin, diclofenac, and lidocaine. Oral NSAIDs may also be used. Mu-agonist agents like tramadol and conventional opiates should be used as a last resort when other medications and therapies have failed. Patients should be assessed for risk factors for medication misuse and abuse and should be counseled on dependence, tolerance, and risk of addiction. Cognitive-behavioral therapy, enhancement of coping skills, and an emphasis on maintaining or restoring function are all tenets of treating a chronic pain syndrome.

PFPS

PFPS is a common cause of localized anterior knee pain, and is seen more frequently in women.[25,26] Overuse, overtraining, and overloading the patellofemoral joint are common causes. Leg-length discrepancy, abnormal foot anatomy, hamstring tightness, hip flexor tightness, angular and rotational deformities of the lower limbs, muscle weakness, and muscle imbalance may also be contributors.[27] Knee pain presents insidiously. Typically, symptoms worsen with using stairs, squatting, and prolonged sitting. Inappropriate patellar tracking or patellar misalignment (patella alta, patella baja) within the femoral trochlea may be seen on exam. Radiographic imaging is usually of limited diagnostic value because the condition is considered a clinical diagnosis. The sunrise radiograph can identify lateral or medial displacement of the patella (Figure 10.1 and Figure 10.4). In some cases, MRI can be useful to detect other problems associated with the patella, such as chondromalacia of the patella, articular

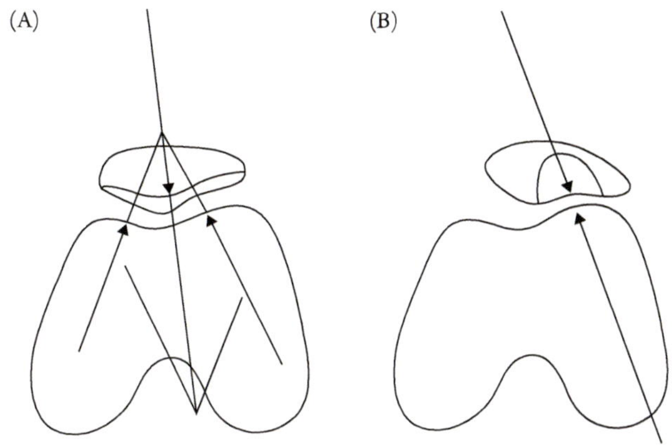

Figure 10.4. A sunrise view diagram of the knee showing the distribution of normal compressive forces (A) and abnormal compressive forces (B) on the knee, resulting in abnormal patellar tracking seen in patellofemoral pain syndrome. Figure 1 shows a radiograph of this finding. Image courtesy of Randy Calisoff.

cartilage injuries, osteochondritis dessicans, or injuries to the patellar retinaculum. Figure 10.5 shows cartilage loss in the patellofemoral joint.

PES ANSERINE SYNDROME (ANSERINE BURSITIS)

The anserine bursa is located at the distal medial aspect of the knee, below the medial joint line and deep to the intersection of the semitendinosus, gracilis, and sartorius tendons. This bursa acts to reduce the friction of these three tendons along the tibia. Due to its location and function, inflammation and pain can develop in runners, athletes, and patients with OA. The condition is associated with diabetes mellitus, rheumatoid arthritis, obesity, and direct trauma.[28–31] Pain in the proximal medial tibial region with palpation is present on exam but local swelling or induration is rarely seen. Saphenous nerve entrapment with tibial

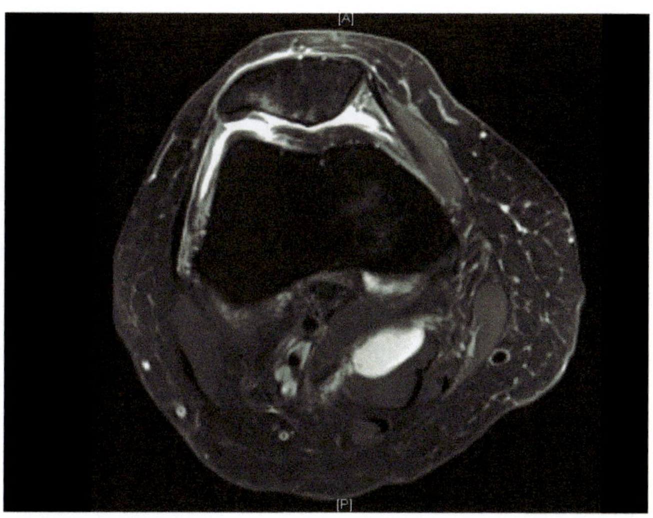

Figure 10.5. Full-thickness cartilage loss in the patellofemoral joint on T2-weighted MRI of the knee. Image courtesy of D. Walega.

pain and paresthesias has been reported. Neither ultrasonography nor MRI is helpful in confirming the diagnosis of pes anserine syndrome. Treatment may include ice, NSAIDs, or local steroid injection. Surgical bursectomy is reserved for severe chronic cases.[32]

CONCLUSIONS

- Primary knee OA is a common source of chronic knee pain.
- Primary knee OA is a common problem in the United States and risk factors for this condition include obesity, prior knee trauma, female sex, and weak quadriceps musculature.
- Evaluation of the knee should include a comprehensive history, physical examination with specific attention to the knee joint, and radiographs. MRI is typically not needed in primary knee OA but may be helpful in diagnosis of ligamentous or soft tissue abnormalities.
- Treatment may range from anti-inflammatories to intra-articular injections of steroid or other therapeutic substances. Knee replacement may eventually be required to restore function. PFPS refers to anterior knee pain that is generally exacerbated with knee joint loading activities, such as squatting, kneeling, prolonged sitting, and ascending/descending stairs. PFPS is a clinical diagnosis, and treatment should be directed toward pain alleviation and restoration of proper biomechanics. Treatment should address muscle weakness or imbalances in the quadriceps, hip abductors, and external rotators.
- Pes anserine syndrome is commonly found in runners, athletes, and individuals with OA of the knee. Female sex and a history of diabetes mellitus, obesity, and arthritis are also risk factors. The clinical presentation usually includes pain along the proximal medial tibia, with exacerbations when ascending and/or descending stairs, rising from a seat, and during the night or early morning.

REFERENCES

1. Garstang S, Stitik T. Osteoarthritis: epidemiology, risk factors, and pathophysiology. *Am J Phys Med Rehabil.* 2006;85(11):S2–S11.
2. Wrightson JD, Malanga GA. Strengthening and other therapeutic exercises in the treatment of osteoarthritis. *Phys Med Rehabil.* 2001;15(1):43–56.
3. Stitik T, Kim JH, Stiskal D, et al. Osteoarthritis. In: Delisa J, Frontera W, eds. *DeLisa's Physical Medicine and Rehabilitation: Principles and Practice.* 5th ed. Philadelphia, PA: Lippincott Williams & Wilkins; 2010:781–810.
4. Lewis GN, Rice DA, McNair PJ, Kluger M. Predictors of persistent pain after total knee arthroplasty: a systematic review and meta-analysis. *Br J Anaesth.* 2014;114(4):551–561.
5. Stitik TP, Kaplan RJ, Kamen L, et al. Rehabilitation of orthopedic and rheumatologic disorders. 2. Osteoarthritis assessment, treatment and rehabilitation. *Arch Phys Med Rehabil.* 2005;86(3)(suppl 1):S48–S55.

6. Sarwark MD. Arthritis of the knee. In: Sarwark JF, ed. *Essentials of Musculoskeletal Care*. 4th ed. Rosemont, IL: American Academy of Orthopedic Surgeons; 2010:650–656.
7. Kraus VB. Pathogenesis and treatment of osteoarthritis. *Med Clin North Am*. 1997;81(1):85–112.
8. Vickers AJ, Cronin AM, Maschino AC, et al. Acupuncture for chronic pain: individual patient data meta-analysis. *Arch Intern Med*. 2012;172(19):1444–1453.
9. Hinman RS, McCrory P, Pirotta M, et al. Acupuncture for chronic knee pain: a randomized clinical trial. *JAMA*. 2014;312(13):1313–1322.
10. Rutjes AW, Juni J, da Costa BR, Trelle S, Nuesch E, Reichenbach S. Viscosupplementation for osteoarthritis of the knee: a systematic review and meta-analysis. *Ann Intern Med*. 2012;157(3):180–191.
11. Laudy AB, Bakker EW, Rekers M, Moen MH. Efficacy of platelet-rich plasma injections in osteoarthritis of the knee: a systematic review and meta-analysis. *Br J Sports Med*. 2015;49(10):657–672.
12. Masala S, Fiori R, Raguso M, Morini M, Calabria E, Simonetti G. Pulse-dose radiofrequency for knee osteoarthritis. *Cardiovasc Intervent Radiol*. 2014;37(2):482–487.
13. Vas L, Pai R, Khandagale N, Pattnaik M. Pulsed radiofrequency of the composite nerve supply to the knee joint as a new technique for relieving osteoarthritic pain: a preliminary report. *Pain Physician*. 2014;17(6):493–506.
14. Cosman ER, Dolensky JR, Hoffman RA. Factors that affect radiofrequency heat lesion size. *Pain Med*. 2014;15(12):2020–2036.
15. Franco CD, Buvanendran A, Petersohn JD, Menzies R, Menzies LP. Innervation of the anterior capsule of the human knee: implications for radiofrequency ablation. *Reg Anesth Pain Med*. 2015;40(4):363–368.
16. Ikeuchi M, Ushida T, Izumi M, Tani T. Percutaneous radiofrequency treatment for refractory anteromedial pain of osteoarthritic knees. *Pain Med*. 2011;12(4):546–551.
17. Choi WJ, Hwang SJ, Song JG, et al. Radiofrequency treatment relieves chronic knee osteoarthritis pain: a double-blind randomized controlled trial. *Pain*. 2011;152(3):481–487.
18. Vallejo R, Benyamin R, Tilley DM, Kelley CA, Cedeno DL. An ex vivo comparison of cooled-radiofrequency and bipolar-radiofrequency lesion size and the effect of injected fluids. *Reg Anesth Pain Med*. 2014;39(4):312–321.
19. Kurtz SM, Ong KL, Lau E, Bozic KJ. Impact of the economic downturn on total joint replacement demand in the United States: updated projections to 2021. *J Bone Joint Surg Am*. 2014;96(8):624–630.
20. Liu SS, Buvanendran A, Rathmell JP, Sawhney M, Manion SC, Sculco TP. A cross-sectional survey on prevalence and risk factors for persistent postsurgical pain 1 year after total hip and knee replacement. *Reg Anesth Pain Med*. 2012;37(4):415–422.
21. Brander V, Gondek S, Martin E, Stulberg D. Pain and depression influence outcome 5 years after knee replacement surgery. *Clin Orthop Relat Res*. 2007;464:21–26.
22. Harden RN, Oaklander AL, Burton AW, et al. Complex regional pain syndrome: practical diagnostic and treatment guidelines, 4th edition. *Pain Med*. 2013;14(2):180–229.
23. Wylde V, Hewlett S, Learmonth ID, Dieppe P. Persistent pain after joint replacement: prevalence, sensory qualities, and postoperative determinants. *Pain*. 2011;152(3):566–572.
24. Puolakka PA, Rorarius MG, Roviola M, Puolakka TJ, Nordhausen K, Lindgren L. Persistent pain following knee arthroplasty. *Eur J Anaesthesiol*. 2010;27(5):455–460.
25. Bolgla L, Malone T, Umberger B, et al. Hip strength and hip and knee kinematics during stair descent in females with and without patellofemoral pain syndrome. *J Orthop Sports Phys Ther*. 2008;38(1):12–18.
26. Malanga GA, Andrus S, Nadler SF, et al. Physical examination of the knee: a review of the original test description and scientific validity of common orthopedic tests. *Arch Phys Med Rehabil*. 2003;84:592–603.
27. Post W. Clinical evaluation of patients with patellofemoral disorders. *Arthroscopy*. 1999;15(9):841–851.
28. Helfenstein M Jr, Kuromoto J. Anserine syndrome. *Rev Bras Reumatol*. 2010;50(3):313–327.
29. Cohen SE, Mahul O, Meir R, Rubinow A. Anserine bursitis and non-insulin dependent diabetes mellitus. *J Rheumatol*. 1997;24:2162.
30. Hemler DE, Ward WK, Karstetter KW, Bryant PM. Saphenous nerve entrapment caused by pes anserine bursitis stress fracture of the tibia. *Arch Phys Med Rehabil*. 1991;72(5):336–337.
31. Pompan DC. Pes anserine bursitis: an underdiagnosed cause of knee pain in overweight women. *Am Fam Physician*. 2016;93(3):170.
32. Ike RW. Chemical ablation as an alternative to surgery for treatment of persistent prepatellar bursitis. *J Rheumatol*. 2009;36:1560.

REVIEW QUESTIONS

1. Which of the following is an accurate description of knee OA?

   A. Synovial fluid collections are not involved.
   B. Articular cartilage is progressively thinned.
   C. Hypotrophic changes in the joint margins are often seen.
   D. Systemic inflammatory mediators are increased in the plasma of patients with knee OA.

2. Which of the following is not a risk factor for developing OA in the knee joint?

   A. Female sex
   B. Obesity
   C. Prior meniscal or ligamentous injury of the knee
   D. Overtraining the quadriceps muscles

3. Which of the following is not one of the criteria used by the American College of Rheumatology in diagnosing OA of the knee?

   A. Morning stiffness less than 30 minutes
   B. Age greater than 50
   C. Crepitus of the knee on active ROM
   D. Radiographs showing subchondral sclerosis

ANSWERS

1. B. Answer A is incorrect because synovial fluid collections may be present in joints that are acutely inflamed. Synovitis and inflammatory markers can also be seen in systemic arthritides like rheumatoid arthritis; therefore, answer D is incorrect. Answer C is incorrect because in OA, a hallmark feature is hypertrophy of joint margins and endplate sclerosis in more severe cases.

2. D. OA is more common in females and the obese, and it appears to be directly related to prior knee trauma and repetitive use injuries, highly physical vocations, and weakness or atrophy of the quadriceps muscles. Strengthening the quadriceps muscles can be protective.

3. D. According to the American College of Rheumatology criteria, in order to make the diagnosis of OA of the knee, X-rays need to show osteophytes only, not subchondral sclerosis. The rest of the answer choices are correct in terms of the criteria used by the American College of Rheumatology in the diagnosis of knee OA.

QUESTIONS AND ANSWERS

This chapter has accompanying questions and answers that are available to subscribers as part of the Oxford eLearning platform. To access the questions, follow the link below, or go to ✔ http://oxfordmedicine.com/painmanagementreview

11.

COMPLEX REGIONAL PAIN SYNDROME OF THE UPPER AND LOWER EXTREMITY

Agnes Stogicza, Bartha Peter Tohotom, Edit Racz, Andrea Trescot, and Alan Berkman

STEM CASE AND KEY QUESTIONS

A 26-year-old, otherwise healthy, high-functioning female was injured when a male business partner shook her hand too hard. Her hand immediately began to hurt, swelled, and turned red, but she thought it would heal in a couple days. A week after the injury, because there was no improvement in the symptoms, she was instructed to wear a brace at night. Symptoms did not improve, and the patient woke up with pain every night for several months.

WHAT IS COMPLEX REGIONAL PAIN SYNDROME (CRPS) AND WHAT ARE THE EARLY SIGNS?

Several months later, her hand was still swollen, sensitive, and red. By that time, she couldn't use her fingers at all because of the severe pain. An X-ray was taken and ruled out a fracture. It showed bone loss of the fifth metacarpal. Rheumatoid arthritis (RA) was suspected, but it was not confirmed by any blood test. The patient was started on anti-inflammatory pain medications (diclofenac sodium) for pain, swelling, and allodynia, with minimal benefit. Meanwhile, the patient tried acupuncture, with no relief.

WHAT DIAGNOSTIC TESTS ARE AVAILABLE FOR CRPS?

A repeat X-ray was ordered to compare the two hands (to see if the problem was isolated to the right hand or if there was a systemic problem), and more blood work, a bone scan, and a CT scan were performed. At that point, a bone tumor was found at the base of the third metacarpal (Figure 11.1)—but not where the pain was located. The bone scan showed increased activity in the third and fifth metacarpals of the affected hand.

WHAT IS THE ETIOLOGY OF CRPS?

The patient's unusual pain was still not understood, but the oncologist recommended radiofrequency ablation (RFA) of her tumor. However, after careful physical exam by a pain physician, the patient was diagnosed with CRPS, since most of her pain was at the fifth finger, not at the third, where the tumor was located. As CRPS is often aggravated by local intervention/surgery, a decision was made to postpone surgery until the CRPS was under better control.

WHAT ARE THE TREATMENT OPTIONS FOR CRPS?

The patient was prescribed alendronate for the bone loss, after which the X-ray showed improvement in the osteopenia, but she had no significant improvement in her symptoms. She also participated in a multidisciplinary treatment program to help minimize the symptoms of CRPS. She underwent several stellate ganglion blocks (SGBs) and local steroid infiltration in her hand, physiotherapy, and occupational therapy (OT). After several months in treatment, she had good return of function in her fingers, and the swelling and pain decreased. She was also prescribed sleep medication, as by then she had barely had any uninterrupted sleep in 2 years because of pain.

WHAT ARE THE ROLES OF, AND THE EVIDENCE FOR, PHYSICAL THERAPY (PT), PSYCHOTHERAPY, MEDICATION, AND INTERVENTIONS?

The patient was still in an unmanageable amount pain; she tried a TENS unit, with minimal benefit. Three years after the initial diagnosis of the tumor in the third metacarpal bone, it showed some growth, so a decision was made to perform surgery. The patient underwent removal of the third metacarpal with bone grafting and plate placement under regional anesthesia (a supraclavicular brachial plexus block). Her CRPS pain dropped by 50% within 24 hours of surgery, and the patient left the hospital without needing any prescription opioids to manage postoperative pain. She still complained of her original pain, but it was reduced.

WHAT INTERVENTIONAL TECHNIQUES ARE AVAILABLE FOR THE TREATMENT OF CRPS?

The patient later returned for a diagnostic thoracic sympathetic block, which resulted in increased temperature of the affected hand. Preprocedure temperatures were 27°C at the

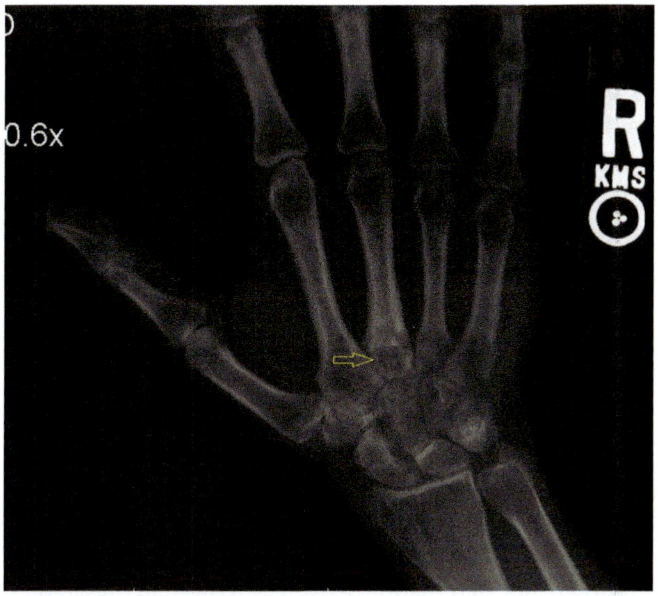

Figure 11.1. X-ray of the hand shows a tumor (arrow) at the base of the third metacarpal bone. Image courtesy of Agnes Stogicza, MD.

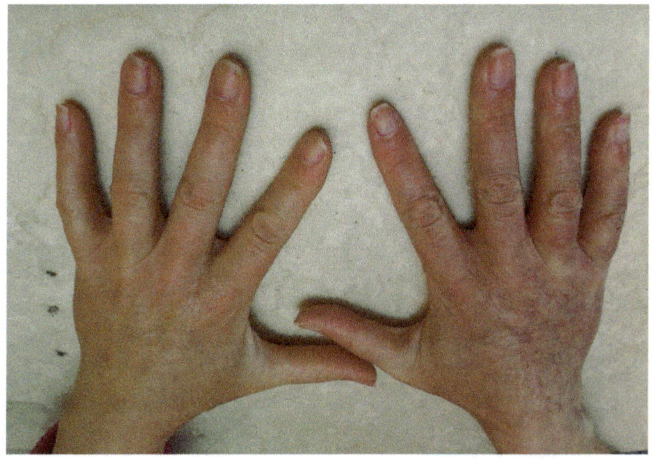

Figure 11.2. Same patient as in Figure 1. Eleven years after the initial hand injury and 2 years after the second radiofrequency ablation, complex regional pain syndrome (CRPS) appears 90% resolved. Right hand is still slightly purplish (Harlequin syndrome). Image courtesy of Agnes Stogicza, MD.

dorsum of the right hand and 34°C on the left hand. The sympathetic block resulted in a 9°C increase in temperature on the right hand, which reached 35°C, while the left hand maintained the same 34°C temperature after the procedure. The procedure also resulted in the complete resolution of her pain. Two weeks after the diagnostic injection, the pain returned, and the patient therefore underwent a therapeutic RFA of the T2-T3 sympathetic ganglia, with almost complete, sustained pain relief and temperature improvement of the hand, along with harlequin syndrome (asymmetric sweating and flushing on the upper thoracic region and face). Two years postprocedure, the patient returned for a repeat RFA, as she noticed an increase in pain and diminished warmth of her hand. Currently, 2 years after the second RFA, the patient takes only occasional acetaminophen, and she uses both hands with full function (Figure 11.2).

DISCUSSION

CRPS is a regional chronic pain syndrome. (It was first called *causalgia* during the Civil War by Silas Weir Mitchell, a US Army physician, and then later it was termed *reflex sympathetic dystrophy*.) CRPS is characterized by vasomotor, sudomotor, and trophic changes, together with pain, allodynia, and hyperalgesia, after the noxious stimulation of a body area. CRPS can affect the limbs, face, and pelvis, or it can spread throughout the whole body.[1,2] In this chapter, the upper and lower extremities are discussed together, because the etiology, pathogenesis, clinical symptoms, diagnosis, and medication management of CRPS are the same in both. However, the specific interventional treatments obviously differ; they are discussed separately in the chapter.

While the exact cause of the disease is still unknown, the role of the central and autonomic nervous system is well documented. Precipitating factors include injury or surgery of the affected body part, or distant insults, such as stroke or myocardial infarction, although there are some cases without any well-established reasons or risk factors. Just like most of the chronic pain syndromes, it has a deleterious effect on the patient's life, causing disability and serious psychosocial problems. Treatment is multidisciplinary, including physiotherapy, psychotherapy, medications, and minimally invasive pain management therapies.

TAXONOMY

During the Orlando conference of 1994, the term *complex regional pain syndrome* was introduced and accepted by the International Association for the Study of Pain (IASP) in order to end the confusion about the different names used for this condition in different countries and by medical schools.[3–5] According to the latest definition, CRPS is a syndrome characterized by a continuing (spontaneous and/or evoked) regional pain that is seemingly disproportionate in time or degree to the usual course of pain after trauma or other lesion. The pain is regional (not in a specific nerve territory or dermatome) and usually has a distal predominance of abnormal sensory, motor, sudomotor, vasomotor/edema, and/or trophic findings. The syndrome shows variable progression over time.

CRPS-I, by definition, occurs after any form of trauma, particularly a fracture or soft tissue lesion. The disease is not limited to the distribution of a single peripheral nerve, and there is no definable nerve injury. However, many experts consider persistent CRPS-I to be a posttraumatic neuralgia associated with distal degeneration of small-diameter peripheral axons. These small-fiber lesions are easily missed on examination and are also undetected by electrophysiologic testing, such as electromyography (EMG) and nerve conduction velocity (NCV).[6] CRPS-I was formerly known as reflex sympathetic dystrophy, algodystrophy, Sudeck's atrophy, and shoulder-hand syndrome. CRPS-II, formerly known as causalgia,[3,4] refers to those cases where a definable nerve lesion is present.

EPIDEMIOLOGY AND PROGNOSIS

The incidence of CRPS-I, as demonstrated by two large retrospective trials, is between 5.5 and 26 new cases per 100,000 persons, depending on the study population and the diagnostic criteria used.[7] Women are about three times more likely to be affected than men, with the highest incidence rate observed in the group of patients 61 to 70 years old. The most common precipitating factor is a bone fracture, accounting for about 44% of all the cases, with the upper limbs more often affected.[7,8] Other risk factors include surgery, strain, crush injury, brain injury, or even myocardial infarction.[5,9] The reported incidence of CRPS-II is much lower, at about 0.8 per 100,000 persons. CRPS-II develops in approximately 1% to 5% of all peripheral nerve injuries.[8,10] Two percent of CRPS cases are relapsing-remitting, with deleterious effect on quality of life and occupation.[11] Six years after disease onset, 30% of patients are recovered, 54% are considered to have stable disease, and 15% experience no improvement. As many as 30% of CRPS patients remain unable to work 6 years after onset, some even after spinal cord stimulation (SCS) therapy.[12]

ETIOLOGY AND PATHOGENESIS

The biologic routes that lead to the development of CRPS, just like the diagnostic measures, have been the subject of debate for a long time. Despite the efforts and investigations made on the topic in the last four decades, the exact pathogenesis of CRPS is still unknown. There are apparently three major pathogenic pathways that are responsible for the initiation and maintenance of CRPS. Treatments that target only one of the pathways can attenuate or decrease symptoms, but such limited treatments work in only a portion of patients or result in a partial resolution, showing that the role of individual pathogenic pathways varies from patient to patient, or may change even in the same patient over time. The different disease pathways and interindividual differences account for the clinical heterogeneity of the disorder, making diagnosis and treatment challenging.

The major pathophysiologic routes are:

1. Aberrant inflammatory mechanisms: Since the classic early signs of CRPS are similar to those seen in inflammation ("dolor, rubor, calor, tumor, functio laesa"), the hypothesis that inflammation plays a role in developing CRPS seems to be supported. Although the inflammation has been proven to be localized, without systemic signs or elevation of classic inflammatory markers, such as leukocyte count, C-reactive protein, or erythrocyte sedimentation rate, the local increases in pro-inflammatory cytokine levels (such as TNF-alpha or bradykinin) seen in CRPS patients seem to confirm this theory. While classic inflammatory processes can be triggered simply by trauma of the affected limb, newer studies show the important role of a so-called neurogenic inflammation.[13,14] This process is driven by neuropeptides, such as calcitonin gene-related peptide (CGRP) and substance P (SP), that are released from C-fiber terminals after nociceptor activation. CGRP and SP are likely to evoke vasodilation and plasma extravasation, creating the classic signs of inflammation. Furthermore, they can trigger local inflammation via the formation of bradykinins. The activation of cutaneous nociceptors can induce retrograde depolarization of small-diameter fibers (axon reflex), causing the release of more CGRP and SP, which is responsible for the stocking/glove, rather than segmental, extension of CRPS. What triggers this system or why it is upregulated in CRPS is still not known, but two theories exist. Coderre et al. initiated CRPS-like symptoms in an animal model after a 3-hour tourniquet ischemia, suggesting that neurogenic inflammation is triggered by hypoxia, acidosis, and free-radical formation.[15] Albrecht et al. showed decreased C-fibers and A-delta fibers in the areas affected by CRPS.[16] An animal model showed the same reduction in nociceptor neuron density after an 18-G needle injury, suggesting that even in CRPS-I, unrecognized nerve injuries could be the initiating factors of the disease.[17] Also, autoimmune markers against alpha-adrenergic and acetylcholine receptors were detected, but the significance of this finding is unclear without any evidence of generalized autonomic failure.[12,18,19]
2. Vasomotor dysfunction: Vasomotor instability is well documented in CRPS patients. In the early "warm," or sometimes called "acute," stage or type of the disease, vasodilatation with an attenuated response to indirect sympathetic stimulation (cold challenge) is present. It is notable that not all CRPS patients pass through this stage of the disease. Measurement of venous norepinephrine concentrations shows decreased levels in the affected limb compared to the nonaffected side or compared to healthy individuals, which could explain the hyperdynamic circulation of the affected extremities. The cause of this diminished sympathetic nervous system (SNS) outflow is not yet known. The role of vasomotor dysfunction in the "cold" type of CRPS seems to be more difficult to explain and is debatable. While the response to indirect sympathetic activation is augmented, and blocking of the sympathetic fibers of the hypodynamically circulated limb improve the symptoms, including pain, in a proportion of patients, the measured levels of venous serum norepinephrine concentration are still low compared to healthy individuals. One

explanation for this is that the density of alpha-adrenergic receptors in the skin of the painful areas is enlarged, which could be a compensatory mechanism for decreased SNS outflow, resulting in hyperreactivity to circulating catecholamines. It should also be mentioned that, besides elevated sensitivity to sympathetic outflow, decreased nitric oxide (NO) production and elevated endothelin levels were detected, probably on the basis of hypoxic endothelial damage, contributing to the vasoconstriction and the hypodynamic circulation of the limb.[12,18,19]

3. Maladaptive neuroplasticity: The term *maladaptive neuroplasticity* refers to the structural and functional changes of the peripheral and central nervous system leading to persistent pain, motor impairments, and higher-order cognitive disorders. Peripheral sensitization and its role in maintaining pain are well documented in chronic pain disorders. Bradykinin, SP, and CGRP release or changes in the nociceptor intracellular signaling system (called hyperalgesic priming) lead to the decreased stimulation threshold and hyperalgesia. The importance of these neuroplastic changes is assumed, although not yet well examined, in CRPS patients. On the same basis, central sensitization plays an important role in maintaining pain among these patients. Continuous firing of nociceptors leads to the upregulation and activation of *N*-methyl-D-aspartate (NMDA) receptors in spinal neurons, causing a decreased stimulation threshold, or even firing of the neurons without peripheral input, which enhances signal transmission in the nociceptive circuitry from the spinal cord to the cerebral cortex. While the above-mentioned changes in the nervous system are not disease specific and are supposed to be found in any chronic pain syndrome, there are some changes that are characteristic for CRPS. In the periphery, for an unknown reason, nociceptive afferent fibers start to express alpha-adrenergic receptors, which lead to sympatho-afferent coupling and the theory of sympathetically maintained pain (SMP). These phenomena are confirmed by indirect sympathetic activation (cold test) or when direct norepinephrine injections to the affected area cause pain, while the pain can be attenuated by sympathetic blockade in some CRPS patients. Disease-specific central changes include dysfunction of GABA-ergic spinal inhibitory pathways, reorganization of motor cortex of the brain with decreased inhibitory mechanism, and increased excitability, leading to tremor and dystonia. Functional imaging of the central nervous system shows a reduction in the area of the S1 primary somatosensory cortex corresponding to the affected limb, which could explain the tactile dysfunction and the spatial neglect experienced in CRPS.

In short, none of the above-mentioned pathophysiologic pathways was confirmed to be the sole initiating or maintaining factor in CRPS, but most of them were proven to be effective as therapeutic targets.[12,18,19]

CLINICAL MANIFESTATIONS OF CRPS

The disease typically manifests within 2 weeks to 1 month after a noxious stimulus, with pain in the affected area as the leading sign. It is a neuropathic-type pain, with allodynia and hyperalgesia. By definition, the pain is out of proportion to the degree or localization of the initiating injury. The sensations include burning, stabbing, grinding, and throbbing. Moving or touching the limb is usually intolerable, but in some cases, sensation can be totally lost, despite normal neural conduction. Patients may also experience local swelling and sweating of the limb, with changes in temperature, which mean a higher temperature compared to the healthy sites in the acute phase in most patients (80%), but that later turns colder, with thinning of the skin due to impaired circulatory activity. Color changes range from bright red to reddish violet. As the disease progresses, muscle spasm or contraction and joint tenderness or stiffness may also occur, with or without the loss of motor function, leading to an impaired ability to move. In the long term, dystrophic changes occur, which include diminished hair growth, with the nails becoming cracked, brittle, grooved, and spotty. Osteoporosis can start early, and can become severe; the joints thicken and muscle atrophy can be recognized. Occasionally, the limb can be displaced from its original position.[11] Pain is usually the leading sign in CRPS, but 7% of all the patients with CRPS present without any pain.[11] Affective symptoms may occur secondary to pain and disability, leading to difficulties that can include neglect syndrome. Altogether, CRPS signs and symptoms may present like many other health conditions, making the correct diagnosis hard to establish.

DIAGNOSIS OF CRPS

The diagnosis of CRPS is mainly based on the signs and symptoms as outlined in the Budapest criteria. This criteria system was developed in 2004 and was approved by the IASP Taxonomy Working Group after validation in 2011.[20,21]

Clinical diagnostic criteria for CRPS are:

1. Continuing pain that is disproportionate to any inciting events
2. One or more symptoms are reported to be present at the time of diagnosis in at least three of the four following categories:
   a. *Sensory*: hyperalgesia, allodynia
   b. *Vasomotor instability*: temperature asymmetry, skin-color changes/asymmetry

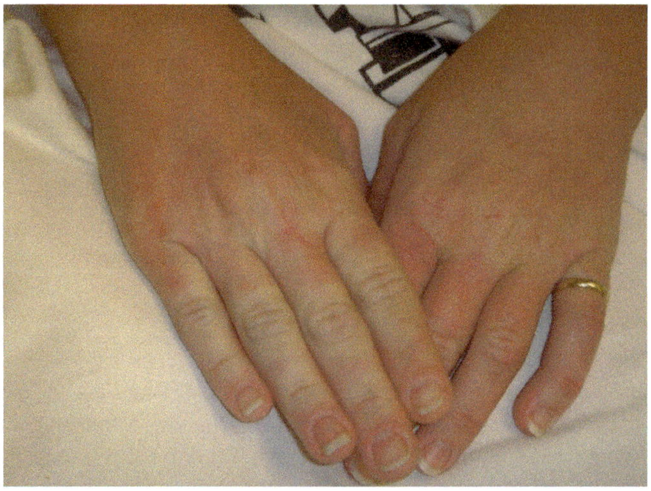

Figure 11.3. Early complex regional pain syndrome (CRPS), with vasoconstriction on the hand. Image courtesy of Andrea Trescot, MD.

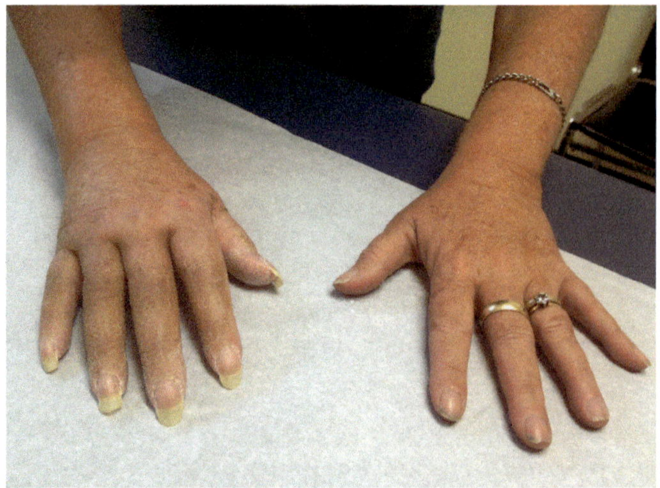

Figure 11.4. Late phase of the hand complex regional pain syndrome (CRPS) with diffuse thickening of the soft tissues. Image courtesy of Andrea Trescot, MD.

   c. *Edema/sudomotor instability*: edema, sweating changes/asymmetry
   d. *Trophic/motor changes*: trophic changes (hair, nails, skin), decreased range of motion, motor dysfunction (weakness, tremor, dystonia)

3. One or more signs are displayed at the time of evaluation in at least two of the four following categories:
   a. *Sensory*: hyperalgesia, allodynia
   b. *Vasomotor instability*: temperature asymmetry, skin-color changes/asymmetry (Figure 11.3)
   c. *Edema/sudomotor instability*: edema, sweating changes/asymmetry
   d. *Trophic/motor changes*: trophic changes (hair, nails, skin; Figure 11.4), decreased range of motion or dystrophy (Figure 11.5), motor dysfunction (weakness, tremor, dystonia)

4. There is no other diagnosis that better explains the signs and symptoms.

For a clinical diagnosis, these more sensitive clinical criteria are used with a specificity of 0.69 and a sensitivity of 0.85, but for research purposes, the Budapest research criteria are used, where all four symptom-categories need to be reported positive among these criteria. This increases the specificity to 0.94, with a sensitivity of 0.70. Better specificity is needed so that there are fewer false-positive results in etiologic and pathophysiologic investigations.[20]

Making the diagnosis of CRPS is purely based on the above-mentioned clinical criteria, as no specific diagnostic test exists yet, meaning that there are no obligatory tests. It is critical to have a high index of suspicion for CRPS when the patient has neuropathic-type pain, especially after trauma or surgery (Figure 11.6). However, the differential diagnosis includes other neuropathic conditions and pain syndromes, as well as some metabolic, vascular, rheumatic, and systemic conditions. Diagnostic testing is useful in three ways, one of which is to exclude any other suspected diagnoses that could better explain the signs and symptoms. The other two uses for diagnostic testing are to quantify the signs of the disease and to follow the results of therapy. No positive or negative test results lead to the diagnosis of CRPS on their own.

Tests that can be useful in the differential diagnosis are:

1. Laboratory studies, such as blood count, inflammatory parameters of the serum, or other disease-specific laboratory examinations
2. Imaging and functional studies, such as ultrasound, MRI, PET, SPECT, NMR spectroscopy and scintigraphy, triple-phase bone scan, plain X-ray, and bone density measurements
3. Neurophysiologic studies, such as EMG, NCV, and somatosensory evoked potentials.

These tests might rule out CRPS; for instance, blood work may show an infection, X-rays may show a stress fracture, and EMG might show a radiculopathy. On the other hand, osteoporosis (Figure 11.7), soft tissue swelling, or diffuse soft tissue atrophy from CRPS can be observed on X-ray, and a bone scan shows increased uptake in all three phases in acute CRPS.[22]

Tests that can be used to quantify/objectify signs and symptoms or to follow the effect of treatment include:

1. Sympathetic skin response and sudomotor function testing for sympathetic dysregulation
2. Volumetric and limb diameter measurement for edema
3. Skin temperature measurements, like infrared thermometry or infrared thermography, for skin temperature differences of at least 1.5°C
4. Quantitative sensory testing for sensory disorders

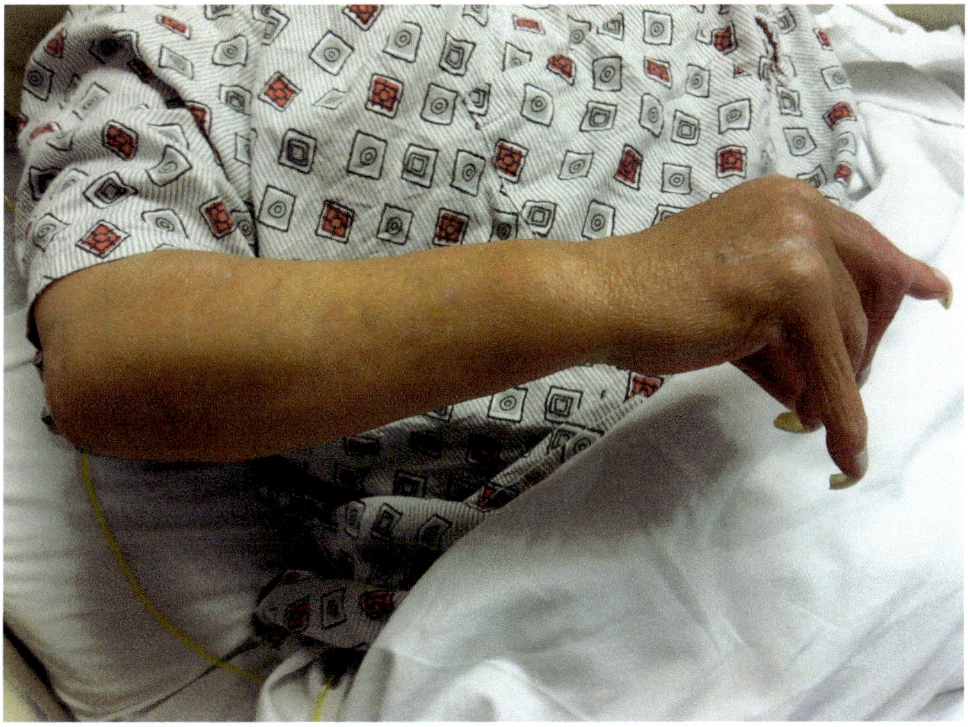

Figure 11.5. End-stage complex regional pain syndrome (CRPS), with atrophy, contractures, and complete loss of function. Image courtesy of Miles Day, MD.

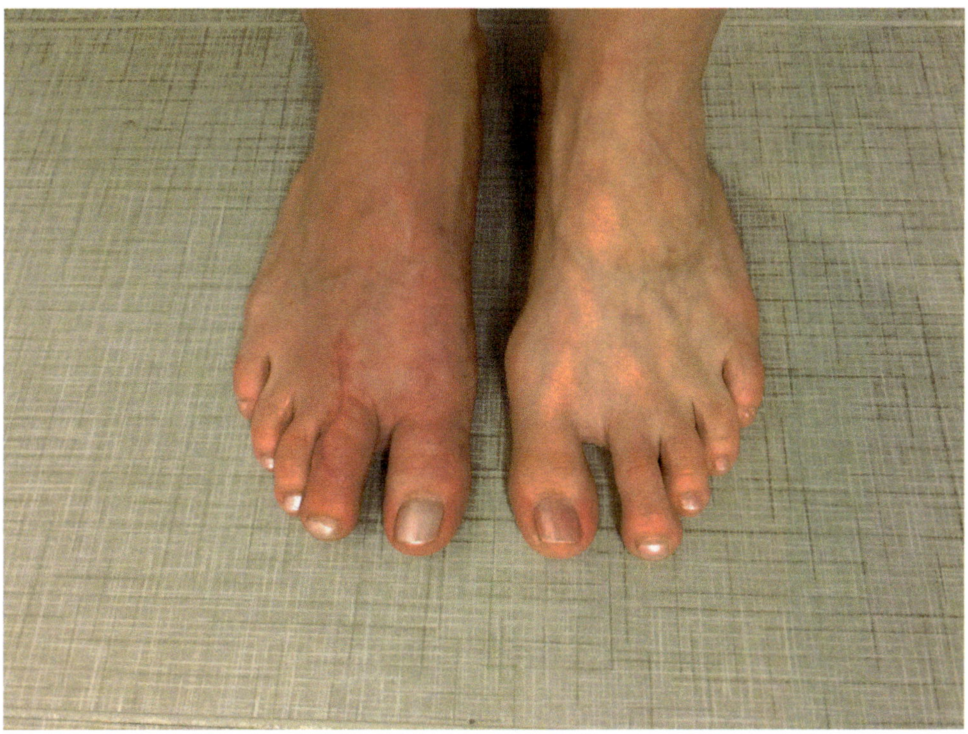

Figure 11.6. Complex regional pain syndrome (CRPS) of the foot, acute phase, with discoloration, swelling, dilated veins, and skin changes on the right foot. Patient complains of burning pain, hyperalgesia, and allodynia. Image courtesy of Agnes Stogicza, MD.

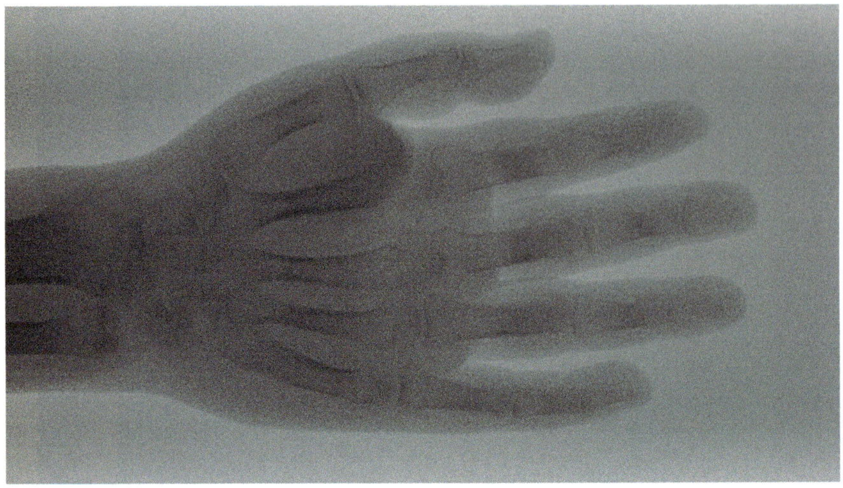

Figure 11.7. Diffuse osteopenia in complex regional pain syndrome (CRPS). Image courtesy of Andrea Trescot, MD.

5. Pain scales, such as Visual Analog Scale (VAS), McGill Questionnaire, or Neuropathic Pain Scale
6. Sphygmomanometer or dynamometer for loss of strength
7. Goniometer for impaired movement.[23]

DIFFERENTIAL DIAGNOSIS

The differential diagnosis of CRPS should consider:

- CNS disorders: stroke, neoplasm, encephalitis, multiple sclerosis, spinal cord trauma, myelitis
- Disk- or osteophyte-related radiculopathy
- Plexopathies and neuropathies: infection, tumor, trauma, entrapment (thoracic outlet syndrome and other tunnel syndromes), diabetes, alcoholism, toxicity, nutritional deficiency, porphyria, Guillain-Barré syndrome
- Vascular disorders: Raynaud phenomena, atherosclerosis, thrombophlebitis, vasculitis
- Systemic disorders: metabolic disorders (renal failure, amyloidosis, diabetes), autoimmune and rheumatologic disorders, infections
- Psychological disorders (e.g., somatoform disorder)

THERAPY

As a general rule, treatment of CRPS primarily focuses on restoration of function of the affected limb and improvement in quality of life. The consequences of the detailed difficulties in diagnosis and complex pathogenic factors of CRPS manifest as a great challenge in the treatment of the disease. Good-quality randomized controlled trials are lacking, in part because of the limiting effect of the last few decades' taxonomic and diagnostic incongruences, so scant evidence exists to guide treatment. Furthermore, CRPS differs from any other neuropathic pain condition in that it involves additional tissues and systems of the body, including microcirculation, inflammatory pathways, central nervous system, and sympathetic efferents in different ways in different individuals, making the right therapeutic choice hard to establish. In addition, a lot of therapeutic modalities used are extrapolated from results of other neuropathic conditions or based on anecdotal efficacy. Nevertheless, therapeutic interventions can be divided into three subgroups: pharmacotherapy, minimally invasive interventions, and interdisciplinary management.

Pharmacotherapy

Pharmacotherapy generally includes medication for chronic pain, circulation disorders, and inflammation, as well as some adjuvants.

Reduction of Pain

1. Antidepressants and/or anticonvulsants should be the first choice for the management of CRPS-associated pain, allodynia, and hyperalgesia. Tricyclic agents like amitriptyline and serotonin-norepinephrine reuptake inhibitors like duloxetine augment descending inhibitory pathways in the dorsal horn by blocking the presynaptic reuptake of monoaminergic neurotransmitters. This effect is well documented in other neuropathic pain conditions, establishing the use of these agents in CRPS, especially in patients with insomnia or other secondary psychologic changes or sensitization symptoms. Anticonvulsants like gabapentin, pregabalin, or phenytoin act by inhibition of sodium or calcium channels, reducing their action potentials. The use of these agents in other neuropathic pain syndromes is also well documented and there is some evidence for the use of gabapentin in CRPS patients.

2. Analgesics are the second-line treatment for CRPS-associated pain; however, most patients have already tried and failed nonsteroidal anti-inflammatory drugs (NSAIDs) and acetaminophen by the time they present to the pain specialist. NSAIDs reduce the synthesis of prostaglandins by inhibiting cyclooxygenase, thus reducing inflammation and hyperalgesia, while paracetamol and acetaminophen act centrally as an analgesic and antipyretic. These medications have no specific benefits in this patient group, although they can be used for a limited period of time, keeping in mind their potentially serious side effects and toxicity. Opioids act on opioid receptors in the brain and spinal cord. They have a well-documented effect in neuropathic pain and nociceptive pain, and are therefore widely used. However, in chronic pain, dose escalation is common because of increasing tolerance, with the growing risks of side effects and overdose, problems that should be understood and prevented. There is no evidence supporting any special benefits of opioids and they should be used cautiously. Strong opioids should be avoided in this patient group.

3. NMDA antagonists act by inhibiting NMDA receptors of the spinal cord and the brain (see maladaptive neuroplasticity), consequently reducing central sensitization and pain. Ketamine is a potent intravenous anesthetic that works via NMDA antagonism, but it can be used with good results in subanesthetic doses to reduce pain in severe (NRS > 7) therapy-resistant cases in appropriate clinical settings. Memantine is an oral NMDA antagonist used for neurodegenerative dementia associated with Alzheimer disease. It reduces pain when used in addition to opioid medication; however, this is currently an off-label use.

Management of Circulation Disorders

1. Vasodilator calcium channel blockers like nifedipine inhibit the calcium influx in smooth muscle cells of the vasculature, causing relaxation of the blood vessels, resulting in vasodilatation. They should be used in non-inflammatory or cold types of CRPS for improving the circulation of the affected limb. The effects and side effects (e.g., hypotension) should be evaluated regularly. An alternative to calcium channel blockers is alpha-receptor blockade by phenoxybenzamine, although evidence is still weak for the use of this medication in CRPS patients. Other agents, such as NO donors or phosphodiesterase inhibitors, are under investigation, and should be used in the context of a trial.

2. TNF-alpha inhibitors like thalidomide have been described to have a positive effect on CRPS but only in open-label studies or case reports, so their use should be restricted to the context of a trial.[24]

Anti-inflammatory Medication

1. Low-quality evidence showed benefits of corticosteroid use in acute cases of CRPS with prominent inflammatory signs, in a dose of 30 mg/day for 2 to 12 weeks, followed by a taper. Corticosteroids act by stimulating mRNA transcription and thus synthesis of a wide range of cellular proteins, including inflammatory pathways. However, corticosteroid usage is one of the most debated issues among CRPS specialists. Given the low-quality supporting data and the wide range of side effects and contraindications, steroid usage should be restricted to short courses only in acute CRPS, with risks carefully weighed against benefits.

2. Free-radical scavengers include dimethyl sulfoxide (DMSO) and *N*-acetyl-cysteine (NAC). These compounds act by reducing reactive oxygen species that contribute to inflammatory processes, thus reducing cell damage. The use of topical DMSO 50% cream five times a day for 3months is advised in CRPS patients with prominent inflammatory symptoms that have existed less than a year. In patients without inflammatory symptoms, NAC can be considered in a dose of 600 mg three times daily for 3 months.

Adjuvants

1. Many clinicians support the use of topical anesthetics like EMLA or 5% lidocaine patches, although evidence supporting their use is low. The reason for using these medications is that they are fully noninvasive with low risk of adverse side effects; unfortunately, they are quite expensive.

2. Bisphosphonates are theoretically useful, lowering osteoclast activity so the acidifying process of the extracellular matrix that releases hydroxyapatite crystals is decreased. They are proven to be useful in decreasing osteoporosis, but not necessarily in treating CRPS-associated pain. The optimal timing of administration, dosage, and duration are still unclear.

3. Muscle relaxants, especially oral baclofen, are useful in treating muscle spasm associated with CRPS. Intrathecal baclofen can also be considered in patients with more than one affected limb if conventional therapy is ineffective, although pharmacologic and mechanical complications are common. Slowly titrated diazepam and clonazepam are acceptable alternatives.[23,25,26]

Minimally Invasive Interventions

Minimally invasive therapeutic interventions like percutaneous stellate, thoracic, and lumbar sympathectomies have been the gold standard in managing CRPS for many years, based on the theory of SMP. However, the efficacy of these interventions has been questioned in double-blind placebo-controlled trials. While some of the actual guidelines strictly forbid the use of percutaneous sympathectomy, others still try to find its correct role in the management of CRPS, or do not make any recommendations on it, showing that data (such as subgroup analysis) and applicable alternatives to these interventions for clinical use are still lacking. Keeping in mind the inhomogeneous pathophysiology and symptoms in CRPS, the decision to perform an invasive intervention should be made on an individual basis, with careful weighing of risks and benefits. An overall rule is to start with the less invasive options and move to the most invasive ones if needed. The goals of invasive interventions are lowering pain and/or improving circulation of the affected limb, leading to better cooperation with physiotherapy and improving quality of life.

Percutaneous sympathectomy has probably been the most widely used invasive intervention to decrease symptoms of CRPS. In spite of the ambiguous study outcomes, most treatment algorithms still consider sympathetic blockade one of the first invasive procedures for cold chronic CRPS, based on largely empirical or traditional practice patterns. It still can be clinically important in individual cases, because it can facilitate amelioration of pain and function in about 50% of the cases. Sympathetic blockade can be done in the stellate ganglion for the face and upper limbs, in the thoracic sympathetic chain for distal upper limbs, or in the lumbar sympathetic chain for the lower limbs, using local anesthetics, phenol, or RFA. The latter two should only be used after successful diagnostic blockade with local anesthetics has resulted in temporary clinical improvement.[25]

SGB

SGB is used for facial and upper extremity pain. The ganglion itself is formed by the fusion of the inferior cervical and the first thoracic sympathetic ganglia and it lies in front of the interspace between the C7 and T1 vertebral bodies. SGB can be performed using landmarks, fluoroscopy via an anterior (Figure 11.8A) or oblique approach, or ultrasound guidance (Figure 11.8B) for identifying anatomy and needle placement. After correct placement of the needle, 3 to 5 mL of local anesthetic should be used to perform the block. RFA and 6% phenol neurolysis have been performed, although it is preferable to do neurolysis at the thoracic level to avoid permanent Horner's syndrome.

PROCEDURE-RELATED COMPLICATIONS Procedure-related complications of SGBs include:

- Neuritis and neuralgia
- Recurrent laryngeal nerve block/damage
- Phrenic nerve block/damage
- Block/damage to the branches of the brachial plexus
- Pneumothorax
- Inadvertent puncture of the vertebral or carotid artery
- Inadvertent epidural or subarachnoid puncture
- Paratracheal hematoma
- Esophageal puncture, infection
- Seizures
- Cardiac emergency

Thoracic Sympathetic Block

The thoracic sympathetic block is performed for CRPS of the upper extremity, especially of the hand. It targets the T2 and T3 paravertebral sympathetic ganglia. The procedure is performed with fluoroscopy guidance, which allows one or two needles to be carefully positioned immediately lateral of the vertebral bodies, between the posterior one-third and anterior two-thirds of the vertebral body (Figure 11.9). The administration of 1 to 2 mL of local anesthetic at each level leads to vasodilation, and subsequent temperature increase on the affected side. Pain is then assessed to decide if there is a sympathetically maintained component. In case of a successful but temporary diagnostic block, a more permanent RFA (80°C for 90 seconds, twice—i.e., two times) can follow (Figure 11.10A).[27]

PROCEDURE-RELATED COMPLICATIONS Procedure-related complications of thoracic sympathetic blocks include:

- Bleeding/nerve damage caused by inadvertent intercostal artery, vein, or nerve puncture
- Pneumothorax
- Exiting nerve root injury, neuralgia
- Inadvertent epidural or subarachnoid puncture
- Inadvertent puncture of azygos vein or thoracic duct
- Esophageal puncture, infection
- Inadvertent puncture of trachea
- Vagus nerve damage
- Inadvertent puncture of the aorta

Lumbar Sympathectomy

The lumbar sympathetic block (LSB) is performed for CRPS of the lower extremity. It targets the L2, L3, and L4 sympathetic ganglia. The procedure is performed with fluoroscopy (Figure 11.11A–C). or ultrasound guidance (Figure 11.11D–E), which allows one to three needles to be carefully positioned immediately anterolateral of the vertebral bodies, between the anterior one-third and posterior two-thirds of the vertebral body Administration of 3 to 5 mL of local anesthetic at each level leads to vasodilation and subsequent temperature increase of the affected limb. Pain is then assessed to decide if there is a sympathetically maintained component. In case of a successful diagnostic block, a more permanent RFA (80°C for

(A)

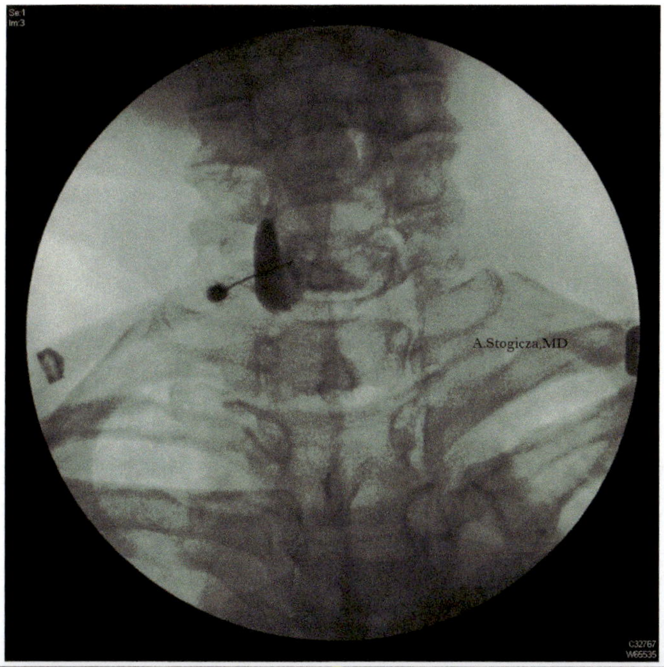

(B)

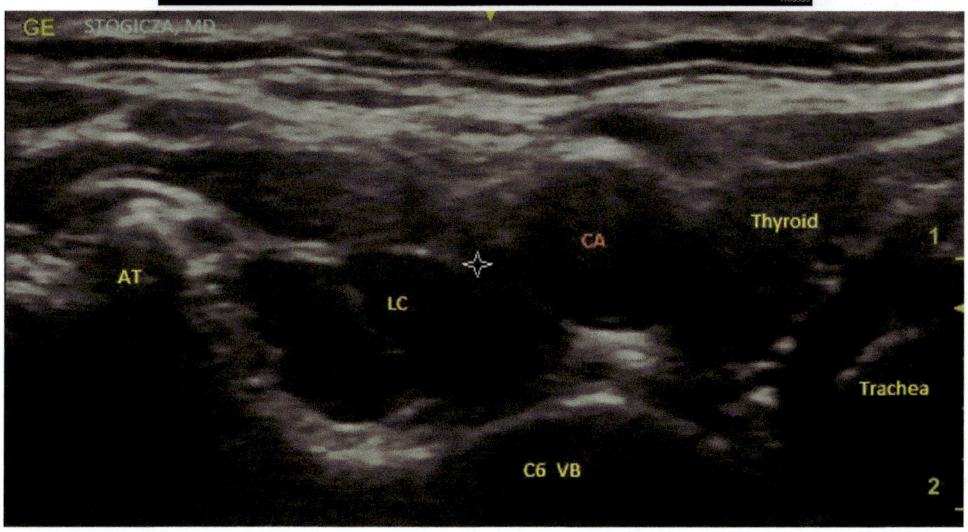

Figure 11.8. (A) AP fluoroscopy image of needle positioned at the C6 level for a stellate ganglion block. The longus colli muscle is outlined by contrast material. (B) Ultrasound-guided stellate ganglion block. The location of the ganglion is marked with a star. Abbreviations: AT, anterior tubercle; CA, carotid artery; LC, longus colli muscle; VB, vertebral body. Images courtesy of Agnes Stogicza, MD.

90 seconds, twice—i.e., two times; Figure 11.12A–C) or phenol 6% 10 mL neurolysis can follow.

PROCEDURE-RELATED COMPLICATIONS Procedure-related complications of lumbar sympathectomy include:

- Neuritis and neuralgia of the exiting nerve roots
- Neuritis and neuralgia of the genitofemoral nerve
- Inadvertent dural or epidural puncture
- Paraplegia due to ischemia of spinal artery
- Inadvertent intradiscal puncture, discitis
- Low back pain and muscle spasm
- Penetration of viscera
- Impotence and retrograde ejaculation
- Inadvertent puncture of vena cava and/or retroperitoneal hematoma
- Hypotension
- Kidney injury

SCS

SCS applies low-voltage electrical stimuli to the spinal cord and nerve roots to block sensation of pain. It has been largely studied in chronic spinal pain patients, with growing evidence supporting its use in CRPS. The neurophysiologic mechanisms of SCS are not completely understood, but

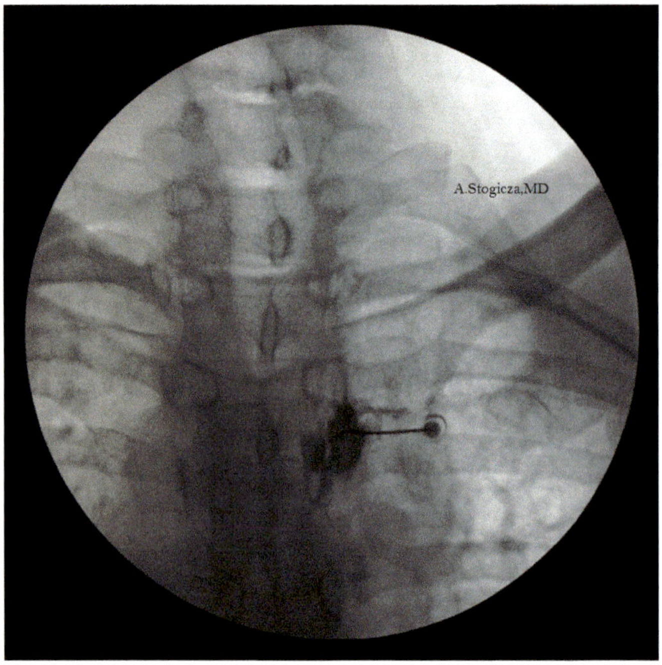

Figure 11.9. Fluoroscopic thoracic sympathetic block with 2 mL of contrast material. Image courtesy of Agnes Stogicza, MD.

seem to include direct electrical inhibition of afferent noxious signals in the dorsal horn (Melzack and Wall's gate-control theory),[28] inhibition of the SNS, activation of supraspinal antinociceptive nuclei, induction of gamma-amino butyric acid (GABA) and serotonin release, and decreased glutamate and aspartame levels. Systematic review of the literature shows 53% to 100% success rate using SCS in CRPS, usually defined as at least a 50% decrease in VAS score. Although the costs of SCS implantation are quite high, new evidence suggests that, with careful patient selection, the overall expenses are decreased because of decreased health care and analgesic requirements. The method should be used on patients with at least a 6-month duration of the disease (chronic CRPS) and with VAS scores of 5 or more after successful trial stimulation (VAS decrease of at least 50%). A minimum of 7 days of trial period is advisable, but practice varies among physicians. Placement of the leads is performed via 14-G Tuohy needle into the posterior epidural space (Figure 11.13). The final position of the electrodes is usually C4-C7 for the arm and T10-T12 for the lower limb, with the electrode passed at least 7 to 8 cm within the epidural space. After fluoroscopic confirmation of correct lead placement, motor stimulation and paresthesia in the desired region should be provoked. Some SCS systems use the same electrodes for trial and permanent stimulation, while others need to be replaced after a successful trial stimulation process. Permanent pulse generators are then implanted.

PROCEDURE-RELATED COMPLICATIONS Early complications of SCS include:

- Bleeding
- Nerve or spinal cord injury
- Dural puncture
- Early infections (meningitis, diskitis, epidural abscess)
- Edema and seroma at the generator site

Late complications include:

- Epidural fibrosis
- Spinal stenosis
- Infection at generator or extension cable sites
- Skin necrosis around generator

Complications related to the device include:

- Migration of the electrodes
- Lead breakage
- Hardware malfunction
- Unwanted stimulation
- Burning of the skin

Regional and Neuraxial Blocks

Standard regional and neuraxial blocks can also be used for the management of intractable pain in CRPS patients. For the upper limb, brachial plexus blocks, and for the lower limb, sciatic, femoral, or more selective nerve blocks and/or catheters with continuous local anesthetic infusion are available. Low-concentration continuous local anesthetic infusions combined with patient-controlled dosing can reduce pain while motor function is conserved, allowing active motion and physiotherapy. Epidural catheters with continuous local anesthetic and clonidine infusions have been proven to relieve CRPS-associated pain. Opioids can be added if needed to decrease local anesthetic concentrations, resulting in spared motor functions and good cooperation with physiotherapy. The most common complication related to long-term epidural catheters is infection, with a rate reported to be as high as 31%. Thus, the catheter insertions should be treated as minor surgical procedures meeting standards of surgical sterility, and catheters should be tunneled away from the entry point to avoid bacterial colonization.[23,25,26,29]

PROCEDURE-RELATED COMPLICATIONS Procedure-related complications of regional and neuraxial blocks include:

- Infection, especially with long-dwelling catheters
- Bleeding
- Intravascular injection
- Intrathecal injection
- Pneumothorax

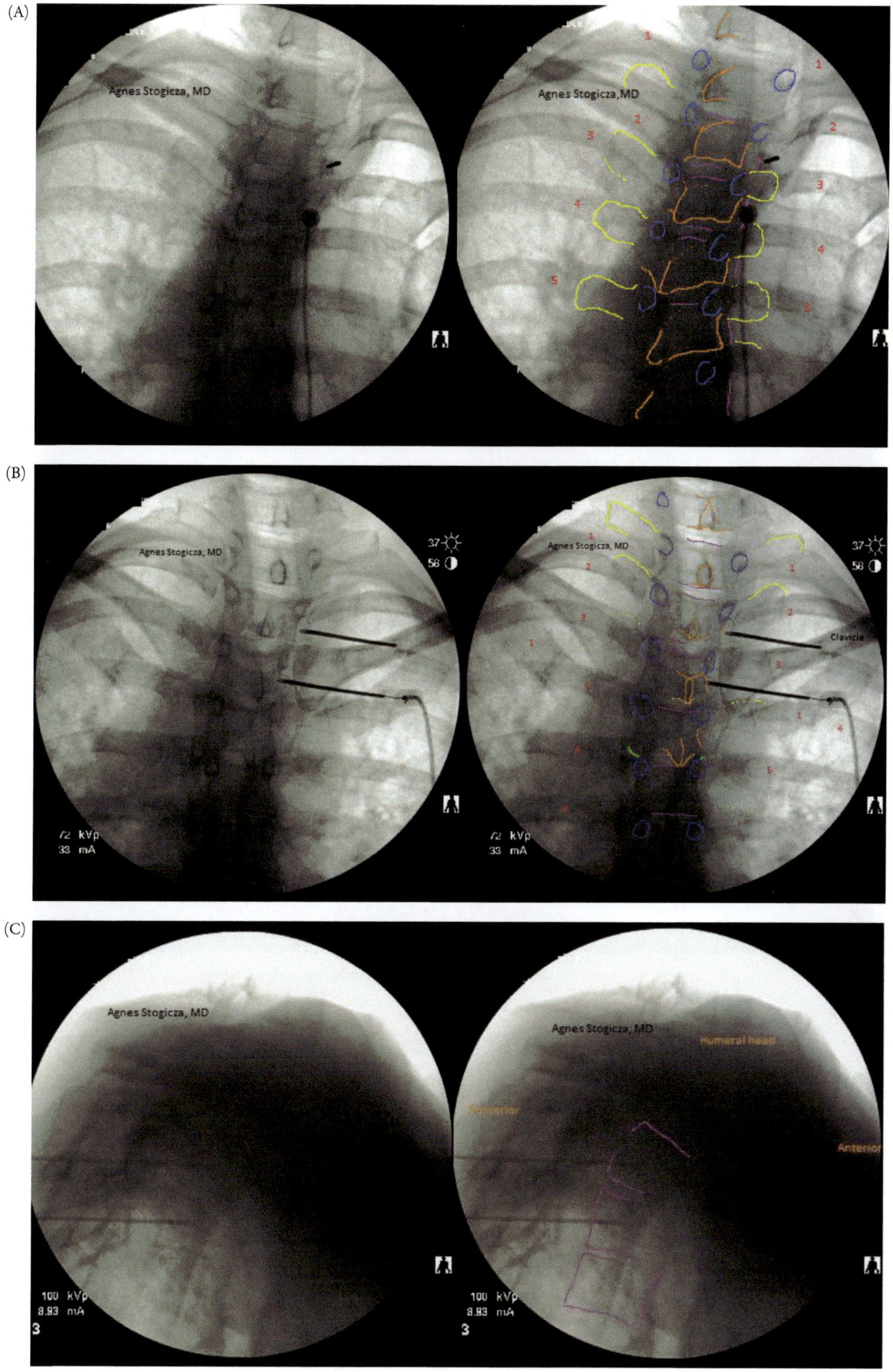

Figure 11.10. (A) Oblique fluoroscopy view of thoracic sympathetic block (radiofrequency ablation). Needles are positioned at T2 and T3 levels. T3 needle in tunnel view. Color key: orange, spinous processes and laminas; yellow, transverse processes; blue, pedicles; purple, vertebral bodies; red, numbers of ribs. (B) AP view of thoracic sympathetic block (radiofrequency ablation). Needles are positioned at T2 and T3 levels. Color key: orange, spinous processes and laminas; yellow, transverse processes; blue, pedicles; purple, vertebral body endplates; red, numbers of ribs; green, inferior articular process. (C) Lateral view of thoracic sympathetic block (radiofrequency ablation). Needles are positioned at T2 and T3 levels between the junction of the posterior one-third and anterior two-thirds of the vertebral body. Color Key: purple, visible vertebral body contours. Images courtesy of Agnes Stogicza, MD.

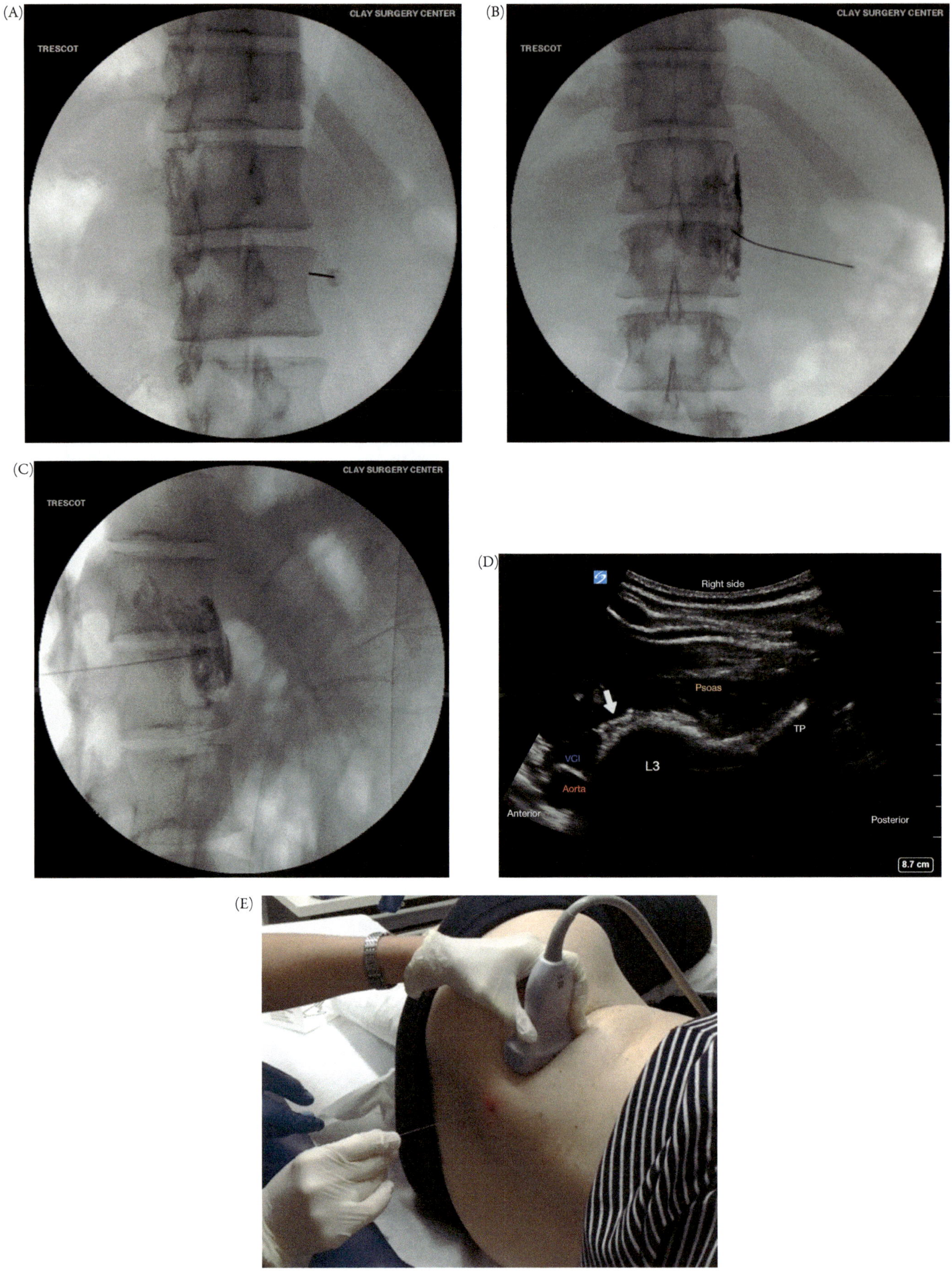

Figure 11.11. (A) Oblique fluoroscopy view of lumbar sympathetic diagnostic block. Needle is positioned at L2 level. (B) AP fluoroscopy view of lumbar sympathetic diagnostic block. Needle is positioned at L2 level. (C) Lateral fluoroscopy view of lumbar sympathetic diagnostic block. Needle is positioned at L2 level. (D–E) Ultrasound guided lumbar sympathetic block. The "gap" between iliac crest and T12 rib allows visualization of L3 or L2 vertebra. After identyfing vertebral body, transverse process (TP), psoas muscle, aorta and inferior vena cava (IVC), the target is just anterior to psoas muscle (arrow). Skin entry 8cm off midline, just like fluoroscopy guided. More lateral entry puts the kidney at risk. Patient size to be considered. Procedure video available here: https://www.youtube.com/watch?v=6R20HBgO7dk&feature=youtu.be. Images courtesy of Andrea Trescot, MD.

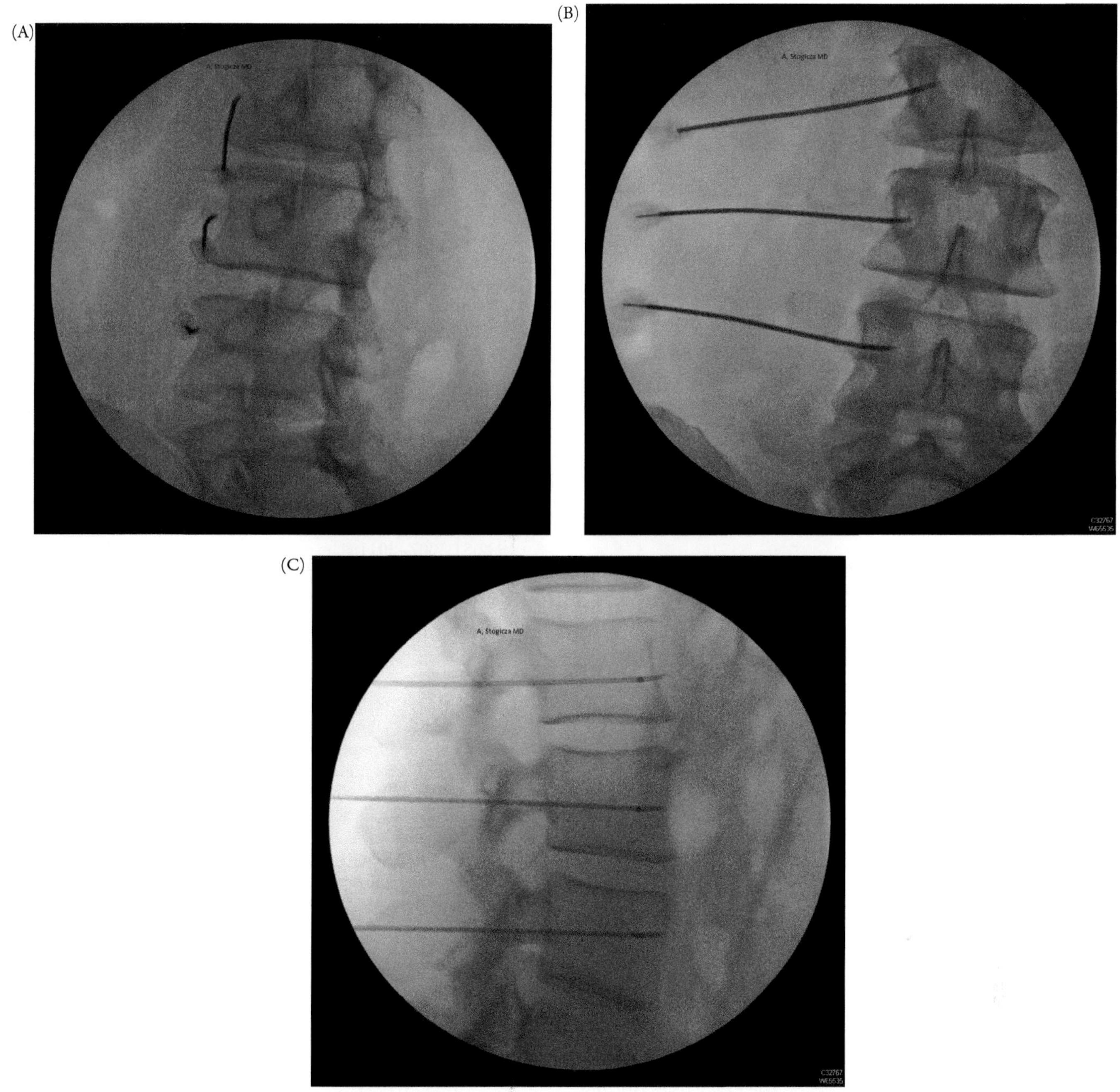

Figure 11.12. (A) Oblique fluoroscopy view of lumbar sympathetic radiofrequency ablation. Needles are positioned at L2, L3, and L4 levels. (B) AP view of lumbar sympathetic radiofrequency ablation. Needles are positioned at L2, L3, and L4 levels. (C) Lateral fluoroscopy image of needle position for lumbar sympathetic radiofrequency ablation. Needles are positioned at L2, L3, and L4 levels. Images courtesy of Agnes Stogicza, MD.

- Plexus injury
- Phrenic nerve paralysis

Interdisciplinary Management

The interdisciplinary management of CRPS focuses on functional restoration of the patient. It encompasses the coordinated use of OT, PT, recreational therapy, and vocational rehabilitation. Using techniques like desensitization, mirror visual feedback, graded motor imagery, and exposure therapy leads to the reactivation of the affected limb, followed by isometric strengthening, stress loading, correction of postural abnormalities, treatment of secondary myofascial pain, aerobic conditioning, and movement therapies.[25]

The basis of using psychologic interventions in CRPS patients is partly extrapolated from the results of other chronic pain conditions, such as fibromyalgia,[30] recognizing that Axis I psychiatric disorders, ongoing life stressors, and cognitive, emotional, or behavioral problems like unrealistic expectations can have a serious negative effect on chronic pain and the success of its therapy. According to the conception of SMP, stress factors originating from the limitation of everyday activities or other life stressors also lead to norepinephrine release

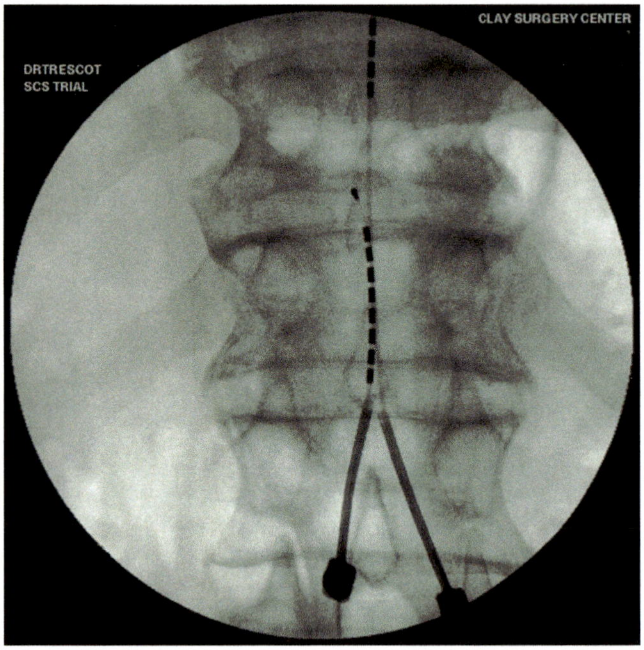

Figure 11.13. Spinal cord stimulator. Epidural needle and dual lead placement. Image courtesy of Andrea Trescot, MD.

and consequent worsening in circulatory symptoms and pain. For these reasons, psychologic interventions should be part of routine CRPS management, including patient and family education, psychologic evaluation, relaxation training with biofeedback strategies, and/or cognitive, behavioral, and family interventions.[25,30]

In addition, several conditions that lead to hyperalgesia, such as chronic opioid use and excessive use of tramadol, may also need to be evaluated.[31]

CONCLUSION

CRPS is a chronic pain disorder that can affect any body area and is accompanied by sensory, motor, circulatory, trophic, and sudomotor changes. The pathogenesis includes neurogenic inflammatory pathways, vasomotor dysfunction, and maladaptive neuroplasticity; however, the exact roles of these factors in initiating and maintaining the disease are not yet fully understood.

Diagnosis is based on clinical signs and symptoms; specific investigations are only used for differential diagnosis or quantifying symptoms. Despite its potential to visualize and analyze local flow, ultrasound is not an established technique for diagnosis of CRPS.[32,33]

Therapy includes the combination of pharmacologic, interventional, paramedical, and psychologic interventions on a personalized case-by-case basis. Supplements, such as vitamin C, may offer benefit.[34,35] Therapeutic goals are relieving pain, restoring function, and improving quality of life.

REFERENCES

1. Janicki TI. Chronic pelvic pain as a form of complex regional pain syndrome. *Clin Obstet Gynecol.* 2003;46(4):797–803.
2. Goenka A, Aziz M, Riley P, Vassallo G. Complex regional pain syndrome involving the face following snowball injury. *Eur J Pediatr.* 2014;173(3):397–400.
3. Merskey H, Bogduk N. *Classification of Chronic Pain.* Seattle, WA: IASP Press; 2002.
4. Wilfred Janig MS-H. *Reflex Sympathetic Dystrophy: A Reappraisal.* Seattle, WA: IASP Press; 1996.
5. Stanton-Hicks M. An updated interdisciplinary clinical pathway for CRPS—report of an expert panel. *Pain Pract.* 2002;2:1–16.
6. Oaklander AL, Fields HL. Is reflex sympathetic dystrophy/complex regional pain syndrome type I a small-fiber neuropathy? *Ann Neurol.* 2009;65(6):629–638.
7. de Mos M, de Bruijn AG, Huygen FJ, Dieleman JP, Stricker BH, Sturkenboom MC. The incidence of complex regional pain syndrome: a population-based study. *Pain.* 2007;129(1-2):12–20.
8. Sandroni P, Benrud-Larson LM, McClelland RL, Low PA. Complex regional pain syndrome type I: incidence and prevalence in Olmsted County, a population-based study. *Pain.* 2003;103(1-2):199–207.
9. Gellman H, Keenan MA, Stone L, Hardy SE, Waters RL, Stewart C. Reflex sympathetic dystrophy in brain-injured patients. *Pain.* 1992;51:3007–3011.
10. Baron R. Mechanisms of disease: neuropathic pain—a clinical perspective. *Nat Clin Pract Neurol.* 2006;2(2):95–106.
11. Veldman PH, Reynen HM, Arntz IE, Goris RJ. Signs and symptoms of reflex sympathetic dystrophy: prospective study of 829 patients. *Lancet.* 1993; 342:1012–1016.
12. de Mos M, Sturkenboom MC, Huygen FJ. Current understandings on complex regional pain syndrome. *Pain Pract.* 2009;9(2):86–99.
13. Schattschneider J, Binder A, Siebrecht D, Wasner G, Baron R. Complex regional pain syndromes: the influence of cutaneous and deep somatic sympathetic innervation on pain. *Clin J Pain.* 2006;22(3):240–244.
14. Cooper MS, Clark VP. Neuroinflammation, neuroautoimmunity, and the co-morbidities of complex regional pain syndrome. *J Neuroimmune Pharm.* 2013;8(3):452–469.
15. Coderre TJ, Bennett GJ. A hypothesis for the cause of complex regional pain syndrome-type I (reflex sympathetic dystrophy): pain due to deep-tissue microvascular pathology. *Pain Med.* 2010;11(8):1224–1238.
16. Albrecht PJ, Hines S, Eisenberg E, et al. Pathologic alterations of cutaneous innervation and vasculature in affected limbs from patients with complex regional pain syndrome. *Pain.* 2006;120(3): 244–266.
17. Klein MM, Lee JW, Siegel SM, Downs HM, Oaklander AL. Endoneural pathology of the needlestick-nerve-injury model of complex regional pain syndrome, including rats with and without pain behaviors. *Eur J Pain.* 2012;16(1):28–37.
18. Marinus J, Moseley GL, Birklein F, et al. Clinical features and pathophysiology of complex regional pain syndrome. *Lancet Neurol.* 2011;10(7):637–648.
19. Bruehl S. An update on the pathophysiology of complex regional pain syndrome. *Anesthesiology.* 2010;113:713–725.
20. Harden RN, Bruehl S, Perez RS, et al. Validation of proposed diagnostic criteria (the "Budapest criteria") for complex regional pain syndrome. *Pain.* 2010;150(2):268–274.
21. Harden RN, Bruehl S, Stanton-Hicks M, Wilson PR. Proposed new diagnostic criteria for complex regional pain syndrome. *Pain Med.* 2007;8(4):326–331.
22. Holder LE, Chew FS. Reflex sympathetic dystrophy imaging. *Medscape.* 2015. Retrieved from http://emedicine.medscape.com/article/394928-overview.

23. Perez RS, Geertzen JHB, Dijkstra PU, et al. Updated guidelines for complex regional pain syndrome type 1, May 2014. http://www.posttraumatischedystrofie.nl/english.html.
24. Dirckx M, Stronks DL, Groeneweg G, Huygen FJ. Effect of immunomodulating medications in complex regional pain syndrome: a systematic review. *Clin J Pain.* 2012;28(4):355–363.
25. Harden RN, Oaklander AL, Burton AW, et al. Complex regional pain syndrome: practical diagnostic and treatment guidelines, 4th edition. *Pain Med.* 2013;14(2):180–229.
26. Goebel A, Barker CH, Turner-Stokes L. Complex regional pain syndrome in adults. UK guidelines for diagnosis, referral and management in primary and secondary care. London: RCP; 2012.
27. Skaebuland C, Racz G. Indications and technique of thoracic(2) and thoracic(3) neurolysis. *Curr Rev Pain.* 1999;3(5):400–405.
28. Melzack R, Wall PD. Pain mechanisms: a new theory. *Science.* 1965;150(3699):971–979.
29. Prithvi R, Serdar E. *Pain-Relieving Procedures.* Chichester, U.K.: Wiley-Blackwell; 2012.
30. Ngian GS, Guymer EK, Littlejohn GO. The use of opioids in fibromyalgia. *Int J Rheum Dis.* 2011;14(1):6–11.
31. Lee SH, Cho SY, Lee HG, Choi JI, Yoon MH, Kim WM. Tramadol induced paradoxical hyperalgesia. *Pain Physician.* 2013;16(1): 41–44.
32. Pekindil G, Pekindil Y, Sarikaya A. Doppler sonographic assessment of posttraumatic reflex sympathetic dystrophy. *J Ultrasound Med.* 2003;22(4):395–402.
33. Nazarian LN, Schweitzer ME, Mandel S, et al. Increased soft-tissue blood flow in patients with reflex sympathetic dystrophy of the lower extremity revealed by power Doppler sonography. *AJR Am J Roentgenol.* 1998;171(5):1245–1250.
34. Zollinger PE, Tuinebreijer WE, Breederveld RS, Kreis RW. Can vitamin C prevent complex regional pain syndrome in patients with wrist fractures? A randomized, controlled, multicenter dose-response study. *J Bone Joint Surg.* 2007;89(7):1424–1431.
35. Zollinger PE, Tuinebreijer WE, Kreis RW, Breederveld RS. Effect of vitamin C on frequency of reflex sympathetic dystrophy in wrist fractures: a randomised trial. *Lancet.* 1999;354(9195):2025–2028.

REVIEW QUESTIONS

1. A 55-year-old patient has had ankle reconstruction surgery after a fall from 20 feet. Which of the following should raise suspicion of CRPS?

A. Four weeks after surgery, the operated foot is still painful and swollen compared to the other foot.
B. Six weeks after surgery, the skin of the whole foot is red, swollen, and tender to touch, veins are dilated, and patient often wakes up with burning pain.
C. Two weeks after surgery, the foot is red and swollen and the veins are dilated compared to the other foot.
D. Eight weeks after surgery, the foot is still tender and function is limited, although weight-bearing is possible. Pain is overall slowly decreasing.

2. Which of the following statements is false?

A. CRPS is always preceded by injury.
B. The symptoms of CRPS can start without any initiating event or trauma.
C. Crush injury of the extremity can trigger CRPS.
D. IV cannula placement at the wrist can injure the superficial branch of the radial nerve.

3. Which of the following patients has CRPS according to the Budapest criteria?

A. A 22-year-old female 3 days after propofol sedation complains about redness and swelling and hyperalgesia in a 10-cm diameter area around the intravenous (IV) cannula.
B. A 45-year-old obese diabetic female with an ulcer on the left lower calf complains of tingling, burning pain that includes the whole foot in a stocking- like distribution.
C. A 65-year-old male patient with arteriosclerosis and prostate cancer complains about pain, tingling, and decreased sensation of the left lower extremity below the knee. He noticed the symptoms just after he hit his knee against the bed. The extremity is colder and whiter then the other extremity.
D. A 25-year-old female hit her lower arm accidently against the doorframe. She felt pain in the lower arm, radiating to the thumb immediately, that got worse over the next few days. The whole hand became swollen and tender. The skin of the involved arm is red, and the temperature is increased compared to the other side.

ANSWERS

1. B. Normal healing after surgery includes increased blood circulation, swelling, and tenderness. The symptoms in A and C are acceptable physiologic changes 2 or 4 weeks after surgery. Also, considering that ankle reconstructive surgery is a relatively major surgery, as long as the pain and swelling decrease overall and function increases, having some pain 8 weeks after surgery is acceptable. However, allodynia at areas where surgery was not performed should certainly raise the suspicion of CRPS after exclusion of other pathologies, like infection.[11]

2. A. CRPS can be triggered by any trauma, even minor trauma, and certainly can be triggered by surgery, IV cannula placement, and crush injuries.[3–5]

3. D. After a minor trauma, the patient developed pain that is disproportionate to the initiating event. She shows the typical early signs of CRPS: allodynia that exceeds the anatomic area of injury, edema, increased circulation, and temperature change. Answer A refers to a normal inflammatory response to propofol accidentally injected subcutaneously. Answer B describes diabetic neuropathy, while answer C is consistent with popliteal artery occlusion. D is the correct

answer because it describes a minor trauma that preceded changes consistent with CRPS.[20,21]

QUESTIONS AND ANSWERS

This chapter has accompanying questions and answers that are available to subscribers as part of the Oxford eLearning platform. To access the questions, follow the link below, or go to ✔ http://oxfordmedicine.com/painmanagementreview

12.

NEUROPATHIC PAIN

Faraz Khursheed and Marc O. Maybauer

STEM CASE AND KEY QUESTIONS

A 38-year-old healthy female, a professional dancer and dance teacher, was referred to the pain clinic for left ankle pain that had persisted since she twisted her ankle 3 months previously. She had gone to a local urgent care center and was placed in an ankle brace for 2 weeks. The pain worsened with time and began to move cephalad toward the outer part of the calf. She described the pain as burning, sharp, and as "a million needles sticking at once." Her pain particularly worsened when anything touched the overlying skin, even light clothing. The pain was intense and adversely affected her functions and daily life. She had been out of dancing class since the injury. She consulted an orthopedic surgeon who ordered plain films and magnetic resonance imaging (MRI) of her left ankle. While the pain physician attempted to obtain her medical records, a provisional diagnosis of complex regional pain syndrome (CRPS) type I was made.

WHAT BROAD CATEGORY OF PAIN IS THIS WOMAN SUFFERING FROM? WHAT IS CRPS?

A review of the patient's MRI and plain films revealed periarticular osteopenia: patchy bone marrow edema and soft tissue swelling with faint enhancement. A comprehensive exam in the clinic revealed a swollen ankle compared to the unaffected side, with mild erythema and warmth around the joint. Passive range of motion was normal but painful. There was also allodynia (unpleasant painful sensation induced by nonpainful stimulus, such as light touch, on the affected area) and hyperalgesia (an extreme pain response to a minimally painful stimulus) around the ankle. A bone scan and nerve conduction study were ordered. The patient was started on meloxicam 15 mg daily and was referred to physical therapy (PT).

HOW IS CRPS DIAGNOSED? WHAT IS THE NECESSARY WORKUP?

The patient returned to the clinic distraught, because meloxicam did not alleviate her pain. She further complained that PT was a "torture" she would never want to go through again. The results of the nerve conduction study were unremarkable. Bone scan showed increased uptake around the left ankle. She was counseled on the importance of PT and a referral was made to a therapist specializing in CRPS. She was prescribed gabapentin with uptitration to 900 mg three times a day over 2 weeks. Meloxicam was discontinued.

WHAT IS THE MAIN CLASS OF MEDICATIONS USED TO TREAT CRPS OR OTHER NEUROPATHIC PAIN? DO NONSTEROIDAL ANTI-INFLAMMATORY DRUGS (NSAIDS) AND STEROIDS HAVE A ROLE?

The patient returned, reporting a slight improvement in pain without significant improvement in her quality of life. She reported that the physical therapist used innovative techniques, including transcutaneous electrical nerve stimulation, progressive weight-bearing, tactile desensitization, massage, and mirror and contrast bath therapy. Because the patient continued to experience significant symptoms, especially at night, when she would often wake up due to allodynia from rubbing her ankle on the sheets, she was prescribed low-dose amitriptyline for use at night. On exam, her ankle remained erythematous, warm to the touch, and swollen. She was scheduled for a series of three lumbar sympathetic blocks over 6 weeks.

WHAT ARE THE DIFFERENT MODALITIES FOR TREATING CRPS?

With ongoing aggressive PT, pharmacotherapy, and a series of lumbar sympathetic blockades, the patient improved clinically and no longer had autonomic changes around the ankle. She progressed well with PT and slowly began to return to her dancing routine. Unfortunately, after a few days, another mild sprain at the ankle caused a recurrence of her symptoms. She returned to the clinic in distress and disappointed. She had been continuing to take gabapentin at the prescribed dose. She was slowly tapered off the gabapentin and was switched to pregabalin. A discussion was then initiated about spinal cord stimulation (SCS). As part of the SCS workup, she was sent for a neuropsychiatric evaluation.

WHAT IS SCS? HOW DOES IT WORK?

Detailed neuropsychiatric testing deemed the patient a good candidate for SCS. She decided to continue with psychotherapeutic interventions, including cognitive-behavioral therapy and biofeedback. Specific psychologic interventions also included comprehensive education about her condition. The patient received detailed information on the known facts of CRPS, the negative effects of disuse, the importance of reactivation, and the need for an active self-management approach. The goal was to prevent the development of dysfunctional behavior patterns that could contribute to the severity, disability, and prolonged chronicity of the condition.

The patient proceeded with the SCS trial, which successfully ameliorated her pain. She later proceeded with a permanent SCS implantation procedure. Twelve months after her implant, she has resumed most of her dancing activities with some restrictions. She runs an online blog to educate and provide support to young patients with CRPS.

DISCUSSION

The International Association for the Study of Pain (IASP) defines neuropathic pain as "pain caused by a lesion or disease of the somatosensory nervous system." This is in contrast to nociceptive pain, which the IASP defines as "pain that arises from actual or threatened damage to non-neural tissue and is due to the activation of nociceptors."[1] However, the two types often present together as a spectrum in many patients. Several studies have demonstrated neurobiologic changes in the central nervous system (CNS) and peripheral nervous system (PNS) resulting from chronic pain of either type.[2,3] Clinically, many patients with chronic nociceptive pain, such as osteoarthritis, demonstrate features of neuropathic pain, likely from damage to peripheral somatosensory fibers and/or from neuroplastic changes that occur in the PNS and CNS.[4–6]

The true prevalence of neuropathic pain is difficult to estimate. It is estimated that one-third of all Americans suffer from chronic pain, with various chronic painful conditions directly and indirectly costing over $600 billion annually.[7,8] In Europe, the prevalence of neuropathic pain syndromes is estimated to be 7% to 8%, which is steadily increasing in concert with the prevalence of chronic medical conditions causing neuropathy, e.g., diabetes.[9]

A thorough understating of neuropathic pain is important because of the significant burden the pain places on the healthcare system and the awareness that conventional methodologies of treatment are not very effective.

PATHOGENESIS

The pathophysiology of neuropathic pain is complex. The initial event is often an insult or an injury to the somatosensory system. This is followed by a cascade of neuroimmunologic processes that lead to central and peripheral sensitization via activation and recruitment of resident macrophages or microglia and invasion of monocytes from the blood. Activated macrophages secreting matrix metalloproteases attack the basal lamina of blood vessels in the endoneurium, causing interruption of the blood–nerve barrier.[10] This leads to local production of proinflammatory factors, including TNF-α, calcitonin gene-related peptide, substance P, bradykinin, nerve growth factors, and other cytokines. The cytokines in turn trigger a pathway of events that leads to the modulation and increased expression of different ion channels, then leading to an increased neural response to a given sensory stimulus. This is what is commonly referred to as "peripheral sensitization."[10,11]

Pathogenic processes of neuropathic pain syndromes are not limited to peripheral nerves. An increasing body of evidence suggests that activation of microglial cells, recruitment of proinflammatory cells from the circulation, and similar glia–neuron interactions are present in the dorsal root ganglion (cell bodies of peripheral sensory neurons) and dorsal horn of the spinal cord (cell bodies of second-degree sensory neurons) as are seen in peripheral nerves.[11] These immune-mediated mechanisms of development of neuropathic pain have opened new doors for the development of targeted therapies to treat neuropathic pain beyond membrane ion channel blockers/modulators (gabapentinoids, carbamazepine) and agents that mimic or enhance endogenous inhibitory mechanisms (opioids, tricyclic antidepressants). Sensitization also occurs at the level of the CNS, where *N*-methyl-D-aspartate (NMDA) receptors play an important role. Central processing implies a phenomenon of spontaneous pulse generations within the CNS and increased gain in central processing circuits. Over the course of time, this leads to atrophy of inhibitory circuits through apoptosis.[10–13]

The perception and modulation of nociception at the level of the brain are even more complicated. The "neuromatrix" of pain comprises areas of brain activity in primary and secondary somatosensory areas and several subcortical structures and their complex interplay with descending pain-modulating pathways. Several studies have demonstrated structural alteration and neurochemistry and activation patterns in the brains of patients suffering from chronic pain.[2,3]

In summary, the neurobiology of chronic neuropathic pain is a complex interplay between neural–glial and immune mechanisms at peripheral and central levels and alteration of the basic pain matrix at the level of the brain.

CLINICAL FEATURES AND DIAGNOSIS

The IASP emphasizes that neuropathic pain is a description and not a diagnosis. Neuropathic pain requires demonstration of a lesion or a disease affecting the somatosensory system. Regardless of etiology, neuropathic pain generally presents with an electric, burning, lancinating, or shocklike character. It can be periodic or constant. The hallmark of neuropathic pain is sensory hypersensitivity, including dysesthesia (abnormal sensations), hyperesthesia (increased sensation for a given stimulus), hyperalgesia (increase pain from a noxious stimulus), and allodynia (pain from a nonnociceptive stimulus). The recognition of various neuropathic pain syndromes is generally clinical.

A thorough patient history often elicits pain distribution in radicular (spinal nerves) or peripheral patterns. Pain may also be distally present in the extremities (diabetic neuropathy) or in patches (leprosy). Distribution may occur around the site of a previous injury, as seen in CRPS. The pain is described as having a peculiar character that is electric, burning, lancinating, or shocklike. There may be signs of sensory dysfunction; therefore, a detailed modality-specific sensory exam is important. It is also important to note that pain/temperature and vibration/proprioception are carried by different peripheral fibers (Aα, Aβ for vibration/proprioception; Aδ, C for pain/temperature), and spinal pathways (dorsal column versus lateral spinothalamic tract) and their dysfunction can be discrete, independently leading to the development of neuropathic pain.

Many clinical tests are carried out to objectively evaluate sensory dysfunction. Electromyography (EMG) and nerve conduction studies (NCS) are very sensitive and can pick up changes in myelinated large-fiber (Aα, Aβ) sensory neuropathy, but will not pick up changes of the unmyelinated or thinly myelinated small fibers (type C and for the most part Aδ). If the suspicion is high for small-fiber neuropathy, a skin biopsy should be done and evaluated for free nerve ending density. It is worth mentioning that a recent study discovered objective evidence of small-fiber neuropathy in many patients who were thought to have fibromyalgia.[14]

Some neuropathic conditions, such as CRPS, lead to localized sympathetic dysregulation. For these patients, tests of autonomic functions like the thermoregulatory sweat test (TST) or the quantitative sudomotor axon reflex test (QSART) are available but are seldom used in clinical practice.

COMMON NEUROPATHIC PAIN SYNDROMES

CRPS

CRPS was first described by Silas Weir Mitchell in 1864 as *causalgia* (Greek *kausis* for burning and *algos* for pain) in Civil War soldiers who suffered from persistent burning pain after their injuries. Later discoveries leading to the recognition of a "sympathetic component" and the utility of sympathetic blockage in these patients prompted a change in nomenclature to *reflex sympathetic dystrophy*. However, the sympathetic component is not always present; hence, in 1993, the IASP renamed the condition *complex regional pain syndrome*.[1,15]

CRPS often presents with pain severity out of proportion to the severity of the inciting event or degree of tissue damage after several weeks in which any symptoms of tissue injury are expected to fully resolve. There may be a striking lack of physical or radiologic findings. CRPS is categorized as type I when it is assumed a nerve or nerves were damaged during the initial injury, often at the cellular level, or as type II when a large nerve injury can be seen.

The two most commonly used criteria for the diagnosis of CRPS are the IASP and Budapest criteria. The former are more inclusive but lead to many false positives and overdiagnoses (Box 12.1).

The symptoms of CRPS have a propensity to spread in the affected limb, often in a nondermatomal or peripheral nerve distribution pattern. Intense neuropathic pain associated with hyperalgesia and allodynia is common. In chronic forms, edema, warmth or cold from changes in skin blood flow, hair loss, and/or motor and trophic changes (muscle atrophy, weakness, skin lichenification, nail changes) are demonstrated.

Box 12.1. **DIAGNOSTIC CRITERIA FOR COMPLEX REGIONAL PAIN SYNDROME**

IASP Criteria

1. Presence of an initiating noxious event or reason for immobilization
2. Disproportional pain, allodynia, or hyperalgesia from a known inciting event
3. Sign or symptom or any evidence showing edema, skin changes, blood flow, or abnormal sudomotor activity in the region of the pain
4. No other condition that would otherwise explain the degree of pain or dysfunction

Budapest Criteria

Presence of continued disproportional pain from the known inciting event

1. Must report at least one symptom in three of the following four categories:
   - Sensory: hyperesthesia, allodynia
   - Vasomotor: temperature asymmetry, changes in skin color
   - Sudomotor/edema: edema, changes in sweating, sweating asymmetry
   - Motor/trophic: decreased range of motion, motor dysfunction (tremor, weakness, dystonia), trophic changes (hair, nail, skin)
2. Must report at least one sign in two or more of the following categories at the time of evaluation:
   - Sensory: hyperalgesia to pinprick, allodynia to touch or joint movement
   - Vasomotor: temperature asymmetry, color asymmetry
   - Sudomotor/edema: edema, asymmetrical sweating, sweating changes
   - Motor/trophic: decreased range of motion, motor dysfunction, trophic changes
3. No other condition that would otherwise explain the degree of pain or dysfunction

Diagnosis is clinical and made through a thorough history and physical exam. Common diagnostic tools used include quantitative sensory testing, tests of autonomic function, and imaging for trophic changes (plain X-ray films, MRI, and bone scans).

Treatment is difficult due to our lack of understanding of common pathophysiologic pathways. The multidisciplinary approach is essential and includes the use of PT modalities, topical and systemic pharmacotherapy, and interventional techniques.

Diabetic Neuropathy (DN)

DN, either subclinical or symptomatic, is a common problem, with neuropathic pain affecting more than 50% of diabetic patients.[16] There are different patterns of DN, with the most common being axonal length-dependent distal symmetric polyneuropathy, leading to neuropathic pain in distal extremities.

The pathophysiology of DN is theorized to have three mechanisms: the polyol pathway, which acts by converting the excess glucose in nerve endings to sorbitol, which interferes with nerve fiber function; microvascular ischemic damage to axons; and glycosylation end products that accumulate in and around axons and affect impulse conduction velocity.[15]

Diagnosis is clinical, through a thorough history and physical exam. Distal sensory loss and loss of ankle jerk reflex are common. Sensory ataxia and falls may occur due to loss of proprioceptive feedback. EMG and NCS are useful in the diagnosis but isolated small-fiber neuropathy leading to neuropathic pain is common.

Tight glycemic control is the single best intervention to halt the progression of DN and improve neuropathic pain. Other conservative and interventional modalities are used in combination to provide symptomatic relief.

Postherpetic Neuralgia (PHN)

PHN is a painful neuropathic condition that affects specific dermatomes following an episode of shingles or herpes zoster (HZ). HZ is a clinical condition involving the reactivation of a varicella-zoster virus infection after a latent period during states of reduced cell-mediated immunity. The viral eruption occurs in a dermatomal fashion, leading to a maculopapular or vesicular rash and an intense burning pain. The condition is treated with appropriate antiviral therapy (acyclovir, valacyclovir) and symptomatic treatment of neuropathic pain using a multimodal approach. Unfortunately, adequate treatment of HZ with antiviral medications does not preclude the later development of PHN.

Spondolytic Radicular Pain

Spondylosis is a collective term denoting degenerative changes in the spine, most often in the cervical and lumbar regions. It comprises facet arthropathy, ligamental thickening, and/or disk degeneration that collectively cause narrowing of the central spinal canal and lateral recess of the neural foramen, leading to spondylotic myelopathy and radiculopathy. Neuropathic pain is common in these conditions, and often occurs in the distribution of the affected spinal nerve root. In some cases of spinal cord compression, the pain is widespread. Often, the pain emerges acutely from disk herniation and causes acute compression of the nerve roots.

Treatment is initially conservative, consisting of PT, analgesics, and rest. Most cases of acute spondylotic radiculopathy (SR) resolve in a few weeks with conservative measures.[17] Chronic radicular pain generally responds well to a multimodal pain management approach, although surgery is needed in some intractable cases.

Central Neuropathic Pain

Chronic pain is a common complaint in patients who have survived a CNS insult (stroke, traumatic brain injury, multiple sclerosis, spinal cord injury). Chronic pain is commonly musculoskeletal and is often related to overuse of unaffected limbs, spasticity, and/or peri-articular weakness. However, many patients suffer from a distinct type of neuropathic pain, often in the distribution of their neurologic deficit. There is a clear distinction between central sensitization from peripheral causes of neuropathic pain and central neuropathic pain from a CNS injury, and the terms should not be used interchangeably.

Thought to occur due to partial or "discomplete" damage to central somatosensory circuits, central neuropathic pain can be disabling and, like any other chronic pain state, can adversely affect sleep and mood.[13] Patients typically complain of neuropathic pain in the distribution of neurologic dysfunction, and it can be constant or intermittent.

Because stroke is by far the most common form of CNS injury, the most frequent form of central neuropathic pain is post-stroke central pain (PSCP), which affects 2% to 8% of all stroke survivors. The onset is variable, from hours after the stroke to years afterward. The location of the brain injury appears to be a more important risk factor than the etiology of the stroke, and approximately one-third of all PSCP is related to thalamic strokes. Lateral medullary strokes also have a high incidence of neuropathic pain (25%), because they affect lateral spinothalamic projections.[13]

Patients with spinal cord injury are a special subset of patients, who are often young, and many of them develop neuropathic pain. The pain can be "below level," which is a pure CPS where pain is present in areas affected by the injury, or "at level," which is dermatomal in distribution, usually due to nerve root or dorsal horn injury.

Treatment is focused on alleviating symptoms and restoration of function. A multidisciplinary approach is employed, with a reported increase in success in recent years using neuromodulation techniques.

HIV-Associated Neuropathic Pain

Like DN, HIV-associated neuropathy is ubiquitous, but it becomes symptomatic in only a minority of patients. It is thought to occur due to accumulation of gp120, an HIV-associated glycoprotein, around neurons and glial cells, affecting ligand–receptor interactions. Patients who take highly active antiretroviral therapy are also prone to getting antiretroviral toxic neuropathy, which has an overlapping phenotype. The most common risk factors for the development of HIV-associated neuropathy before initiating highly active antiretroviral therapy are older age and advanced disease states.

Patients usually complain of neuropathic pain in symmetrical distal extremities that is associated with sensory deficits, allodynia, and hyperesthesia. A thorough history, an exam, and laboratory tests to rule out toxins and nutrient deficiencies should take place. Treatment is symptomatic, using various modalities, although small-scale studies have shown amitriptyline, topical lidocaine, and pregabalin to be ineffective.[15]

TREATMENT

The treatment of neuropathic pain is challenging and often does not result in complete resolution of symptoms. Some acute neuropathic pain conditions, such as acute radiculopathy from herniated disks, resolve well with time. Considering the complex and varied pathophysiology of neuropathic pain syndromes and their secondary effects on mood, sleep, and overall psychosocial well-being, a truly multidisciplinary approach should be employed. Because several mechanisms could be at play, the use of different pharmacologic agents with different mechanisms of action (e.g., antidepressants, gabapentinoids, topicals) has a higher chance of success in difficult-to-treat cases.

In general, conservative and nonpharmacologic therapies, such as massage therapy, biofeedback, and relaxation techniques, have all been proven to be effective in chronic neuropathic pain and should be widely employed.

Occupational Therapy (OT) and PT

Various PT and OT modalities, such as isometric strengthening, active range of motion, myofascial release, tactile desensitization, progressive weight-bearing, transcutaneous electrical nerve stimulation, and contrast bath therapy, have all been proven to be effective in the treatment of various conditions with neuropathic pain, notably CRPS.[15,18,19] Stretching exercises, core-strengthening and traction techniques, and active range of motion have been shown to ameliorate acute neuropathic pain in lumbar and cervical disk and spondylotic disease.[17]

PT should be goal-directed, meaning initiation of therapy at minimally tolerable levels with goals to increase activity each week or session. Therapy is geared toward facilitating the patient's physical activity and movement, and toward stimulation of the painful areas.

In patients unable to tolerate PT in the beginning, graded motor imagery and mirror therapy are particularly useful.[18]

Pharmacotherapy

Membrane Stabilizers

The so-called gabapentinoids, pregabalin and gabapentin, are generally regarded as first-line agents in the treatment of most conditions that lead to neuropathic pain by various societies, including the European Federation of Neurological Societies and the American Academy of Neurology.[20,21] A notable exception is trigeminal neuralgia, where the first-line agent is carbamazepine. The gabapentinoids work through the inhibition of voltage-gated calcium channels and are generally very well tolerated at therapeutic doses.

Antidepressants

Tricyclic antidepressants and selective serotonin-norepinephrine reuptake inhibitors (e.g., duloxetine, venlafaxine) have been widely used in the treatment of neuropathic pain with good success. They have the additional therapeutic effect of treating concomitant mood symptoms. Tricyclics, although generally more effective, are accompanied by anticholinergic and anti-adrenergic adverse effects (see Table 12.1).

Anticonvulsants

Carbamazepine, oxcarbazepine, and lamotrigine have been widely prescribed as adjunctive treatments for various neuropathic pain conditions. They work by blocking peripheral and central sodium channels. Caution should be exercised due to their systemic adverse effects, particularly with carbamazepine.

Opioids

Opioids are generally used after all other options have been tried and pain is functionally so incapacitating that the short-term benefits outweigh the potential risks. Long-term opioid therapy, however, is generally discouraged for nonmalignant

Table 12.1. **ADVERSE EFFECTS OF TRICYCLIC ANTIDEPRESSANTS**

Commonly Reported Adverse Effects (AEs)	Fewest AEs ↑ Most AEs	Tricyclic Antidepressants
• Blurred vision	Fewest AEs	• Desipramine
• Cognitive changes		• Nortriptyline
• Constipation		• Imipramine
• Dry mouth		• Doxepin
• Orthostatic hypotension		• Amitriptyline
• Sedation		
• Sexual dysfunction		
• Tachycardia		
• Urinary retention	Most AEs	

chronic pain. If opioids are prescribed, universal opioid prescription guidelines should be followed.

Topical Agents

The benefits of using topical agents include limiting systemic toxicity and side effects and ease of use. However, their absorption can be inadequate and may require frequent applications, thereby affecting compliance. Commonly used agents include anesthetics (e.g., lidocaine), capsaicin, menthol, camphor, and NSAIDs, such as diclofenac.

Other Agents

Steroids are widely prescribed in some acute painful neuropathic conditions, such as CRPS, carpal tunnel syndrome, and radiculopathy. The best evidence for their use is in CRPS, where studies have shown their effectiveness in alleviating symptoms in some patients.

Bisphosphonates have been found to be effective in treating patients with CRPS.[22]

Systemic and topical ketamine has shown much promise in the treatment of neuropathic pain. Other oral NMDA antagonists, such as memantine and dextromethorphan, are currently under investigation and have shown promise in early small-scale studies.[15]

Interventional Techniques

Interventional therapy should be considered part of a multidisciplinary approach to treating chronic neuropathic pain. Interventions vary based on specific clinical conditions. The most commonly employed techniques are neuraxial blocks (epidural injections), sympathetic blockage and/or ablative procedures, intrathecal pumps, and SCS.

Epidural injections are used to treat neuropathic pain associated with various conditions affecting spinal nerves and nerve roots (e.g., radiculopathy, PHN). Sympathetic blockage, radiofrequency ablation, and chemical neurolysis have been shown to be effective in treating symptoms in some patients with CRPS. There is fair evidence for their effectiveness in the short term, but they must be used in conjunction with other modalities geared toward long-term functional rehabilitation, including PT.[15]

SCS (dorsal column stimulation) has shown promise in the treatment of various neuropathic pain disorders, specifically CRPS and postlaminectomy syndrome (SR). Several studies have demonstrated its efficacy and cost-effectiveness.[23]

Intrathecal pumps should be used only after all other modalities have been exhausted. Intrathecal ziconotide, a potent calcium channel blocker extracted from sea snail venom, in particular, is very effective in treating refractory neuropathic pain, but it is almost always associated with unpleasant side effects.

CONCLUSIONS

- Neuropathic pain is a common condition and a major source of increasing healthcare costs.
- Most patients who have nociceptive pain syndromes also develop varying degrees of neuropathic pain.
- Neuropathic pain has a burning, shocklike, or lancinating character and is often present in a nerve distribution or in distal extremities.
- Peripheral and central sensitization and neuroimmunologic processes seem to play a large role in the pathogenesis of neuropathic pain.
- Common neuropathic pain conditions include CRPS, DN, PHN, SR, and CPS.
- Because neuropathic pain is often difficult to treat, a multimodality approach is required to improve patients' quality of life.

REFERENCES

1. International Association for the Study of Pain. IASP taxonomy. Available at: http://www.iasp-pain.org/Taxonomy?navItemNumber=576#Neuropathicpain. Last updated May 22, 2012. Accessed April 10, 2016.
2. Apkarian AV, Hashmi JA, Baliki MN. Pain and the brain: specificity and plasticity of the brain in clinical chronic pain. *Pain.* 2011;152:S49–S64.
3. Tracey I. Can neuroimaging studies identify pain endophenotypes in humans? *Nat Rev Neurol.* 2011;7:173–181.
4. Koop SM, ten Klooster PM, Vonkeman HE, Steunebrink LM, van de Laar MA. Neuropathic-like pain features and cross-sectional associations in rheumatoid arthritis. *Arthritis Res Ther.* 2015;17:237.
5. Moreton BJ, Tew V, das Nair R, Wheeler M, Walsh DA, Lincoln NB. Pain phenotype in patients with knee osteoarthritis: classification and measurement properties of painDETECT and self-report Leeds Assessment of Neuropathic Symptoms and Signs scale in a cross-sectional study. *Arthritis Care Res.* 2015;67:519–528.
6. Soni A, Batra RN, Gwilym SE, et al. Neuropathic features of joint pain: a community-based study. *Arthritis Rheum.* 2013;65:1942–1949.
7. Gaskin DJ, Richard P. The economic costs of pain in the United States. *J Pain.* 2012;13:715–724.
8. Johannes CB, Le TK, Zhou X, Johnston JA, Dworkin RH. The prevalence of chronic pain in United States adults: results of an Internet-based survey. *J Pain.* 2010;11:1230–1239.
9. Torrance N, Smith BH, Bennett MI, Lee AJ. The epidemiology of chronic pain of predominantly neuropathic origin. Results from a general population survey. *J Pain.* 2006;7:281–289.
10. Scholz J, Woolf CJ. The neuropathic pain triad: neurons, immune cells and glia. *Nat Neurosci.* 2007;10:1361–1368.
11. Krames ES. The role of the dorsal root ganglion in the development of neuropathic pain. *Pain Med.* 2014;15:1669–1685.
12. Bouhassira D, Attal N. Translational neuropathic pain research: a clinical perspective. *Neuroscience.* 2016;338:27–35.
13. Watson JC, Sandroni P. Central neuropathic pain syndromes. *Mayo Clin Proc.* 2016;91(3):372–385.
14. Oaklander AL, Herzog ZD, Downs HM, Klein MM. Objective evidence that small-fiber polyneuropathy underlies some illnesses currently labeled as fibromyalgia. *Pain.* 2013;154:2310–2316.
15. Hurley RW, Henriquez OH, Wu CL. Neuropathic pain syndromes. In: Benzon HT, Rathmell JP, Wu CL, Turk DC, Argoff CE, Hurley RW, eds. *Practical Management of Pain.* 5th ed. Maryland Heights, MO: Mosby; 2013.
16. Sadosky A, McDermott AM, Brandenburg NA, Strauss M. A review of the epidemiology of painful diabetic peripheral neuropathy,

postherpetic neuralgia, and less commonly studied neuropathic pain conditions. *Pain Pract.* 2008;8:45–56.

17. Saal JA, Saal JS. Nonoperative treatment of herniated lumbar intervertebral disc with radiculopathy. An outcome study. *Spine.* 1989;14:431–437.
18. Daly AE, Bialocerkowski AE. Does evidence support physiotherapy management of adult complex regional pain syndrome type one? A systematic review. *Eur J Pain.* 2009;13:339–353.
19. van de Meent H, Oerlemans M, Bruggeman A, et al. Safety of "pain exposure" physical therapy in patients with complex regional pain syndrome type 1. *Pain.* 2011;152:1431–1438.
20. Attal N, Cruccu G, Baron RA, et al. EFNS guidelines on the pharmacological treatment of neuropathic pain: 2010 revision. *Eur J Neurol.* 2010;17(9):1113.
21. Bril V, England J, Franklin GM, et al. Evidence-based guideline: treatment of painful diabetic neuropathy: report of the American Academy of Neurology, the American Association of Neuromuscular and Electrodiagnostic Medicine, and the American Academy of Physical Medicine and Rehabilitation. *PM&R.* 2011;3(4):345–352.
22. Giusti A, Bianchi G. Treatment of complex regional pain syndrome type I with bisphosphonates. *RMD Open.* 2015;1(suppl 1):e000056.
23. Hurley RW, Burton AW. Spinal cord and peripheral nerve stimulation. In: Benzon HT, Rathmell JP, Wu CL, Turk DC, Argoff CE, Hurley RW, eds. *Practical Management of Pain.* 5th ed. Maryland Heights, MO: Mosby; 2013.

REVIEW QUESTIONS

1. Which of the following scenarios represents a predominantly neuropathic painful condition?

A. A 42-year-old woman with a bandlike headache
B. A 76-year-old man with severe retrosternal burning chest pain after meals
C. A 38-year-old man with electric shocklike facial pain
D. An 81-year-old man with crushing low back pain upon standing straight

2. Which of the following agents, if used in treatment of neuropathic pain, is most likely to interfere with sodium channel function in the dorsal root ganglia?

A. Lamotrigine
B. Pregabalin
C. Doxepin
D. Topical lidocaine

3. A 67-year-old woman has burning pain in her feet. Molecular analysis of her nerve endings shows high levels of sorbitol. The single most important intervention that could change the course of her disease is:

A. Initiation of pregabalin
B. Tight glycemic control
C. Consultation with a podiatrist
D. Genetic testing

ANSWERS

1. C. A man with shocklike facial pain is most likely suffering from trigeminal neuralgia, which is a neuropathic pain condition. Bandlike headaches are likely to be tension headaches; therefore, answer A is not correct. Retrosternal burning chest pain is most likely pain from esophageal reflux disease, so answer B is not correct. The elderly patient with low back pain has spondylotic axial back pain associated with degenerative joint disease, also known as facet arthropathy, and may respond well to medial branch nerve block and radiofrequency denervation. His pain is not neuropathic, and therefore answer D is incorrect.

2. A. Lamotrigine is an antiepileptic drug that exerts its analgesic effect in neuropathic pain by blocking sodium channels. Pregabalin is a voltage-gated calcium channel blocker and doxepin is a tricyclic antidepressant. Lidocaine blocks sodium channels in peripheral nerve endings and will not have an effect in the dorsal root ganglia. Therefore, the only correct answer is A

3. B. The patient has DN, as evidenced by sorbitol accumulation in the axons. Several studies have shown that tight glycemic control halts, and in some cases improves, symptoms related to DN; therefore, answer B is correct.[15,16,21] Her pain can be treated with pregabalin but it is not known to affect the underlying pathologic process. Podiatry consult and genetic testing will not change the course of disease.

QUESTIONS AND ANSWERS

This chapter has accompanying questions and answers that are available to subscribers as part of the Oxford eLearning platform. To access the questions, follow the link below, or go to ✔ http://oxfordmedicine.com/painmanagementreview

13.

PHANTOM LIMB PAIN

Kenneth D. Candido, Teresa M. Kusper, Alexei Lissounov, and Nebojsa Nick Knezevic

STEM CASE AND KEY QUESTIONS

A 37-year-old Operation Iraqi Freedom veteran with no prior medical history comes to a pain clinic for an initial evaluation of his chronic right lower extremity pain, which severely interferes with his lifestyle. The patient lost his leg from the hip joint distally during his last deployment 8 months earlier. Since that time, he has been feeling a severe aching, sometimes burning, pain in the area of the right foreleg and the dorsum of the foot. He is also experiencing an occasional less severe pain in the stump of the same extremity. He wears a prosthesis and has already had it replaced twice thinking that it might be too tight or improperly built. The patient appears despondent and states that he "is losing his mind." He appears to be severely depressed.

WHAT ARE THE PHANTOM PAIN SYNDROMES AND HOW DO THEY DIFFER FROM EACH OTHER? WHICH ONES DO YOU SUSPECT IN THIS PATIENT?

You evaluate the patient and attempt to explain to him that he may suffer from a phantom pain syndrome. Phantom pain syndromes include phantom sensation, phantom limb pain (PLP), and residual (stump) pain. PLP (post-amputation pain, PAP) is a feeling of pain in the missing extremity, while phantom sensation is the experience of nonpainful sensations emanating from the missing body part, and residual pain is a painful sensation in the remaining portion of the body part. PAP most frequently involves the extremities, but it can also be associated with other body parts (e.g., a breast after a mastectomy). The patient's symptoms are most consistent with PLP and residual (stump) pain.

WHAT ARE THE RISK FACTORS FOR PLP? WILL THE PAIN EVER GO AWAY?

In evaluating PLP you recognize that it is a common occurrence after the loss of an extremity. During the interview with the patient, you evaluate him for some of the multiple risk factors that might predispose one to developing PLP, such as pain in the body part before the amputation, presence of phantom sensations after the amputation, stump pain, use of a prosthesis, and increased time from the amputation. You reassure the patient that phantom pain can resolve or decrease in intensity over time; however, it is not uncommon for it to persist for several months or even for years after the amputation.

WHAT IS THE BEST INITIAL APPROACH IN MANAGING PLP?

Analyzing the best treatment option for your patient, you decide to begin with multimodal therapy incorporating antidepressants and anticonvulsants for the neuropathic pain, nonsteroidal anti-inflammatory drugs (NSAIDs) or opioid medications for the achy type pain, and physical and behavioral therapy. The patient is started on nortriptyline, gabapentin, and tramadol and is referred for cognitive-behavioral therapy and physical therapy. On subsequent visits, a significant improvement is noted in the patient's affect and he reports improved sleep quality; however, his pain is only slightly improved. Over the course of several weeks, the patient underwent multiple nerve blocks and he has been using a transcutaneous electrical nerve stimulator (TENS unit), but the results are still barely noticeable. The patient inquires about the benefits of electrostimulation therapy.

WHAT KINDS OF INTRACRANIAL STIMULATION ARE AVAILABLE, AND HOW DO THEY DIFFER?

Available methods of intracranial stimulation include deep brain stimulation (DBS) and motor cortex stimulation (MCS). MCS involves placing electrodes connected to an implantable battery-operated stimulator. DBS is more extensive because it entails implanting electrodes deeper in the brain. Because your patient failed both conservative and interventional management and is still experiencing intractable pain, he is a candidate for neurostimulation. The patient consents to MCS. He reports an initial 60% pain reduction 1 month after the surgery, and at the 6-month follow-up visit, he reports 80% reduction of both phantom and residual stump pain.

DISCUSSION

PAP has challenged clinicians for centuries. The first written record of this perplexing condition came from the

16th-century French military surgeon Ambrose Paré.[1] The term *phantom limb pain* was coined by Silas Weir Mitchell, who provided a comprehensive description of the condition during the 19th century.[2]

EPIDEMIOLOGY

PAP is a dreaded and yet prevalent consequence of an amputation. There are multiple risk factors for PAP, such as pain in the body part before the amputation, presence of phantom sensations after the amputation, stump pain, use of a prosthesis, and increased time from the amputation.[3] Furthermore, PAP is not limited to the extremities: it has been described after loss of the tongue,[4] a breast,[5,6] and parts of the GI[7] and urinary tracts.[8] The pain can occur within weeks, months, or even several years after the amputation. The incidence of PAP at 8 days, 6 months, and 2 years after amputation is reported to be as high as 72%, 65%, and 59%, respectively.[9] Prevalence of PLP ranges among different authors from 44.6% to 79.9%; the differences can be attributed to a variation in timing of the pain onset and reasons for the amputations.[10–13] According to the Healthcare Cost and Utilization Project (1988–1996) data on reasons for amputations, vascular disease is the most likely pathology (Figure 13.1), accounting for 82% of all nonmilitary limb amputations, followed by trauma (16.4%), cancer (0.9%), and congenital anomalies (0.8%).[14]

A population-based study of Medicare claims between 1996 and 1997 revealed an annual rate of 3.83 amputations per 1,000 individuals with diabetes, compared to an annual rate of 0.38 per 1,000 nondiabetic individuals.[15] Among surveyed military veterans (N = 2,750), PLP was reported by 78%, and only 1% reported lasting pain relief from a multitude of attempted treatments.[16] These data correspond with a survey of 298 Vietnam War and 283 Operation Iraqi Freedom/Operation Enduring Freedom (OIF/OEF) veterans, which revealed PLP prevalence rates of 72.2% and 76%, respectively.[17] It is predicted that the number of limbs lost in the United States will grow from 1.6 million in 2005 to 3.6 million by the year 2050.[18]

PATHOGENESIS

Theories explaining the emergence of PLP have greatly evolved, from the theory that it is primarily a psychiatric condition with origins in the patient's brain, to a theory that encompasses complex, and perhaps intertwined, mechanisms in the peripheral, spinal, and supraspinal neural circuitry. Peripherally, tissue injury causes neuroma formation characterized by loss of myelin from large-diameter axons and axonal sprouting, leading to the upregulation of the voltage-gated sodium channels in the neural membrane, and subsequently causing an increased sensitivity to external stimuli, as well as generation of ectopic impulses in the primary afferents.[19] Axonal sprouting of the severed peripheral nerve, which forms synaptic connections with the neurons within the spinal cord, and sprouting of the Aβ mechanoreceptors into lamina 2 of the dorsal horn of the spinal cord, lead to central sensitization characterized by increased neuronal activity and an increase in the neuronal receptive field.[20–22] This process also leads to increased activity of the *N*-methyl-D-aspartate (NMDA) receptors mediated by substance P, tachykinins, and neurokinins, followed by the "windup phenomenon"—a facilitation of dorsal horn activity with upregulation of the NMDA receptors, increased firing of the nociceptive neurons, and diminished inhibitory input of the descending pathways.[23] The supraspinal mechanism involves a reorganization of the sensory and motor cortices in the amputee's brain, where the area representing the lost body part is replaced by the adjacent cortical areas.[24–27] Thalamic changes might also be implicated, since phantom sensation

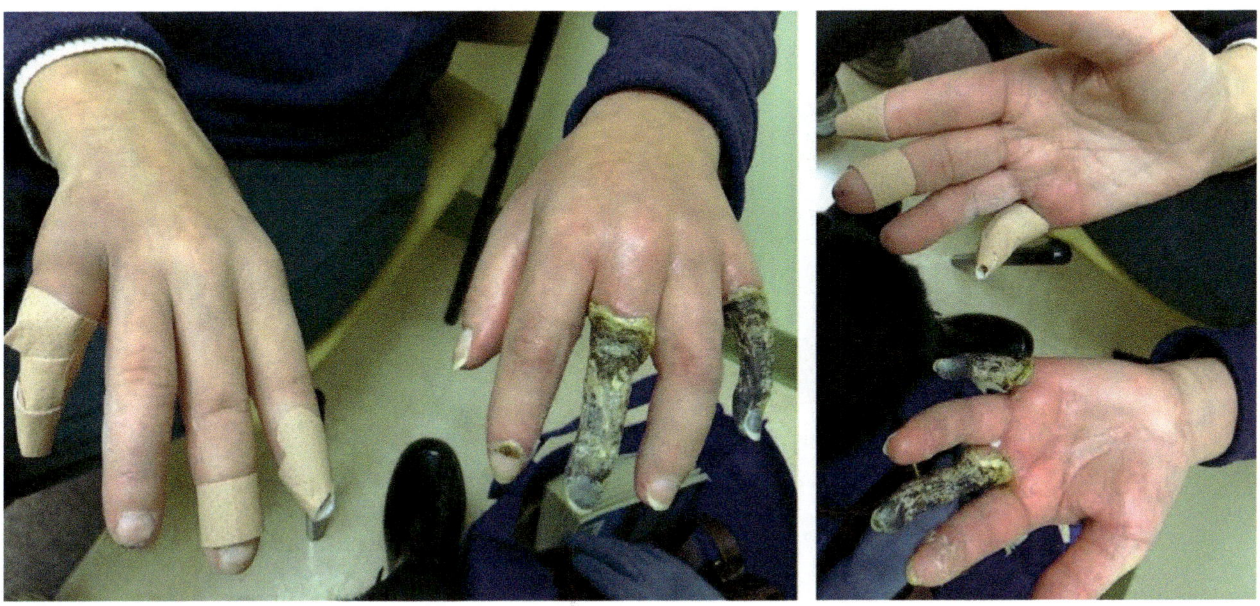

Figure 13.1. Digital photographs of dry gangrene of the phalanges due to prolonged ischemia. Vascular disease is one of the most common pathologies accounting for nontraumatic amputations. Photo courtesy of Kenneth D. Candido, MD.

and pain have been elicited in amputees during stimulation of the thalamus.[28] Le Feuvre and Aldington based their observation on the lack of a single therapy and the lack of preventive tools on the interplay of multiple mechanisms in development of PLP.[29]

CLINICAL MANIFESTATION AND DIAGNOSIS

Phantom pain syndromes include three separate entities: phantom sensation, phantom pain, and residual (stump) pain. These syndromes might occur independently of each other or coexist in a given individual after a limb loss.[30] The characteristics of PLP vary: common pain descriptors include sharp, throbbing, piercing, dull, squeezing, tingling, burning, or cramping. The concept of "telescoping" described in the literature is characterized by a loss of sensation in the middle portion of the limb, which produces an illusion that the lost limb is shorter than its normal counterpart.[31] Physical examination has limited utility in diagnosing PLP and at the present time, there is no established diagnostic test that aids in reaching the diagnosis. An important aspect of the initial evaluation is to carefully examine the amputee and to inspect the affected part for skin abrasions, local infections, or bony exostosis—this assessment helps to avoid misdiagnosis and to identify factors that can aggravate PLP. Other serious pathologies must be ruled out, such as residual limb ischemia, joint sepsis, vasculitis, or complex regional pain syndrome (Figure 13.2).

PREVENTION

Preemptive analgesia implemented during the pre- and postoperative period has been utilized in an attempt to diminish the noxious stimuli that trigger hyperplastic changes at the amputation site and central sensitization, which are believed to serve as amplifiers of future noxious stimuli.[32] The success of peripheral neural blockade in reducing PLP was assessed in 71 patients scheduled for lower extremity amputation. The patients were started on a continuous epidural infusion of 0.5% ropivacaine pre- or intraoperatively and the infusion was continued for 4 to 83 days after the surgery.[33] The authors reported that 73% of the amputees experienced severe to intolerable pain on postoperative day 1, while only 3% experienced it 12 months later.[33] In a different study, 30 patients were randomized to receive either preoperative epidural bupivacaine or intra- and postoperative perineural bupivacaine.[34] Although there was no evidence that either of the treatments was superior to the other, the study revealed decreasing severity of pain in both groups over time (63% and 88% at 6 months, and 38% and 50% at 12 months).[34] The results of these two trials contrast with the study by Nikolajsen et al., who examined the long-term effect on PLP in 60 limb amputees who were randomly assigned to receive either pre- and postoperative epidural bupivacaine and morphine or epidural saline with oral or IM morphine.[35] No changes in the response was noted between the two study groups at 1 week, and 3, 6, 9, or 12 months.[35] Although perioperative epidural infusions might appear to be of value for some patients in preventing or terminating phantom pain, based on the disparity of study results, the applicability of this approach in routine care is uncertain.

Studies assessing the effect of regional anesthetic techniques on PLP prevention have also yielded dichotomous results. A few separate studies looked at perineural and intraneural bupivacaine blocks administered intra- or postoperatively, and found no significant differences between the treatment group and the controls.[36,37] A chart review of 39 amputees showed a lower incidence of PLP in patients who received continuous nerve sheath catheter analgesia.[38]

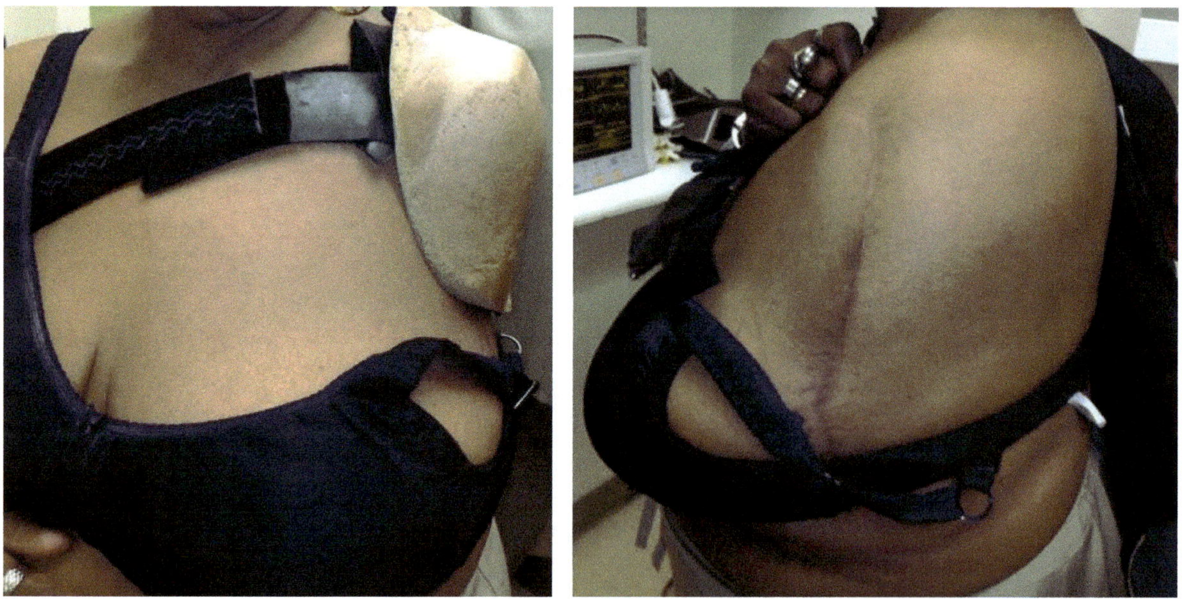

Figure 13.2. Digital photographs of a complete left upper extremity amputation at the shoulder joint in a patient treated for chronic phantom limb pain. Photo courtesy of Kenneth D. Candido, MD.

TREATMENT

Pharmacologic Management

Although a variety of treatments have been proposed to address phantom pain, there is little evidence from randomized, placebo-controlled trails to guide clinicians with a standardized treatment.[39] McCormick et al. analyzed current therapeutic modalities that are based on the three pathophysiologic targets: peripheral/afferent, central, and efferent pathways, and indicated a lack of level 1 evidence for a specific treatment of PLP.[40] In 2011, a Cochrane review suggested only a short-term analgesic efficacy for morphine, gabapentin, and ketamine.[41]

Acetaminophen and NSAIDs are among the most commonly used pharmacologic agents but demonstrated only mild pain relief in patients with PLP when compared to opioids.[42] Studies examining the efficacy of opioids for PLP have shown a significant, albeit short-term, reduction of pain after oral and intravenous morphine.[43,44] Analgesic benefits were also noted after tramadol and methadone treatments.[45,46]

Tricyclic antidepressants (TCAs) and anticonvulsants have been used efficaciously in a number of neuropathic pain states.[47] The primary goal of targeting the neuropathic component of PLP has led to early use of pregabalin, gabapentin, and/or amitriptyline, which are considered efficacious despite contradictory study results.[41,48,49] Additional case series have shown equivalent efficacy and fewer side effects for nortriptyline and desipramine.[50] Mirtazapine, an α_2-receptor antagonist, demonstrated therapeutic benefit in a small case series, and it is associated with fewer side effects than TCAs.[51]

Infusion of the NMDA receptor antagonist ketamine perioperatively and continued for 72 hours postoperatively might reduce the incidence of PLP at 6 months postoperatively.[52] Additionally, ketamine infusion has been associated with a reduction in the pain scores in various amputees at different postoperative time points.[53,54] However, oral memantine had no effect on the intensity of PLP.[55,56] Other medications, such as calcitonin[57,58] and propranolol,[59,60] have shown mixed results in PLP therapy.

Injections

Although several interventional techniques have been investigated, the available data failed to confirm lasting benefit. Nerve blocks and trigger-point injections have yielded short-term pain reduction, but the results are insufficient to support any definitive conclusions.[61–64] A case report of successful coblation of the femoral and sciatic nerves describes a remarkable 80% pain reduction in both phantom and stump pain at 1, 3, and 6 months after the procedure.[65] Studies on botulinum toxin type A injections have demonstrated promising results in relieving residual limb pain (RLP) and PLP in a small number of amputees.[66–68]

Complementary Modalities

The effectiveness of noninvasive complementary modalities is described mostly in case reports. Transcutaneous electrical nerve stimulation (TENS), which delivers a mild electrical current to cutaneous nerve fibers, provided approximately 50% pain reduction for the studied individuals.[69,70] Despite these positive results, a recent Cochrane review found no good-quality randomized controlled trials (RCTs) that assess the effectiveness of TENS for PLP.[71]

First accounts of mirror therapy date back to 1996, when it was used to help amputee patients to resolve the visual-proprioceptive dissociation in their brains.[72,73] This strategy interferes with somatosensory inputs and blocks protopathic pain perception in the phantom limb.[74,75] The effectiveness of the approach has been confirmed in an RCT with 22 patients assigned to a mirror, a covered mirror, and mental visualization groups during a 4-week period. The study showed pain reduction in the first group (uncovered mirror), but not in the other two groups.[76] In an RCT (N = 26) comparing mirror therapy with TENS, no statistically significant difference was found in the efficacies of the two modalities, although both study groups derived pain relief.[77]

Additional noninvasive therapies currently explored for PLP treatment include biofeedback,[78] acupunture,[79] behavioral techniques,[80,81] and electroconvulsive therapy (ECT).[82] Transcranial magnetic stimulation (TMS) produces a relevant clinical improvement of as much as 63% in neuropathic and deafferentation pain syndromes.[83–87] However, in studies of TMS of the cortex in patients with PLP, only transient pain relief was noted, and it could not be sustained for a longer period of time.[88] Due to a paucity of data, further investigation is required to assess the usefulness of TMS in providing significant, long-lasting pain reduction.

Invasive Interventions

Invasive therapies are indicated for individuals who fail conservative treatment. Destructive interventions, such as neuroablative neuroma resection, dorsal root entry zone lesioning (DREZ), anterolateral cordotomy, thalamotomy, and sympathectomy, are typically considered in cases of severe refractory PLP. Electrostimulation therapy has been successfully used in a number of cases of chronic neuropathic pain, which prompted its use in treating PLP. A meta-analysis of 11 studies using noninvasive therapy and 22 studies of invasive brain stimulation showed 72.6% and 45.3% response rates, respectively.[89] A substantial clinical improvement was described in case reports of ECT use in PLP patients with refractory pain.[82,90] Bitar et al. assessed the clinical outcome with DBS of the periventricular gray and somatosensory thalamus in three individuals with PLP, and found 62% pain reduction (range 55% to 70%) in all three patients.[91]MCS, which targets the precentral gyrus, is considered an acceptable procedure for PLP, with therapeutic efficacy comparable to DBS. Sol et al. used MCS in three amputees with refractory pain and reported initial pain relief in all three individuals, and continuing pain reduction in two of the three patients at 2-year follow-up.[92]

Spinal cord stimulation (SCS) is the most commonly performed invasive procedure for treatment of PLP (Figure 13.3). SCS requires regular maintenance and

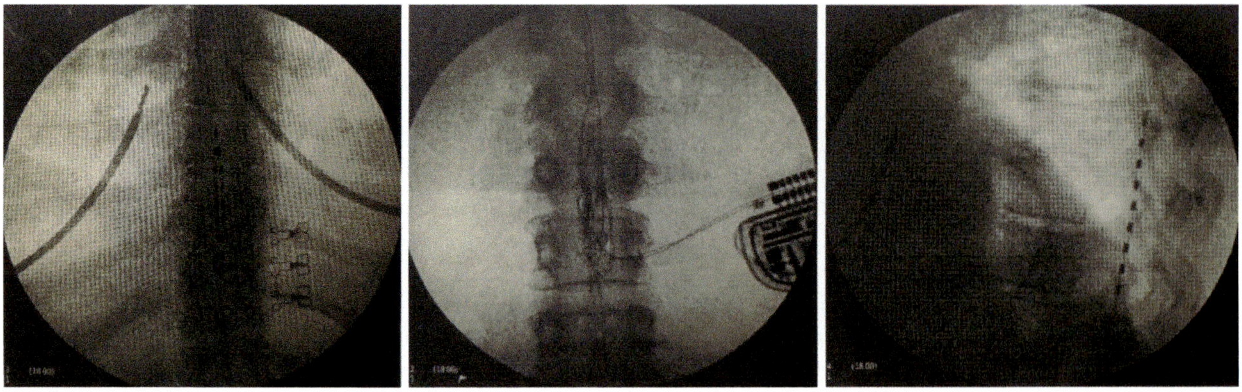

Figure 13.3. Radiographic images of the spinal cord stimulator showing leads placed at the T7 level, as well as implantable pulse generator (IPG). Photo courtesy of Kenneth D. Candido, MD.

reprogramming visits, which is why careful patient selection followed by psychologic evaluation is of paramount importance. SCS use ameliorates PLP to a significant degree, and in one particular study with four participants, all experienced > 80% pain reduction.[93] Unfortunately, a decline in the effectiveness over time has been reported, as evidenced in a study of 84 patients (63 amputees), where the therapeutic benefit decreased from 52.4% at the 2-year follow-up to 39% 5 years after placement.[94] A novel approach, high-frequency electrical nerve block, where an electrode is wrapped around the nerve of interest, has been analyzed in a pilot study of seven PLP patients, and 75% pain reduction was observed 3 months after the procedure.[95]

CONCLUSIONS

- PLP is a common consequence of limb amputation, with high prevalence among traumatic and nontraumatic amputees.
- The most frequent pathologies leading to limb loss are vascular disease, trauma, cancer, and congenital anomalies.
- Pathophysiology of PLP involves the peripheral, spinal, and supraspinal levels of the nervous system.
- Tissue injury at the periphery leads to neuroma formation and accumulation of voltage-gated sodium channels.
- Central sensitization and windup phenomenon cause increased activity of the nociceptive fibers in the spinal cord.
- Cortical reorganization and thalamic plasticity are observed at the supraspinal levels.
- A wide range of treatment options are available, with varying effectiveness.
- TCAs, anticonvulsants, and opioids are the mainstays of the conservative treatment approach.
- Injections might be of value for a select group of patients.
- Electrostimulation therapy and neuromodulation are indicated in refractory cases of PLP.

REFERENCES

1. Weinstein SM. Phantom limb pain and related disorders. *Neurol Clin.* 1998;16(4):919–936.
2. Louis ED, York GK. Weir Mitchell's observations on sensory localization and their influence on Jacksonian neurology. *Neurology.* 2006;66(8):1241–1244.
3. Manchikanti L, Singh V. Managing phantom pain. *Pain Physician.* 2004;7(3):365–375.
4. Hanowell ST, Kennedy SF. Phantom tongue pain and causalgia: case presentation and treatment. *Anesth Analg.* 1979;58(5):436–438.
5. Jamison K, Wellisch DK, Katz RL, Pasnau RO. Phantom breast syndrome. *Arch Surg.* 1979;114(1):93–95.
6. Rothemund Y, Grusser SM, Liebeskind U, Schlag PM, Flor H. Phantom phenomena in mastectomized patients and their relation to chronic and acute pre-mastectomy pain. *Pain.* 2004;107(1-2):140–146.
7. Fingren J, Lindholm E, Carlsson E. Perceptions of phantom rectum syndrome and health-related quality of life in patients following abdominoperineal resection for rectal cancer. *J Wound Ostomy Continence Nurs.* 2013;40(3):280–286.
8. Biley FC. Phantom bladder sensations: a new concern for stoma care workers. *Br J Nurs.* 2001;10(19):1290–1296.
9. Jensen TS, Krebs B, Nielsen J, Rasmussen P. Immediate and long-term phantom limb pain in amputees: incidence, clinical characteristics and relationship to pre-amputation limb pain. *Pain.* 1985;21(3):267–278.
10. Ehde DM, Czerniecki JM, Smith DG, et al. Chronic phantom sensations, phantom pain, residual limb pain, and other regional pain after lower limb amputation. *Arch Phys Med Rehabil.* 2000;81(8):1039–1044.
11. Ephraim PL, Wegener ST, MacKenzie EJ, Dillingham TR, Pezzin LE. Phantom pain, residual limb pain, and back pain in amputees: results of a national survey. *Arch Phys Med Rehabil.* 2005;86(10):1910–1919.
12. Kooijman CM, Dijkstra PU, Geertzen JH, Elzinga A, van der Schans CP. Phantom pain and phantom sensations in upper limb amputees: an epidemiological study. *Pain.* 2000;87(1):33–41.
13. Schley MT, Wilms P, Toepfner S, et al. Painful and nonpainful phantom and stump sensations in acute traumatic amputees. *J Trauma.* 2008;65(4):858–864.
14. Dillingham TR, Pezzin LE, MacKenzie EJ. Limb amputation and limb deficiency: epidemiology and recent trends in the United States. *South Med J.* 2002;95(8):875–83.
15. Wrobel JS, Mayfield JA, Reiber GE. Geographic variation of lower-extremity major amputation in individuals with and without diabetes in the Medicare population. *Diabetes Care.* 2001;24(5):860–864.
16. Sherman RA, Sherman CJ, Parker L. Chronic phantom and stump pain among American veterans: results of a survey. *Pain.* 1984;18(1):83–95.

17. Reiber GE, McFarland LV, Hubbard S, et al. Service members and veterans with major traumatic limb loss from Vietnam War and OIF/OEF conflicts: survey methods, participants, and summary findings. *J Rehab Res Dev.* 2010;47(4):275–297.
18. Ziegler-Graham K, MacKenzie EJ, Ephraim PL, Travison TG, Brookmeyer R. Estimating the prevalence of limb loss in the United States: 2005 to 2050. *Arch Phys Med Rehabil.* 2008;89(3): 422–429.
19. Devor M, Govrin-Lippmann R, Angelides K. Na^+ channel immunolocalization in peripheral mammalian axons and changes following nerve injury and neuroma formation. *J Neurosci.* 1993;13(5): 1976–1992.
20. Flor H, Nikolajsen L, Staehelin Jensen T. Phantom limb pain: a case of maladaptive CNS plasticity? *Nat Rev Neurosci.* 2006;7(11):873–81.
21. Dickinson BD, Head CA, Gitlow S, Osbahr AJ III. Maldynia: pathophysiology and management of neuropathic and maladaptive pain—a report of the AMA Council on Science and Public Health. *Pain Med.* 2010;11(11):1635–1653.
22. Woolf CJ, Shortland P, Coggeshall RE. Peripheral nerve injury triggers central sprouting of myelinated afferents. *Nature.* 1992;355(6355):75–78.
23. Baron R. Mechanisms of disease: neuropathic pain—a clinical perspective. *Nat Clin Pract Neurol.* 2006;2(2):95–106.
24. Karl A, Birbaumer N, Lutzenberger W, Cohen LG, Flor H. Reorganization of motor and somatosensory cortex in upper extremity amputees with phantom limb pain. *J Neurosci.* 2001;21(10): 3609–3618.
25. Flor H, Elbert T, Knecht S, et al. Phantom-limb pain as a perceptual correlate of cortical reorganization following arm amputation. *Nature.* 1995;375(6531):482–484.
26. Birbaumer N, Lutzenberger W, Montoya P, et al. Effects of regional anesthesia on phantom limb pain are mirrored in changes in cortical reorganization. *J Neurosci.* 1997;7(14):5503–5508.
27. Reilly KT, Sirigu A. The motor cortex and its role in phantom limb phenomena. *Neuroscientist.* 2008; 14(2): 195–202.
28. Davis KD, Kiss ZH, Luo L, Tasker RR, Lozano AM, Dostrovsky JO. Phantom sensations generated by thalamic microstimulation. *Nature.* 1998;391(6665):385–387.
29. Le Feuvre P, Aldington D. Know pain know gain: proposing a treatment approach for phantom limb pain. *J R Army Med Corps.* 2014;160(1):16–21.
30. Flor H. Phantom-limb pain: characteristics, causes, and treatment. *Lancet Neurol.* 2002;1(3):182–189.
31. Jensen TS, Krebs B, Nielsen J, Rasmussen P. Phantom limb, phantom pain and stump pain in amputees during the first 6 months following limb amputation. *Pain.* 1983;17(3):243–256.
32. Reuben SS, Buvanendran A. Preventing the development of chronic pain after orthopaedic surgery with preventive multimodal analgesic techniques. *J Bone Joint Surg Am.* 2007;89(6):1343–1358.
33. Borghi B, Bugamelli S, Stagni G, Missiroli M, Genco R, Colizza MT. Perineural infusion of 0.5% ropivacaine for successful treatment of phantom limb syndrome: a case report. *Minerva Anestesiol.* 2009;75(11):661–664.
34. Lambert A, Dashfield A, Cosgrove C, Wilkins D, Walker A, Ashley S. Randomized prospective study comparing preoperative epidural and intraoperative perineural analgesia for the prevention of postoperative stump and phantom limb pain following major amputation. *Reg Anesth Pain Med.* 2001;26(4):316–321.
35. Nikolajsen L, Ilkjaer S, Christensen JH, Kroner K, Jensen TS. Randomised trial of epidural bupivacaine and morphine in prevention of stump and phantom pain in lower-limb amputation. *Lancet.* 1997;350(9088):1353–1357.
36. Fisher A, Meller Y. Continuous postoperative regional analgesia by nerve sheath block for amputation surgery—a pilot study. *Anesth Analg.* 1991;72(3):300–303.
37. Pinzur MS, Garla PG, Pluth T, Vrbos L. Continuous postoperative infusion of a regional anesthetic after an amputation of the lower extremity. A randomized clinical trial. *J Bone Joint Surg Am.* 1996;78(10):1501–1505.
38. Morey TE, Giannoni J, Duncan E, Scarborough MT, Enneking FK. Nerve sheath catheter analgesia after amputation. *Clin Orthop Relat Res.* 2002;397:281–289.
39. Halbert J, Crotty M, Cameron ID. Evidence for the optimal management of acute and chronic phantom pain: a systematic review. *Clin J Pain.* 2002;18(2):84–92.
40. McCormick Z, Chang-Chien G, Marshall B, Huang M, Harden RN. Phantom limb pain: a systematic neuroanatomical-based review of pharmacologic treatment. *Pain Med.* 2014;15(2):292–305.
41. Alviar MJ, Hale T, Dungca M. Pharmacologic interventions for treating phantom limb pain. *Cochrane Database Syst Rev.* 2011;12:CD006380.
42. Hanley MA, Ehde DM, Campbell KM, Osborn B, Smith DG. Self-reported treatments used for lower-limb phantom pain: descriptive findings. *Arch Phys Med Rehabil.* 2006;87(2):270–277.
43. Huse E, Larbig W, Flor H, Birbaumer N. The effect of opioids on phantom limb pain and cortical reorganization. *Pain.* 2001;90(1-2):47–55.
44. Wu CL, Tella P, Staats PS, et al. Analgesic effects of intravenous lidocaine and morphine on postamputation pain: a randomized double-blind, active placebo-controlled, crossover trial. *Anesthesiology.* 2002;96(4):841–848.
45. Wilder-Smith CH, Hill LT, Laurent S. Postamputation pain and sensory changes in treatment-naive patients: characteristics and responses to treatment with tramadol, amitriptyline, and placebo. *Anesthesiology.* 2005;103(3):619–628.
46. Bergmans L, Snijdelaar DG, Katz J, Crul BJ. Methadone for phantom limb pain. *Clin J Pain.* 2002;18(3):203–205.
47. Finnerup NB, Otto M, McQuay HJ, Jensen TS, Sindrup SH. Algorithm for neuropathic pain treatment: an evidence based proposal. *Pain.* 2005;118(3):289–305.
48. Nikolajsen L, Finnerup NB, Kramp S, Vimtrup AS, Keller J, Jensen TS. A randomized study of the effects of gabapentin on postamputation pain. *Anesthesiology.* 2006;105(5): 1008–1015.
49. Spiegel DR, Lappinen E, Gottlieb M. A presumed case of phantom limb pain treated successfully with duloxetine and pregabalin. *Gen Hosp Psychiatry.* 2010;32(2):228–227.
50. Jefferies K. Treatment of neuropathic pain. *Semin Neurol.* 2010;30(4):425–432.
51. Kuiken TA, Schechtman L, Harden RN. Phantom limb pain treatment with mirtazapine: a case series. *Pain Pract.* 2005;5(4):356–360.
52. Hayes C, Armstrong-Brown A, Burstal R. Perioperative intravenous ketamine infusion for the prevention of persistent post-amputation pain: a randomized, controlled trial. *Anaesth Intensive Care.* 2004;32(3):330–338.
53. Nikolajsen L, Hansen CL, Nielsen J, Keller J, Arendt-Nielsen L, Jensen TS. The effect of ketamine on phantom pain: a central neuropathic disorder maintained by peripheral input. *Pain.* 1996;67(1):69–77.
54. Eichenberger U, Neff F, Sveticic G, et al. Chronic phantom limb pain: the effects of calcitonin, ketamine, and their combination on pain and sensory thresholds. *Anesth Analg.* 2008;106(4): 1265–1273.
55. Wiech K, Kiefer RT, Topfner S, et al. A placebo-controlled randomized crossover trial of the *N*-methyl-D-aspartic acid receptor antagonist, memantine, in patients with chronic phantom limb pain. *Anesth Analg.* 2004;98(2):408–413.
56. Maier C, Dertwinkel R, Mansourian N, et al. Efficacy of the NMDA-receptor antagonist memantine in patients with chronic phantom limb pain—results of a randomized double-blinded, placebo-controlled trial. *Pain.* 2003;103(3):277–283.
57. Jaeger H, Maier C. Calcitonin in phantom limb pain: a double-blind study. *Pain.* 1992;48(1):21–27.
58. Simanski C, Lempa M, Koch G, Tiling T, Neugebauer E. [Therapy of phantom pain with salmon calcitonin and effect on postoperative patient satisfaction.] *Chirurg.* 1999;70(6):674–681.
59. Scadding JW, Wall PD, Parry CB, Brooks DM. Clinical trial of propranolol in post-traumatic neuralgia. *Pain.* 1982;14(3):283–292.
60. Marsland AR, Weekes JW, Atkinson RL, Leong MG. Phantom limb pain: a case for beta blockers? *Pain.* 1982;12(3):295–297.

61. Borghi B, D'Addabbo M, Borghi R. Can neural blocks prevent phantom limb pain? *Pain Manag.* 2014;4(4):261–266.
62. Wassef MR. Phantom pain with probable reflex sympathetic dystrophy: efficacy of fentanyl infiltration of the stellate ganglion. *Reg Anesth.* 1997;22(3):287–290.
63. Lierz P, Schroegendorfer K, Choi S, Felleiter P, Kress HG. Continuous blockade of both brachial plexus with ropivacaine in phantom pain: a case report. *Pain.* 1998;78(2):135–137.
64. Reiestad F, Kulkarni J. Role of myofascial trigger points in post-amputation pain: causation and management. *Prosthet Orthot Int.* 2013;37(2):120–123.
65. Zeng Y, Wang X, Guo Y, He L, Ni J. Coblation of femoral and sciatic nerve for stump pain and phantom limb pain: a case report. *Pain Pract.* 2016;16(2):E35–E41.
66. Kern U, Martin C, Scheicher S, Muller H. [Long-term treatment of phantom- and stump pain with botulinum toxin type A over 12 months. A first clinical observation.] *Nervenarzt.* 2004;75(4):336–340.
67. Kern U, Martin C, Scheicher S, Muller H. [Treatment of phantom pain with botulinum-toxin A. A pilot study.] *Schmerz.* 2003;17(2):117–124.
68. Jin L, Kollewe K, Krampfl K, Dengler R, Mohammadi B. Treatment of phantom limb pain with botulinum toxin type A. *Pain Med.* 2009;10(2):300–303.
69. Giuffrida O, Simpson L, Halligan PW. Contralateral stimulation, using TENS, of phantom limb pain: two confirmatory cases. *Pain Med.* 2010;11(1):133–141.
70. Mulvey MR, Radford HE, Fawkner HJ, Hirst L, Neumann V, Johnson MI. Transcutaneous electrical nerve stimulation for phantom pain and stump pain in adult amputees. *Pain Pract.* 2013;13(4):289–296.
71. Johnson MI, Mulvey MR, Bagnall AM. Transcutaneous electrical nerve stimulation (TENS) for phantom pain and stump pain following amputation in adults. *Cochrane Database Syst Rev.* 2015;8:CD007264.
72. Ramachandran VS, Rogers-Ramachandran D. Synaesthesia in phantom limbs induced with mirrors. *Proc Biol Sci.* 1996;263(1369):377–386.
73. Feinberg TE. Brain and self: bridging the gap. *Conscious Cogn.* 2011;20(1):2–3.
74. Ramachandran VS, Rogers-Ramachandran D. Sensations referred to a patient's phantom arm from another subject's intact arm: perceptual correlates of mirror neurons. *Med Hypotheses.* 2008;70(6):1233–1234.
75. Rossi S, Tecchio F, Pasqualetti P, et al. Somatosensory processing during movement observation in humans. *Clin Neurophysiol.* 2002;113(1):16–24.
76. Chan BL, Witt R, Charrow AP, et al. Mirror therapy for phantom limb pain. *N Engl J Med.* 2007;357(21):2206–2207.
77. Tilak M, Isaac SA, Fletcher J, et al. Mirror therapy and transcutaneous electrical nerve stimulation for management of phantom limb pain in amputees—a single blinded randomized controlled trial. *Physiother Res Int.* 2016;21(2):109–115.
78. Harden RN, Houle TT, Green S, et al. Biofeedback in the treatment of phantom limb pain: a time-series analysis. *Appl Psychophysiol Biofeedback.* 2005;30(1):83–93.
79. Bradbrook D. Acupuncture treatment of phantom limb pain and phantom limb sensation in amputees. *Acupunct Med.* 2004;22(2):93–97.
80. MacIver K, Lloyd DM, Kelly S, Roberts N, Nurmikko T. Phantom limb pain, cortical reorganization and the therapeutic effect of mental imagery. *Brain.* 2008;131(pt 8):2181–2191.
81. Ramachandran VS, Brang D, McGeoch PD. Size reduction using mirror visual feedback (MVF) reduces phantom pain. *Neurocase.* 2009;15(5):357–360.
82. Rasmussen KG, Rummans TA. Electroconvulsive therapy for phantom limb pain. *Pain.* 2000;85(1-2):297–299.
83. Andre-Obadia N, Peyron R, Mertens P, Mauguiere F, Laurent B, Garcia-Larrea L. Transcranial magnetic stimulation for pain control. Double-blind study of different frequencies against placebo, and correlation with motor cortex stimulation efficacy. *Clin Neurophysiol.* 2006;117(7):1536–1544.
84. Lefaucheur JP, Hatem S, Nineb A, et al. Somatotopic organization of the analgesic effects of motor cortex rTMS in neuropathic pain. *Neurology.* 2006;67(11):1998–2004.
85. Hirayama A, Saitoh Y, Kishima H, et al. Reduction of intractable deafferentation pain by navigation-guided repetitive transcranial magnetic stimulation of the primary motor cortex. *Pain.* 2006;122(1-2):22–27.
86. Khedr EM, Kotb H, Kamel NF, Ahmed MA, Sadek R, Rothwell JC. Longlasting antalgic effects of daily sessions of repetitive transcranial magnetic stimulation in central and peripheral neuropathic pain. *J Neurol Neurosurg Psychiatry.* 2005;76(6):833–838.
87. Saitoh Y, Hirayama A, Kishima H, et al. Stimulation of primary motor cortex for intractable deafferentation pain. *Act Neur S.* 2006;99:57–59.
88. Topper R, Foltys H, Meister IG, Sparing R, Boroojerdi B. Repetitive transcranial magnetic stimulation of the parietal cortex transiently ameliorates phantom limb pain-like syndrome. *Clin Neurophysiol.* 2003;114(8):1521–1530.
89. Lima MC, Fregni F. Motor cortex stimulation for chronic pain: systematic review and meta-analysis of the literature. *Neurology.* 2008;70(24):2329–2337.
90. Fukui S, Shigemori S, Yoshimura A, Nosaka S. Chronic pain with beneficial response to electroconvulsive therapy and regional cerebral blood flow changes assessed by single photon emission computed tomography. *Reg Anesth Pain Med.* 2002;27(2):211–213.
91. Bittar RG, Otero S, Carter H, Aziz TZ. Deep brain stimulation for phantom limb pain. *J Clin Neurosci.* 2005;12(4):399–404.
92. Sol JC, Casaux J, Roux FE, et al. Chronic motor cortex stimulation for phantom limb pain: correlations between pain relief and functional imaging studies. *Stereot Funct Neuros.* 2001;77(1-4):172–176.
93. Viswanathan A, Phan PC, Burton AW. Use of spinal cord stimulation in the treatment of phantom limb pain: case series and review of the literature. *Pain Pract.* 2010;10(5):479–484.
94. Krainick JU, Thoden U, Riechert T. Pain reduction in amputees by long-term spinal cord stimulation. Long-term follow-up study over 5 years. *J Neurosurg.* 1980;52(3):346–350.
95. Soin A, Shah NS, Fang ZP. High-frequency electrical nerve block for postamputation pain: a pilot study. *Neuromodulation.* 2015;18(3):197–205.

REVIEW QUESTIONS

1. All of the following are considered risk factors for development of PLP, except:

A. Pain in the limb before it is amputated
B. Use of a prosthesis
C. Presence of diabetes mellitus
D. Residual pain

2. Which of the following processes characterizes the windup phenomenon?

A. Reorganization of the somatomotor cortex in response to amputation
B. Sprouting of axons at proximal peripheral afferent fibers
C. Facilitation of dorsal horn activity and exaggerated firing of dorsal neurons
D. Loss of the descending inhibitory pathway

3. An elderly diabetic patient develops PLP after below-knee amputation of his left lower extremity. He is subsequently placed on a medication that is supposed to reduce

the neuropathic pain that he experiences. During a follow-up visit, the patient mentions dry mouth, flushing, and urinary retention. Physical exam is notable for dry skin and dilated pupils. Which of the following medications is the most likely culprit?

A. Pregabalin
B. Imipramine
C. Tramadol
D. Fluoxetine

ANSWERS

1. C. The most common risk factors for developing PLP are: pain in the limb before amputation (A), use of a prosthesis (B), and residual pain (D).[3] While diabetes mellitus is one of the leading causes of amputation, no direct relationship has been established between the disease and PLP; therefore, the correct answer is C.

2. C. Windup phenomenon is a process of facilitation of dorsal horn activity characterized by an upregulation of the NMDA receptors, increased firing of nociceptive neurons, and diminished inhibitory input of the descending pathways.[23] Answer A is incorrect because reorganization of the somatomotor cortex involves replacement of the area that represents the lost limb with the neighboring areas of the cortex.[24–27] Sprouting of axons at the proximal peripheral afferent fibers results from tissue injury at the periphery,[20–22] and is one of the preceding steps in the development of the windup phenomenon; therefore, answer B is incorrect. Loss of the descending inhibitory pathway occurs after amputation at the time of facilitation of dorsal horn activity, but does not explain the windup process; therefore, answer D is incorrect.

3. B. The patient presents with signs and symptoms suggestive of anticholinergic toxidrome, which can include any of the following signs and symptoms: dry skin, mydriasis, fever, flushing, hallucinations, psychosis, urinary retention, seizures, and coma. TCAs (nortriptyline, amitriptyline, imipramine, and desipramine), albeit efficacious in this condition, might result in the anticholinergic syndrome.[47] Pregabalin, tramadol, and fluoxetine are not known to cause anticholinergic symptoms; therefore, answers A, C, and D are incorrect.

QUESTIONS AND ANSWERS

This chapter has accompanying questions and answers that are available to subscribers as part of the Oxford eLearning platform. To access the questions, follow the link below, or go to

✔ http://oxfordmedicine.com/painmanagementreview

14.

CHRONIC CHEST WALL PAIN IN POSTHERPETIC NEURALGIA

Kenneth D. Candido, Teresa M. Kusper, and Nebojsa Nick Knezevic

STEM CASE AND KEY QUESTIONS

A 52-year-old female with a history of rheumatoid arthritis (treated with chronic methotrexate therapy) and atopic dermatitis (treated with frequent topical steroid use) presented to a pain management center with a complaint of a constant stinging pain across the chest wall and spreading to the back of several months' duration. She rated the pain as "10/10" on a 0 to 10 visual analog scale. The patient reported an exquisite sensitivity to light touch, and stated that touch by clothing worsened the pain. The pain resulted in a significant decline in her quality of life. She had not slept well in weeks, was avoiding intimacy with her partner, and stopped using public transportation to work due to excruciating pain upon skin contact. She tried Tylenol and ibuprofen, which didn't relieve her pain, and hydrocodone prescribed by her primary doctor gave her no relief while causing headaches and constipation. On physical examination, exquisite tenderness was elicited by palpating the chest wall, with tactile allodynia and hyperalgesia to pinprick noted in the right T5 dermatome. Mild skin hypopigmentation was noted along the affected skin area.

WHAT IS POSTHERPETIC NEURALGIA (PHN)? DOES HERPES ZOSTER (HZ) OCCUR IN ALL INDIVIDUALS WITH A HISTORY OF CHICKENPOX? WHICH RISK FACTORS INCREASE SUSCEPTIBILITY TO PHN?

Upon physical examination, you suspect that the patient suffers from PHN, which is a known complication of acute HZ virus reactivation. It is also called *shingles*, and results from the reactivation of the varicella-zoster virus (VZV), the etiologic agent of chickenpox. As is typical in PHN, the patient complained of constant burning or stinging pain, with intermittent lancinating or shooting sensations in a unilateral dermatomal pattern, and that persisted beyond the healing period of the skin eruption. *Zoster sine herpete* is a comparable entity that is also characterized by a neuropathic pain in a dermatomal distribution, but which is not preceded by the typical herpetic rash. Upon further questioning, the patient mentioned having had a painful rash across her chest about 8 months ago. She hadn't been evaluated by her PCP because she attributed the skin changes to eczema that she had been struggling with her entire life. Both her atopic dermatitis and her rheumatoid arthritis required immunomodulating therapy that predisposed the patient to acute HZ. Additionally, the fact that she did not take antivirals during the acute phase of the disease increased the likelihood of progression to PHN.

WHAT SHOULD BE INCLUDED IN THE DIFFERENTIAL DIAGNOSIS?

The differential diagnosis of radiating chest wall pain includes angina, myocardial infarction, pleurodynia, pericarditis, costochondritis (Tietze's syndrome), spinal nerve compression, thoracic facet joint arthropathy, intercostal nerve entrapment, myofascial pain, peptic ulcer disease, biliary colic, and other acute abdominal processes. All life-threatening conditions must be ruled out before full attention is given to non-emergent causes of the pain.

HOW IS HZ DIAGNOSED? IS LABORATORY WORKUP NECESSARY TO DIAGNOSE HZ?

The diagnosis of HZ is almost exclusively clinical when the pain is accompanied by the distinctive vesicular rash or skin changes resulting from the healed skin eruption. The challenge arises in the absence of any cutaneous manifestations of the disease, such as in *zoster sine herpete*. In those instances, VZV reactivation is confirmed with laboratory testing involving evaluation of the serum anti-VZV IgG level, direct immunofluorescent antigen staining, or polymerase chain reaction for VZV DNA. Elevated levels of antibodies to VZV in patients without a prior vaccination against VZV are indicative of the reactivation of the virus. In this patient, hypopigmentation was noted along the affected dermatome, raising suspicion for a recent herpes infection. Therefore, her pain was attributed to VZV reactivation, and confirmatory testing was not indicated.

WHAT OPTIONS ARE AVAILABLE FOR TREATMENT OF PHN, AND WHICH ONES WOULD BENEFIT THIS PATIENT THE MOST?

The overarching focus of PHN treatment is to break the pain cycle and to prevent the development of a chronic pain syndrome, which can be achieved with a number of pharmacologic agents, including tricyclic antidepressants (TCAs), anticonvulsants, topical analgesics, and opioids. An individual's needs and response to therapy must be considered when formulating the best treatment strategy. The goals of treatment for this individual were fivefold: alleviate the spontaneous neuropathic pain, reduce hypersensitivity and allodynia, restore sleep, improve psychologic health, and facilitate a return to normal activities. With those objectives in mind, the patient was started on a regimen consisting of nortriptyline, gabapentin, and tramadol in place of hydromorphone. On her follow-up visit, the patient reported minimal pain improvement and severe drowsiness that impaired her performance at work. The pain continued despite switching to pregabalin, dose escalation of the TCA and opioid, and initiation of a Lidoderm patch. Over a 1-year period, the patient underwent multiple injections, including intercostal and sympathetic nerve blocks, which provided inadequate and short-term pain relief.

Box 14.1. **RISK FACTORS FOR PHN IN PATIENTS WITH ACUTE HZ**

- Increasing age
- Female sex
- Presence of a prodrome
- Greater rash severity
- Greater acute pain severity
- Immunosuppressive therapy
- Neoplasms
- Organ transplantation
- HIV infection and other diseases resulting in impaired cell-mediated immunity

WHAT ARE THE INDICATIONS FOR NEUROMODULATION? WHAT ARE THE MOST COMMON COMPLICATIONS OF THE PROCEDURE?

An implantable neurostimulation device is recommended for intractable pain of the trunk and/or limbs refractory to other forms of treatment. It is indicated for a number of chronic pain syndromes, including post-laminectomy syndrome, radiculopathies, complex regional pain syndrome type I or type II, peripheral neuropathy, and PHN, among many others. Possible adverse effects include infection, hematoma, CSF leakage, lead migration, unpleasant stimulation, and pain at the insertion site. Given the treatment failure with oral and topical analgesics, and a suboptimal response to multiple nerve blocks, the patient could be considered a reasonable candidate for spinal cord stimulation (SCS). After a detailed and frank discussion about the risks and benefits of SCS, the patient decided to proceed with a percutaneous SCS dual lead trial, followed by permanent SCS device placement. At the 6-month follow-up visit, she reported 80% pain reduction, which enabled her to resume her everyday activities and to eliminate use of most of her oral pain medications.

DISCUSSION

EPIDEMIOLOGY AND PATHOGENESIS

The incidence of HZ in the United States is 3.2 cases per 1,000 person-years, with 60% of cases reported in females, and the majority occurring in individuals between the ages of 50 and 79.[1] PHN is the most frequently occurring complication of HZ, with an estimated incidence of 120,000 to 200,000 cases per year.[2] There are several risk factors that predispose patients to development of PHN (Box 14.1).[3,4]

Primary VZV infection, commonly called chickenpox, usually occurs in childhood in nonimmune individuals, after which the virus remains latent in the sensory ganglia (dorsal root ganglion; DRG). Increased age, stress, immunosuppression, or impaired cell-mediated immunity may lead to reactivation of the virus, during which the virus travels to the epidermis, triggering the acute phase of HZ. Increased age is the most common risk factor for development of HZ, and age > 60 is the most commonly reported association, possibly due to reduced cell-mediated immunity.

Although multiple theories have emerged to explain the pathogenesis of PHN, an exact mechanism has not been fully elucidated. Two separate processes have been described that might be implicated in the emergence of PHN. First, peripheral sensitization may be induced by the inflammatory mediators substance P, histamine, and cytokines due to HZ, which leads to a heightened sensitivity of the dorsal horn neurons to incoming signals from the periphery, and consequently culminates in allodynia and hyperalgesia.[5,6] The second process involves deafferentation of central neurons or alteration of the central nociceptive circuitry, leading to a state of intense spontaneous pain with or without allodynia.[7] The latter process stems from the neural damage that occurs either as a direct sequela of the VZV in the DRG or indirectly from tissue inflammation induced by the infection, causing swelling, ischemia, and demise of the nerve cells.[2,5] Pathologic abnormalities observed in patients with PHN include a loss of innervation in the epidermis, an axonal degeneration in the primary afferents, atrophied dorsal horn, and fibrosis of the DRG.[8]

CLINICAL MANIFESTATIONS OF HZ AND PHN

The most common initial symptoms of HZ infection are pain (41%), itching (27%), and paresthesias (12%).[9] Other prodromal symptoms include headache, photophobia, malaise, and occasional fever. A characteristic rash erupts within 1 to 2 days (Figure 14.1) in a unilateral dermatomal distribution. The rash starts out as maculopapular and transforms into fluid-filled vesicles.

The vesicles crust over after 7 to 10 days and the rash generally resolves within 3 to 4 weeks. Scarring or hypopigmentation

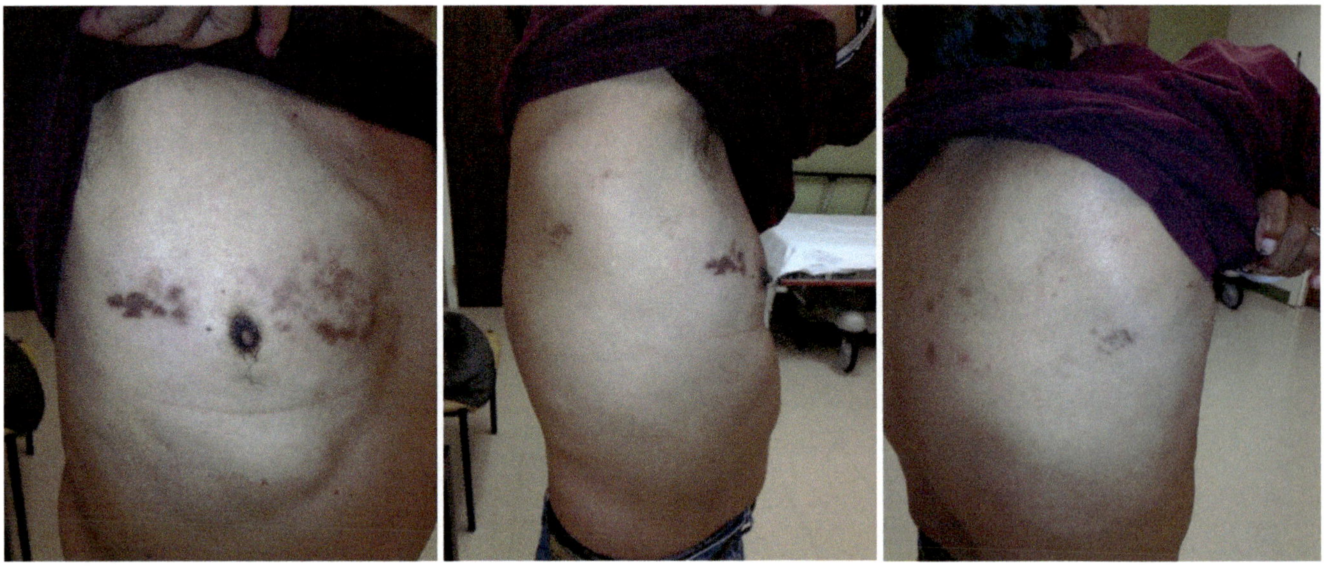

Figure 14.1. Cutaneous manifestation of varicella-zoster virus. Clusters of vesicular herpes zoster rash are distributed along a thoracic dermatome. Photo courtesy of Kenneth D. Candido, MD.

after the rash resolves might ensue. A variety of potential complications have been reported in patients with acute HZ, including neurologic complications (Ramsay Hunt syndrome), ophthalmic involvement (acute retinal necrosis), dermatologic involvement (secondary bacterial infections), and visceral complications (esophagitis, hepatitis).[10] PHN is the most commonly encountered complication, manifested by an intense, unrelenting, spontaneous, deep, aching or burning pain, with intermittent shooting or electrical-type sensations, and evoked allodynia (pain in response to an innocuous stimulus), dysesthesias (abnormal sensation without a stimulus), or hyperalgesia (exaggerated pain with a painful stimulus).[11] Thoracic dermatomes are the most frequently affected (45%), followed by the cervical dermatomes (23%).[9] PHN is a highly debilitating condition that negatively affects all life domains: physical, psychologic, functional, and social.[10]

PREVENTION OF HZ AND PHN

Zostavax is a live attenuated VZV vaccine approved by the FDA for the prevention of HZ in individuals > 50 years old.[12] The effectiveness of the vaccine has been demonstrated by various investigators.[13–15] According to the Shingles Prevention Study, the vaccine is 51.2% and 66.5% effective in preventing HZ and PHN, respectively.[15] The incidence of PHN is decreased by 39% in patients with HZ who received the vaccination.[13] An advisory committee on immunization practices recommends routine vaccination of individuals > 60 years old, unless otherwise contraindicated.[13]

TREATMENT OF HZ AND PREVENTION OF PHN

The goals in treating HZ are to terminate the symptoms of the acute infection, prevent secondary infections, and avert possible sequelae, such as including PHN. Antiviral medications (acyclovir, famciclovir, or valacyclovir), which inhibit viral DNA replication, are considered the first-line treatment options (Table 14.1).

Prompt treatment with antivirals initiated within 72 hours after eruption of the rash has been shown to hasten recovery and diminish pain during the acute zoster infection.[16–18] Concomitant use of prednisone with antivirals has been shown to diminish pain during the active infection.[19] Studies assessing the effect of antivirals on PHN yielded conflicting evidence, with some studies showing no benefit in preventing PHN,[20] and others reporting decreased symptom duration.[21,22] Eighty-five patients diagnosed with PHN were assessed 6 months after acute HZ, and only 2.6% of patients treated with antivirals within 72 hours of rash onset reported neuropathic pain, compared to 18.6% of those who did not receive antiviral treatment.[23]

Sympathetic blocks, such as stellate ganglion blocks, are one of the main interventional techniques used to treat the pain due to HZ (Figure 14.2). Winnie and Hartwell investigated the correlation between the time of treatment of acute HZ infection with sympathetic blocks and the prevention of PHN.[24] Sympathetic blockade was performed at various times after the onset of the symptoms in 122 patients. The pain of acute HZ resolved and PHN was prevented or alleviated in 80% of patients who received treatment within a 2-month window.[24] After that time, the effectiveness of the treatment was markedly reduced and more sympathetic blocks were required to obtain a favorable response. The authors postulated that, if administered early, the block restores intraneural blood flow before irreversible ischemic damage occurs, thereby preventing the death of large nerve fibers within the affected nerves, and ultimately preventing the emergence of PHN.[24]

Table 14.1. PHARMACOTHERAPY FOR ACUTE HZ AND PHN

TREATMENT OF ACUTE HERPES ZOSTER		TREATMENT OF POSTHERPETIC NEURALGIA		
MEDICATION	DOSE	MEDICATION	DOSE	SIDE EFFECTS
Antivirals		Tricyclic antidepressants		Dry mouth, blurry vision, urinary retention, constipation, sweating, drowsiness, dysrhythmia
– Acyclovir	800 mg 5x/day for 7–10 days	– Amitriptyline	10–25 mg at bedtime; Max: 150 mg/day	
– Famciclovir	500 mg 3x/day for 7 days	– Nortriptyline		
		– Imipramine		Somnolence, blurred vision, dizziness, fatigue, ataxia, peripheral edema
– Valacyclovir	1,000 mg 3x/day for 7 days	– Desipramine		
– Brivudine	125 mg once/day for 7 days			
		Anticonvulsants	100–300 mg 3x/day;	Nausea, emesis, constipation, diarrhea, headache, dizziness, vertigo, anxiety
Prednisone	60 mg once/day for 7 days; taper down for 2 more weeks	– Gabapentin	Max: 1800 mg/day	
		– Pregabalin	150–300 mg/day; Max: 600 mg/day	
		Atypical opioid	50–100 mg 4x/day	
		Tramadol		
		Topical analgesics		
		5% lidocaine patch	1 patch/day 12 h (up to 3 patches/time)	Local skin irritation
		Capsaicin	Apply to skin 3–5x/day (cream) 8% patch: Apply every 12 h	Burning sensation and skin irritation

Modified from Sampathkumar et al.[36] and Stankus et al.[37]

TREATMENT OF CHEST WALL PAIN IN PHN

Conservative Management

Conservative management involves the use of TCAs, antiepileptics (AEDs), opioids, lidocaine transdermal patch, and capsaicin lotion or patch (Table 14.1). Their analgesic efficacy is supported by a meta-analysis of 35 randomized controlled trials (RCTs).[25] TCAs and AEDs are considered the first-line treatment, while narcotics are usually utilized for a breakthrough pain. Gabapentin and pregabalin are the two most extensively studied anticonvulsant medications. They both bind the $\alpha_2\delta$ subunit of the voltage-gated calcium channel, thereby inhibiting the release of excitatory neurotransmitters, but pregabalin has the advantage of better absorption and linear kinetics, allowing easier titration. The efficacy of gabapentin in PHN has been established in a RCT of 229 patients randomized to either gabapentin or placebo groups, with a maximum dose of 3600 mg/day of gabapentin titrated over a 4-week period.[26] The success of pregabalin in reducing neuropathic pain and improving sleep and mood with PHN has been demonstrated by two large independent RCTs.[27,28] In one trial, pain reduction of > 50% was attained by 26% of patients on 150 mg/day and 28% on 300 mg/day.[27] Freynhagen et al. corroborated these results by showing > 50% pain reduction in 48.2% of patients on a flexible 12-week schedule (150, 300, 450, and 600 mg/day of pregabalin titrated weekly), and 52.3% of patients on a fixed-dose regimen of 300 mg/day for 1 week followed by 600 mg/day for 11 more weeks.[28] The role of opioids in treatment of neuropathic pain has been debated by some investigators,[29,30] but the efficacy of opioids in treatment of PHN has been supported by a few distinct clinical trials.[31–33] A comparison of opioids and TCAs carried out by Raja et al. demonstrated greater pain reduction with opioids compared to TCAs in 76 patients suffering from PHN (38% and 32%).[31] This finding correlates with other reports that showed a favorable response after tramadol[33] and oxycodone treatments.[32] Topical analgesics represent a viable treatment option due to the ease of application and low risk of systemic toxicity. Lidocaine transdermal patch has been studied extensively and it has shown effectiveness in reducing postherpetic pain. A literature review of 20 studies on 5% lidocaine patch has revealed a positive effect, especially on allodynia, without anesthesia or diminished cutaneous sensitivity.[34] Similarly, the value of capsaicin topical preparations in treating neuropathic pain has been presented in a Cochrane review of six studies ($N = 389$) on the cream, and two studies ($N = 709$) on the 8% patch formulation.[35]

Interventional Techniques

The literature indicates that an injection of corticosteroids, with or without a local anesthetic, and sympathetic blockade might be valuable treatment options for a select group of patients. Sympathetic nerve blocks have been routinely used

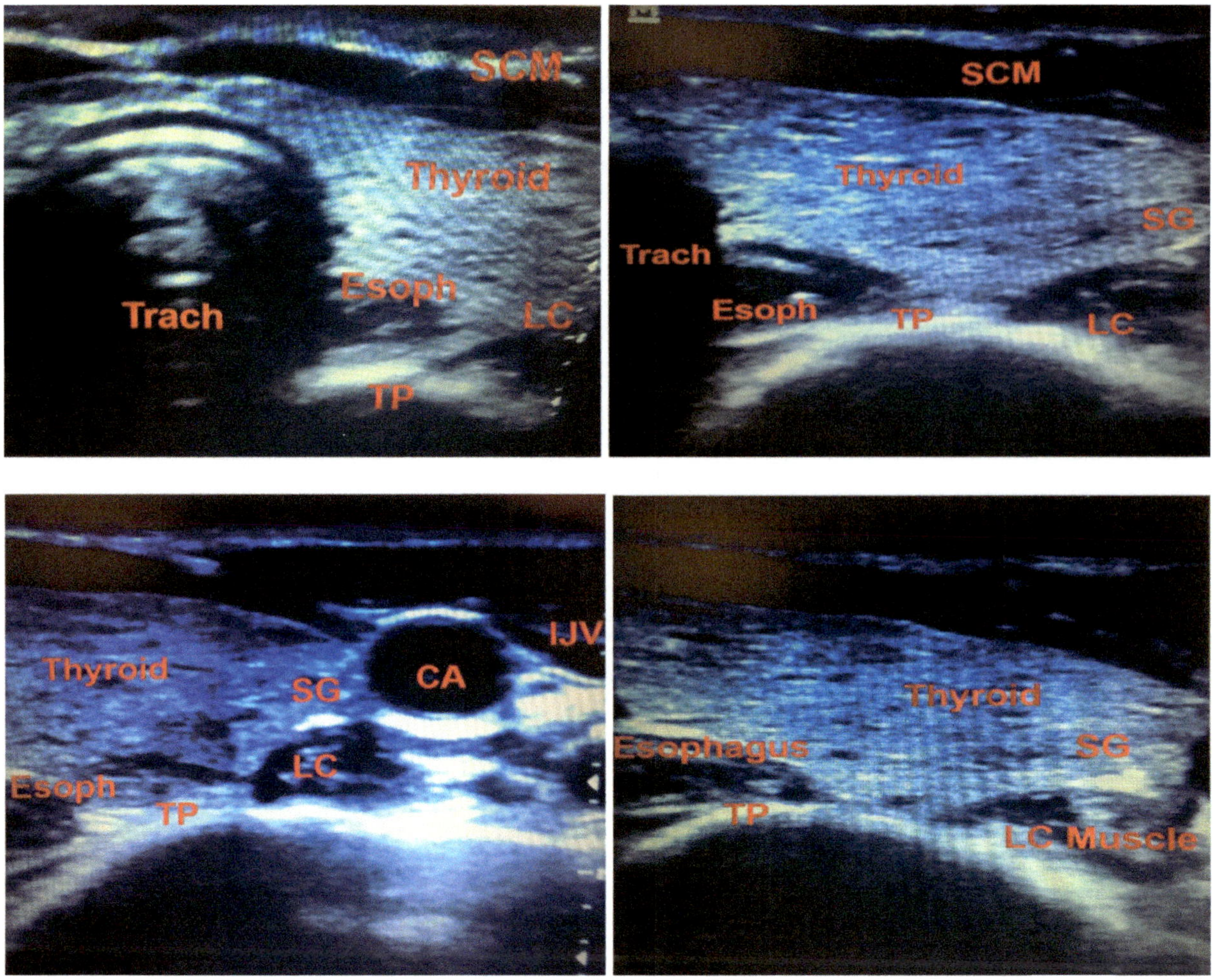

Figure 14.2. Ultrasonographic images of stellate ganglion blocks used for relief of pain in acute herpes zoster neuritis. Abbreviations: CA, carotid artery; Esoph, esophagus; IJV, internal jugular vein; LC, longus colli; SCM, sternocleidomastoid muscle; SG, stellate ganglion; TP, transverse process; Trach, trachea. Photo courtesy of Kenneth D. Candido, MD.

to treat both acute HZ and PHN. Significant pain reduction, with complete pain resolution during the acute phase of HZ, has been observed in several independent studies, although the ability of sympathetic blocks to prevent PHN remains controversial.[24,38–40] Unfortunately, the same response to sympathetic block could not be replicated in PHN, where the majority of patients derived only transient pain relief.[38] The available evidence in support of transforaminal epidural steroid injections (TESI) for PHN is conflicting (Figure 14.3). The benefits of TESI have been documented by some in case reports of PHN involving cervical,[2] thoracic,[41] and lumbar[5] dermatomes. TESI was performed at the left T10 level in a patient who failed conservative treatment with oral and topical medications and who did not respond to intercostal nerve blocks.[41] The patient reported 100% pain relief at 2-week follow-up and 1 out of 10 VAS pain rating at 12-week follow-up, which enabled him to return to his previous activities without any functional limitations.[41] Opstelten et al. could not substantiate the long-term benefits in PHN reported by the other investigators.[42] In their large study, 598 patients with acute HZ rash below dermatome C6 of < 7 days' duration were randomized into a control group (standard therapy with antivirals and analgesics) and a treatment group, consisting of the standard therapy

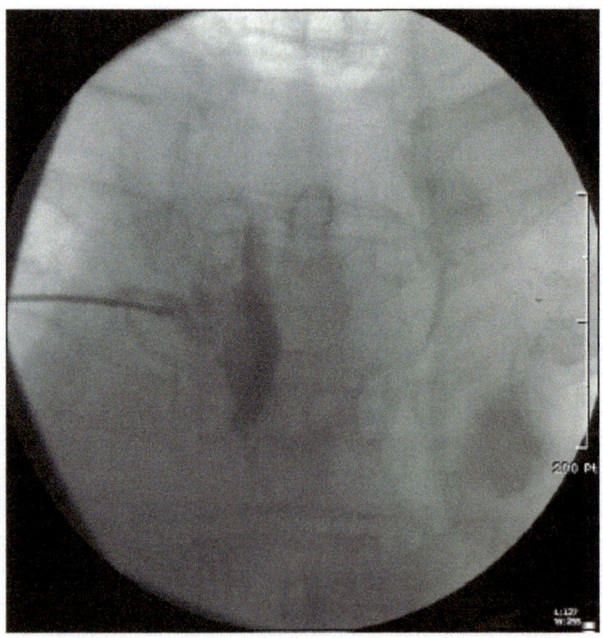

Figure 14.3. Spread of contrast media at left T3 nerve root during transforaminal epidural steroid injection in a patient treated for postherpetic neuralgia. Reproduced with permission from Yu et al.[43]

plus an epidural injection of 10 mg methylprednisolone and 10 mg bupivacaine.[42] While steroid treatment was superior to standard therapy in alleviating the pain during the acute phase of the illness at 1-month follow-up (52% in the treatment group and 42% in the control group), no statistical differences were found in the pain intensity at 3 months (79% in the treatment group and 75% in the control group) and at 6 months (85% in the treatment group and 83% in the control group).[42]

Neuromodulation

SCS has been investigated in patients with PHN refractory to conservative treatment and/or interventional approaches. In a prospective study of 28 patients with intractable pain due to PHN, SCS conferred long-lasting pain relief (with a median decrease from 9 to 1 on the VAS) in 82% of patients.[44] SCS of the DRG shows great promise in treating neuropathic pain of various etiologies, including that secondary to PHN. A positive outcome was observed in a trial with 51 subjects, 76.5% of whom reported substantial pain relief, with an average of 74.2% after a 12-month period.[45]

CONCLUSIONS

- The incidence of HZ and PHN increases with age.
- Decreased cell-mediated immunity increases the risk of HZ.
- Acute infection manifests by an eruption of a painful rash in dermatomal distribution.
- Thoracic dermatomes are the most commonly affected followed by the first division of the trigeminal (V1) nerve.
- Antiviral therapy should be initiated within 72 hours of onset of the rash in order to decrease the disease burden and prevent PHN.
- TCAs, anticonvulsants, and a 5% lidocaine patch are considered first-line treatment for PHN.
- Interventional pain management has proven helpful in reducing or terminating the pain from PHN.

REFERENCES

1. Insinga RP, Itzler RF, Pellissier JM, Saddier P, Nikas AA. The incidence of herpes zoster in a United States administrative database. *J Gen Intern Med.* 2005;20(8):748–753.
2. Shakir A, Kimbrough DA, Mehta B. Postherpetic neuralgia involving the right C5 dermatome treated with a cervical transforaminal epidural steroid injection: a case report. *Arch Phys Med Rehabil.* 2007;88(2):255–258.
3. Dworkin RH, Johnson RW, Breuer J, et al. Recommendations for the management of herpes zoster. *Clin Infect Dis.* 2007;44(suppl 1):S1–S26.
4. Jung BF, Johnson RW, Griffin DR, Dworkin RH. Risk factors for postherpetic neuralgia in patients with herpes zoster. *Neurology.* 2004;62(9):1545–1551.
5. Opstelten W, van Wijck AJ, Stolker RJ. Interventions to prevent postherpetic neuralgia: cutaneous and percutaneous techniques. *Pain.* 2004;107(3):202–206.
6. van Wijck AJ, Wallace M, Mekhail N, van Kleef M. Evidence-based interventional pain medicine according to clinical diagnoses. 17. Herpes zoster and post-herpetic neuralgia. *Pain Pract.* 2011;11(1):88–97.
7. Fields HL, Rowbotham M, Baron R. Postherpetic neuralgia: irritable nociceptors and deafferentation. *Neurobiol Dis.* 1998;5(4):209–227.
8. Watson CP, Deck JH, Morshead C, Van der Kooy D, Evans RJ. Post-herpetic neuralgia: further post-mortem studies of cases with and without pain. *Pain.* 1991;44(2):105–117.
9. Goh CL, Khoo L. A retrospective study of the clinical presentation and outcome of herpes zoster in a tertiary dermatology outpatient referral clinic. *Int J Dermatol.* 1997;36(9):667–672.
10. Johnson RW, Bouhassira D, Kassianos G, Leplege A, Schmader KE, Weinke T. The impact of herpes zoster and post-herpetic neuralgia on quality-of-life. *BMC Med.* 2010;8:37.
11. Dworkin RH, Gnann JW Jr, Oaklander AL, Raja SN, Schmader KE, Whitley RJ. Diagnosis and assessment of pain associated with herpes zoster and postherpetic neuralgia. *J Pain.* 2008;9(1)(suppl 1):S37–S44.
12. FDA approves Zostavax vaccine to prevent shingles in individuals 50 to 59 years of age http://www.fda.gov/NewsEvents/Newsroom/PressAnnouncements/ucm248390.htm. Accessed April 23, 2016.
13. Harpaz R, Ortega-Sanchez IR, Seward JF; Advisory Committee on Immunization Practices, Centers for Disease Control and Prevention. Prevention of herpes zoster: recommendations of the Advisory Committee on Immunization Practices (ACIP). *MMWR Recomm Rep.* 2008;57(RR-5):1–30.
14. Marin M, Yawn BP, Hales CM, et al. Herpes zoster vaccine effectiveness and manifestations of herpes zoster and associated pain by vaccination status. *Hum Vaccin Immunother.* 2015;11(5):1157–1164.
15. Oxman MN, Levin MJ, Johnson GR, et al. A vaccine to prevent herpes zoster and postherpetic neuralgia in older adults. *N Engl J Med.* 2005;352(22):2271–2284.
16. Tyring SK, Beutner KR, Tucker BA, Anderson WC, Crooks RJ. Antiviral therapy for herpes zoster: randomized, controlled clinical trial of valacyclovir and famciclovir therapy in immunocompetent patients 50 years and older. *Arch Fam Med.* 2000;9(9):863–869.
17. Tyring S, Barbarash RA, Nahlik JE, et al. Famciclovir for the treatment of acute herpes zoster: effects on acute disease and postherpetic neuralgia. A randomized, double-blind, placebo-controlled trial. Collaborative Famciclovir Herpes Zoster Study Group. *Ann Intern Med.* 1995;123(2):89–96.
18. Wood MJ, Kay R, Dworkin RH, Soong SJ, Whitley RJ. Oral acyclovir therapy accelerates pain resolution in patients with herpes zoster: a meta-analysis of placebo-controlled trials. *Clin Infect Dis.* 1996;22(2):341–347.
19. Whitley RJ, Weiss H, Gnann JW Jr, et al. Acyclovir with and without prednisone for the treatment of herpes zoster. A randomized, placebo-controlled trial. The National Institute of Allergy and Infectious Diseases Collaborative Antiviral Study Group. *Ann Intern Med.* 1996;125(5):376–383.
20. High KP. Preventing herpes zoster and postherpetic neuralgia through vaccination. *J Fam Pract.* 2007;56(10)(suppl A):51A–57A.
21. Gnann JW Jr, Whitley RJ. Clinical practice. Herpes zoster. *N Engl J Med.* 2002;347(5):340–346.
22. Alper BS, Lewis PR. Does treatment of acute herpes zoster prevent or shorten postherpetic neuralgia? *J Fam Pract.* 2000;49(3):255–264.
23. Pica F, Gatti A, Divizia M, et al. One-year follow-up of patients with long-lasting post-herpetic neuralgia. *BMC Infect Dis.* 2014;14:556.
24. Winnie AP, Hartwell PW. Relationship between time of treatment of acute herpes zoster with sympathetic blockade and prevention of post-herpetic neuralgia: clinical support for a new theory of the mechanism by which sympathetic blockade provides therapeutic benefit. *Reg Anesth.* 1993;18(5):277–282.
25. Hempenstall K, Nurmikko TJ, Johnson RW, A'Hern RP, Rice AS. Analgesic therapy in postherpetic neuralgia: a quantitative systematic review. *PLoS Med.* 2005;2(7):e164.

26. Rowbotham M, Harden N, Stacey B, Bernstein P, Magnus-Miller L. Gabapentin for the treatment of postherpetic neuralgia: a randomized controlled trial. *JAMA*. 1998;280(21):1837–1842.
27. Sabatowski R, Galvez R, Cherry DA, et al. Pregabalin reduces pain and improves sleep and mood disturbances in patients with post-herpetic neuralgia: results of a randomised, placebo-controlled clinical trial. *Pain*. 2004;109(1-2):26–35.
28. Freynhagen R, Strojek K, Griesing T, Whalen E, Balkenohl M. Efficacy of pregabalin in neuropathic pain evaluated in a 12-week, randomised, double-blind, multicentre, placebo-controlled trial of flexible- and fixed-dose regimens. *Pain*. 2005;115(3):254–263.
29. Arner S, Meyerson BA. Lack of analgesic effect of opioids on neuropathic and idiopathic forms of pain. *Pain*. 1988;33(1):11–23.
30. Portenoy RK, Foley KM, Inturrisi CE. The nature of opioid responsiveness and its implications for neuropathic pain: new hypotheses derived from studies of opioid infusions. *Pain*. 1990;43(3):273–286.
31. Raja SN, Haythornthwaite JA, Pappagallo M, et al. Opioids versus antidepressants in postherpetic neuralgia: a randomized, placebo-controlled trial. *Neurology*. 2002; 59(7): 1015–1021.
32. Watson CP, Babul N. Efficacy of oxycodone in neuropathic pain: a randomized trial in postherpetic neuralgia. *Neurology*. 1998;50(6):1837–1841.
33. Hollingshead J, Duhmke RM, Cornblath DR. Tramadol for neuropathic pain. *Cochrane Database Syst Rev*. 2006(3):CD003726.
34. Wolff RF, Bala MM, Westwood M, Kessels AG, Kleijnen J. 5% lidocaine-medicated plaster vs other relevant interventions and placebo for post-herpetic neuralgia (PHN): a systematic review. *Acta Neurol Scand*. 2011;123(5):295–309.
35. Derry S, Lloyd R, Moore RA, McQuay HJ. Topical capsaicin for chronic neuropathic pain in adults. *Cochrane Database Syst Rev*. 2009(4):CD007393.
36. Sampathkumar P, Drage LA, Martin DP. Herpes zoster (shingles) and postherpetic neuralgia. *Mayo Clin Proc*. 2009;84(3):274–280.
37. Stankus SJ, Dlugopolski M, Packer D. Management of herpes zoster (shingles) and postherpetic neuralgia. *Am Fam Physician*. 2000;61(8):2437–2444, 2447–2448.
38. Colding A. Treatment of pain: organization of a pain clinic: treatment of acute herpes zoster. *Proc R Soc Med*. 1973;66(6):541–543.
39. Riopelle JM, Naraghi M, Grush KP. Chronic neuralgia incidence following local anesthetic therapy for herpes zoster. *Arch Dermatol*. 1984;120(6):747–750.
40. Yanagida H, Suwa K, Corssen G. No prophylactic effect of early sympathetic blockade on postherpetic neuralgia. *Anesthesiol*. 1987; 66(1): 73–76.
41. Mehta P, Maher P, Singh JR. Treatment of postherpetic neuralgia using a thoracic transforaminal epidural steroid injection. *PM R*. 2015;7(4):443–446.
42. Opstelten W, van Wijck AJ, Moons KG, et al. [Treatment of patients with herpes zoster by epidural injection of steroids and local anaesthetics: less pain after 1 month, but no effect on long-term postherpetic neuralgia—a randomised trial.] *Ned Tijdschr Geneeskd*. 2006;150(48):2649–2655.
43. Yu HK, Lee JH, Cho SH, Kim YI. Relief of postherpetic neuralgia with transforaminal epidural injection of magnesium—a case report. *Korean J Pain*. 2011;24(1):53–56.
44. Harke H, Gretenkort P, Ladleif HU, Koester P, Rahman S. Spinal cord stimulation in postherpetic neuralgia and in acute herpes zoster pain. *Anesth Analg*. 2002;94(3):694–700.
45. Liem L, Russo M, Huygen FJ, et al. One-year outcomes of spinal cord stimulation of the dorsal root ganglion in the treatment of chronic neuropathic pain. *Neuromodulation*. 2015;18(1):41–48, discussion 48–49.
46. Babu R, Hazzard MA, Huang KT, et al. Outcomes of percutaneous and paddle lead implantation for spinal cord stimulation: a comparative analysis of complications, reoperation rates, and health-care costs. *Neuromodulation*. 2013;16(5):418–426, discussion 426–427.

REVIEW QUESTIONS

1. A pain service consult is requested for a 55-year-old overweight female with a complaint of intense burning pain below the left breast radiating outward to the posterior back. She states that the fabric of her shirt irritates her skin and aggravates the pain. The patient has a history of hypertension, high cholesterol, and diabetes, for which she takes a thiazide, an ACE inhibitor, a statin, and metformin. She denies neck, jaw, or arm pain, dizziness, and visual disturbances. The most appropriate step at this time would be:

A. Intercostal nerve block with bupivacaine
B. Administration of valacyclovir
C. Obtain an electrocardiogram
D. Initiate therapy with nortriptyline

2. Which of the following statements is the most accurate in relation to herpes zoster?

A. Cervical nerve roots are the most commonly affected site.
B. The pain arises as a result of ganglionitis and peripheral neuritis due to virus reactivation.
C. A laboratory analysis of fluid from the vesicles is required for diagnosis of the virus.
D. Immune status, but not age, determines the risk of HZ.

3. What are some of the common adverse effects limiting the utility of anticonvulsants in the treatment of PHN?

A. Constipation and headaches
B. Unsteady gait and weight gain
C. Dry mouth and urinary retention
D. Peripheral edema and QTc prolongation

ANSWERS

1. C. The patient has multiple risk factors for acute coronary syndrome, thus ECG should be obtained before commencing treatment for HZ. Angina and myocardial infarction should be included in the differential of any chest wall pain. Older females with comorbidities like diabetes might have an atypical presentation, which explains the absence of symptoms suggestive of myocardial infarction. While intercostal nerve block is a viable treatment option, it usually is employed after conservative measures have been attempted; therefore, answer A is not correct. Answer B is incorrect, because would be an appropriate step after the ACS workup is instituted. TCAs might benefit patients with PHN, but they are not a drug of choice for acute HZ; therefore, answer D is incorrect.

2. B. Pain experienced during the acute phase of the infection is due to inflammation of the nerve ganglion

and peripheral nerves induced by the reactivated virus.[8] Thoracic nerve roots, not cervical, are the most frequently affected.[9] HZ is usually diagnosed clinically by recognizing the symptoms and presence of the rash, and fluid analysis is not required. Although impaired immunity increases susceptibility to the infection, the risk increases substantially with age; therefore, both factors determine the occurrence of HZ.

3. B. Unsteady gait and weight gain are commonly reported side effects of gabapentin and pregabalin. Other noteworthy adverse reactions include drowsiness, dizziness, blurry vision, peripheral edema, and mental cloudiness.[26] Constipation and headaches are common with opioids (answer A), dry mouth and urinary retention characterize the anticholinergic effects of TCAs (answer C). While peripheral edema is seen in patients on anticonvulsants, QTc prolongation is likely with TCAs; therefore, answer D is incorrect.

QUESTIONS AND ANSWERS

This chapter has accompanying questions and answers that are available to subscribers as part of the Oxford eLearning platform. To access the questions, follow the link below, or go to ✔ http://oxfordmedicine.com/painmanagementreview

15.

POSTMASTECTOMY NEUROPATHIC PAIN

Heena Pranav and Dalia H. Elmofty

STEM CASE AND KEY QUESTIONS

A 32-year-old female with left breast cancer underwent a modified radical mastectomy and reconstructive surgery with breast implants. She suffers from anxiety and is taking klonopin 0.5 mg twice daily. The patient experienced severe postoperative pain and could not tolerate several medications. She continued to have significant discomfort 3 months after surgery. The breast surgeon referred her to the pain clinic for evaluation of ongoing chest wall pain. She reports numbness and severe burning, with paroxysms of lancinating shocklike pain in the left chest wall over the breast scar that radiates into the axilla. The pain is worsened by activity. Examination of the chest wall reveals a healed left breast scar, hypersensitive to light touch and associated with an area of numbness in the right upper inner arm. The skin is pigmented from radiation therapy. Sensation to coldness is reduced over the T2-T4 dermatomes. Range of motion of the left shoulder is limited by pain. Motor strength of the left upper extremity is intact.

WHAT IS THE DIFFERENTIAL DIAGNOSIS OF HER PAIN? IS ADDITIONAL DIAGNOSTIC WORKUP INDICATED?

Breast MRI is negative for tumor recurrence, hematoma, and infection. Laboratory findings, blood count, and serologic markers for inflammation are normal. The diagnosis is postmastectomy pain syndrome.

WHAT ARE COMMON VARIABLES ASSOCIATED WITH HIGHER RISK FOR POSTMASTECTOMY PAIN SYNDROME?

The patient is emotional and does not understand why she continues to have pain and discomfort. She fears recurrence of the disease, although her workup has been negative.

HOW WOULD YOU MANAGE HER PAIN?

A multimodal approach is initiated, with physical therapy, consultation with a pain psychologist for coping, topical lidocaine over the painful scar, and gabapentin 300 mg three times a day. At follow-up 4 weeks later the patient reports 20% improvement of pain but continues to be severely limited in daily activities. Duloxetine 30 mg every day is added to the medication regimen. If she experiences no side effects from the medication, she is to increase the dose to 60 mg every day after 1 week.

WHAT INTERVENTIONAL PROCEDURES SHOULD BE CONSIDERED?

The patient cannot tolerate the medication regimen because of its cognitive effects. She undergoes left-sided T3, T4, and T5 diagnostic intercostal nerve blocks. She reports significant relief of pain and improvement in function. She subsequently undergoes T3, T4, and T5 intercostal nerve radiofrequency ablations. At the 3-month follow-up visit, she reports some discomfort, but her pain has been significantly improved from baseline.

DISCUSSION

DEFINITION OF NEUROPATHIC PAIN

The International Association for the Study of Pain (IASP) defines neuropathic pain as pain that arises from a lesion or disease of the somatosensory nervous system.[1,2] Neuropathic pain is not a single disease, but a syndrome caused by a range of different diseases and lesions, which manifests as an array of symptoms and signs.[3] The pathogenesis of neuropathic pain can be categorized both anatomically (peripheral vs central) and etiologically (generative, traumatic, infectious, and toxic).[4] Numerous etiologies underlie neuropathic pain, each of which corresponds to a different underlying mechanism. As a result, it is important to diagnose the underlying etiology of neuropathic pain for mechanism-based treatment. Ideally, a multidisciplinary approach that utilizes preventative, pharmacologic, and interventional treatment options is preferred.

Neuropathic pain is generally a chronic and disabling disease process that has been associated with a negative impact on mental and physical health along with decreased quality of life (QoL).[5,6] Health-related quality of life (HRQoL) is significantly impaired in patients with neuropathic pain in comparison to patients with chronic nonneuropathic pain.[7] According to one population-based study, respondents who reported pain with neuropathic characteristics had higher impairment in all markers relating to QoL and sleep.[8] They also were found to have higher anxiety and depression scores than chronic nonneuropathic pain patients.[8]

PREVALENCE

Based on a recent systematic review of epidemiologic studies on neuropathic pain, the prevalence of neuropathic pain varies between 1% and 17.9%.[9] To find prevalence, some studies used population-based questionnaires, such as the Leeds Assessment of Neuropathic Symptoms and Signs and the Douleur Neuropathique 4 Questions. These tools identify neuropathic pain in the general population using symptoms and self-examined signs.[10] The Study of the Prevalence of Neuropathic Pain, a French population-based study, estimated the prevalence of chronic pain with neuropathic characteristics to be 6.9%.[11] A similar cross-sectional postal survey in the United Kingdom estimated a prevalence of 8.2%.[12] A postal survey in the United States determined the prevalence to be 8.8%.[13] Although the rates appear similar, a telephone-based survey completed in Canada determined a greater prevalence rate of 17.9%.[14] Factors in population-based studies associated with neuropathic pain include sex (higher risk in females), manual occupation, inability to work, and living in a rural area.[11,12,15] Variability in prevalence may be attributed to lack of consensus on diagnostic criteria and definition as well as lack of appropriate and consistent use of screening tools.[9]

With regard to postmastectomy pain syndrome, the prevalence is reported to be 25% to 50%.[16] In a prospective cohort study of women who had breast cancer surgery in Brazil, 52% of patients reported persistent postsurgical pain at the 6-month follow-up visit.[17] Additionally, in a population-based study in Denmark, a prevalence rate of 24% was determined from questionnaires mailed to patients 1.5 years after breast cancer surgery.[18] There is variability in etiology among the different types of postmastectomy pain syndrome, including neuroma pain (23%–49%), phantom breast pain (13%–44%) and intercostobrachial neuralgia.[19]

PATHOPHYSIOLOGY

Neuropathic pain is pain that results from injury to, or dysfunction of, the somatosensory nervous system.[20] Neuropathic pain can be classified by the etiology of the lesion and the location of insult in the nervous system. Lesions may be a central nervous system (CNS) lesion, a peripheral nervous system lesion, or a mixed lesion. For example, poststroke or phantom limb pain arises from abnormal activity in the CNS. Postherpetic neuralgia (PHN) or diabetic neuropathy stems from lesions in the peripheral nervous system.

The broadness of the chronic pain syndrome and its coexistence with other types of pain make the underlying mechanism of neuropathic pain complex. It is generally accepted that, in neuropathic pain, tissue damage affects the nervous system directly, resulting in ectopic discharges that bypass the transduction of pain.[21] Although the specific mechanisms are yet to be elucidated, animal models of neuropathic pain and research in humans have provided valuable information in the past decade.[22,23] Once tissue is injured, inflammatory processes ensue, leading to a hyperexcitable state in the primary afferent nociceptors known as peripheral sensitization. In most patients, this state resolves with healing; however, when the noxious stimulus persists because of repeated stimulation from ongoing injury (as in diabetes), the changes in the primary afferent neurons may persist.[24] Injury to a sensory nerve can lead to eventual neuronal death and fewer intraepidermal nociceptors. With fewer receptors, local nerve growth factors are released, and collateral nerve fibers sprout, producing hyperalgesia and increased pain (deafferentation pain).[24,25] As a consequence of peripheral nociceptor hyperactivity, responsiveness of nociceptive neurons in the CNS increases, which is known as central sensitization.[26,27]

Postmastectomy pain, in particular, can arise from a number of contributing factors. Both surgical and nonsurgical treatment options for breast cancer can predispose to postmastectomy pain syndrome. Postmastectomy pain originates from tissue or nerve trauma (Table 15.1).[28] Tissue trauma, nociceptive in nature, results from muscle injury; nerve trauma from a surgical or nonsurgical insult creates neuropathic pain. Neuropathic pain after breast cancer surgery can be neuroma pain, phantom breast, intercostobrachial neuralgia, or pain from injury to motor nerves.[19] Injury to small cutaneous sensory nerves produces cutaneous scar neuromas.[29] In one study, patients who had a lumpectomy were more likely to have neuroma pain than patients who had modified radical mastectomy.[30] Phantom breast pain is the sensation that the removed breast is present and painful after modified radical mastectomy. The most common mastectomy pain syndrome is intercostobrachial neuralgia caused by damage to the intercostobrachial nerve during axillary node dissection. Forceful traction during surgery may injure the medial and lateral pectoral nerve or long thoracic and thoracodorsal nerve.

DIAGNOSIS

The assessment of pain in general can be challenging because pain is subjective. Nonetheless, a thorough history and physical examination are fundamental to the assessment. A gold standard for diagnosing neuropathic pain does not exist. The diagnosis of neuropathic pain depends on the clinician's judgment and the interpretation of test results.[31] According to the criteria of the Neuropathic Pain Specialists Interest Group (NeuPSIG), pain is neuropathic if the patient's clinical history is compatible with the presence of a neurologic lesion or disease and if the physical examination reveals a sensory deficit in the same plausible neuroanatomic area of the body.[31,32]

Research over the past decade has shown a set of sensory signs likely to be associated with neuropathic pain.[33,34] Clinical symptoms of neuropathic pain can be positive or negative. The positive symptoms are pain, paresthesias, and dysesthesias (tingling, numbness, or pins and needles). The negative symptoms are neurologic sensory deficits in the painful area.[35]

In a study of 482 patients with neuropathic pain, the three most frequently reported symptoms were ongoing burning pain (65.4%), paroxysmal shocklike pain (57%) and brush-evoked pain (54.9%).[36] Symptom-based questionnaires have been developed for screening and identification of

Table 15.1. ETIOLOGY AND CLINICAL CHARACTERISTICS OF POSTMASTECTOMY PAIN SYNDROME

TISSUE TRAUMA (NOCICEPTIVE)	CLINICAL CHARACTERISTICS	NERVE TRAUMA (NEUROPATHIC)	CLINICAL CHARACTERISTICS
Muscle injury (Myofascial pain)	Aching muscle pain associated with stiffness and limited range of motion, with palpable trigger points	Neuroma	Hyperalgesia or allodynia over breast scar
		Phantom breast	Knifelike, shooting, or pricking pain in area of surgically removed breast
		Inter-costo brachiallis nerve (ICBN)	Aching, burning, or stabbing pain, numbness, and other sensory changes in the upper medial aspect of the arm
		Injury to Motor Nerves	
		Medial and lateral pectoral nerve	Paralysis and atrophy of pectoral muscle
		Long thoracic nerve—notalgia paresthetica	Burning pain between the medial border of the scapula and spine on the affected side, with winging of the scapula
		Thoracodorsal nerve	Paralysis of the latissimus dorsi muscle and weakness with adduction and internal rotation of the shoulder

neuropathic pain. The questionnaires identify patients with possible neuropathic pain based on sensory descriptors. Some sensory quality descriptors in the questionnaires are tingling, burning, and shooting.[30,32,35] Standardized neuropathic screening tools include the Leeds Assessment of Neuropathic Symptoms and Signs, the Neuropathic Pain Questionnaires, Douleur Neuropathique 4 Questions, PainDETECT, and the ID Pain Scale.

Physical examination is primarily focused on the sensory aspect to detect possible abnormalities suggestive of a lesion of the somatosensory system, mostly thermal or mechanical deficits.[37] Simple bedside methods are used to assess hypesthesia (reduced sensation to touch or cold), hypalgesia (reduced pain sensation to noxious stimuli), hyperalgesia (increased pain to pinprick, pressure, heat/cold), and allodynia (pain sensation with non-noxious stimuli).[4]

Imaging, neurophysiologic tecgniques, punch biopsies, and quantitative sensory testing (QST) can potentially give more information about a neurologic lesion underlying pain, but tests cannot confirm a causal relationship.[31]

QST complements the traditional neurologic bedside examination in the analysis of the somatosensory anomalies.[38] It measures perception of mechanical, thermal, and painful stimuli delivered at a controlled intensity.[38] Punch biopsies are a quick, minimally invasive technique with a high diagnostic yield for patients suspected of having small-fiber neuropathy.[39] Investigators report a significant decrease in intraepidermal nerve fiber density in patients with neuropathy compared to healthy controls.[40] Other neurophysiologic techniques are nerve conduction studies and measurement of evoked potentials.[41] In laser-evoked potentials (LEPs), pulses of laser-generated heat excite free nerve endings in superficial skin layers.[42] Suppression of LEPs suggests neuropathic pain. LEPs are more sensitive than any other neurophysiologic test for the detection of peripheral and central lesions causing neuropathic pain.[43,44]

PREVENTION

The first step in prevention of neuropathic pain is identifying patients at risk. Some risk factors for postmastectomy pain are anxiety, depression, young age, high body mass index (BMI), pain in the breast before surgery, axillary lymph node dissection, radiation therapy, and uncontrolled postoperative pain.[45–47]

The goal of prevention is to limit primary damage completely or to minimize the nerve damage in place. Preemptive analgesia is beneficial in preventing postsurgical neuropathic pain because it inhibits surgery-induced central sensitization. In a randomized, double-blind clinical trial, perioperative administration of extended-release venlafaxine reduced the incidence of postsurgical mastectomy pain at 6 months.[48] In animal studies, early increasing-intensity treadmill exercise after nerve injury reduced collateral nerve sprouting and subsequent hyperalgesia associated with neuropathic pain.[49]

TREATMENT

One of the most important factors in the treatment of neuropathic pain is the physician–patient relationship. The quality of this relationship determines not only the patient's and doctor's satisfaction but also the patient's compliance. Realistic goals should be discussed and the measures to achieve the goals must be defined clearly. The treatment plan should consider prevention and nonpharmacologic, pharmacologic, and interventional options.

Nonpharmacologic Treatment

Nonpharmacologic methods, such as transcutaneous electrical nerve stimulation (TENS) and psychotherapy, have not been well studied for neuropathic pain. Their role remains unclear at this time. Among the psychotherapeutic approaches for chronic pain are cognitive behavioral therapy, biofeedback, hypnosis, operant-behavioral therapy, and meditation. The goal of these therapies is to help the patient function in spite of pain.[50]

Pharmacologic Treatment

Even with pharmacologic treatment, patients continue to experience moderate or severe pain.[5] Many patients experience intolerable adverse effects from pharmacologic agents. Combination therapy has been more beneficial in the treatment of neuropathic pain than single-agent therapy.[51,52] The NeuPSIG of the IASP, the Canadian Pain Society, and the European Federation of Neurological Societies (EFNS) have published evidence-based clinical guidelines for the pharmacologic treatment of neuropathic pain (Table 15.2).[53–55]

The choice of pharmacologic agent for treatment depends on the potential benefit. Most physicians will introduce medications at separate times to determine efficacy and to observe side effects. With a multimodal analgesic approach, different receptors are targeted to maximize analgesia and minimize doses of individual drugs. Common agents for the treatment of neuropathic pain include antidepressants, anticonvulsants, and opioids.

Antidepressants

Tricyclic antidepressants (TCAs) were introduced in the 1950s as antipsychotics. TCAs were effective in numerous, randomized, blinded and placebo-controlled studies for the treatment of neuropathic pain.[56] The exact mechanism of action for the analgesic effect is still unclear. TCAs act primarily by inhibiting reuptake of norepinephrine and serotonin. They are also antagonistic at the *N*-methyl-D-aspartate (NMDA) receptor. TCAs may block sodium channels. Their side effects include anticholinergic (altered mental status, dry mouth, mydriasis), CNS (myoclonus, syncope), cardiac (tachycardia, orthostatic hypotension), and gastrointestinal (deceased bowel motility) symptoms. Caution is necessary

Table 15.2. **PHARMACOLOGIC TREATMENT OF NEUROPATHIC PAIN: RECOMMENDATIONS OF THE NEUROPATHIC PAIN SPECIALISTS INTEREST GROUP (NEUPSIG), THE CANADIAN PAIN SOCIETY, AND THE EUROPEAN FEDERATION OF NEUROLOGICAL SOCIETIES (EFNS)**

LINE OF TREATMENT	NEUPSIG 2007	CANADIAN PAIN SOCIETY 2007
First	Antidepressants (secondary amine TCAs, SNRIs) Anticonvulsants (gabapentin, pregabalin) Topical lidocaine	Antidepressants Anticonvulsants (gabapentin, pregabalin) Carbamazepine only for trigeminal neuralgia
Second	Tramadol Opioids (oxycodone, methadone, morphine)	SNRIs (duloxetine, venlafaxine) Topical lidocaine
Third	NMDA antagonists Topical capsaicin Mexiletine Other anticonvulsants (carbamazepine, lamotrigine, topiramate, valproic acid, oxycarbazepine) Other antidepressants (bupropion, citalopram, paroxetine)	Tramadol Extended-release opioids
Fourth	Not applicable	Cannabinoids Methadone Other anticonvulsants (topiramate, lamotrigine, valproic acid)

LINE OF TREATMENT	EFNS 2010			
First	Painful polyneuropathy (DPN, non-DPN) Antidepressants (TCAs, SNRIs) Anticonvulsants (gabapentin, pregabalin)	Postherpetic neuralgia Antidepressants (TCAs) Anticonvulsant (gabapentin, pregabalin) Topical lidocaine	Trigeminal neuralgia Carbamazepine and oxycarbazepine (if intolerable side effects, consider lamotrigine or surgical intervention)	Central neuropathic pain Antidepressants (TCAs) Anticonvulsants (gabapentin)
Second	Tramadol	Opioids Capsaicin cream		Tramadol
Third	Strong opioids			Strong opioids

Abbreviations: DPN, diabetic peripheral neuropathy; NMDA, *N*-methyl-D-aspartate; SNRI, serotonin and norepinephrine reuptake inhibitors; TCA, tricyclic antidepressants.

when TCAs are prescribed for the elderly or for patients with cardiovascular comorbidities. An electrocardiogram is recommended before initiating therapy. There are two classes of TCAs, tertiary and secondary amines. The tertiary amines (e.g., amitriptyline) inhibit serotonin reuptake more than the secondary amines do. Tertiary amines have a tendency to cause sedation, anticholinergic side effects, and orthostatic hypotension. Secondary amines (e.g., nortriptyline and desipramine) enhance inhibition of norepinephrine reuptake and have a more favorable side-effect profile than the tertiary amines, but they can cause irritability and disturbed sleep. Tertiary amines may be beneficial in a patient who has insomnia, while secondary amines may benefit a patient with chronic fatigue.

Serotonin and Norepinephrine Reuptake Inhibitors (SNRIs)

SNRIs (venlafaxin, milnacipran, duloxetine) exert balanced inhibition of reuptake of serotonin and norepinephrine that can be dose-dependent. Venlafaxin was as effective in the treatment of neuropathic pain as TCAs.[56]

Selective Serotonin Reuptake Inhibitors (SSRIs)

SSRIs (fluoxetine, paroxetine, citalopram, escitalopram, sertraline, fluvoxamine) inhibit serotonin reuptake without affecting norepinephrine reuptake. These agents do not appear to be as efficacious as TCAs for treatment of neuropathic pain.[57,58]

Norepinephrine and Dopamine Reuptake Inhibitors

Bupropion is a norepinephrine and dopamine reuptake inhibitor. In a placebo-controlled crossover trial, bupropion sustained release was effective in the treatment of neuropathic pain.[59]

Anticonvulsants

Gabapentin and pregabalin are commonly used agents for the treatment of neuropathic pain. Both bind to the $\alpha_2\delta$ subunit of the voltage-gated calcium channel to reduce the release of excitatory neurotransmitters. Their efficacy in the treatment of neuropathic pain has been demonstrated in randomized controlled trials.[60,61]

Opioids

The use of opioids for the treatment of neuropathic pain remains controversial. Opioids can be administered to patients severely incapacitated from pain until antidepressant and anticonvulsant therapies are titrated to efficacy. Opioid agonists are also initiated if patients cannot tolerate antidepressant or anticonvulsant therapy. In a systematic review of randomized controlled trials of opioid agonists for the treatment of neuropathic nonmalignant pain, short-term trials (opioid administered less than 24 hours) and intermediate-term trials (opioid administered 8 to 56 days) were identified. Results of short-term studies were equivocal; intermediate-term studies demonstrated significant efficacy for the treatment of neuropathic pain.[62]

Intravenous Infusion Therapies

Intravenous lidocaine and ketamine infusions have been used in the treatment of neuropathic pain.[63,64] Lidocaine is a sodium channel blocker that acts centrally. Ketamine is an NMDA receptor antagonist. NMDA receptor activation is associated with neuropathic pain.

Interventional Options

Interventional options should be considered in patients with refractory neuropathic pain. Yet, there are few randomized, controlled trials assessing their efficacy. Many of the interventions used in practice to treat refractory pain are supported by weak, if any, evidence. In 2013, the IASP evaluated systematic reviews, clinical trials, and existing guidelines for the management of neuropathic pain.[65] They evaluated neural blockade, spinal cord stimulators, intrathecal drug delivery systems, and neurosurgical interventions in patients with peripheral and central pain, such as herpes zoster, PHN, diabetic peripheral neuropathy (DPN), spinal cord injury (SCI,) poststroke pain, failed back surgery syndrome (FBSS), complex regional pain syndrome (CRPS), and trigeminal neuralgia. Strong recommendations could not be made for any interventional procedure. Weak recommendations were given for epidural injections for herpes zoster and radiculopathy, and for spinal cord stimulation (SCS) for FBSS and CRPS type I.

Intercostal nerve, stellate ganglion, and paravertebral blocks have been described as interventional options for the treatment of postmastectomy pain. Their efficacy is inconclusive.[66]

Epidural Steroid Injections (ESI)

Most practitioners agree that radicular symptoms are likely to be neuropathic in etiology. There is ongoing controversy in the literature regarding the efficacy of ESI for the treatment of radiculopathy. The clinical practice guidelines of the American Pain Society gave a weak recommendation for the injections, given lack of long-term benefits and inconsistencies in the evidence.[67] The guidelines of the American Society of Interventional Pain Physicians group ESI for disk herniation with or without radiculopathy into three categories: caudal, interlaminar, and transforaminal ESI. They give strong recommendations for caudal, lumbar transforaminal, and cervical ESI. Strong recommendations were given for short-term relief with interlaminar ESI and weak recommendations were given for long-term relief.[68] The IASP guidelines give a weak recommendation for ESI for short-term benefits.[65]

Sympathetic Blocks

In certain types of neuropathic pain, the sympathetic nervous system is dysfunctional. Sympathetic nerve fibers sprout into the dorsal root ganglia, resulting in sympathetically maintained pain. Sympathetic blocks have been studied for the treatment of neuropathic pain. Stellate ganglion blocks have been described in the literature as a possible therapeutic intervention for postmastectomy pain syndrome.[69] In patients with CRPS, excessive sympathetic activity may provoke neuropathic pain. There is an ongoing debate regarding the contribution of the sympathetic nervous system to this clinical syndrome. Sympathetic blocks are relatively safe and are still considered a sensible treatment option for patients in whom pharmacologic and nonpharmacologic options have failed.

SCS

SCS can be an alternative treatment for certain types of neuropathic pain. It was first used in 1967 to treat neuropathic cancer pain.[70] In 2007, the EFNS proposed guidelines for the use of neurostimulation for neuropathic pain.[71] The mechanism of action of SCS still remains unclear. The gate-control theory of pain proposed by Melzack and Wall provides some of the basic concepts behind stimulation treatment.[72] Cost-effectiveness studies have favored SCS.[73] In the PROCESS study, SCS improved HRQoL at 3 and 6 months better than conventional medical management in patients with neuropathic pain from FBSS.[74] The 24-month follow-up study reported sustained improvement of HRQoL.[75]

Intrathecal Drug Delivery

The first administration of an intrathecal medication is credited to Leonard Corning in 1885.[76] The identification of opioid receptors in the substantia gelatinosa of the dorsal horn of the spinal cord led to the use of intrathecal opioid analgesia. Intrathecal treatment for neuropathic pain should be considered when conservative measures have failed.[77] Opioids suitable for intrathecal administration include morphine, hydromorphone, and fentanyl. The main advantage of intrathecal opioids is that the dose needed is lower than that for opioids taken orally, resulting in fewer adverse effects. One disadvantage is the formation of granulomas at the catheter tip, which can lead to spinal cord compression. In animals, granuloma formation has been associated with escalating doses and concentrations of intrathecal opioids.[78] Intrathecal local anesthetics, however, such as bupivacaine, are effective in the treatment of neuropathic pain.[79] Dosage is adjusted to prevent numbness and weakness. Ziconotide, an intrathecally administered calcium channel blocker, has been beneficial in the treatment of refractory neuropathic pain.[80] Other agents that can be administered intrathecally include alpha-2 agonists (clonidine) and gamma-aminobutyric acid agonists (baclofen). Dosing recommendations for intrathecal infusions were made at the polyanalgesic consensus conference held in 2012.[81]

CONCLUSION

Neuropathic pain syndrome is complex and multifactorial. Success in the treatment of neuropathic pain depends on evidence-based medicine and individualized patient care. Collaborative efforts are needed to implement a multimodal analgesic plan. Preventative, nonpharmacologic, pharmacologic, and interventional options are recommended.

REFERENCES

1. IASP Taxonomy. International Association for the Study of Pain. http://www.iasp-pain.org/Taxonomy. Accessed December 31, 2016.
2. Definitions of Chronic Pain Syndromes. International Association for the Study of Pain. http://www.iasp-pain.org/Advocacy/icd.aspx?ItemNumber=5354. Accessed December 31, 2016.
3. Jensen TS, Baron R, Haanpää M, et al. A new definition of neuropathic pain. *Pain.* 2011;152(10):2204–2205.
4. Gilron I, Baron R, Jensen T. Neuropathic pain: principles of diagnosis and treatment. *Mayo Clin Proc.* 2015;90(4):532–545.
5. O'Connor A. Neuropathic pain. Quality-of-life impact, costs, and cost effectiveness of therapy. *Pharmacoeconomics.* 2009;27(2):95–112.
6. Jensen MP, Chadroff MJ, Dworkins RH. The impact of neuropathic pain on health-related quality of life. Review and implications. *Neurology.* 2007;68:1178–1182.
7. Smith B, Torrance N, Bennett M, Lee AJ. Health and quality of life associated with chronic pain of predominantly neuropathic origin in the community. *Clin J Pain.* 2007;23(2):142–149.
8. Attal N, Lanteri-Minet M, Laurent B, et al. The specific disease burden of neuropathic pain: results of a French nationwide survey. *Pain.* 2011;152:2836–2843.
9. van Hecke O, Austin SK, Khan RA, Smith BH, Torrance N. Neuropathic pain in the general population: a systematic review of epidemiological studies. *Pain.* 2014;155(4):654–662.
10. Smith BH, Torrance N. Epidemiology of neuropathic pain and its impact on quality of life. *Curr Pain Headache Rep.* 2012;16(3):191–198.
11. Bouhassira D, Lantéri-Minet M, Attal N, Laurent B, Touboul C. Prevalence of chronic pain with neuropathic characteristics in the general population. *Pain.* 2008;136(3):380–387.
12. Torrance N, Smith BH, Bennett MI, Lee AJ. The epidemiology of chronic pain of predominantly neuropathic origin. Results from a general population survey. *J Pain.* 2006;7(4):281–289.
13. Yawn BP, Wollan PC, Weingarten TN, Watson JC, Hooten WM, Melton LJ. The prevalence of neuropathic pain: clinical evaluation compared with screening tools in a community population. *Pain Med.* 2009;10(3):586–593.
14. Toth C, Lander J, Wiebe S. The prevalence and impact of chronic pain with neuropathic pain symptoms in the general population. *Pain Med.* 2009;10(5):918–929.
15. Dieleman JP, Kerklaan J, Huygen FJ, Bouma PA, Sturkenboom MC. Incidence rates and treatment of neuropathic pain conditions in the general population. *Pain.* 2008;137(3):681–688.
16. Gertner R, Jensen MB, Nielsen J, Ewertz M, Kroman N, Kehlet H. Prevalence of and factors associated with persistent pain following breast cancer surgery. *JAMA.* 2009;302(18):1985–1992.
17. Alves Nogueira Fabro E, Bergmann A, do Amaral E Silva B, et al. Post-mastectomy pain syndrome: incidence and risk. *Breast.* 2012;12(3):321–325.
18. Villholm OJ, Cold S, Rasmussen L, Sindrup SH. The post-mastectomy pain syndrome: epidemiology study on the prevalence of chronic pain after surgery for breast cancer. *Br J Cancer.* 2008;99:604–610.
19. Jung B, Ahrendt G, Oaklander A, Dworkin R. Neuropathic pain following breast cancer surgery: proposed classification and research update. *Pain.* 2003;104:1–13.
20. Treede R, Jensen TS, Campbell JN, et al. Neuropathic pain: redefinition and a grading system for clinical and research purposes. *Neurology.* 2007;70(18):1630–1635. doi:10.1212/01.wnl.0000282763.29778.59
21. Devor M. Neuropathic pain and injured nerve: peripheral mechanisms. *Br Med Bull.* 1991;47(3):619–630.
22. Sang CN, Gracely RH, Max MB, Bennett GJ. Capsaicin-evoked mechanical allodynia and hyperalgesia cross nerve territories. *Anesthesiology.* 1996;85(3):491–496.
23. Ørstavik K, Weidner C, Schmidt R, et al. Pathological C-fibres in patients with a chronic painful condition. *Brain.* 2003;126:567–578.
24. Cohen SP, Mao J. Neuropathic pain: mechanisms and their clinical implications. *BMJ.* 2014;348:f7656.

25. Schüning J, Scherens A, Haussleiter IS, et al. Sensory changes and loss of intraepidermal nerve fibers in painful unilateral nerve injury. *Clin J Pain.* 2009;25(8):683–690.
26. Baron R. Neuropathic pain: a clinical perspective. *Handbook of Experimental Pharmacology.* New York, NY: Springer; 2009:3–30.
27. Curatolo M, Arendt-Nielsen L, Petersen-Felix S. Central hypersensitivity in chronic pain: mechanisms and clinical implications. *Phys Med Rehabil Clin N Am.* 2006;17(2):287–302.
28. Wallace A, Wallace M. Post-mastectomy and post thoracotomy pain. *Anesthesiol Clin North Am.* 1997;15(2):353–370.
29. Barelka P, Carroll IR. Chronic pain after surgery for breast cancer. In: Dirbas F, Scott-Conner C, eds. *Breast Surgical Techniques and Interdisciplinary Management.* New York, NY: Springer; 2011:1029–1037.
30. Tasmuth T, Smitten von, Hietanen P, Kataja M, Kalso E. Pain and other symptoms after different treatment modalities of breast cancer. *Ann Oncol.* 1995;6(5):453–459.
31. Bouhassira D, Attal N. Translational neuropathic pain research: a clinical perspective. *Neuroscience.* 2016;338:27–35.
32. Finnerup NB, Haroutounian S, Kamerman P, et al. Neuropathic pain. *Pain.* 2016;157(8):1599–1606.
33. Gilron I. Neuropathic pain: a practical guide for the clinician. *CMAJ.* 2006;175(3):265–275.
34. Bennett MI, Attal N, Backonja MM, et al. Using screening tools to identify neuropathic pain. *Pain.* 2007;127(3):199–203.
35. Baron R, Binder A, Wasner G. Neuropathic pain: diagnosis, pathophysiological mechanisms, and treatment. *Lancet Neurol.* 2010;9(8):807–819.
36. Attal N, Fermanian C, Fermanian J, Lanteri-Minet M, Alchaar H, Bouhassira D. Neuropathic pain: are there distinct subtypes depending on the aetiology or anatomical lesion? *Pain.* 2008;138(2):343–353.
37. Bouhassira D, Attal N. Diagnosis and assessment of neuropathic pain: the saga of clinical tools. *Pain.* 2011;152(suppl):S74–S83.
38. Backonja MM, Attal N, Baron R, et al. Value of quantitative sensory testing in neurological and pain disorders: NeuPSIG consensus. *Pain.* 2013;154(9):1807–1819.
39. Devigili G, Tugnoli V, Penza P, et al. The diagnostic criteria for small fibre neuropathy: from symptoms to neuropathology. *Brain.* 2008;131(7):1912–1925.
40. Vlckova-Moravcova E, Bednarik J, Belobradkova J, Sommer C. Small-fibre involvement in diabetic patients with neuropathic foot pain. *Diabet Med.* 2008;25(6):692–699.
41. Garcia-Larrea L. Objective pain diagnostics: clinical neurophysiology. *Neurophysiol Clin.* 2012;42(4):187–197.
42. Leandri M, Saturno M, Spadavecchia L, Iannetti GD, Cruccu G, Truini A. Measurement of skin temperature after infrared laser stimulation. *Neurophysiol Clin.* 2006;36(4):207–218.
43. Cruccu G, Sommer C, Anand P, et al. EFNS guidelines on neuropathic pain assessment: revised 2009. *Euro J Neurol.* 2010;17(8):1010–1018.
44. Garcia-Larrea L. Laser-evoked potential abnormalities in central pain patients: the influence of spontaneous and provoked pain. *Brain.* 2002;125(12):2766–2781.
45. Kudel I, Edwards RR, Kozachik S, et al. Predictors and consequences of multiple persistent postmastectomy pains. *J Pain Symptom Manage.* 2007;34:619–627.
46. Andersen KG, Kehlet H. Persistent pain after breast cancer treatment: a critical review of risk factors and strategies for prevention. *J Pain.* 2011;12(7):725–746.
47. Peintinger F, Reitsamer R, Stranzl H, Ralph G. Comparison of quality of life and arm complaints after axillary lymph node dissection vs sentinel lymph node biopsy in breast cancer patients. *Br J Cancer.* 2003;89:648–652.
48. Amr YM, Yousef AAA-M. Evaluation of efficacy of the perioperative administration of venlafaxine or gabapentin on acute and chronic post-mastectomy pain. *Clin J Pain.* 2010;26(5):381–385.
49. López-Álvarez VM, Modol L, Navarro X, Cobianchi S. Early increasing-intensity treadmill exercise reduces neuropathic pain by preventing nociceptor collateral sprouting and disruption of chloride co-transporter homeostasis after peripheral nerve injury. *Pain.* 2015;156(9):1812–1825.
50. Songer D. Psychotherapeutic approaches in treatment of pain. *Psychiatry.* 2005;2(5):19–24.
51. Gilron I, Bailey JM, Tu D, Holden RR, Weaver DF, Houlden RL. Morphine, gabapentin, or their combination for neuropathic pain. *N Engl J Med.* 2005;352:1324–1334.
52. Hanna M, O'Brien C, Wilson MC. Prolonged-release oxycodone enhances the effects of existing gabapentin therapy in painful diabetic neuropathy patients. *Eur J Pain.* 2008;12:804–813.
53. Dworkin RH, O'Connor AB, Backonja M, et al. Pharmacologic management of neuropathic pain: evidence-based recommendations. *Pain.* 2007;132:237–251.
54. Moulin DE, Clark AJ, Gilron I, et al. Pharmacological management of chronic neuropathic pain—consensus statement and guidelines from the Canadian Pain Society. *Pain Res Manage.* 2007;12(1):13–21.
55. Attal N, Cruccu G, Baron R, et al. EFNS guidelines on the pharmacological treatment of neuropathic pain: 2010 revision. *Eur J Neurol.* 2010;17:1113–1123.
56. Saarto T, Wiffen PJ. Antidepressants for neuropathic pain. *Cochrane Database Syst Rev.* 2007;4CD:005454.
57. Finnerup NB, Otto M, Jensen TS, Sindrup SH. Algorithm for neuropathic pain treatment: an evidence based proposal. *Pain.* 2005;118:289–305.
58. Max MB, Lynch SA, Muir J, Shoaf S, Smoller B, Dubner R. Effects of desipramine, amitriptyline, and fluoxetine on pain in diabetic neuropathy. *N Engl J Med.* 1992;326:1250–1256.
59. Semenchuk MR, Sherman S, Davis B. Double-blind, randomized trial of bupropion SR for the treatment of neuropathic pain. *Neurology.* 2001;57:1583–1588.
60. Caraceni A, Zecca E, Bonezzi C, et al. Gabapentin for neuropathic cancer pain; a randomized controlled trial from the gabapentin cancer pain study group. *J Clin Oncol.* 2004;22:2909–2917.
61. Freynhagen R, Strojek K, Griesing T, Wahlen E, Balkenohl M. Efficacy of pregabalin in neuopathic pain evaluated in a 12-week, randomized, double-blind, multicenter, placebo-controlled trial of flexible- and fixed-dose regimens. *Pain.* 2005;115:254–263.
62. Eisenberg E, McNicol ED, Carr DB. Efficacy and safety of opioid agonists in the treatment of neuropathic pain of nonmalignant origin. Systematic review and meta-analysis of randomized controlled trials. *JAMA.* 2005;293(24):3043–3052.
63. Park CH, Jung SH, Han CG. Effects of intravenous lidocaine on the neuropathic pain of failed back surgery syndrome. *Korean J Pain.* 2012;25(2):94–98.
64. Kvarnstrom A, Karsten R, Quiding H, Emanuelsson BM, Gordh T. The effectiveness of intravenous ketamine and lidocaine on peripheral neuropathic pain. *Acta Anaesthesiol Scand.* 2003;47:868–878.
65. Dworkin RH, O'Connor AB, Kent J, et al. Interventional management of neuropathic pain: NeuPSIG. *Pain.* 2013;154:2249–2261.
66. Wijayasinghe N, Anderson KG, Kehlet H. Neural blockade for persistent pain after breast surgery. *Reg Anesth Pain Med.* 2014;39(4):1–7.
67. Chou R, Loeser JD, Owns DK, et al. Interventional therapies, surgery, and interdisciplinary rehabilition for low back pain: an evidence-based clinical practice guideline from the American Pain Society. *Spine.* 2009;34(10):1066–1077.
68. Manchikanti L, Boswell MV, Singh V, et al. Comprehensive evidence-based guidelines for interventional techniques in the management of chronic spine pain. *Pain Physician.* 2009;12:699–802.
69. Abbas DN, Abd el Ghafar EM, Ibrahim WA, Omran AF. Fluoroscopic stellate ganglion block for post-mastectomy pain: a comparison of the classic anterior approach and the oblique approach. *Clin J Pain.* 2011;27:207–213.
70. Shealy CN, Mortimer JT, Reswick JB. Electrical inhibition of pain by simulation of the dorsal columns: preliminary clinical report. *Anesth Analg.* 1997;46(4):489–491.
71. Cruccu G, Aziz TZ, Garcia-Larrea L, et al. EFNS guidelines on neurostimulation therapy for neuropathic pain. *Eur J Neurol.* 2007;14(9):952–970.

72. Melzack R, Wall PD. Pain mechanisms: a theory. *Science.* 1965;150(699):971–979.
73. North R, Kidd D, Shipley J, Taylor R. Spinal cord stimulation versus reoperation for failed back surgery syndrome: a cost effectiveness and cost utility analysis based on a randomized, controlled trial. *Neurosurgery.* 2007;61(2):361–369.
74. Manca A, Kumar K, Taylor R, et al. Quality of life, resource consumption and cost of spinal cord stimulation versus conventional medical management in neuropathic pain patients with failed back surgery syndrome (PROCESS trial). *Eur J Pain.* 2008;12(8):1047–1058.
75. Kumar K, Taylor R, Jacques L, et al. The effects of spinal cord stimulation in neuropathic pain are sustained: a 24-month follow-up of the prospective randomized controlled multicenter trial of the effectiveness of spinal cord stimulation. *Neurosurgery.* 2008;63:762–770.
76. Corning JL. Spinal anesthesia and local medication of the cord. *NY Med J.* 1885;42:483–485.
77. Jamison DE, Wilkinson IM, Cohen SP. Intrathecal drug delivery for neuropathic pain. *US Neurology.* 2011;7(2):154–162.
78. Gradert TL, Baze WB, Satterfield WC, Hildebrand KR, Johansen MJ, Hassenbusch SJ. Safety of chronic intrathecal morphine infusion in a sheep model. *Anesthesiology.* 2003;99:188–198.
79. Osenbach R. Intrathecal drug delivery in the management of pain. In: Fishman SM, Ballantyne JC, Rathmell JP, eds. *Bonica's Management of Pain.* 4th ed. Philadelphia, PA: Lippincott Williams and Wilkins; 2010:1437–1458.
80. Rauck RL, Wallace MS, Burton AW, Kapural L, North JM. Intrathecal ziconotide for neuropathic pain: a review. *Pain.* 2009;9(5):327–337.
81. Deer TR, Prager J, Levy R, et al. Polyanalgesic consensus conference 2012: recommendations for the management of pain by intrathecal (intraspinal) drug delivery: report of an interdisciplinary expert panel. *Neuromodulation.* 2012;15(5):436–466.

REVIEW QUESTIONS

1. Compared to patients with chronic nonneuropathic pain, patients with chronic neuropathic pain tend to have a higher incidence of:

   A. Depression
   B. Schizophrenia
   C. Bipolar disorder
   D. Conversion disorder

2. All the following are considered positive symptoms of neuropathic pain except:

   A. Numbness in the affected area
   B. Tingling in the affected area
   C. Sensory loss in the affected area
   D. Burning sensation in the affected area

3. A higher prevalence of chronic neuropathic pain was associated with all of the following except:

   A. Female sex
   B. Manual occupation
   C. Urban population
   D. Inability to work

ANSWERS

1. A. Patients with chronic neuropathic pain tend to have higher depression and anxiety scores than patients with chronic nonneuropathic pain.[8] Answer A is therefore correct. Schizophrenia, bipolar disorder, and conversion disorder are psychiatric entities that are not associated with chronic neuropathic pain.

2. C. Clinical symptoms of neuropathic pain can be positive or negative. The positive symptoms are pain, paresthesias, or dysesthesias (tingling, numbness, or "pins and needles"); negative symptoms are neurologic sensory deficits in the painful area.[35]

3. C. The prevalence of chronic pain with neuropathic characteristics is associated with middle age (50–64 years), manual occupation, female sex, and living in rural areas.[11]

QUESTIONS AND ANSWERS

This chapter has accompanying questions and answers that are available to subscribers as part of the Oxford eLearning platform. To access the questions, follow the link below, or go to ✔ http://oxfordmedicine.com/painmanagementreview

16.

POSTTHORACOTOMY PAIN SYNDROME

Melinda Aquino

STEM CASE AND KEY QUESTIONS

The patient, a 67-year-old male with a 100-pack/year smoking history, was referred to the pain clinic complaining of right chest pain radiating to his back. He had a right thoracotomy and right upper lobectomy for lung cancer 3 months earlier. His past medical history is significant for type 2 diabetes mellitus, hypertension, deep vein thrombosis, and atypical angina. Current medications include insulin 25 units every morning, metoprolol, losartan, Plavix, Percocet 5/325 mg every 4 to 6 hours as needed for pain, and ibuprofen 400 mg every 6 to 8 hours as needed for pain. The patient states that he is having severe pain, and that the Percocet "doesn't really help." His thoracic surgeon referred him to the pain clinic for suspected postthoracotomy pain syndrome (PTPS).

WHAT IS PTPS?

Essentially all patients who undergo thoracotomy will suffer from acute postoperative pain. Current recommendations for acute perioperative pain management include preemptive analgesia and regional anesthetic techniques. PTPS is relatively common and is seen in approximately 50% of patients after thoracotomy.[1] The condition becomes chronic, and up to 30% of patients still experience pain 4 to 5 years after surgery. Most patients experience mild to moderate pain that doesn't interfere with daily life. A small subset of patients have severe, debilitating pain. The exact mechanism of the pathogenesis is not clear, but it is thought to be a combination of neuropathic and nonneuropathic (myofascial) pain.

WHAT ARE THE SIGNS AND SYMPTOMS OF PTPS?

The patient says that he has severe pain in the right side of his chest, under the breast, which radiates to the axilla and his back on the right side. He rates the pain 8 out of 10 on the Numerical Analog Scale. The pain is described as burning and shooting, and is constant. Pain is made worse by wearing tight shirts and by lying on the right side. Percocet gives minimal relief. Ibuprofen gives no relief. He states that he has had the pain for the past 3 months since he had surgery.

WHAT ELSE SHOULD WE CONSIDER IN THE DIFFERENTIAL DIAGNOSIS AND WHAT TESTS SHOULD WE ORDER TO RULE THEM OUT?

The pain of PTPS may be mistaken for pain of cardiac or gallbladder origin and can lead to visits to the emergency department and unnecessary cardiac and gastrointestinal workups.[2] Tietze's syndrome, pleural disease, pulmonary embolus, and rib and sternal fractures can all confuse the diagnosis. Neuropathic pain involving the chest wall, including acute herpes zoster and painful diabetic neuropathy, also should be considered. A chest X-ray, CBC, HgA_{1c}, and electrocardiogram (ECG) should be ordered for the patient to rule out these diseases.

WHAT ARE THE TREATMENT OPTIONS FOR THIS PATIENT?

Several modalities of pain management have been shown to be successful in PTPS. Oral medications, physical therapy, and regional blocks are discussed with the patient. He is fearful of needles, and opts for medical management.

The patient is advised to discontinue Percocet, because it is not relieving the pain and is causing constipation and drowsiness. Ibuprofen is discontinued as well. Meloxicam 7.5 mg is recommended. Gabapentin is started at a bedtime dosage of 300 mg and the patient is instructed to increase it to 300 mg three times a day each week as tolerated. Follow-up is scheduled for 1 month's time. The patient declines physical therapy at this time.

WHAT OTHER TREATMENTS ARE AVAILABLE FOR PTPS?

The patient returns for follow-up in 1 month. He states that the Meloxicam is not helping. He discontinued the gabapentin because it made him "sick" and sleepy and he didn't like the way it made him feel. He wants to know what other medications he can try. He is still refusing injections.

Lengthy discussion ensues, and the patient still prefers medical management. After reviewing his ECG, you decide to initiate therapy with nortriptyline 25 mg in the morning and to increase the Meloxicam to 15 mg every day. You perform a trial with a transcutaneous nerve stimulator (TENS) unit, and patient will use it daily at home. Follow-up is scheduled for 1 month's time.

WHAT INVASIVE PROCEDURES ARE AVAILABLE FOR THIS PATIENT?

The patient returns for follow-up saying the pain is worse, and that he is ready to consider invasive treatment options. Trigger-point injections (TPI) are considered for the scar pain he is experiencing. There are several invasive treatment options for PTPS. Thoracic paravertebral nerve blocks are becoming widely used. In thoracic paravertebral nerve block, local anesthetic is injected alongside the thoracic vertebra close to where the spinal nerves emerge from the intervertebral foramen.[3] Thoracic paravertebral nerve block is an effective way of providing analgesia in PTPS. Intercostal nerve blocks are also beneficial for PTPS. Intercostal nerve blocks provides excellent analgesia for chest trauma, such as rib fractures, and for postsurgical pain after chest and upper abdominal surgery, such as thoracotomy, thoracoscopy, mastectomy, gastrectomy, and cholecystectomy.[4]

After discussion with the patient, he agrees to having an injection, and thoracic paravertebral block is chosen. Consultation with the patient's primary care physician follows, and he allows the patient to hold Plavix for the procedure.

The patient returns after having the paravertebral injection. He reports approximately 50% pain relief.

The patient will return for repeat injection. He will continue to escalate the nortriptyline as tolerated.

DISCUSSION

Postthoracotomy pain is pain persisting in the area of thoracotomy lasting for at least 2 months after the surgery. Patients complain of achy, sharp, and shooting pain in the distribution of the surgical incision. There is usually tenderness, sensory loss, and numbness along the thoracotomy scar. Trigger points may be present, usually secondary to neuroma formation.

Multiple factors contribute to PTPS. The most common cause is direct surgical trauma to the intercostal nerves. The nerves can take up to 1 year to heal, and if they heal abnormally, chronic neuropathic pain ensues. Pain may also be caused by rib fractures due to use of rib spreaders intraoperatively. There can also be compressive neuropathy of the intercostal nerves due to direct compression of the intercostal nerves by retraction. There can be incisional scar pain due to cutaneous neuroma formation. Stretch injuries to the intercostal nerves can occur at the costovertebral junction. The pain from the rib fractures produces characteristic localized pain that is increased with deep inspiration, movement of the affected ribs, and coughing. The pain of PTPS is usually described as burning, achy, and deep, sharp, and shooting, neuritic and dysesthetic, and is moderate to severe in intensity.

Virtually all patients who have a thoracotomy will experience postoperative pain. Many treatment modalities can help with this pain. These include preemptive analgesia, intraoperative management with regional anesthetic techniques, and postoperative pain management with continuous catheters and/or systemic opioids. Many theories exist that controlling pain in the perioperative period can lessen the incidence of the development of chronic pain syndromes, in this case, PTPS.

A thorough history and physical exam should be performed. In the patient described, the physical examination revealed a well-healed incision extending from the right anterolateral chest wall to the right posterior paraspinal area. There was tenderness to palpation along the scar. There was also a paresthesia elicited, which suggested neuroma formation. Sensory examination of the affected dermatomes revealed decreased sensation to pinprick and decreased temperature sensation. There was also allodynia (sensitivity to a stimulus that is normally not painful), and the patient reported that wearing a shirt exacerbated the pain. In some cases, there is subcostal nerve involvement, and significant motor nerve impairment may be noted. The patients complain that their abdomen bulges out. Also, in rare cases, patients may develop a chronic regional pain syndrome of the ipsilateral upper extremity, and evaluation for this should be a component of the patient's evaluation. If upper extremity chronic regional pain syndrome is left undiagnosed and untreated, a frozen shoulder may develop.

RECOMMENDED TESTING FOR PATIENTS WITH POSTTHORACOTOMY PAIN

First and foremost, a chest radiography should be ordered. If the pain is thought to be coming from the intercostal nerve, one needs to rule out bony pathology, including fractures and tumor, from the differential diagnosis. Radionuclide bone scanning may be useful to rule out occult fractures of the ribs and sternum. A CT scan of the thoracic contents is indicated if an occult mass or pleural disease is suspected. Electromyography is helpful in distinguishing injury of the intercostal nerve from stretch injury of the intercostal nerve at the costovertebral junction. Depending on the clinical presentation of the patient, additional testing may be indicated, including complete blood count, coagulation profile, prostate-specific antigen, erythrocyte sedimentation rate (ESR), and antigen-specific antibody testing.

DIFFERENTIAL DIAGNOSIS

The pain of PTPS can be mistaken for several medical entities. It may be mistaken for pain of cardiac origin, patients present at the emergency department, and the clinician has to rule out myocardial infarction. If pain radiates to the right upper quadrant, then gallbladder issues can be erroneously considered. If a trauma has occurred, then rib and sternal fractures should be ruled out. Continuous pain after a chest traumatic event with negative radiographic images should be investigated further with radionuclide bone scanning for proper identification of missed fractures. Tietze's syndrome can be confused with PTPS. Tietze's syndrome is a common cause of chest pain distinct from costochondral syndrome. It is characterized by painful swelling of the costal cartilages. The second and third cartilages are most commonly involved. There is tenderness to palpation and pain is increased with coughing and shrugging of the shoulders. There is an association with viral infections.[10]

Neuropathic pain syndrome of the upper chest wall can also be confused with PTPS. The two entities may co-exist as well. Examples of neuropathic chest wall pain include acute herpes zoster/postherpetic neuralgia and diabetic neuropathy. Diseases that cause inflammation of the pleura must be considered in the differential diagnosis as well. Pulmonary embolus and infection may cloud the diagnosis.

INITIAL PAIN MEDICATIONS USED FOR TREATMENT OF POSTTHORACOTOMY PAIN

Initially, the recommended pain medications are nonsteroidal anti-inflammatory drugs (NSAIDs). NSAIDs are among the most widely used analgesics in the world because of their ability to reduce pain and inflammation.[5] They work by inhibiting prostaglandin production from arachidonic acid, by either reversible or irreversible acetylation of cyclooxygenase. The side-effect profile of NSAIDs includes gastrointestinal upset and bleeding, decreased renal function and renal failure, and cardiovascular events, including stroke and myocardial infarction. Caution must be used in elderly patients and patients with comorbidities.

ANALGESIC ADJUNCTS FOR PTPS

The most widely used medication for neuropathic pain is gabapentin. Gabapentin is similar in structure to GABA (gamma-aminobutyric acid), and has been shown to bind to the alpha$_2$-subunit of the voltage-gated calcium channels that contribute to pain attenuation in neuropathic states. Gabapentin also interacts with NMDA receptors, protein kinase C, and inflammatory cytokines.[6] The standard initial dosage is 100 to 300 mg at bedtime, which is then titrated up to administration three times per day. The maximum dosage is 3600 mg per day divided into three doses. The most common side effects of gabapentin include dizziness, fatigue, and drowsiness. Peripheral edema, nystagmus, and tremor can also occur. Gabapentin should be used with caution in patients with renal failure, due to increased accumulation and toxicity. Studies have shown that in patients with neuropathic pain (diabetic neuropathy and postherpetic neuralgia), there is a decrease in pain scores, more restful sleep at night, and an overall improvement in functioning when gabapentin is administered in therapeutic doses. Pregabalin (Lyrica) is a therapeutic agent close in structure to the neurotransmitter GABA. It is a potent gabapentinoid and is similar in mechanism of action to gabapentin and baclofen. It is thought to exert its effect at the calcium channels. Pregabalin has been shown to have benefit for fibromyalgia pain and diabetic neuropathy. It is also a potent anxiolytic and has high abuse potential, and thus is a Schedule V controlled substance. Side effects include sleepiness, confusion, trouble with memory, poor coordination, dry mouth, problems with vision, and weight gain. The starting dose is 50 mg twice to three times a day, with a maximum recommended dosage of 300 mg per day.

Traditionally, the tricyclic antidepressants (TCAs) have been used for PTPS. Controlled studies have demonstrated the efficacy of amitriptyline for this indication.[7] Amitriptyline blocks both serotonin and norepinephrine receptors. It has a significant unfavorable side-effect profile, including sedation, orthostasis, and anticholinergic side effects (dry mouth, dry eyes, urinary retention, and constipation). Amitriptyline must be avoided in patients with known cardiac conduction delays, because it can cause tachydysrhythmias. Amitriptyline can worsen narrow-angle glaucoma and should be avoided in patients with this issue. Urinary retention is also a problem that can arise with its usage. Although amitriptyline has an extensive side-effect profile, due to its low cost, high efficacy, and availability in both liquid and pill form, it is a good choice for pain management. In order to minimize its sedative side effect, the recommended starting dose is 10 to 25 mg at bedtime, with careful monitoring for side effects as the dosage is escalated. Patients should be cautioned about the risk of orthostatic hypotension, and should be counseled to use caution when getting up from bed. If analgesia is not achieved when the 150-mg dosage is reached, then another medication should be used. Nortriptyline (Pamelor) and desipramine (Norpramin) are excellent choices when the sedative effects of amitriptyline are too intense. These medications are given as a morning dose of 10 to 25 mg and may be titrated up to 150 mg per day. Most patients tend to see an effect at 50 to 75 mg per day. Because it usually takes 2 to 3 weeks to see the effect, the patients must be counseled to not give up if benefit is not noticed immediately. The TCAs should be used with caution in patients who have cardiac arrhythmias. Furthermore, patients prone to psychiatric activation or agitation can have exacerbation if these medications are co-administered with steroids.

Selective serotonin reuptake inhibitors (SSRIs) can also be useful in neuropathic pain management. They have a more benign side-effect profile than the TCAs and are better tolerated. However, they are more expensive, and certain medications are not covered by insurance carriers. The SSRIs selectively block the reuptake of serotonin by blockade of the sodium/potassium ATP pump, which results in increased levels of serotonin in the synaptic junction. They also affect other serotonin receptors, most notably in the gut, which probably accounts for their propensity to cause gastrointestinal side effects, especially during initiation of therapy.[2] Fluoxetine (Prozac, Sarafem), paroxetine (Paxil), and sertraline (Zoloft) are the most commonly available. They all have a benign side-effect profile, and patients complain mainly of lack of energy and constipation.

Local anesthetics can be used in neuropathic pain states to block the aberrant firing of abnormal nerves as well as to block the normally firing nerves. They have been studied and have been found to be effective in the treatment of postherpetic neuralgia, peripheral neuropathies, and radiculopathies. Lidoderm patch (5% concentration) is worn 12 hours on and 12 hours off. Mexilitene, the oral form of lidocaine, can be used after pain relief is achieved during a lidocaine infusion test. Data have shown it to be helpful in diabetic neuropathy, thalamic stroke pain, and other neuropathic pain states.

Muscle relaxants may be of use in several cases of muscle spasm associated with the PTPS; many classes do exist with varied mechanisms of action. Low dose of any of those agents may be used as adjuvants as part of multimodal analgesic treatment of the PTPS.

INVASIVE MODALITIES AVAILABLE TO MANAGE POSTTHORACOTOMY PAIN

When scar neuroma is suspected, one treatment option recommended is TPI. A trigger point is an area of spasm and inflammation in the muscles. Tender points and/or palpable nodules can also be felt in scar tissues, reflecting the presence of neuromas. A combination of local anesthetic (lidocaine or bupivacaine) and corticosteroid can be injected into these areas. Sometimes a needle alone inserted into the trigger point can give relief via the technique called "dry needling": Upon insertion of a small (25-G) needle, multiple passages are initiated within the taut band of the trigger point; the purpose of the maneuver is inactivation of the trigger point and subsequent pain relief. Complications include bleeding, infection, pain at the site, and pneumothorax. The injections may need to be repeated several times for prolonged effect.

There are several injections that can be beneficial for postthoracotomy pain. For inpatients, thoracic sympathetic block with a thoracic epidural or thoracic paravertebral catheter may be utilized.[8] More commonly, the patients with pain syndromes are treated as outpatients, and intercostal nerve blocks and single-shot thoracic paravertebral nerve blocks are utilized.

The intercostal nerves arise from the anterior division of the thoracic paravertebral nerves. Intercostal nerves have four branches—anterior cutaneous, posterior cutaneous, postganglionic fibers of gray rami communicantes that join the sympathetic chain, and the lateral cutaneous division. For the intercostal block, the patient is positioned prone, with the arms hanging off the side of the bed, or in the sitting or lateral position. The levels of the ribs to be blocked are identified in the posterior axillary line. The injection must be performed in this area, because the lateral cutaneous branch may be missed if the injection is not posterior enough. Ultrasound guidance is commonly used, to decrease the risk of pneumothorax. If ultrasound not available, a walk-off technique inferiorly can be used. Fluoroscopy has also been used, and, by using radiopaque dye, has the advantage of assessing appropriate medication spread along the intercostal nerves. Three to five mL of local anesthetic (lidocaine or bupivacaine) are injected to each intercostal nerve.[9] Corticosteroids, such as methylprednisolone, triamcinolone, or dexamethasone, can be added. Caution must be used in this area because intercostal nerves have the highest reuptake of local anesthetics due to the proximity of the intercostal nerve and artery.[10] Pneumothorax (less than 1%), bleeding, infection, and pain at the injection site are other complications. Due to the overlap of cutaneous nerves in this area, one rib above and one rib below the suspected level of concern should be blocked. Although there is a risk of pneumothorax and local anesthetic toxicity, the risk can be reduced with good technique, consideration given to the maximum allowable drug dose, and the patient's clinical condition.[7]

An alternative to the intercostal nerve block is the thoracic paravertebral nerve block. The thoracic paravertebral nerves exit the intervertebral foramen just below the transverse process of the vertebra. Once it exits the intervertebral foramen, the thoracic paravertebral nerve gives off the four branches. The twelfth thoracic nerve courses beneath the twelfth rib and is called the subcostal nerve. The subcostal and intercostal nerves supply the skin, muscles, parietal pleura, and ribs. In a paravertebral nerve block, all four branches of the nerve are blocked, and excellent analgesia of the chest wall and posterolateral thoracic areas can be achieved. The patient is placed in the sitting or lateral decubitus position. Spinal levels are identified and marked. Ultrasound guidance is used to locate the transverse processes, costotransverse ligament, and pleura. For a successful block, the injectate should be below the costotransverse membrane, and visualization of the pleura moving downward confirms adequate spread. A single-level injection with 15 mL of 0.5% marcaine or three separate injections at three levels with 5 mL each is recommended. As with the intercostal nerve block, the procedure can be performed under fluoroscopic guidance or via blind technique.

CONCLUSIONS

- PTPS is a relatively common entity that occurs in patients undergoing thoracotomy and other chest surgery. The pain is neuropathic and nonneuropathic, and the causes are multifactorial.
- Many of the patients affected by this pain syndrome have multiple co-existing diseases that can confound the diagnosis. Careful history and physical examination are necessary. Judicious use of testing, including laboratory tests, ECGs, and X-rays, are necessary to rule out other causes of chest pain. Consultation with the patient's primary care provider may be necessary in order to facilitate treatment.
- Analgesic adjuvants have been successful in treatment of the neuropathic component of PTPS. NSAIDS, gabapentin, Lyrica, TCAs, SSRIs, serotonin-norepinephrine reuptake inhibitors (SNRIs), and muscle relaxants have been widely used. Care must be taken upon initiation of these medications to avoid potential side effects and to encourage patient compliance.
- Invasive techniques have been successful for the management of this pain syndrome. TPIs have been utilized for scar pain due to neuromas and associated muscle pains. Thoracic paravertebral injections, with

or without ultrasound guidance, and intercostal nerve blocks may be of benefit and decrease the need for oral medications.

REFERENCES

1. Karmarkar MK, Ho AM. Post-thoracotomy pain syndrome. *Thorac Surg Clin.* 2004;14(3):345–352.
2. Waldman SD. *Pain Review: Expert Consult.* 1st ed. Philadelphia, USA: W. B. Saunders; 2009.
3. Gerner P. Post-thoracotomy pain management problems. *Anesthesiol Clin.* 2008;26(2):355–367.
4. Karmarker MK, Gin T, Ho AH. Ipsilateral thoraco-lumbar anesthesia and paravertebral spread after low thoracic paravertebral injection. *Br J Anaesth.* 2001;87(2):312–316.
5. Benzon Raj, and Lui et al. *Essentials of Pain Medicine.* 3rd ed. Elsevier; 2011.
6. Kukkar A, Bali A, Singh N, Jaggi AS. Implications and mechanisms of action of gabapentin in neuropathic pain. *Arch Pharmacol Res.* 2013;36(3):237–251.
7. Hadzic A. *Textbook of Regional Anesthesia and Acute Pain Management.* 2nd ed. McGraw-Hill Education/Medical; 2017.
8. Karmarkar MK. Thoracic paravertebral nerve block. *Anesthesiology.* 2001;95:771–780.
9. Wall, Melzack, McMahon, et al. *Textbook of Pain.* 6th ed. Philadelphia, PA: W. B. Saunders; 2013.
10. Benzon H, Rathmell JP, Wu CL, Turk D, Argoff CE, Hurley RW. *Practical Management of Pain E-Book.* Elsevier Health Sciences; 2013.

REVIEW QUESTIONS

1. In costochondritis, the following signs and symptoms are present except:

   A. Tenderness occurring at the costochondral junction
   B. Pain radiating widely
   C. Pain in a band from the spine to sternum along the intercostal nerves, mimicking intercostal neuralgia
   D. Symptoms occurring with musculoskeletal pain

2. All of the following help distinguish chest pain of acute herpes zoster from PTPS except:

   A. Presence of rash
   B. Dermatomal distribution
   C. Response to antibiotics
   D. Burning, dysesthetic-type pain

3. The nerves that have the highest uptake of local anesthetic are:

   A. Sciatic nerve
   B. Intercostal nerves
   C. Axillary nerve
   D. Lumbosacral plexus

ANSWERS

1. C. Pain associated with costochondritis is generally localized, over the costochondral junction; it may radiate widely but does not typically align with the intercostal nerves in a band distribution, as is the case in intercostal neuralgia. Costochondritis may occur in patients suffering from musculoskeletal pain. A special form of costochondral inflammation is Tietze's syndrome, which occurs primarily in the second and third ribs. Based on the explanations above, only answer C is correct, beacuse the condition described does not usually mimic intercostal neuralgia.

2. D. The correct answer is D because both conditions are associated with burning pain. Acute herpes zoster is associated with a specific rash and responds to antibiotics, while the PTPS does not; therefore, answers A and C are incorrect. Answer B is incorrect because while acute herpes zoster may be localized to only one intercostal nerve, PTPS may involve more than one nerve in a wider distribution.

3. B. From the possible answers, the highest uptake of local anesthetic is seen in intercostal nerve blocks; therefore, dosages of local anesthetic should be carefully considered to avoid local anesthetic systemic toxicity (LAST).[7]

QUESTIONS AND ANSWERS

This chapter has accompanying questions and answers that are available to subscribers as part of the Oxford eLearning platform. To access the questions, follow the link below, or go to ✔ http://oxfordmedicine.com/painmanagementreview

17.

CHRONIC STERNAL PAIN AFTER CARDIAC SURGERY

Afzaal Iqbal and Joel Kent

STEM CASE AND KEY QUESTIONS

A 56-year-old male presents with sharp, stabbing, burning, pins-and-needles type, non-radiating pain in his central chest. He underwent an uneventful four-vessel coronary artery bypass graft (CABG) 8 months ago. The pain started initially as a throbbing pain directly at the sternotomy site that never fully resolved after his cardiac surgery. He tolerated the pain for 6 weeks; it then gradually transformed into a burning sensation over the following 6 months. An electrocardiogram showed signs of an old anterior myocardial infarction with first-degree atrioventricular block but no signs of acute ischemia. Cardiac enzymes and stress echocardiography were also within normal limits. He has tried acetaminophen and topical analgesics with no benefit.

HOW DO YOU DEFINE CHRONIC POST-STERNOTOMY PAIN (PSP)? WHAT SHOULD WE CONSIDER IN THE DIFFERENTIAL?

The patient is started on gabapentin and duloxetine, with mild improvement of his pain over 1 month of titrating the medications upward. He has also found lidocaine patches helpful and intermittently applies capsaicin cream with minimal benefit. He denies any allodynia, swelling, erythema, temperature changes, or skin changes.

WHAT INCREASES THE RISK OF DEVELOPING PSP? WILL YOU CONSIDER OPIOIDS FOR THESE PATIENTS?

The patient states that nonsteroidal anti-inflammatory drugs (NSAIDs) do help his pain but he was told not to take them with his blood thinners. His risk for misuse of opioid analgesics is objectively assessed via standardized screening instruments, including the Opioid Risk Tool (ORT) and Diagnosis, Intractability, Risk, Efficacy (DIRE) score, which were both favorable. A decision is made to start the patient on 5 mg of oxycodone three times daily as needed to help curb his pain, to allow him to sleep through the night, and to facilitate his rehabilitation exercises during the week.

IS THERE ANYTHING THAT CAN BE DONE INTRAOPERATIVELY DURING CABG TO MINIMIZE THE DEVELOPMENT OF CHRONIC PSP?

A review of the anesthetic record shows that the patient underwent uneventful anesthesia, with sufentanil and midazolam induction and sufentanil boluses dosed throughout the case. He did not receive any regional anesthesia before, during, or after the procedure. Review of the surgical operative note shows that median sternotomy was made in a standard fashion and the left internal mammary artery (IMA) was dissected for one of the grafts. The patient received hydromorphone via a patient-controlled analgesia (PCA) device afterward, which he used for 2 days. He was then transitioned to an oral regimen of oxycodone and acetaminophen and was discharged on postoperative day 6. He continued the oxycodone and acetaminophen for 3 weeks after discharge.

ARE THERE IMMEDIATE POSTOPERATIVE TREATMENTS THAT HELP PREVENT PSP?

The patient has noted that he tends to be more anxious overall and has a "short fuse" with his wife. He has a history of anxiety that predated his cardiac disease and surgery. He does not remember being told that cardiac surgery would cause this level of chest pain. He feels his wife does not understand his pain. He is now wondering if he should have been more aggressive with pursuing coronary stents rather than surgery. He also wonders whether there is a less invasive method of undergoing CABG surgery.

WHAT ARE THE EFFECTS OF PSYCHOSOCIAL FACTORS ON PAIN PERCEPTION IN PATIENTS UNDERGOING CARDIAC SURGERY?

The patient is considering the usefulness of steroid injections and whether the anticipated side effects are acceptable. A transcutaneous electrical nerve stimulation (TENS) unit does provide him with some transient relief (about 10%).

WHAT PROCEDURAL/INTERVENTIONAL TREATMENTS EXIST FOR TREATING PSP?

The patient returned to see his surgeon, who suggested that the sternal wires may be worsening his pain and that removing the wires might help him. Eventually, he underwent surgical sternal wire removal. His pain worsened immediately afterward, but did subside about 20% 2 months later.

He agreed to try a neuroma injection with local anesthetic and steroid, which helped decrease his pain about 60% for 4 months. He repeated the injections two more times and is satisfied with coming back every 4 to 5 months.

DISCUSSION

INCIDENCE AND RISK FACTORS

Chronic PSP, defined as noncardiac thoracic pain after median sternotomy, has a relatively high incidence after cardiac surgery—about 28%.[1]

Factors that appear to be associated with persistent pain include young age, female sex, IMA harvest, and an increased requirement for postoperative analgesics during the immediate postoperative period.[2]

Studies have found that patients less than 60 years old had higher pain intensities than older patients in the early postoperative period after cardiac surgery.[2] Poorly controlled postoperative pain is a risk factor for developing chronic pain after surgery.[3] Therefore, younger age has been linked to increased chronic pain. In addition, women have been reported to experience more pain in the early postoperative phase after cardiac surgery as well as more chronic pain after thoracotomy and median sternotomy.[2]

It is well established that chronic pain is more common in patients who undergo IMA grafting as part of CABG surgery. A specific syndrome of chronic pain after IMA grafting was first described in a case series of 11 Canadian patients in 1989.[4] Mailis et al. ascribed the pain to severing of the intercostal nerves during dissection of the IMA. In a retrospective study, Eng and Wells reported a higher incidence of chronic left-sided chest pain in patients who had the left IMA harvested (23%) compared to those who had vein grafts only (4.5%).[5] A longer cohort study conducted over 3 months with 188 patients showed similar results, with an increased rate and severity of chronic chest pain with those who had the IMA harvested versus those who did not.[6] IMA harvesting may thus contribute to the milieu that leads to chronic PSP.

Anesthetic factors may also play a role in the postoperative pain experience. Fechner et al. found that higher doses of intraoperative sufentanil were associated with elevated postoperative pain scores and higher postoperative morphine requirements in cardiac surgery patients. In a similar manner, higher postoperative morphine consumption was observed after high intraoperative dosing of remifentanil.[7] These observations, in conjunction with animal models of acute pain, suggest opioid-induced hyperalgesia may be one factor in increasing acute postoperative pain. Since poorly controlled acute pain can lead to chronic pain, this may represent another modifiable risk factor for developing chronic PSP.[7]

PATHOPHYSIOLOGY

PSP results from a complex interchange of nociceptive input and a widespread inflammatory response. Trauma to skin, subcutaneous tissue, and bone is responsible for initially activating nociceptors; the ensuing inflammatory response leads to sensitization of peripheral and central pathways, resulting in the experience of pain.

Primary afferent pain fibers (Aδ and C) conduct impulses from peripheral nociceptors to the dorsal horn of the spinal cord. From here, sensory information is relayed primarily via the spinothalamic tract to the supraspinal structures, including the brainstem, thalamus, and finally the cortex, where the perception of pain takes place.[8]

A number of inflammatory mediators are released after injury, including sodium, potassium, and calcium ions, bradykinin, substance P, histamine, 5-hydroxytryptamine (5-HT), adenosine triphosphate, nitric oxide, prostanoids, and leukotrienes.[8] These molecules work via both direct and indirect mechanisms on nociceptors and play an important role in the sensitization of both peripheral and central neurons to subsequent stimuli.

Injury to multiple sets of nerves may contribute to PSP. Intercostal nerves arising from thoracic nerve roots innervate the sternum, ribs, and surrounding subcutaneous tissue. The primary thoracic nerves supplying the sternum are T2 to T6. The parietal pleura and visceral pleura also contain nerves that may be complicit in PSP. While the parietal pleura is innervated by a dense network of pain fibers that can be activated by either mechanical or chemical stimuli, the visceral pleura, in contrast, does not have significant sensory innervation. Another source may be the pericardium, which is innervated with pain fibers that arise from the vagus nerve, phrenic nerve, and sympathetic trunks.[8]

Studies have shown that acute tissue injury occurs after sternotomy not only at the site of surgical incision but also at more distant sites due to prolonged sternal retraction, manual manipulation, and use of electrocautery to dissect the IMA.[8] These factors may lead to a range of painful local injuries, such as rib fractures, costochondritis, rib joint dislocation, or nerve injury. Painful sternal pseudoarthroses have also been described around the sites of sternal wire entry into bone.[9] Previous studies have suggested that allergy to the steel wire materials, especially nickel, may cause sternal pain and skin reactions.[10] The presence of chest tubes and mediastinal tubes, which irritate the parietal pleura and pericardium, are also a significant source of pain for patients. Finally, pericarditis can occur after pericardiotomy, leading to significant pain.[8]

Neuromas may play a major role in chronic PSP. Bromley et al. found that patients with exquisitely tender and hard nodules around the sternotomy incision could achieve immediate and complete pain relief after bupivacaine injections. This suggested that the pain was caused by scar-entrapped neuromas of small terminal rami of the anterior branches of the upper intercostal nerves.[11] The neuromas are of two types: those that emerge from transection of nerve rami, known as terminal neuromas, or those that occur with damage to nerve rami, known as neuromas-in-continuity.[11] It is likely that tight sternal wires inserted at the interchondral spaces induce a marked scar reaction, which leads to neuroma formation.

Poorly controlled chest pain after surgery has been associated with numerous adverse outcomes, including pulmonary complications, cardiac ischemic events, cardiac arrhythmias, hypercoagulability, and increased rates of wound infection.[8] Specifically, with regard to pulmonary function, there is a restrictive deficit that occurs within the first three postoperative days, with a decrease in vital capacity and other spirometric values of approximately 33%.[8] Also, there are increases in intrapulmonary shunting and the alveolar-arterial oxygen tension gradient as well as reductions in arterial oxygen tension.[8]

TREATMENT

The treatment paradigms for chronic PSP range from medical management to procedural intervention. As described, anatomically distinct factors may contribute to cases of PSP. Thus, a careful history and physical are important to properly diagnose the pain generator and tailor treatment to the patient's presentation. Individualized care will yield the best results. It is important to realize that efficient pain control intraoperatively and postoperatively is also important to prevent the development of chronic PSP (Table 17.1). Typically, medical management is attempted first; procedural interventions are reserved for more advanced cases. In certain patients with comorbidities or decreased medication tolerance, interventional procedures may be attempted first (Table 17.2).

Finally, careful preoperative patient preparation can mitigate need for medication and/or procedures and improve analgesia. Perception of pain in certain patients can be significanty influenced by psychological factors, especially catastrophization states, perceived support and communications related to satisfactory pain treatments. Setting realistic postoperative expectations during preoperative period is essential to an adequate and timely recovery time.[12] Moreover, this can translate to decreased hospital length of stay, decreased medication/procedure burden on both the patient and healthcare system, and overall mitigation of healthcare costs.[12]

CONCLUSION

- Chronic PSP, defined as noncardiac thoracic pain after median sternotomy, has an incidence of 28% and is associated with young age, female sex, IMA harvest, and an increased requirement for analgesics during the immediate postoperative period.
- PSP results from both activation of nociceptors and an ensuing inflammatory response. The spinothalamic tract relays information from nociceptors to the brainstem, thalamus, and cortex. Major inflammatory mediators include sodium, potassium, and calcium ions, bradykinin, substance P, histamine, 5-HT, adenosine triphosphate, nitric oxide, prostanoids, and leukotrienes. These work via both direct and indirect mechanisms on nociceptors and sensitize both peripheral and central neurons.

Table 17.1. **MODALITIES FOR THE PREVENTION OF POST-STERNOTOMY PAIN**

PERIOPERATIVE MODALITIES		
TECHNIQUE	**ADVANTAGES**	**DISADVANTAGES AND RISKS**
IV opioids (PCA)	Patient autonomy Rapid onset Patient satisfaction	Respiratory depression Pruritus, constipation, nausea/vomiting, ileus, urinary retention, sedation, delirium, dysphoria Similar complication rate to oral opioids No significant change in hospital length of stay Opioid-induced hyperalgesia[7] Build-up of metabolites in renal insufficiency (morphine/meperidine)
Thoracic epidural/paravertebral analgesia	Mitigates stress response to surgery May improve pulmonary function postoperatively[13,14] Decreased opioid use Faster recovery[14]	Epidural—Potential for epidural hematoma, abscess, post-dural-puncture headache, hypotension Paravertebral—Potential for pneumothorax
Intrathecal analgesia	May improve pulmonary function postoperatively Decreased opioid use[15]	Potential for infection, epidural hematoma, headache Opioid side effects as above

Table 17.2. **MODALITIES FOR TREATMENT OF CHRONIC POST-STERNOTOMY PAIN**

	CHRONIC PAIN MODALITIES	
TECHNIQUE	ADVANTAGES	DISADVANTAGES AND RISKS
Local infiltrative techniques—Scar neuroma injections and trigger- point injections	Generally low risk with local anesthetic (LA)	LA—Intravascular injection Neurolytic block—Tissue, skin damage Steroid—Skin discoloration, infection Pneumothorax (all)
Paravertebral block	Low risk of epidural hematoma May improve pulmonary function postoperatively[13]	Pneumothorax
Intercostal block/Pulsed radiofrequency ablation[16]	Quick onset of relief Repeatable	Potential for pneumothorax or hemothorax, hematoma, tissue damage
NSAIDs	Peripheral and central mechanism of action	Risk of cardiovascular events and thrombosis (COX-2 inhibitors and nonselective NSAIDs) Risk of worsening renal disease Risk of bleeding (if anticoagulated)
Opioids	Well tolerated in liver/renal dysfunction.	Respiratory depression, tolerance, dependence, addiction, others as above
Serotonin/norepinephrine-reuptake inhibitors and tricyclic antidepressants—duloxetine, venlafaxine, nortriptyline, amitriptyline	Address neuropathic pain component Mood-enhancing qualities May help with sleep	Sedation, serotonin syndrome, tachycardia/orthostasis, weight gain, sexual side effects Delirium—Older patients
Antiepileptics[17]—gabapentin, topiramate, oxcarbazepine, carbamazepine	May prevent chronic sternotomy pain[17] Addresses neuropathic pain component	Slow onset of analgesia Dizziness or sedation Paresthesias Hyponatremia/aplastic anemia
Acetaminophen	Generally low risk	Contraindicated in patients with significant liver disease
Ketamine[18]	Strong analgesia via NMDA antagonism Does not cause respiratory depression	Dysphoria, hallucinations, excessive salivation, tachycardia
TENS	Decreased medication use Low risk of skin damage with moderate use	Muscle twitching Possible electromagnetic interference in patients with pacemakers/defibrillators[8] Cannot be used when operating machinery/vehicles

- Sensory innervation to the sternum comes from intercostal nerves T2 to T6. Other sites may also be involved, including the pericardium, parietal pleura, and ribs. Some patients may develop allergies causing pain. Scar-entrapped neuromas from the anterior branches of intercostal nerves may play a major role in PSP.
- Poorly controlled chest pain after surgery has been associated with numerous cardiopulmonary adverse outcomes.
- Treatment, whether medical, procedural. or psychologic, should be individualized to each patient's unique presentation.

REFERENCES

1. Meyerson J, Thelin S, Gordh T, Karlsten R. The incidence of chronic post-sternotomy pain after cardiac surgery—a prospective study. *Acta Anaesthesiol Scand.* 2001;45(8):940–944.
2. van Gulik L, Janssen LI, Ahlers SJ, et al. Risk factors for chronic thoracic pain after cardiac surgery via sternotomy. *Eur J Cardiothorac Surg.* 2011;40(6):1309–1313.
3. Katz J, Jackson M, Kavanagh BP, Sandler AN. Acute pain after thoracic surgery predicts long-term post-thoracotomy pain. *Clin J Pain.* 1996;12(1):50–55.
4. Mailis A, Chan J, Basinski A, et al. Chest wall pain after aortocoronary bypass surgery using internal mammary artery graft: a new pain syndrome? *Heart Lung.* 1989;18(6):553–558.
5. Eng J, Wells FC. Morbidity following coronary artery revascularisation with the internal mammary artery. *Int J Cardiol.* 1991;30(1): 55–59.

6. Kamalipour H, Vafaei A, Parviz Kazemi A, Khademi S. Comparing the prevalence of chronic pain after sternotomy in patients undergoing coronary artery bypass grafting using the internal mammary artery and other open heart surgeries. *Anesth Pain Med.* 2014;4(3):e17969.
7. Fechner J, Ihmsen H, Schüttler J, Jeleazcov C. The impact of intra-operative sufentanil dosing on post-operative pain, hyperalgesia and morphine consumption after cardiac surgery. *Eur J Pain.* 2013;17(4):562–570.
8. Mazzeffi M, Khelemsky Y. Poststernotomy pain: a clinical review. *J Cardiothorac Vasc Anesth.* 2011;25(6):1163–1178.
9. Goy JJ, Poncioni L, Morin D. Chest pain due to severe sternal pseudoarthrosis post-coronary artery bypass surgery. *Circulation.* 2010;122(11):1134–1135.
10. Rashidi S, Elenbaas TW, Hamad MA, van Suijlekom HJ, van Straten AH. Does removal of steel wires relieve post-sternotomy pain after cardiac surgery? *Asian Cardiovasc Thorac Ann.* 2013;21(4):409–413.
11. Defalque RJ, Bromley JJ. Poststernotomy neuralgia: a new pain syndrome. *Anesth Analg.* 1989;69(1):81–82.
12. Leal EN, Ribeiro JL, Oliveira MM, Roquette J. Psychosocial aspects associated with pain perception in individuals undergoing coronary surgery. *Rev Port Cardiol.* 2005;24(10):1221–1231.
13. Komatsu T, Sowa T, Takahashi K, Fujinaga T. Paravertebral block as a promising analgesic modality for managing post-thoracotomy pain. *Ann Thorac Cardiovasc Surg.* 2014;20(2):113–116.
14. Ronald A, Abdulaziz KA, Day TG, Scott M. In patients undergoing cardiac surgery, thoracic epidural analgesia combined with general anaesthesia results in faster recovery and fewer complications but does not affect length of hospital stay. *Interact Cardiovasc Thorac Surg.* 2006;5(3):207–216.
15. Roediger L, Joris J, Senard M, Larbuisson R, Canivet JL, Lamy M. The use of pre-operative intrathecal morphine for analgesia following coronary artery bypass surgery. *Anaesthesia.* 2006;61(9):838–844.
16. Sihoe AD, Lee TW, Wan IY, Thung KH, Yim AP. The use of gabapentin for post-operative and post-traumatic pain in thoracic surgery patients. *Eur J Cardiothorac Surg.* 2006;29(5):795–799.
17. Maher DP, Loyferman R, Yumul R, Louy C. Initial experience with IV ketamine infusion for treatment of post sternotomy pain in a patient with a total artificial heart. *Pain Physician.* 2015;18(3):E425–E427.

REVIEW QUESTIONS

1. A 64-year-old female is scheduled to undergo an aortic valve replacement. What is the likelihood she will develop chronic PSP after the procedure?

   A. 6%
   B. 13%
   C. 28%
   D. 66%

2. Which is not known as an anatomic cause of chronic PSP?

   A. Use of the IMA for graft in cardiac bypass surgery
   B. Wound infection
   C. Sternal pseudoarthroses
   D. Development of neuromas

3. Which opioid has been associated with hyperalgesia in patients undergoing CABG surgery?

   A. Morphine
   B. Fentanyl
   C. Hydromorphone
   D. Sufentanil

ANSWERS

1. C. The literature has cited an overall incidence of PSP, defined as noncardiac thoracic pain after sternotomy, to be roughly 28%.[1] This takes into account all comers and does not adjust for age, gender, or other population factors. The literature has shown that age less than 60 and female sex are both associated with increased incidence of PSP.[2]

2. B. Scar-entrapped neuromas, use of the IMA for a graft during cardiac bypass surgery, and the formation of sternal pseudoarthroses have all been implicated in PSP. Use of the IMA has shown a fivefold increase in incidence of pain.[5] Scar-entrapped neuromas formed from the terminal rami of the anterior branches of the upper intercostal nerves are thought to underlie a significant portion of PSP.[11] Painful sternal pseudoarthroses have been reported to form around the entry site of sternal wires.[9] Wound infection has not been shown to be strongly associated with causing PSP, although certainly persistent pain can lead to chronic infections, which in turn can be painful.

3. D. Both sufentanil and remifentanil in high intraoperative doses during cardiac surgery have been associated with increased morphine consumption postoperatively. Given that increased acute pain can lead to chronic pain, opioid-induced hyperalgesia is likely a risk factor for developing chronic PSP.[7] Fentanyl, hydromorphone, and morphine have not been definitively linked to hyperalgesia in the cardiac surgery population.

QUESTIONS AND ANSWERS

This chapter has accompanying questions and answers that are available to subscribers as part of the Oxford eLearning platform. To access the questions, follow the link below, or go to ✔ http://oxfordmedicine.com/painmanagementreview

18.

CHRONIC ABDOMINAL PAIN IN THE ELDERLY: ISCHEMIC PAIN

Ashley Reed and Tariq M. Malik

STEM CASE AND KEY QUESTIONS

An 80-year-old female with a history of hypertension, type 2 diabetes mellitus, previous myocardial infarction (10 years earlier with placement of two coronary artery stents), and gastroesophageal reflux disease (GERD) comes to your clinic for evaluation of 6 months' duration postprandial abdominal pain. She is accompanied by her daughter, who is concerned about her mother's weight loss of 20 kg (44 lb) over the last 6 months. The patient's abdominal pain begins within an hour after eating and resolves after several hours of not eating. She describes the pain as generalized cramping over her entire abdomen. Because of pain, she consumes only small meals of soup and crackers. Lately, she feels abdominal pain even after these small meals, and she is distressed by her symptoms. Multiple visits to her primary care physician and the emergency department have failed to determine a cause for her abdominal pain.

WHAT WOULD YOUR NEXT STEPS BE? WHAT IS THE DIFFERENTIAL DIAGNOSIS?

Physical examination is remarkable only for weight loss. You review the imaging from another workup (CT) from 3 months ago and are reassured by negative findings: no evidence of bowel obstruction, masses, pancreatitis, or cholelithiasis. Urinary analysis and culture are negative; an abdominal ultrasound and an abdominal CT scan with oral contrast are unremarkable. You are concerned that chronic mesenteric ischemia (CMI) may be causing the symptoms and want to rule out this condition.

WHAT IS CMI? HOW WOULD YOU ADDITIONALLY EVALUATE THIS PATIENT?

Given its high sensitivity and specificity, you send the patient for a CT angiogram (CTA). The patient's daughter wants to know if anything can alleviate her mother's pain until the imaging results are completed. You prescribe a course of low-dose gabapentin and amitriptyline to see if these interventions will improve her symptoms. One week later the results of the CTA are positive for 75% stenosis of the celiac artery and 80% stenosis of the superior mesenteric artery (SMA).

WHEN THE PATIENT RETURNS TO THE CLINIC, YOU INFORM HER OF THE DIAGNOSIS OF CMI. WHAT SHOULD YOU TELL HER ABOUT HOW THE CONDITION IS MANAGED?

Pharmacologic approaches to management with opioids, vasodilators, antiepileptic drugs for neuropathic pain, and NSAIDs (nonsteroidal anti-inflammatory drugs) have unpredictable results and will not slow the disease progression. Primary treatment is surgical intervention, and you recommended a consult with a vascular surgeon. The patient expresses concern about undergoing surgery. She states that she "is too old for surgery" and will "die on the table." The patient's daughter asks if there are alternatives to surgical management.

WHAT NONSURGICAL OPTIONS ARE AVAILABLE TO THE PATIENT?

Celiac plexus and splanchnic nerve neurolysis are effective in treatment of chronic abdominal pain originating from the liver, gallbladder, pancreas, spleen, adrenal glands, kidneys, distal esophagus, and bowel to the level of the distal transverse colon.[1] Targeting these nerves prevents transmission of nociceptive signals from the target organs to the brain. You recommend that the patient undergo a diagnostic celiac plexus block with local anesthetic and steroid. Depending on her response, you may recommend celiac plexus neurolysis for prolonged pain control.

SHE RETURNS TO CLINIC A WEEK LATER FOR THE CELIAC PLEXUS BLOCK. WHICH CONTRAINDICATIONS TO CELIAC PLEXUS BLOCK SHOULD BE CONSIDERED BEFORE PROCEEDING?

Contraindications to celiac plexus block are severe coagulopathy, thrombocytopenia, abdominal aortic aneurysm, local infection or sepsis, bowel obstruction, and hypotension. Although abdominal malignancy is not a contraindication, tumor location should be identified because direct invasion of a tumor into the plexus is associated with worse outcomes.

The patient has no contraindications and agrees to proceed. She is taken into the procedure room and placed in the prone position. A transcrural approach is selected. Under fluoroscopic guidance, 22-G needles are advanced bilaterally to the anterior portion of the T12-L1 intervertebral space to deposit a bupivacaine and triamcinolone solution. The patient suffers hypotension in the recovery area that resolves after a bolus of intravenous fluid. She is discharged without other any complication.

The patient returns for follow-up 4 weeks later. She states that her pain resolved almost completely during the first week after the procedure. Her appetite improved, and she believes that she may have gained weight. Now, however, the pain has returned and she feels no improvement. She expresses concern that the pain was controlled only for a short time.

WHAT WOULD YOUR NEXT STEP BE?

You discuss a neurolytic celiac block option with the patient and her daughter. The possibility of paralysis dissuades them from that option. You suggest a splanchnic nerve block, which, if equally effective in relieving pain, can then be followed by radiofrequency ablation of the nerves.

The patient agrees to undergo the procedure a week later. Under fluoroscopic guidance, a 22-G needle is again advanced at the T12 vertebral level bilaterally. A bupivacaine and triamcinolone solution is deposited retrocrural at the junction between the anterior one-third and posterior two-thirds of the vertebral body. The patient tolerates the procedure without complication and is discharged from the clinic. At her 6-week follow-up appointment, the patient reports feeling "better than ever." The postprandial pain has improved from an 8/10 to 2/10. She is now able to consume larger meals and has gained 2 kg. Six weeks later she returns for her second follow-up appointment. Her pain is now worse than before the splanchnic nerve block. She has returned to a soup and crackers diet but feels the pain is worse than ever. She refuses to undergo radiofrequency ablation of the splanchnic nerves because she now has back pain at the injection site. You again recommend a referral to vascular surgery, but the patient insists she does not want to undergo an invasive procedure.

WHAT INTERVENTION WOULD BE APPROPRIATE FOR THE PATIENT AT THIS POINT?

You offer her spinal cord neuromodulation therapy. After the procedure is explained to the patient and her daughter, they decide to pursue that option. Upon discontinuation of her anticoagulants, spinal cord stimulation leads are placed under fluoroscopic guidance. The patient is sent home and is asked to keep a diary of pain and food intake.

The trial period lasts for 7 days, during which her pain completely resolves. Permanent leads are subsequently implanted. At the time of discharge, and subsequent follow-up appointments, the patient is tolerating full meals and her energy level and sleep times have improved. She visits your office for a 6-month follow-up appointment and happily reports that she has experienced continued pain relief.

DISCUSSION

Mesenteric ischemia is a rare but debilitating cause of abdominal pain in elderly patients. In the acute form, sudden blockage of blood flow to the bowel is a potentially life-threatening vascular emergency. The less common chronic presentation, however, follows a more benign course, and decisions regarding pain management and quality of life become important. Open surgical or endovascular repair remains the mainstay of treatment. Pain specialists often manage pain for these patients as a bridge to surgical intervention or as destination therapy for those deemed to be poor operative candidates. The ability to recognizing the differences in pain presentation among the elderly and to identify these rare chronic pain conditions that increase in prevalence with older age helps prevent the deleterious consequences of chronic pain in the elderly.

EVALUATION OF AN ELDERLY PATIENT WITH CHRONIC PAIN

Elderly patients with chronic pain can pose a particularly difficult diagnostic and management challenge for physicians. As many as half of elderly patients in the community and 45% to 80% of those in nursing homes suffer from chronic pain.[2] Although the prevalence of persistent pain increases with age, pain in elderly patients is often underreported and is attributed to normal aging.[3,4] The consequences of chronic pain in elderly patients are many. Deconditioning, sleep disturbance, immobility, impaired cognition, and depression have been associated with chronic pain in the elderly.[5–7]

Older patients may be reluctant to report pain from fear of need to undergo diagnostic testing, hospitalization, or loss of independence. Geriatric patients may report atypical symptoms instead of pain: gait disturbance, anorexia, and cognitive impairment. Easily administered pain assessment tools, the McGill Pain Questionnaire, Visual Analog Scale (VAS), and Numeric Rating Scale, have been proven reliable and valid across multiple settings and independent of patient age.[7] Even patients with mild to moderate cognitive impairment can be assessed with these aforementioned screening tools. The atypical nature of geriatric pain and the high prevalence of dementia, sensory impairment, and disability call for a comprehensive assessment with these assessment tools, a physical examination, and collateral information from caregivers, family members, and others participating in the patient's care.

CMI OVERVIEW

First described in 1918 as "abdominal angina," CMI is characterized by intermittent episodes of acute postprandial abdominal pain, weight loss, and an epigastric bruit.[8] Pain results from decreased blood flow to the bowel during periods of increased metabolic demand. CMI is the rarest manifestation of intestinal ischemia; colonic ischemia is the most common.[9] Women are disproportionately affected, making up 70% of those diagnosed with the condition; patients are usually over the age of 60. As the association of pain with eating is evident later in the course of disease, patients may suffer initially with nonspecific abdominal pain and weight loss that lead to diagnostic delays and extensive workups.

When symptoms are present, the pain is generalized in the abdomen, starts shortly after a large meal, and can persist for 1 to 3 hours. At first, pain is felt only after large meals. As the disease progresses, pain is experienced with any oral intake. The patient then becomes fearful of food. Patients will gradually reduce food intake and become reluctant to eat. Weight loss can be severe, leading to malnutrition. A few patients have nausea, vomiting, or diarrhea.[10] The disorder should be suspected in any elderly patient with prolonged abdominal pain and weight loss where standard diagnostic testing has failed to identify a specific etiology.

ETIOLOGY AND PATHOGENESIS

CMI is almost always caused by atherosclerosis. Most patients will have a history of pre-existing atherosclerotic disease. Up to 50% of patients have had surgery for atherosclerosis.[11] Factors that predispose patients to atherosclerotic disease, such as smoking, hypertension, diabetes mellitus, and hyperlipidemia, put patients at increased risk for CMI. Atherosclerotic plaques make mesenteric vessels unable to support increased blood flow during the postprandial period. One study documented blood flow changes from a decrease of 25% in the fasting CMI patient to 35% after eating.[12] Less frequently identified causes include fibromuscular dysplasia, mesenteric artery dissection, median arcuate ligament syndrome, aortic dissection, and retroperitoneal fibrosis.

A majority of the atherosclerotic plaques are found in the splanchnic vessels, specifically the proximal parts of the celiac artery, SMA, and inferior mesenteric artery (IMA). Proximal occlusion of one vessel is generally common in the elderly patient population and well tolerated, with no clinically apparent symptoms. A review of Medicare beneficiaries over 65 found that about 17.5% of the cohort had statistically significant stenosis of one of the major mesenteric vessels.[13] Only 1.3% of cohort patients had involvement of more than one vessel. Patients with known atherosclerosis of the aorta or the iliac or femoral vessels had increased incidence of mesenteric stenosis ranging from 25% to 40%.[14]

Although mesenteric artery disease is relatively common, the incidence of CMI is considerably less. The abundant blood supply to the abdominal viscera and slow development of atherosclerotic plaques expand collateral circulation and compensate for single-vessel disease. The atherosclerotic burden does not lead to symptoms until two or even all three of the major vessels have clinically significant stenosis.[15] Angiography of the mesenteric vessels of symptomatic individuals supports this theory. Over 90% of patients had occlusion of two vessels; 55%, all three. Of patients with single-vessel disease, isolated pathology involving the SMA was more likely. Symptomatic single-vessel disease also was found in patients with prior abdominal surgeries, division of integral collateral circulation, or median arcuate ligament syndrome.[11]

DIAGNOSTIC IMAGING MODALITIES

Clinicians should have a low threshold for imaging elderly patients with abdominal pain. Nonclassic syndrome presentation, unreliable findings on physical examination, and less predictable changes in vital signs and laboratory data make imaging a vital part of the diagnostic process for older patients.[16] CMI is a diagnosis of exclusion based on classic symptoms and positive imaging for mesenteric stenosis.

Angiography remains the most sensitive (74%–100%) and specific (100%) imaging modality for assessment of the mesenteric vessels.[17] Both diagnosis and intervention are possible with a single procedure. For patients with chronic disease, angiography followed by therapeutic angioplasty is associated with prompt resolution of symptoms.

Noninvasive imaging techniques with a sensitivity and specificity similar to that of an angiogram have emerged as popular initial imaging choices. There is general agreement that CTA and magnetic resonance angiography (MRA) are first-line alternatives to angiography. Practice guidelines recommend use of CTA, MRA, or duplex ultrasound as initial imaging modalities and use of angiography when noninvasive imaging is unavailable or indeterminate.[11] CTA with contrast has a sensitivity of up to 96% and specificity of 94% for detecting stenotic changes consistent with CMI. CTA is fast, convenient, and often readily available. MRA with contrast has a sensitivity of 100% and specificity of 95%. Imaging of smaller peripheral vessels with MRA is reduced and the IMA is captured along only 25% of its course.[18] Both modalities allow clinicians to rule out other causes of abdominal pain and weight loss, such as pancreatitis, appendicitis, abscess, perforation, or obstruction. Duplex scanning of mesenteric vessels has approximately 90% accuracy for detection of 70% or greater stenosis or occlusion of the celiac artery or SMA.[11] Differences in postprandial arterial flow also can be assessed.

SURGICAL RESTORATION OF INTESTINAL BLOOD FLOW

The mainstay of treatment for CMI is surgical revascularization. In patients with multiple comorbidities and prolonged malnutrition, perioperative risk is greater. Physicians must weigh the possible morbidity and mortality from surgical intervention against the outcome without treatment. It is thought that intervention for CMI will prevent progression to acute mesenteric ischemia. Acute mesenteric ischemia is a medical emergency, which threatens bowel viability and places patients at high risk for perforation, sepsis, and death. The most common cause of acute mesenteric ischemia is arterial embolus or thrombus, the latter associated with insidious onset and atherosclerosis.[19] Mortality estimates for acute mesenteric ischemia range from 30% to 90%. Case reports exist describing patient progression from chronic to acute mesenteric ischemia.[20] The actual proportion of patients with CMI that will progress to acute ischemia is unknown.

Instead, recommendations for treatment are based on the clinical findings that early diagnosis and treatment have high success rates at reducing pain and preventing additional weight loss. Surgical management may be open or percutaneous endovascular repair. Both treatment modalities have a high rate of technical success and symptom relief. Pain is resolved in 93% to 100% of patients following open repair and for a similar to slightly lower proportion of patients after endovascular repair.[21–24] Patients whose symptoms fail to improve after endovascular repair are often later diagnosed with external causes of compression, like median arcuate ligament syndrome.[25]

Open repair is associated with a 30-day mortality of 0% to 17% and morbidity between 19% and 54%. Although mortality rates after open repair have improved drastically over the last several years, in some studies they remain up to five times higher than after endovascular repair (1% to 3.7%).[25,26] The incidence of restenosis necessitating re-intervention with percutaneous endovascular repair with or without stenting is higher.[25] Repeat percutaneous intervention is typically successful at controlling symptoms. With the trend toward fewer open procedures, it is now generally accepted that they should be reserved for patients whose condition does not improve after percutaneous procedures, who have had multiple restenoses, or who require multivessel repair in a technically challenging anatomy.

ALTERNATIVES TO SURGICAL MANAGEMENT

To date, no documented cases of spontaneous resolution have been reported. Secondary prevention through smoking cessation and better control of diabetes, hypertension, and hyperlipidemia should be implemented in all patients. These measures may halt the disease's progression and make patients suitable surgical candidates. Results with vasodilators, opioids, NSAIDs, or neuropathic pain medications vary.

Celiac plexus and splanchnic nerve blockade and neurolysis are effective adjuncts for management of intractable abdominal pain. Located in the upper abdomen anterior to the T12-L1 vertebral body and the aorta, the celiac plexus receives nerve contributions from sympathetic efferent, parasympathetic efferent, and sensory afferent fibers of the upper abdominal viscera.[1] Consisting of two ganglia groups, the nerve plexus transmits nociceptive information from the distal esophagus and alimentary tract to the splenic flexure, liver, spleen, and retroperitoneal structures like the pancreas and kidney. Autonomic innervation of the abdominal blood vessels arises in the celiac plexus. The greater, lesser, and least splanchnic nerves are paired nerves originating from the thoracic sympathetic trunk that pierce the diaphragm and enter the abdominal cavity to join the celiac plexus.

Celiac plexus blockade can be performed through an anterior or posterior approach. The posterior approach can be retrocrural, antecrural, or transaortic (Figure 18.1 and Figure 18.2).

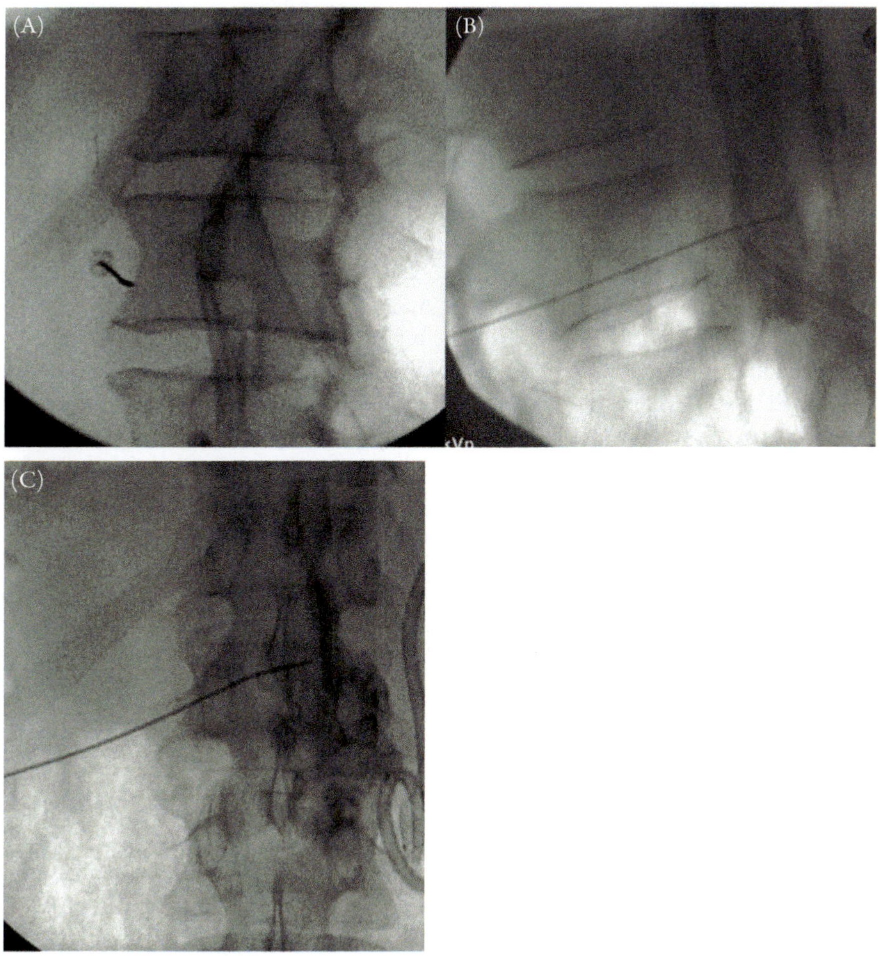

Figure 18.1. Transaortic approach to the celiac plexus in a pancreatic cancer patient. Needle placed anterior to the diaphragm and in front of aorta with the entry point on the left. (A) shows initial needle placement in oblique view, and (B) (lateral) and (C) (posteroanterior) show excellent spread of the dye.

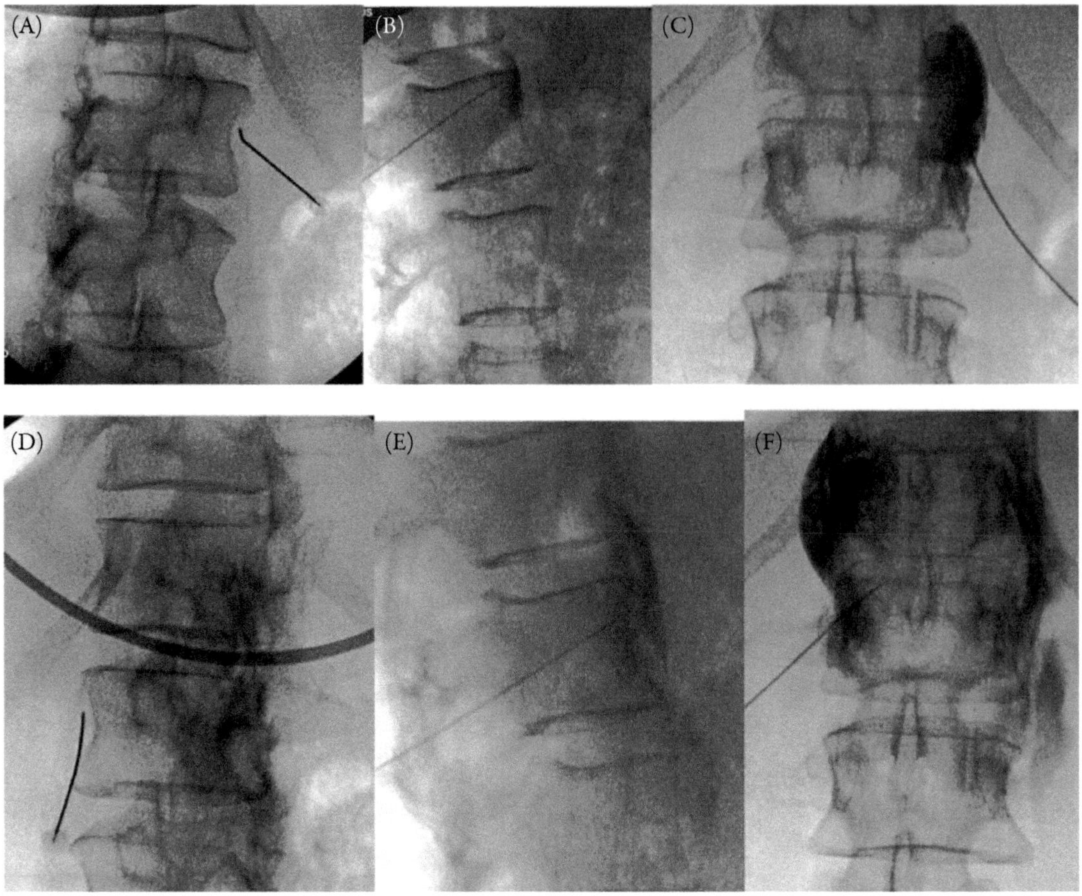

Figure 18.2. Retrocrural approach to the celiac plexus. Bilateral needle placement starting in oblique view on the right (A) and on the left (D). Final needle placement behind diaphragm fibers on the right (B) and on the left (E) confirmed on lateral and posteroanterior (C and F) fluoroscopic image.

The retrocrural approach blocks the thoracic splanchnic, vagal, and sensory afferents that form the celiac plexus.[27] Permanent ablation of the celiac plexus is accomplished with alcohol or phenol. Various imaging modalities, including fluoroscopy, CT, and most recently endoscopic ultrasound, can facilitate the procedure. Common adverse effects are pain at the local site (98%), hypotension (38%), and diarrhea (44%), which are transient.[28] Rare neurologic complications include paraplegia, epidural or subarachnoid injection, and nerve root injury. Rare nonneurologic complications are pneumothorax, vascular trauma, shoulder or chest pain, and visceral injury. Major complications are estimated to affect less than 2% of patients.[27] Splanchnic nerve blocks and radiofrequency ablation via a retrocrural approach at the T12 vertebral body are also available options (Figure 18.3 and Figure 18.4).

The advantages of celiac plexus neurolysis are well documented for patients with chronic abdominal pain and abdominal malignancies. Improved pain relief over pharmacologic therapy is observed in almost 89% of patients at 2 weeks after neurolysis. A majority of patients with initial pain relief maintained the benefit with follow-up of 3 months or greater.[28,29] Consumption of opioids also decreases after celiac plexus neurolysis, and again a statistically significant difference in opioid use has been documented at 3-month follow-up.

Patients whose condition does not improve with the aforementioned therapies are considered for more permanent interventional management. Because spinal cord stimulator implants have promising results in the treatment of refractory coronary angina, peripheral vascular disease, and chronic neuropathic pain, some have suggested that they are a viable option for patients with CMI.[30,31] Patients with intractable angina who were treated with spinal cord stimulation had increased exercise tolerance, decreased frequency of angina episodes, reduced hospitalization, and improved quality of life.[32] In these patients, spinal cord stimulation not only provided symptomatic relief but also increased myocardial blood flow and decreased sympathetic tone, which improved myocardial oxygen supply/demand and reduced myocardial ischemia. Spinal cord stimulation in peripheral vascular disease increased local blood flow, produced warmer extremities, and yielded long-term pain relief. In some patients, ischemic ulcers were healed and limbs were saved.[33]

Spinal cord stimulation has also been applied in patients with refractory abdominal visceral pain. Refractory postprandial abdominal pain of nonischemic origin has been successfully treated with spinal cord modulation.

VAS scores improved, opioid medication requirements were reduced, and daily activities were resumed.[34,35] Although spinal cord stimulation in CMI is not well documented, there

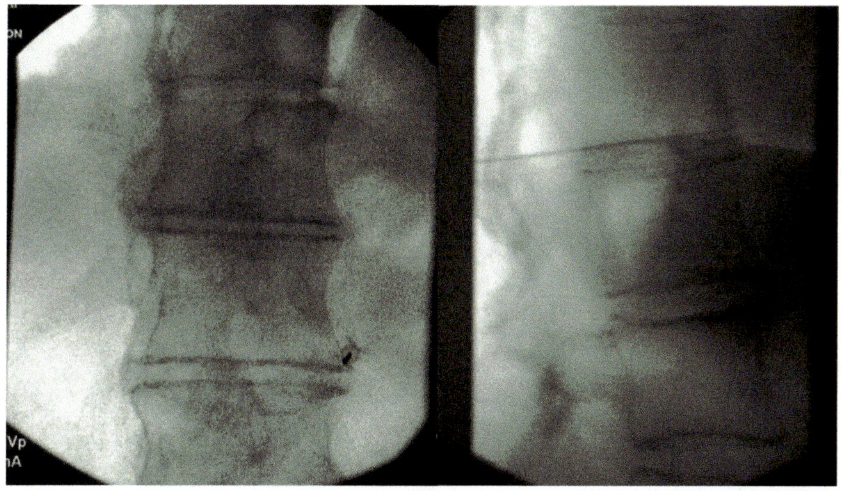

Figure 18.3. Splanchnic block, PA and oblique fluoroscopic view of needle placement; diagnostic block done with local anesthetic at the T11-T12 vertebral body level.

are a few cases with promising results. A 78-year-old male with progressive CMI who was deemed a poor operative candidate had complete relief from pain after a thoracic spinal cord stimulator was implanted. The patient remained symptom-free over the 12-month follow-up and was able to consume meals without fear of pain and returned to normal daily activities.[36] In another case, a patient whose endovascular repair was unsuccessful found pain relief without opioids after spinal cord stimulator implantation.[37]

CONCLUSIONS

- CMI is a rare but debilitating cause of chronic abdominal pain in the elderly.
- Symptoms are postprandial abdominal pain, weight loss, and an abdominal bruit.
- The disease results from atherosclerotic plaques that reduce the bowel's ability to increase blood flow after meals.
- Management is through surgical intervention. Both endovascular and open techniques have high rates of relieving pain.
- Interventional management with celiac plexus or splanchnic nerve neurolysis is an effective adjunct for chronic abdominal pain.
- In patients with refractory abdominal pain, placement of a spinal cord stimulator has shown promising results for reducing pain and opioid requirements.

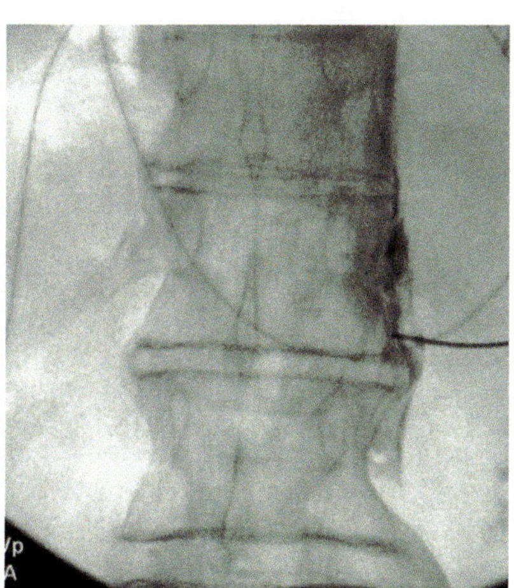

Figure 18.4. Splanchnic nerves radiofrequency ablation. The cannula is placed at the level of T11-T12 under direct fluoroscopic view.

REFERENCES

1. Nitschke AM, Ray CE Jr. Percutaneous neurolytic celiac plexus block. *Semin Intervent Radiol.* 2013;30(3):318–321.
2. American Geriatric Society Panel on Persistent Pain in Older Persons. The management of persistent pain in older persons. *J Am Geriatr Soc.* 2002;50(6)(suppl):S205–S224.
3. Kaye AD, Baluch A, Scott JT. Pain management in the elderly population: a review. *Ochsner J.* 2010;10(3):179–187.
4. Crook J, Rideout E, Browne G. The prevalence of pain complaints in a general population. *Pain.* 1984;18(3):299–314.
5. Manchikanti L, Singh V, Datta S, et al. Comprehensive review of epidemiology, scope, and impact of spinal pain. *Pain Physician.* 2009;12(4):E35–E70.
6. Parmelee PA, Smith B, Katz IR. Pain complaints and cognitive status among elderly institution residents *J Am Geriatr Soc.* 1993;41(5):517–522.
7. Herr KA, Garand L. Assessment and measurement of pain in older adults. *Clin Geriatr Med.* 2001;17(3):457–478.
8. Hohenwalter EJ. Chronic mesenteric ischemia: diagnosis and treatment. *Semin Intervent Radiol.* 2009;26(4):345–351.
9. Greenwald DA, Brandt LJ, Reinus JF. Ischemic bowel disease in the elderly. *Gastroenterol Clin North Am.* 2001;30(2):445–473.
10. Barret M, Martineau C, Rahmi G, et al. Chronic mesenteric ischemia: a rare cause of chronic abdominal pain. *Am J Med.* 2015;128(12):1363.e1–1363.e8
11. American Gastroenterological Association medical position statement: guidelines on intestinal ischemia. *Gastroenterology.* 2000;118(5): 951–953.
12. Chang RW, Chang JB, Longo WE. Update in management of mesenteric ischemia. *World J Gastroenterol.* 2006;12(20):3243–3247.
13. Hansen KJ, Wilson DB, Craven TE, et al. Mesenteric artery disease in the elderly. *J Vasc Surg.* 2004;40(1):45–52.

14. Valentine RJ, Martin JD, Myers SI, Rossi MB, Clagett GP. Asymptomatic celiac and superior mesenteric artery stenoses are more prevalent among patients with unsuspected renal artery stenoses. *J Vasc Surg.* 1991;14(2):195–199.
15. Biebl M, Oldenburg WA, Paz-Fumagalli R, McKinney JM, Hakaim AG. Surgical and interventional visceral revascularization for the treatment of chronic mesenteric ischemia—when to prefer which? *World J Surg.* 2007;31(3):562–568.
16. Paranjape C, Dalia S, Pan J, Horattas M. Appendicitis in the elderly: a change in the laparoscopic era. *Surg Endosc.* 2007;21(5):777–781.
17. Oliva IB, Davarpanah AH, Rybicki FJ, et al. ACR appropriateness criteria imaging of mesenteric ischemia. *Abdom Imaging.* 2013;38(4):714–719.
18. Laissy JP, Trillaud H, Douek P. MR angiography: noninvasive vascular imaging of the abdomen. *Abdom Imaging.* 2002;27(5):488–506.
19. Oldenburg WA, Lau LL, Rodenberg TJ, Edmonds HJ, Burger CD. Acute mesenteric ischemia: a clinical review. *Arch Intern Med.* 2004;164(10):1054–1062.
20. Abe S, Yamakawa T, Kawashima H, et al. Surgery for acute exacerbation of chronic mesenteric ischemia: a case report. *Surg Case Rep.* 2016;2(1):146.
21. Cho JS, Carr JA, Jacobsen G, Shepard AD, Nypaver TJ, Reddy DJ. Long-term outcome after mesenteric artery reconstruction: a 37-year experience. *J Vasc Surg.* 2002;35(3):453–460.
22. Jimenez JG, Huber TS, Ozaki CK, et al. Durability of antegrade synthetic aortomesenteric bypass for chronic mesenteric ischemia. *J Vasc Surg.* 2002;35(6):1078–1084.
23. Park WM, Cherry KJ Jr, Chua HK, et al. Current results of open revascularization for chronic mesenteric ischemia: a standard for comparison. *J Vasc Surg.* 2002;35(5):853–359.
24. Assar AN, Abilez OJ, Zarins CK. Outcome of open versus endovascular revascularization for chronic mesenteric ischemia: review of comparative studies. *J Cardiovasc Surg.* 2009;50(4):509–514.
25. Kougias P, El Sayed HF, Zhou W, Lin PH. Management of chronic mesenteric ischemia. The role of endovascular therapy. *J Endovasc Ther.* 2007;14(3):395–405.
26. Schermerhorn ML, Giles KA, Hamdan AD, Wyers MC, Pomposelli FB. Mesenteric revascularization: management and outcomes in the United States, 1988–2006. *J Vasc Surg.* 2009;50(2):341–348.
27. McCartney CJ, Chambers WA. Coeliac plexus block. *Curr Anaesth Crit Care.* 1998;9(6):318–324.
28. Eisenberg E, Carr DB, Chalmers TC. Neurolytic celiac plexus block for treatment of cancer pain: a meta-analysis. *Anesth Analg.* 1995;80(2):290–295.
29. Nagels W, Pease N, Bekkering G, Cools F, Dobbels P. Celiac plexus neurolysis for abdominal cancer pain: a systematic review. *Pain Med.* 2013;14(8):1140–1163.
30. Klomp HM, Spincemaille GH, Steyerberg EW, et al. Spinal-cord stimulation in critical limb ischaemia: a randomised trial. *Lancet.* 1993;353(9158):1040–1044.
31. Mannheimer C, Eliasson T, Augustinsson LE, et al. Electrical stimulation versus coronary artery bypass surgery in severe angina pectoris. *Circulation.* 1998; 97(12):1157–1163.
32. Latif OA, Nedeukovic SS., Stevenson LW. Spinal cord stimulation for chronic intractable angina pectoris: a unified theory on its mechanism. *Clin Cardiol.* 2001;24(8):533–541.
33. Cameron T. Safety and efficacy of spinal cord stimulation for the treatment of chronic pain: a 20-year literature review. *J Neurosurg Spine.* 2004;100(3):254–267.
34. Tiede JM, Ghazi SM, Lamer TJ, Obray JB. The use of spinal cord stimulation in refractory abdominal visceral pain: case reports and literature review. *Pain Pract.* 2006;6(3):197–202.
35. Khan, YN, Raza SS, Khan EA. Application of spinal cord stimulation for the treatment of abdominal visceral pain syndromes: case reports. *Neuromodulation.* 2005;8(1):14–27.
36. Ceballos A, Cabezudo L, Bovaira M, Fenollosa P, Moro B. Spinal cord stimulation: a possible therapeutic alternative for chronic mesenteric ischaemia. *Pain.* 2000;87(1):99–101.
37. Caruso C, Lo Sapio D, Ragosa V, Lo Sapio S, Cafora C, Romano L. Abdominal angina due to obstruction of mesenteric artery treated with spinal cord stimulation: a clinical case. *Neuromodulation.* 2011;14(2):146–150.

REVIEW QUESTIONS

1. At what vertebral level is the celiac plexus most commonly located?

   A. T4-T5
   B. T9-T10
   C. T12-L1
   D. L3-L5

2. Chronic pain in elderly patients is

   A. Unlikely to present with cognitive dysfunction
   B. Present in over 40% of nursing home residents
   C. Considered a normal part of the aging process
   D. Not appropriately assessed by the McGill Pain Questionnaire

3. CMI is most commonly caused by

   A. Emboli
   B. Atherosclerosis
   C. Inflammation
   D. Vasospasm

ANSWERS

1. C. The celiac plexus is a group of sympathetic ganglia located around the celiac trunk of the aorta. The preganglionic fibers come from the T5-L1 level and are grouped into greater, lesser, and least splanchnic nerves before they synapse at the ganglia. The celiac plexus is located between T12 and L2 vertebral levels, and is most commonly found at the L1 in front of the aorta.[1]

2. B. It is estimated that between 40% and 80% of elderly patients in nursing homes experience chronic pain,[2] and they sometimes present with atypical symptoms, including sleep disturbance, cognitive impairment, and failure to thrive. While a comprehensive approach to pain assessment in the elderly is necessary, simple-to-administer questionnaires have been shown to be valid across demographics.

3. B. Atherosclerosis is the most common cause of CMI.[11] Approximately 50% of patients presenting with CMI have had surgery for atherosclerosis. Less frequently identified causes

include aortic dissection, median arcuate ligament syndrome, and fibromuscular dysplasia.

QUESTIONS AND ANSWERS

This chapter has accompanying questions and answers that are available to subscribers as part of the Oxford eLearning platform. To access the questions, follow the link below, or go to ✔ http://oxfordmedicine.com/painmanagementreview

19.

CHRONIC ABDOMINAL PAIN IN CHILDREN

Alina Lazar

STEM CASE AND KEY QUESTIONS

A 14-year-old female patient is scheduled for laparoscopic release of the median arcuate ligament (MAL). For the previous 6 months she has experienced abdominal pain, nausea, and unintentional weight loss. She was admitted to the hospital a week ago with worsening pain (pain scores 8/10 at baseline, and 10/10 postprandially). As part of an extensive gastrointestinal workup, duplex ultrasound and CT angiography revealed celiac artery compression. Pain management was complicated by severe nausea after intravenous (IV) opioids. The patient was given scheduled doses of gabapentin, amitriptyline, and acetaminophen, and tramadol, lorazepam, and hydromorphone as needed, with subsequent improvement in pain. She has no other medical problems or allergies, weighs 42 kg, and is 5′3″ tall. She is now in the preoperative holding area accompanied by her parents.

WHAT ARE THE MANAGEMENT STRATEGIES FOR SEVERE ACUTE-ON-CHRONIC PAIN? DISCUSS HOW THE PATIENT'S CHRONIC PAIN HISTORY AND OPIOID-INDUCED NAUSEA MAY AFFECT YOUR PREOPERATIVE PLANNING AND INTRAOPERATIVE MANAGEMENT.

Various options for pain management and their risks and benefits are discussed with the patient and her parents, including patient-controlled epidural analgesia (PCEA). Although the patient herself seems interested in an epidural, she is quickly dissuaded by her mother, a medical professional. The mother knows of patients with epidurals who experienced excruciating pain because of delays in response to pain complaints. She thinks that the small laparoscopy incisions will not create a lot of additional pain.

HOW DO YOU MANAGE THIS SITUATION? DO YOU TRY TO CONVINCE THE MOTHER THAT THE EPIDURAL IS A VALUABLE OPTION IN THIS CASE? DO YOU ENLIST THE SURGEON'S HELP IN "PITCHING" THE EPIDURAL? THE SURGEON IS FULLY SUPPORTIVE OF AN EPIDURAL.

A decision is made to proceed with general anesthesia, intraoperative opioids, low-dose ketamine and propofol infusions, postoperative hydromorphone via patient-controlled analgesia (PCA), and postoperative nausea and vomiting prophylaxis with scopolamine, dexamethasone, and ondansetron.

WHAT ARE THE OPTIONAL STRATEGIES FOR COMPREHENSIVE PERIOPERATIVE PAIN MANAGEMENT FOR THIS PATIENT? DISCUSS THE RISKS, BENEFITS, AND MEDICAL EVIDENCE FOR EACH OPTION.

Surgery is complicated by bleeding from a branch of the celiac artery that cannot be adequately controlled laparoscopically. An emergent laparotomy is performed with an incision from the xyphoid process to the umbilicus, and the patient is resuscitated with 1.5 L lactated Ringer's, 1 L of 5% albumin, and 1 unit of packed red blood cells. The patient remains hemodynamically stable.

HOW WILL THE CONVERSION TO LAPAROTOMY AFFECT YOUR PAIN MANAGEMENT PLAN? WOULD YOU REVISIT THE EPIDURAL OPTION? HOW WOULD OTHER ALTERNATIVES, SUCH AS A TRANSVERSUS ABDOMINIS PLANE (TAP) BLOCK, INTRATHECAL MORPHINE, OR PARAVERTEBRAL BLOCK COMPARE TO THE THORACIC EPIDURAL TECHNIQUE? WHAT ARE THE RISKS AND BENEFITS OF EACH MODALITY?

Upon consultation with the surgeon, you call the parents and discuss the recent turn of events. They agree with the placement of an epidural catheter.

At the end of surgery, with the patient asleep, an epidural catheter is placed at the T6-T7 level via a midline approach and is tested with 3 mL of 1.5% lidocaine and 1:200,000 epinephrine, with no signs of intravascular injection. Next, a bolus of 6 mL 0.25% bupivacaine is injected through the epidural catheter, and the patient is allowed to emerge from anesthesia.

WHICH LOCAL ANESTHETIC WOULD YOU CHOOSE FOR CONTINUOUS INFUSION? WHAT IS YOUR STRATEGY FOR THE ADMINISTRATION OF OPIOIDS (IV OR EPIDURAL)? WHAT ARE THE RISKS AND BENEFITS OF ADDING CLONIDINE TO YOUR CONTINUOUS EPIDURAL INFUSION? WOULD YOU CONTINUE THE IV KETAMINE INFUSION IN THE POSTOPERATIVE PERIOD? WHERE SHOULD THE PATIENT RECOVER?

Upon arrival in her room, the patient is awake and complaining of pain she rates as 8/10. The tested sensory level is T3-T11 on the left side and T5-T8 on the right side. The epidural catheter is slightly pulled back and rebolused with the epidural infusion (bupivacaine 0.1% and fentanyl 5 μg/mL). The epidural infusion rate is increased. Despite these changes, the patient continues to experience pain and is very anxious and tearful. The parents demand that something be done!

WHAT WOULD BE YOUR NEXT COURSE OF ACTION? REPLACE THE EPIDURAL? SWITCH TO A PLAIN LOCAL ANESTHETIC EPIDURAL INFUSION AND ADMINISTER OPIOIDS IV? WHAT FORM OF OPIOID ADMINISTRATION WOULD BE BEST (PCA, CONTINUOUS INFUSION, ADMINISTRATION OF MEDICATION AS NEEDED)? WOULD YOU CONSIDER SEDATING THE PATIENT? WHAT AGENTS WOULD YOU CHOOSE? WOULD YOU CONSIDER ADMINISTERING KETOROLAC?

Over the next few days, the patient's pain is better controlled, and she is eventually discharged home on hydrocodone/acetaminophen 5/325 and amitriptyline. However, 6 weeks later, after a period of initial improvement, her pain is back to the baseline (8/10). Her discomfort is similar to that in the preoperative period but less associated with eating. She has a tender epigastrium. When she elevates her head off the examination table with arms crossed over the chest while the examiner presses on the tender area, her pain does not worsen (negative Carnett's sign). Vascular ultrasound tests performed intraoperatively and at 6 weeks show normalized celiac artery velocities. The CT angiogram is negative.

WHAT IS CAUSING THE PAIN NOW? WHAT DOES A NEGATIVE CARNETT'S SIGN MEAN? HOW WOULD YOU DIFFERENTIATE BETWEEN FUNCTIONAL PAIN, CHRONIC POSTSURGICAL PAIN (CPSP), AND RECURRENT MEDIAN ARCUATE LIGAMENT SYNDROME (MALS)? COMPARE AND CONTRAST THE INCIDENCE, MECHANISMS, RISK FACTORS, AND MANAGEMENT OF THESE THREE CONDITIONS

After evaluation in the pain clinic, the patient receives a celiac plexus block with bupivacaine, triamcinolone, and clonidine, which markedly improves pain relief. The pain relief lasts for the next 5 months. One month later, she receives a second celiac plexus block, resulting in complete and sustained pain relief.

DISCUSSION

Chronic pain, defined as recurrent or continuous pain for more than 3 months, may affect up to a 25% of children.[1] The most common types of pain in children are limb, abdominal, and headache pain. Chronic pain has a profound impact on the development of children and on family dynamics. Children with chronic pain frequently miss school and have difficulties maintaining and developing social contacts. The necessity to stay home with a sick child and the emotional burden imposed by witnessing their children's pain struggles significantly affect their parents.

Chronic abdominal pain occurs in 10% to 19% of children.[2] Its prevalence, increased in children 4 to 6 years old and in young adolescents, is significantly higher in girls.[1] Chronic abdominal pain is classified as functional (Box 19.1) and organic (Table 19.1). Overlap and interaction exist between the two types of disorders.[3]

FUNCTIONAL ABDOMINAL PAIN

Functional abdominal pain (FAP) is a type of functional gastrointestinal disorder (FGID). FGID also includes functional nausea and vomiting disorders and functional defecation disorders. Based on the Rome IV criteria, there are four subtypes of FAP: functional dyspepsia, abdominal migraine, irritable bowel syndrome, and unspecified FAP (children not meeting criteria for irritable bowel syndrome, functional dyspepsia, or abdominal migraine).[4] Rome IV criteria define FAP as pain that occurs more than 4 times a month for at least 2 consecutive months and cannot be fully explained by other medical conditions. The pain is severe enough to interfere with the child's normal activities. Excessive school absence is a significant problem for many children with recurrent abdominal pain.

Worldwide, 13% of children suffer from FAP.[5] Girls are affected more than boys. The prevalence is increased in young children and young adolescents. There is a known association between childhood FAP and long-term comorbidity, including depression, anxiety, lifetime psychiatric disorders, social phobia, and somatic complaints.[6] FAP frequently coexists with other types of recurrent pain, such as chronic headaches and migraines.

The pathophysiology of FAP is thought to involve abnormalities in the enteric nervous system, leading to altered bowel motility, low-grade inflammation, and visceral hyperalgesia—that is, a decreased threshold for pain in response to changes in the intraluminal pressure.[4] Peripheral sensitization, neuropathic pain mechanisms, and abnormal central processing of afferent signals at the level of the central nervous system (CNS) affect the pathophysiology of visceral hyperalgesia.[7] Predisposing factors for this condition are female sex, genetic predisposition, and maladaptive coping

Box 19.1. **ROME IV DIAGNOSTIC CRITERIA FOR FUNCTIONAL ABDOMINAL PAIN DISORDERS IN THE CHILD/ADOLESCENT**

Universal Criterion: Symptoms cannot be fully explained by another medical condition

Functional Dyspepsia

In addition to the universal criterion, at least 2 months with ≥ 1 of the following symptoms on ≥ 4 days per month:

- Postprandial fullness
- Early satiation
- Epigastric pain or burning not associated with defecation

Irritable Bowel Syndrome

In addition to the universal criterion, ≥ 2 months with abdominal pain associated with one of the following on ≥ 4 days per month:

- Related to defecation
- Change in frequency of stool
- Change in form (appearance) of stool

Abdominal Migraine

In addition to the universal criterion, all of the following:

- Paroxysmal episodes of intense, acute, periumbilical, midline, or diffuse abdominal pain lasting ≥ 1 hr (abdominal pain is the most severe and distressing symptom) at least twice within a 6-month period
- Episodes are separated by weeks or months
- The pain is incapacitating and interferes with normal activities
- Stereotypical pattern and symptoms in the individual patient
- The pain is associated with ≥ 2 of the following: anorexia, nausea, vomiting, headache, photophobia, pallor

Functional Abdominal Pain—Not Otherwise Specified

In addition to the universal criterion, all of the following:

- Occurs ≥ 4 times per month for ≥ 2 months
- Episodic or continuous abdominal pain that does not occur solely during physiologic events (e.g., eating, menses)
- Insufficient criteria for irritable bowel syndrome, functional dyspepsia, or abdominal migraine

Adapted from: Hyams JS, Di Lorenzo C, Saps M, et al. Childhood functional gastrointestinal disorders: child/adolescent. *Gastroenterology.* 2016;150:1456–1468.

Table 19.1. **ORGANIC CAUSES OF CHRONIC ABDOMINAL PAIN IN CHILDREN AND ADOLESCENTS (SELECTED)**

COMMON	LESS COMMON
Celiac disease	Inflammatory bowel disease
Acid peptic disorders	Sickle cell disease
Carbohydrate malabsorption	Pelvic inflammatory disease
Musculoskeletal pain	Endometriosis
	Gallstones, chronic cholecystitis, choledochal cyst
	Mesenteric ischemia
	Vasculitis (e.g., Henoch-Schönlein purpura, polyarteritis nodosa)

mechanisms, such as catastrophizing. Psychosocial stress, such as parental divorce, hospitalization, bullying, and childhood abuse, are contributing factors. Pain generated by the altered gastrointestinal physiology with predisposing factors and psychosocial stressors may lead to a state of chronic pain (the biopsychosocial model) in pediatric patients.[8,9]

The pain is poorly localized or periumbilical, usually lasts less than 1 hour, and never lasts longer than 3 hours. It may be accompanied by autonomic symptoms, such as nausea, vomiting, dizziness, and pallor. It is usually triggered or exacerbated by stressful events. There are no alleviating factors. The pain resolves by itself and never wakes a child from sleep.

The initial evaluation of children with recurrent abdominal pain includes a detailed pain history (quality, pattern, intensity, triggers, accompanying symptoms, disability, and current management methods), a physical examination focused on the gastrointestinal and genitourinary system, and stool testing for occult blood. Psychologic problems, such as family conflict or difficulties with peers and school, also are documented. Additional testing is not recommended in the absence of atypical pain or positive findings on physical examination.

Most patients with FAP report substantial and sustained improvement in symptoms over time. In one-third of the patients, the pain persists, and in another third, it is replaced by another pain symptom. Among the factors associated with persistent FAP are parental modeling and reinforcement of the sick role, family history of chronic pain disorders, age younger than 6 years at presentation, more than 6 months of chronic pain before presentation, traumatic life events, and a significant history of anxiety and depression.[10]

The goal of management of FAP in children and adolescents is to restore overall normal function, not to completely eliminate pain. Once an organic cause for abdominal pain has been eliminated, treatment is tailored primarily toward psychiatric modalities. Behavioral interventions are implemented by psychologists and social workers, who focus on modifying the perception of pain, teaching effective coping skills, and addressing reinforcing factors, such as school anxiety and parental behaviors that encourage the expression of pain. Parents may affect a child's pain behavior through inadvertent encouragement of pain by rewarding complaints, by relieving the child of responsibilities, or by modeling pain behaviors themselves. Therapy is largely supportive and includes cognitive-behavioral therapy, biofeedback and relaxation, acupuncture, hypnosis, and meditation. In a prospective, randomized trial, 12 months after a three-session social learning and cognitive-behavioral therapy intervention, 200 children with FAP reported greater decreases in pain severity and greater improvements in pain coping responses than the control group.[11] A follow-up study of patients who underwent gut-directed hypnotherapy found that 5 years after the intervention, two-thirds of the patients were still in remission.[12]

Avoiding dietary triggers and taking prokinetic and antispasmodic agents may be helpful in selected patients. Antidepressants and anxiolytics are reserved for patients with significant associated depression and anxiety. The understanding that a large proportion of pain in FAP is associated with abnormal perception of visceral sensations has led to an interest in the effects of antidepressants on the central and enteric nervous neurotransmitters and their role in mediating FAP. Studies of using these agents for FAP in children are limited. Establishing a therapeutic relationship, patient and family education, and a plan for return to school are important components of management.

ANTERIOR CUTANEOUS NERVE ENTRAPMENT SYNDROME

A frequently overlooked cause of chronic abdominal pain originates from the abdominal wall. Anterior cutaneous nerve entrapment syndrome (ACNES) is the most common cause of parietal pain. Within the pediatric age group, it most frequently occurs in adolescent girls. In ACNES, the entrapment of superficial branches of the intercostal thoracic nerves between the abdominal muscles or in an area of surgical scar produces abdominal pain that may mimic an intra-abdominal source of pain, such as appendicitis. Carnett's test helps to distinguish visceral from abdominal wall pain; the abdomen of a supine patient is palpated to elicit the area of tenderness. The patient is then asked to contract the abdominal muscles by raising the head off the examination table. Pressure is then reapplied to the area of tenderness. If the cause of the pain is intra-abdominal, the tensed musculature protects the viscera and the pain diminishes. If, however, the pain is at least as severe with tensing, this implies the source of the pain resides in the abdominal wall (a positive Carnett's test).

The diagnostic criteria consist of the presence of localized abdominal pain, a positive Carnett's sign, and resolution of pain after trigger-point injection with a local anesthetic. The duration of pain relief after trigger-point injection varies from several hours to complete pain relief.[13]

Management is initially conservative: physical therapy and avoiding activities that require tensing the abdominal muscles. The injection of local anesthetic alone or in combination with a glucocorticoid may be repeated up to three times within a year. For persistent pain, chemical neurolysis or surgical neurectomy may be considered.

MALS

MALS, also referred to as celiac artery compression syndrome or Dunbar syndrome, is a less common cause of chronic abdominal pain. The median arcuate ligament (a fibrous arch formed by the left and right diaphragmatic crura) compresses the celiac artery and plexus, producing ischemic and sympathetic autonomically maintained pain. The condition was first described more than 50 years ago,[14] but its pathophysiology remains controversial. The mechanism suggested is intestinal angina caused by occlusion of the celiac artery. Alternative hypotheses include a steal phenomenon resulting in a watershed effect on the celiac plexus, and disruption of neuroenteric pain pathways affecting visceral hypersensitivity mediated through the celiac ganglion, the latter perhaps similar to the pathogenesis of functional gastrointestinal disorders.[15]

The pain is chronic, typically with a postprandial or exercise-induced component, and commonly associated with nausea, vomiting, and weight loss. Similar to patients with FAP, patients with MALS are young females who have a high prevalence of psychopathology. In one report,[16] nearly one-half of patients with MALS met criteria for an axis I psychiatric disorder: anxiety, mood disorder, and adjustment disorders, according to the *Diagnostic and Statistical Manual of Mental Disorders* (DSM-IV-TR) criteria.[17] Chronic pain can be triggered by psychologic problems or could itself increase the risk of mental illness. In a sample of adult patients with MALS, those with a history of psychiatric disorder tended to have poorer clinical outcomes.[18] Patients suffering from MALS classically exhibit chronic, difficult-to-control pain for years before the diagnosis is made.

Patients typically undergo extensive diagnostic tests before a vascular component is suspected. The diagnosis is one of exclusion of other etiologies of chronic abdominal pain. The screening test of choice is duplex ultrasound, which shows increased peak velocities (> 200 cm/s) in the celiac artery. Angiography, CT angiography, or MRA confirms the diagnosis. A typical "hook sign" is revealed in lateral views (Figure 19.1).

The presence of collaterals and narrowed native vessels suggests a diagnosis of chronic mesenteric ischemia. Because of respiratory variations, both inspiratory and expiratory phases are required for all imaging tests.

The management consists of open or laparoscopic release of the MAL and endovascular or surgical revascularization.[19] Overall success rates of 70% to 80% have been reported after laparoscopic release of the celiac artery compression with or without concomitant neurolysis.[15] A careful psychosocial evaluation is needed to inform appropriate surgical, psychologic, and pain interventions.

The rates of recurrent pain after surgical intervention are between 0 and 50%, but usually less than 10%.[18] Possible causes of recurrent pain are an incomplete release of the MAL, fixed residual stenoses not relieved by external decompression,

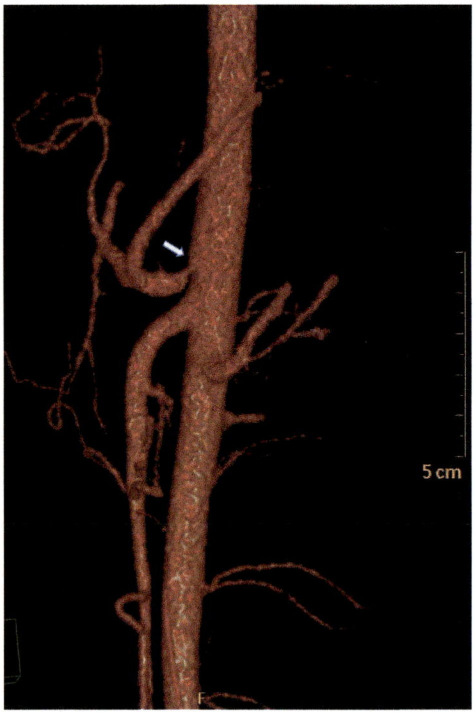

Figure 19.1. CT angiogram 3D reconstruction. The arrow shows the narrowing of the celiac artery origin from aorta by the median arcuate ligament (the "hook sign").

nerve compression that was inadequately released at the time of surgery, and the presence of chronic FAP concomitant with the MALS.[15] Patients with persistent symptoms in the postoperative period, primarily from incomplete ganglionectomy, may benefit form celiac plexus block. A combination of local anesthetic and corticosteroids may relieve pain through anti-inflammatory properties and direct blockade of the sympathetic nerve terminal. Potential management options in patients with MALS-related pain not amenable to surgical intervention include neurolytic celiac plexus block[20] and spinal cord stimulation.[21]

INFLAMMATORY BOWEL DISEASE

Inflammatory bowel disease (IBD), such as Crohn's disease and ulcerative colitis, is associated with chronic abdominal pain that can be debilitating. The prevalence of opioid use in children with IBD is less than in adults (5.6% and 13%, respectively).[22] Although narcotics may be used for short-term treatment of flare-ups or after surgery, long-term narcotic analgesia is discouraged because of gastrointestinal side effects, tolerance, and possibility of addiction. Opioid-induced gastrointestinal dysfunction may induce confusion regarding the status of IBD activity, overtreatment, and further escalation of narcotic doses, resulting in significant physical and psychologic disability. In children, chronic opioid use may cause growth failure, malnutrition, opportunistic infections, and hepatosplenic lymphoma.[22] A retrospective study of 4,344 children with IBD found that psychologic impairment (anxiety, depression), older age, increased health care utilization, and fractures were strongly associated with chronic use of narcotics.[22]

PERIOPERATIVE PAIN MANAGEMENT IN PATIENTS WITH CHRONIC ABDOMINAL PAIN

Chronic pain patients represent a challenge in the perioperative period. Higher levels of pain immediately before surgery and chronic pain are independent predictors for moderate-to-intense pain after abdominal surgery.[23] Preoperative pain may induce diverse central neuroplastic changes, which increase vulnerability to higher postoperative pain levels and postsurgical chronic pain complications.[24]

Pediatric pain assessment is notoriously difficult because young children lack cognitive and emotional maturity and have difficulty in articulating symptoms. It may be difficult to discriminate between pain behaviors and behaviors resulting from other sources of distress or anxiety. Among pain assessment tools are the Children's Hospital of Eastern Ontario Pain Scale (CHEOPS) and the Wong-Baker FACES pain scale for preschool children, and FACES or a numeric or a visual analog scale for older children (Figure 19.2).

Comprehensive pain management with regional anesthesia (epidural and peripheral nerve blocks) and systemic multimodal analgesia (e.g., opioids, nonsteroidal anti-inflammatory drugs [NSAIDs], cyclooxygenase-2 [COX-2] inhibitors, ketamine, gabapentin, and dexmedetomidine or clonidine) is essential in protecting against intense postoperative pain. Multimodal analgesic techniques target pain along various pathways involving transduction, transmission, modulation, and perception by the CNS. Multimodal analgesic techniques decrease opioid consumption, opioid-related adverse effects, postoperative pain, and hospital stay and increase patient satisfaction. In addition to facilitating the recovery process after surgery, nonopioid anesthetics also reduce the risk of long-term opioid dependency and abuse in patients with chronic pain syndromes.

Ketamine

Ketamine works primarily by the noncompetitive inhibition of the *N*-methyl-D-aspartate (NMDA) receptor in the CNS and spinal cord. It is particularly useful in opioid-tolerant patients and those with a history of chronic pain.[25] Even a single perioperative subanesthetic dose (0.5 mg IV) can decrease postoperative pain, nausea, and morphine consumption for 24 hours or longer.[26] As part of a multimodal analgesic regimen, ketamine can be initiated as an infusion at 0.1 to 0.3 mg/kg/hr after a bolus of 0.1 to 0.5 mg/kg. The protocol for administration of low-dose ketamine outside the intraoperative period at our institution is presented in Box 19.2. Low-dose infusions perioperatively have an opioid-sparing effect and decrease hyperalgesia and tolerance without an increase in side effects. Postoperative ketamine administration has been shown to decrease morphine consumption after major abdominal surgery.[27] A systematic review of 70 studies of IV ketamine for perioperative analgesia found that ketamine significantly reduced postoperative opioid consumption and increased the time to first postoperative analgesic requirement, most profoundly in upper abdominal and thoracic

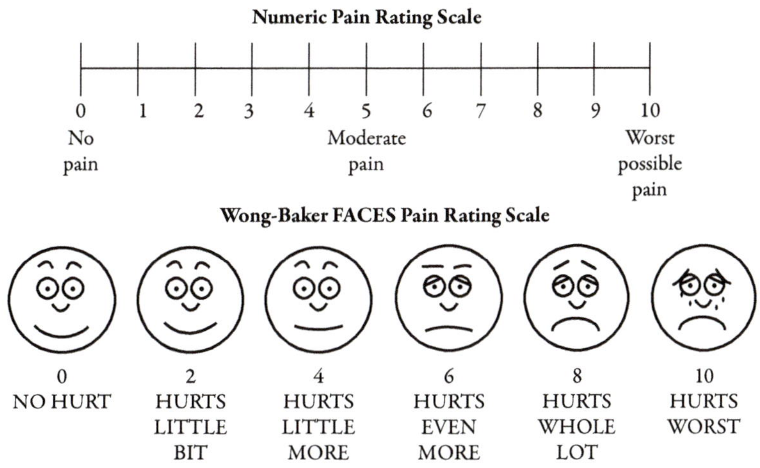

Figure 19.2. Pain scales used in pediatric patients.

Box 19.2. THE UNIVERSITY OF CHICAGO PROTOCOL FOR LOW-DOSE CONTINUOUS IV KETAMINE INFUSION FOR POSTOPERATIVE PAIN CONTROL

All low-dose ketamine orders for the management of pain will be written by a member of the Acute Pain Service following consultation and utilizing the analgesic, subanesthetic, low-dose ketamine order set.

Common Indications

- Opioid tolerance: typically for those ingesting greater than 100 mg of oral morphine equivalents per day.
- Uncontrolled postoperative pain from orthopedic, bowel, or spine surgery.
- Severe intractable pain not controlled by escalating doses of opioids.
- Opioid rotation has failed to improve side effects or intolerance of opioid analgesics.
- Severe neuropathic pain, including central sensitization.
- Evidence of opioid-related hyperalgesia.

Contraindications and Warnings against Ketamine

ABSOLUTE

- Hypersensitivity to ketamine
- Uncontrolled/active seizures
- Uncontrolled/active psychotic disorder(s)
- Renal failure: oliguria
- Liver failure

RELATIVE

- Elevated intracranial pressure (ICP) or intraocular pressure (IOP)
- Uncontrolled hypertension
- Severe ischemic heart disease or severe congestive heart failure (increased myocardial oxygen demand)
- Thyrotoxicosis (ketamine causes hypertension and supraventricular tachycardia)
- Aneurysms
- Hemorrhagic cystitis (ketamine causes hemorrhagic cystitis after long-term use)

Dosing

- For IV administration of ketamine, continuous pulse oximetry is required
- No bolus doses of IV ketamine are allowed
- IV ketamine is limited to 1 to 5 μg/kg/min based on ideal body weight

STARTING DOSE

- Normal renal or hepatic function: typically 2 μg/kg/min based on ideal body weight. Consider starting at 1 μg/kg/min in patients with a BMI ≤ 18. Consider a lower dose in patients with renal or hepatic dysfunction because of reduced ketamine and norketamine (active metabolite) clearance
- Renal failure: ketamine contraindicated at our center
- Liver failure: ketamine contraindicated at our center

DOSE CHANGES

Ketamine infusion cannot be titrated; infusion rate changed only with a pain physician's order. Opioid doses are maintained at the current dose level while ketamine infusion is initiated. Opioid dose is not escalated simultaneously with ketamine infusion initiation, due to risk of sedation and respiratory depression.

Monitoring

- Continuous pulse oximetry
- Routine vital signs
- Pain and sedation scores every 2 hr for 4 hr, then every 4 hr for the duration of the infusion
- At the start of an infusion or after an increase in dose, monitoring should be more frequent: every 2 hr for 4 hr (pain score, sedation level) then every 4 hr

Nursing documents total drug amount infused every 12 hr.

The Acute Pain Service monitors the patient receiving a ketamine infusion for side effects.

Monitoring is not required of a patient ambulating or outside of his room.

Management of Complications

The following medications should be ordered for every patient started on ketamine. Although it is unlikely that low doses of ketamine will cause adverse effects, these medications may be scheduled if necessary.

- Lorazepam 1 mg PO/IV every 6 hr as needed for hallucinations/agitation.
- Prochlorperazine 10 mg PO every 6 hr as needed for nausea/vomiting.

If systolic blood pressure changes more than 20% from baseline, systolic blood pressure is > 160 mm Hg, respirations are < 10 breaths/min, or mental status changes, or the patient is slow to arouse with continuous stimulation:

- Assess vital signs
- Administer oxygen and provide positive-pressure ventilation if necessary
- Prepare for reversal with naloxone

Holding Parameters

If any of the following occur, notify a physician on the pain service.

- Change (increase/decrease) in systolic blood pressure by more than 20% of baseline
- Respiratory rate is <10 breaths/min
- Acute change in mental status (i.e., blunted affect, emotional withdrawal, thought disorders, delirium)
- Difficult to arouse despite continuous stimulation

procedures.[28] Ketamine was effective, although less so, in orthopedic and lower abdominal surgery. The opioid-sparing effect was greatest in patients with high VAS scores, suggesting that ketamine is more useful for the most painful operations.[29] IV infusions of subanesthetic doses of ketamine may significantly improve pain scores in patients with severe intractable pain syndromes refractory to conventional treatments, particularly in neuropathic pain syndromes, such as complex regional pain syndrome, intractable headache, and chronic back pain.[29] In one study, the pain relief after ketamine infusion lasted more than 3 weeks in 38% of the patients, and more than 1 to 2 days in 73% of the patients.[30] The protocol for outpatient ketamine infusion for chronic pain at our institution is described in Box 19.3.

There is less support in the literature for the use of ketamine for pediatric patients. A meta-analysis of pediatric ketamine studies concluded that, although ketamine was associated with lower postanesthesia care unit (PACU) pain scores and opioid requirements, it did not reduce postoperative opioid consumption after ambulatory surgeries, such as tonsillectomy.[31] Pharmacokinetic differences relating to age suggest that children require higher ketamine doses to maintain the same plasma concentrations as adults and that there is a shorter context sensitive half-life.[32] The incidence of psychomimetic symptoms associated with ketamine is lower in children than in adults.[33] Some adult studies highlighted better postoperative analgesia when IV ketamine was associated with epidural analgesia.[34,35] In pediatric patients, a regimen of IV ketamine and caudal anesthesia was not found to be superior to caudal anesthesia alone.[36] No such studies exist in pediatric patients undergoing major surgery.

Gabapentin and Pregabalin

Gabapentin and pregabalin have been used in clinical practice for the treatment of neuropathic pain and as preemptive agents perioperatively. They act as membrane stabilizers and reduce neuronal hyperexcitability. In a meta-analysis of randomized trials, Dahl showed a significant reduction of postoperative morphine requirements with gabapentinoid agents in a variety of surgeries, including mastectomy, hysterectomy, spinal surgery, and laparoscopic cholecystectomy.[37] Moderate (600 mg) doses of preoperative Neurontin reduced the occurrence of postoperative nausea and vomiting (PONV) associated with general anesthesia in adults in a meta-analysis of studies with PONV as primary end point.[38] A preoperative oral loading dose of gabapentin (15 mg/kg), before 5 mg/kg three times per day for 5 days, improved analgesia and reduced morphine use in pediatric patients undergoing spinal fusion surgery up to 2 days after surgery.[39]

Dexmedetomidine and Clonidine

Dexmedetomidine and clonidine are alpha-2 agonists with analgesic and opioid-sparing effects. Alpha-2 agonists produce analgesia by inhibiting transmission of noxious information in the dorsal horn of the spinal cord and locus ceruleus and by inhibiting sympathetic outflow in the intermediolateral cell column, or by inhibiting norepinephrine release by sympathetic nerve terminals.[40]

Epidurally administered clonidine (300 μg) to patients with complex regional pain syndrome provided effective

Box 19.3. **UNIVERSITY OF CHICAGO PROTOCOL FOR OUTPATIENT LIDOCAINE INFUSION FOR CHRONIC PAIN**

Consultation

Obtain baseline EKG and cardiac history
Evaluate the patient for arrhythmias before scheduling procedure

Day of Procedure

Assess the patient for fasting and alertness
Determine effects of previous infusion, if any, on pain reduction
Duration of effects
Patient function after infusion
Decrease in use of pain medication since infusion
Verify that patient has companion to accompany patient home
Obtain signed consent on the consent form

Procedure

Apply standard monitors: blood pressure, EKG, pulse oximeter, capnograph
Start IV access and administer 1 mg/kg lidocaine bolus over 3 to 5 min
Follow with 4 mg/kg lidocaine (or 2–4 mg) administered slowly over 30 min (or 20–30 min)
Record at 1, 5, 10, 15, 20, 25, and 30 min the following:
Time of administration
Blood pressure
Heart rate
Pulse oximetry
Pain score
Stop the infusion in the event of seizure activity or cardiac instability.

Recovery

Patients recover within 30 to 60 min after the procedure.
Vital signs are monitored over 15 min during recovery.
At the end of the recovery period, the patient is discharged from the clinic to the accompanying caregiver.

Follow-up

In 4 weeks, patient returns for evaluation of treatment or repeat infusion.
The dose of lidocaine is not increased if the initial infusion was performed with 4 mg/kg over 20 min.

pain relief with mild sedation.[40] In the same study, epidural clonidine infused for a mean of 43 days at a mean rate of 32 μg/hr provided sustained analgesia.[40] Epidural infusion of clonidine at 0.2 μg/kg/hr after a bolus of 2 μg/kg, alone or in combination with ropivacaine 0.1%, provided good postoperative analgesia at rest, but not during coughing, in children undergoing major abdominal surgery.[41] Sedation and hypotension were observed only in the group that received the bolus. Replacing epidural fentanyl with clonidine resulted in comparable analgesia, but fewer side effects.[42] In addition to the IV and neuraxial routes, clonidine may be administered orally and transdermally. One clinical report describes successful opioid-free postoperative analgesia in a patient with chronic abdominal and opioid-induced delirium by alternating various routes of administration of alpha-2 agonists.[43]

Intravenously administered dexmedetomidine at 0.4 μg/kg/hr for 4 hours after an initial loading dose of 1 μg/kg over 10 min reduced the early need for morphine by 66% after major inpatient surgery in adults.[44] A meta-analysis of randomized, controlled trials showed that the most effective postoperative analgesia using intraoperative infusions of dexmedetomidine in adults was obtained with doses of 1 μg/kg, followed by a continuous infusion of 0.5 to 1 μg/kg/hr.[44] The study showed a stronger opioid-sparing effect at 24 hours for dexmedetomidine, compared to acetaminophen and COX-2 inhibitors.[45] The doses for continuous infusion in pediatric patients are similar to doses for adults; however, the initial loading dose is increased in children less than 2 years old because of a larger volume of distribution. Prolonged use (days to weeks) of IV dexmedetomidine infusions may lead to a state of physiologic dependence. Gradual weaning (by 0.1 μg/kg/hr every 8 hr) is warranted to prevent tachycardia and hypertension associated with withdrawal.[46]

Limiting side effects of alpha-2 agonists include hypotension, bradycardia, and sedation. Although alpha-2 agonists do have sedation potential, respiratory drive and airway tone are preserved, and the patients are able to respond to verbal instructions, thus enhancing clinical safety.

Lidocaine

Perioperative systemic lidocaine infusions reduce postoperative pain, opioid requirements, intestinal ileus, and duration of hospitalization without significant systemic anesthetic toxicity.[47] Peri-incisional lidocaine patches are also effective in diminishing postoperative pain.[48]

Acetaminophen

Acetaminophen centrally inhibits prostaglandins via the COX-3 pathway, reinforces the descending serotoninergic pathways, triggers indirect activation of cannabinoid receptors, and inhibits nitric oxide pathways to reverse hyperalgesia induced by NMDA. Peripherally, it exerts an anti-inflammatory action. Acetaminophen can be administered via oral, rectal, and IV routes. The combination of acetaminophen and opioids reduces pain, sedation, and PONV.[49] Risk factors for hepatotoxicity include prolonged fasting, dehydration, chronic malnutrition, and hepatic impairment. In obese children, the dosage should be based on ideal body weight. IV acetaminophen achieves peak plasma concentrations in ~ 15 min, compared to 40 to 50 min after oral administration and 3 to 4 hours after rectal administration. Duration of action is up to 4 hours. For management of acute postoperative pain, patients weighing at least 50 kg may receive an oral or IV acetaminophen dose of 650 mg every 4 hours, or 1 g every 6 hours, to a maximum of 4 g/day. For patients weighing less than 50 kg, the dose is 12.5 mg/kg every 4 hours or 15 mg/kg every 6 hours, with a maximum dose of 75 mg/kg/day. When acetaminophen is administered rectally, doses of 25 to 40 mg/kg are required.

NSAIDs and COX-2 Inhibitors

IV NSAIDs or COX-2 inhibitors have an opioid-sparing effect and consequently decrease the risk of respiratory depression, sedation, nausea, pruritus, and postoperative ileus. NSAIDs inhibit cyclooxygenase (COX), reduce the production of prostaglandins at the site of tissue injury, and diminish the inflammatory cascade. In addition, NSAIDs have a direct spinal effect by blocking the hyperalgesic response induced by activation of spinal glutamate and substance P receptors. Selective COX-2 inhibition has less effect on gastric mucosal function and platelet aggregation, resulting in fewer side effects. Caution should be exercised when administering NSAIDs to patients with a history of gastric discomfort, asthma, renal dysfunction, or bleeding disorders. Diclofenac and ibuprofen are most commonly used because of their safer toxicity profile. When acetaminophen and an NSAID were combined, the benefit was synergistic.[50] When not contraindicated, these agents should be administered concurrently for maximal benefit. Ibuprofen is administered orally in a dose of 5 to 10 mg/kg, with a maximum dose of 40 mg/kg/day in patients weighing less than 50 kg, and 200 to 800 mg every 6 hr in patients weighing more than 50 kg. The dose of ketorolac is 0.5 mg/kg every 6 hours IV or intramuscularly for up to a maximum of 72 hours. Ketorolac is contraindicated in renal insufficiency. American Society of Regional Anesthesia and Pain Medicine (ASRA) guidelines state that there is grade 1A evidence that NSAIDs alone add no significant risk for the development of spinal hematoma in patients undergoing neuraxial blocks.[51]

Opioids

IV PCA with opioids is the preferred method for the management of moderate and severe acute and chronic pain associated with cancer or sickle cell disease in children more than 5 to 6 years old. The education of children and their parents on the usage of PCA is paramount. It should be made clear that children are to activate the pump whenever they feel pain and not wait for severe pain, and that they cannot give themselves too much medication because of the lockout interval. Surrogate control of PCA by parents or nurses increases the risk of respiratory depression. Its use is allowed only in special circumstances: chronic pain, palliative pain, and repeated or extensive surgery. Well-developed policies regarding the selection of suitable caregivers, communication, and monitoring mechanisms are required.

PCA opioid dosages for opioid-naïve patients are shown in Table 19.2. A basal infusion rate may be used to replace a patient's baseline opioid requirement in patients who are taking opioids regularly. Morphine is the most common opioid administered via PCA, with hydromorphone and fentanyl reserved for children who cannot tolerate morphine. Hydromorphone induces less itching and nausea than morphine; fentanyl may be associated with a higher incidence of apnea and hypoxemia. For patients receiving PCA or neuraxial or intermittent doses of opioids, continuous respiratory monitoring is required (at a minimum, pulse oximetry and respiratory rate).

Epidural Analgesia

Epidural analgesia provides significant pain relief with improved gastrointestinal function after laparotomy. Data are inconclusive with regard to epidural analgesia after a laparoscopic procedure. The epidural catheter is ideally placed at the dermatomal level of the surgical incision. Most children are anesthetized or heavily sedated before administration of epidural anesthesia. There has been an intense debate on the safety of performing regional anesthesia in anesthetized children. The consensus of pediatric anesthesiologists is that there is a long record of safety in performing regional blocks in anesthetized children, and it may be safer to perform these blocks in an anesthetized child rather than a struggling child.[52] There is more controversy over direct needle placement of thoracic epidurals in anesthetized children, particularly in infants. Because children's ligaments are softer and easier to penetrate, caution and a slow, deliberate approach should be exercised to avoid dural puncture. Loss of resistance to saline is preferred in pediatric patients. The side effects and complications from epidural anesthesia are the same for children as for adults. Post-dural-puncture headache is rarely seen in children less than 8 years old. Typical infusions are a combination of local anesthetic and opioid and/or clonidine (Table 19.3). For abdominal pain, when the epidural catheter is placed at the correct thoracic spinal level, the bupivacaine or ropivacaine infusions are 0.1 to 0.15 mg/kg/hr. When the epidural catheter tip is at the low lumbar level, the infusion rate is 0.2 to 0.3

Table 19.2. TYPICAL DOSES FOR PATIENT-CONTROLLED ANALGESIA

DRUG	DEMAND DOSE (MG/KG)	LOCKOUT INTERVAL (MIN)	CONTINUOUS BASAL INFUSION (MG/KG/HR)	4-HR LIMIT (MG/KG)
Morphine	10–20	6–15	0–20	250–400
Hydromorphone	2–4	6–15	0–4	50–80
Fentanyl	0.5	6–10	0–0.5	7–10

Table 19.3. **RECOMMENDED RATES OF ADJUVANTS FOR CONTINUOUS EPIDURAL INFUSION IN PEDIATRIC PATIENTS**

DRUG	DOSE* (MG/KG/HR)	TYPICAL CONCENTRATION (MG/ML)
Fentanyl	0.1–0.5	5 (2–5)
Hydromorphone	1.5–2.5	10–20
Morphine	3–5	25–50
Clonidine**	0.1–0.2	0.4–1 (lumbar epidural tip) 0.4–0.6 (thoracic epidural tip)

*Larger doses of opioids are indicated for opioid-tolerant patients.

** When clonidine is added to an epidural solution, the epidural opioid dose should be reduced by 50%.

mg/kg/hr for a site of pain below the umbilicus (T10), and 0.3 to 0.4 mg/kg/hr for a site of pain above the umbilicus, with a maximum of 15 mL/hr. The maximal infusion rate of 0.4 mg/kg/hr of bupivacaine should not be exceeded to prevent local anesthetic toxicity. PCEA can be used in children as young as 5 years old. A common PCEA regimen is a basal rate of 0.2 mg/kg/hr, bolus of 0.1 mg/kg/hr, a lockout interval 15 min, and a maximum hourly rate of 0.4 mg/kg/hr.

Lack of parental or patient consent and infection at the insertion site are absolute contraindications for using epidural analgesia. Coagulopathy, anatomic anomalies, and hypovolemia are relative contraindications. In general, epidural analgesia is not offered to patients who have an ongoing coagulopathy. However, data suggest a relatively low complication rate in performing lumbar punctures in cancer patients with mild thrombocytopenia. An international normalized ratio (INR) value ≤ 1.5 correlates with excellent perioperative hemostasis. Epidural analgesia may be performed in select cases with infusion of platelets, fresh frozen plasma, or other blood products, in situations in which the benefits outweigh the risks. The concurrent use of other medications that affect the clotting mechanism, such as aspirin, NSAIDs, and heparin, increases the risk of bleeding complications without affecting the INR.

Intrathecal morphine is an option to reduce both pain scores and opioid requirements after laparoscopic abdominal surgery; however, the reduction in pain scores is observed only early in the postoperative period when compared to IV PCA.[53] An intrathecal morphine dose of 5 to 10 μg/kg provides prolonged (12–24 hr) postoperative analgesia. Because morphine travels cephalad to the brain and persists in the CSF for 24 hours, delayed respiratory depression can occur after concurrent administration of parenteral opioids. All patients who received neuraxial opioids require postoperative respiratory monitoring for 24 hours after the opioid administration. If rescue opioids are needed, a mixed agonist-antagonist, such as nalbuphine, is preferred. Pruritus is a common side effect of intrathecal morphine administration and may be treated with diphenhydramine or a low-dose naloxone infusion.

Thoracic Paravertebral Block

Thoracic paravertebral block, as a single shot or continuous infusion, provides equal or superior analgesia for abdominal surgery compared to thoracic epidural analgesia via a direct somatic nerve and sympathetic nerve blockade and by spilling into the epidural space. Bilateral catheters for paravertebral block resulted in equivalent opioid consumption and pain scores when compared to a thoracic epidural for postoperative pain management in pediatric patients undergoing the Nuss procedure.[54] In pediatric patients undergoing cardiac surgery, the paravertebral block was associated with similar analgesia but significantly less failure rate and side effects (nausea, vomiting, hypotension, and urinary retention) compared to epidural analgesia.[55]

TAP Block

The TAP block provides analgesia only to the abdominal wall (incisional), and fails to address the visceral component of pain. A TAP block minimized postsurgical pain in adults[56] and children.[57] In data from the Pediatric Regional Anesthesia Network, of 1,994 TAP blocks, only two were associated with minor complications.[58]

In patients with FAP, depression, anxiety, stress, negative affect, and maladaptive coping mechanisms may contribute to postoperative pain. Preoperative pain catastrophizing (a tendency to magnify or exaggerate the threat value or seriousness of pain sensations) predicts heightened postsurgical pain, independent of anxiety or depression. Identification of catastrophizers, through various validated measuring tools, can help optimize patient care. More aggressive analgesia may be needed for those who catastrophize more.[59] Reducing the levels of catastrophizing can be achieved through cognitive-behavioral therapy, by distraction techniques, and by removing the social reinforcers of catastrophizing.[59,60] Preemptive cognitive and behavioral interventions aimed at decreasing anxiety before and after surgery also reduce postoperative pain intensity and analgesic use. Educating patients and their parents and managing expectations about pain intensity and duration encourage a positive attitude to pain relief. As much as possible, patients should be involved in their pain management strategy.

MANAGEMENT OF POSTSURGICAL ABDOMINAL PAIN

The diagnosis and treatment of postsurgical abdominal pain are challenging. The differential diagnosis consists of new or residual pathology, CPSP, and functional pain. A careful history of the characteristics of pain before and after surgery and associated symptoms can differentiate between a preexisting pain condition, persistent postsurgical pain, and new pathology. A positive Carnett's sign (increased abdominal pain in response to palpation when the muscles of the abdominal wall are voluntarily tensed) suggests that the pain originates in the abdominal wall. A negative Carnett's sign indicates that the source of pain is visceral. Patient risk factors, such as young age, anxiety, female sex, preexisting abdominal pain, and less-than-optimal postoperative pain control, increase the likelihood of persistent postsurgical pain. A differential neuraxial block, TAP block, and celiac plexus block may help differentiate between the somatosensory (incisional) and visceral or neuropathic origin of pain.[61] Diagnostic tests should be performed to rule out residual pathology and surgical-site infection; coexistent functional pain remains a diagnosis of exclusion.

Box 19.4. PREVENTIVE STRATEGIES FOR PERSISTENT POSTSURGICAL PAIN

- Minimize tissue trauma during surgery
- Control postoperative pain (particularly dynamic pain) aggressively
- Antianxiety interventions
- Preventive analgesia
- Multimodal analgesia (regional anesthesia, COX-2 inhibitors, opioids)
- NMDA antagonists, alpha-2 agonists, and anticonvulsants

CPSP

Persistent postsurgical pain is pain that lasts more than 2 months after surgery without other explanation (preexisting pain condition, chronic infection, recurrent malignancy).[62] In adults, the incidence varies from 10% to 50% depending on the operation (thoracotomy 29%, amputation 50%–85%, abdominal surgery 20%, laparoscopic cholecystectomy 5%).[63] Studies of pediatric CPSP are mostly retrospective and subject to recall bias. The reported prevalence of CPSP in children is lower than in adults (between 5% and 50% depending on the type of surgery).[64] The reported pain is frequent and interferes with activities at home, at school, and with friends. One study showed that almost one-quarter of children who underwent major surgery developed CPSP, and of these, 14% had severe pain 6 months after surgery.[65]

Hypothetical mechanisms are ongoing inflammation, nerve injury or neuropathic pain, and a genetic predisposition. Peripheral sensitization of nociceptors results in hyperexcitability in dorsal horn neurons and central sensitization, leading to a reduced pain threshold and the amplification of the pain response. There is evidence that early-life pain and surgery can produce long-term changes in sensory processing and increase the degree and duration of hyperalgesia when repeat surgery is performed later in life.[66]

The risk factors associated with CPSP in adults are younger age, female sex, pain before the operation, surgery longer than 3 hours, surgical approach with risk of nerve damage, high-intensity pain in the first days following surgery (especially movement-evoked pain), preoperative anxiety, catastrophizing, and fear of surgery.[63] Pediatric-specific risk factors are anxiety, sensitivity, and pain unpleasantness, but not pain intensity.[65] As with adults,[63] higher baseline preoperative pain, depression, anxiety (both patient's and parent's), catastrophizing (especially by parents), intensity of acute postoperative pain, and duration of surgery are predictive factors for CPSP. In adults, acute postoperative pain is one of the strongest predictors of chronic pain after surgery. Some studies suggest that in children, younger age at the time of surgery was associated with a lower risk of developing CPSP. For example, the prevalence of phantom pain in patients who lost their limb before and after the age of 6 years is 20.5% and 85.7%, respectively.[67] One study found that early visceral pain, but not somatic or referred pain, was an independent risk factor for chronic pain after laparoscopic cholecystectomy.[68] Preoperative pain in adults is likely to increase the risk of chronic pain after surgery. Keller and colleagues found that 48% of patients who received narcotics before thoracotomy developed chronic postthoracotomy pain, compared to a mere 5% of those who received no narcotics.[69]

Prevention is paramount in the management of persistent postoperative pain (Box 19.4). Achieving control of pain at rest is not sufficient; relief for movement-evoked pain is necessary to prevent persistent postsurgical pain. Several studies demonstrated superiority of neuraxial anesthesia (especially spinal anesthesia) to general anesthesia in the prevention of CPSP.[70] Adequate acute pain control with multimodal strategies (including appropriately dosed preoperative opioids, anti-inflammatory drugs, local and regional analgesia, gabapentinoids, and NMDA receptor antagonists) has been recommended but has not been well studied in children. Nerve blocks, such as TAP block[61] and celiac plexus block, have been reported as therapeutic tools for patients with chronic pain after abdominal surgery. Preemptive epidural analgesia has a significant benefit for postoperative pain; however, the benefit of other types of analgesia provided preemptively is not so clear. Preventive analgesia should focus on effective control of pain over the entire time that there is an inflammatory stimulus and not just at skin incision. The goal is to prevent sensitization of the nervous system, postsurgical hyperalgesia, and CPSP. Interventions directed toward decreasing the levels of psychosocial predictors of chronic pain, such as anxiety, depression, stress, and poor coping mechanisms, are likely to be effective in the prevention and management of CPSP. Such interventions include cognitive-behavioral therapy, family-oriented interventions, biofeedback, and relaxation techniques.

CONCLUSIONS

Chronic pain in pediatric patients has a high prevalence, and FAP is the most common cause. Patients with higher preoperative pain scores who are opioid tolerant, or who display anxiety and maladaptive coping mechanisms, have a higher risk of severe and difficult-to-manage postoperative pain. Aggressive and comprehensive pain management with multimodal pain strategies and psychologic intervention are required for optimal outcomes. Although the incidence of chronic postoperative pain in children is believed to be lower than in adults, its consequences are costly, affecting both children and their parents.

REFERENCES

1. Perquin CW, Hazebroek-Kampschreur AA, Hunfeld JA, et al. Pain in children and adolescents: a common experience. *Pain.* 2000;87(1):51–58.
2. Apley J. *The Child with Abdominal Pains.* 2nd ed. Oxford: Blackwell Scientific Publications; 1975.
3. Zimmerman LA, Srinath AI, Goyal A, et al. The overlap of functional abdominal pain in pediatric Crohn's disease. *Inflamm Bowel Dis.* 2013;19:826–831.
4. Hyams JS, Di Lorenzo C, Saps M, et al. Childhood functional gastrointestinal disorders: child/adolescent. *Gastroenterology.* 2016;150:1456–1468.
5. Korterink JJ, Diederen K, Benninga MA, Tabbers MM. Epidemiology of pediatric functional abdominal pain disorders: a meta-analysis. *PLoS One.* 2015;10(5):e0126982.
6. Hotopf M, Carr S, Mayou R, et al. Why do children have chronic abdominal pain, and what happens to them when they grow up? Population based cohort study. *BMJ.* 1998;316:1196–1200.
7. Tack J, Masaoka T, Janssen P. Functional dyspepsia. *Curr Opin Gastroenterol.* 2011;27:549–557.
8. Zernikow B, Wager J, Hechler T, et al. Characteristics of highly impaired children with severe chronic pain: a 5-year retrospective study on 2249 pediatric pain patients. *BMC Pediatr.* 2012;12:54–66.
9. Bonilla S, Saps M. Early life events predispose the onset of childhood functional gastrointestinal disorders. *Rev Gastroenterol Mex.* 2013;78:82–91.
10. Mulvaney S, Lambert EW, Garber J, Walker LS. Trajectories of symptoms and impairment of pediatric patients with functional abdominal pain: a 5-year longitudinal study. *J Am Acad Child Adolesc Psychiatry.* 2006;45:737.
11. Levy RL, Langer SL, Walker LS, et al. Twelve-month follow-up of cognitive behavioral therapy for children with functional abdominal pain. *JAMA Pediatr.* 2013;167(2):178.
12. Vlierger AM, Rulten JM, Govers AM. Long-term follow-up of gut-directed hypnotherapy vs. standard of care in children with functional abdominal pain or irritable bowel disease. *Am J Gastroenterol.* 2012;107(4):627–631.
13. Akhnikh S, de Korte N, de Winter K. Anterior cutaneous nerve entrapment syndrome (ACNES): the forgotten diagnosis. *Eur J Pediatr.* 2014;173:445–449.
14. Harjola PT. A rare obstruction of the coeliac artery. *Ann Chi Gynaec.* 1963;52:547.
15. Mak GZ, Speaker C, Anderson K, et al. Median arcuate ligament syndrome in the pediatric population. *J Pediatr Surg.* 2013;48(11):2261–2270.
16. Mak GZ, Lucchetti AR, Drossos T, et al. Pediatric chronic abdominal pain and median arcuate ligament syndrome: a review and psychological comparison. *Pediatr Ann.* 2016;45(7):257–264.
17. American Psychiatric Association. *Diagnostic and Statistical Manual of Mental Disorders.* 4th ed. Washington, DC: American Psychiatric Publishing; 2000.
18. Reilly SM, Ammar AD, Stoney RJ, Ehrenfeld WK. Late results following operative repair for celiac artery compression syndrome. *J Vasc Surg.* 1985; 2(1):79–91.
19. Jimenez JC, Harlander-Locke M, Dutson EP. Open and arthroscopic treatment of median arcuate ligament syndrome. *J Vasc Surg.* 2012;56(3):869–873.
20. de Oliveira R, dos Reis MP, Prado WA. The effect of early and late neurolytic sympathetic plexus block on the management of abdominal or pelvic cancer pain. *Pain.* 2004;110:400–408.
21. Caruso C, Lo Sapio D, Ragosa V, et al. Abdominal angina due to obstruction of mesenteric artery treated with spinal cord stimulation: a clinical case. *Neuromodulation.* 2011;14:146–150.
22. Buckley JP, Cook SF, Allen JK, Kappelman MD. Prevalence of chronic narcotic use among children with inflammatory bowel disease. *Clin Gastroenterol Hepatol.* 2015;13(2):310–315.
23. Caumo W, Schmidt AP, Schneider CN, et al. Preoperative predictors of moderate to intense acute postoperative pain in patients undergoing abdominal surgery. *Acta Anaesthesiol Scand.* 2002;46:1265–1271.
24. Wilder-Smith OHG, Tassoni E, Arendt-Nielsen L. Preoperative back pain is associated with diverse manifestations of central neuroplasticity. *Pain.* 2002;97:189–194.
25. Barreveld AM, Corell DJ, Liu X, et al. Ketamine decreases postoperative pain scores in patients taking opioids for chronic pain: results of a prospective, randomized, double-blind study. *Pain Med.* 2013;14(6):925–934.
26. Bell RF, Dahl JB, Moore RA, et al. Perioperative ketamine for acute postoperative pain. *Cochrane Database Syst Rev.* 2006;(1):CD004603.
27. Zakine J, Samarcq D, Lorne E, et al. Postoperative ketamine administration decreases morphine consumption in major abdominal surgery: a prospective, randomized, double-blind, controlled study. *Anesth Analg.* 2008;106(6):1856–1861.
28. Laskowski K, Stirling A, McKay WP, Lim HJ. A systematic review of intravenous ketamine for postoperative analgesia. *Can J Anaesth.* 2011;58:911–923.
29. Niesters M, Martini C, Dahan A. Ketamine for chronic pain: risks and benefits. *Br J Clin Pharmacol.* 2014;77(2):357–367.
30. Patil S, Anitescu M. Efficacy of outpatient ketamine infusions in refractory chronic pain syndromes: a 5-year retrospective analysis. *Pain Med.* 2102;13(2):263–269.
31. Dahmani S, Michelet D, Abback PS, et al. Ketamine for perioperative pain management in children: a meta-analysis of published studies. *Paediatr Anaesth.* 2011;21(10):1080–1082.
32. Dallimore D, Anderson B. Ketamine anesthesia in children–exploring infusion regimens. *Paediatr Anaesth.* 2008;18(8):708–714.
33. Grant IS, Nimmo WS, McNicol LR, Clements JA. Ketamine disposition in children and adults. *Br J Anaesth.* 1983;55:1107–1111.
34. Karakamaz A, Kaya S, Karaman H, et al. Intraoperative intravenous ketamine in combination with epidural analgesia: postoperative analgesia after renal surgery. *Anesth Analg.* 2003;97:1092–1096.
35. Kaye AD, Ali SI, Urman RU. Perioperative analgesia: ever-changing technology and pharmacology. *Best Pract Res Clin Anaesthesiol.* 2014;28:3–14.
36. Bazin V, Bollot J, Asehnoune K, et al. Effects of perioperative intravenous low dose of ketamine on postoperative analgesia in children. *Eur J Anaesthesiol.* 2010;27(1):47–52.
37. Dahl JB, Mathiesen O, Moiniche S, et al. "Protective premedication": an option with gabapentin and related drugs? A review of pregabalin in the treatment of postoperative pain. *Acta Anaesthesiol Scand.* 2004;48:1130–1136.
38. Grant MC, Lee H, Page AJ, et al. The effect of preoperative gabapentin on postoperative nausea and vomiting: a meta-analysis. *Anesth Analg.* 2016;122:976–985.
39. Rusy LM, Hainsworth KR, Nelson TJ, et al. Gabapentin use in pediatric spinal fusion patients: a randomized, double-blind, controlled trial. *Anesth Analg.* 2010;110(5):1393–1398.
40. Rauck RL, Eisenack JC, Jackson K, et al. Epidural clonidine treatment for refractory reflex sympathetic dystrophy. *Anesthesiology.* 1993;79:1163–1169.
41. Klamt JG, Garcia LV, Stocche RM, et al. Epidural infusion of clonidine or clonidine plus ropivacaine for postoperative analgesia in children undergoing major abdominal surgery. *J Clin Anesth.* 2003;15(7):510–514.
42. Cucchiaro G, Adzick SN, Rose JB, et al. A comparison of epidural bupivacaine-fentanyl and bupivacaine-clonidine in children undergoing the Nuss procedure. *Anesth Analg.* 2006;103(2):322–327.

43. Patil SK, Anitescu M. Opioid-free perioperative analgesia for hemicolectomy in a patient with opioid-induced delirium: a case report and review of the analgesic efficacy of the alpha-2 agonist agents. *Pain Pract.* 2012;8:656–662.
44. Arain SR, Ruehlow RM, Uhrich TD, et al. The efficacy of dexmedetomidine versus morphine for postoperative analgesia after major inpatient surgery. *Anesth Analg.* 2004;98:153–158.
45. Schnabel A, Reichl SU, Poepping DM, et al. Efficacy and safety of intraoperative dexmedetomidine for acute postoperative pain in children: a meta-analysis of randomized controlled trials. *Paediatr Anaesth.* 2013;23(2):170–179.
46. Weber MD, Thammasitboon S, Rosen DA. Acute discontinuation syndrome from dexmedetomidine after protracted use in a pediatric patient. *Paediatr Anaesth.* 2008;18:87–88.
47. Sun Y, Li T, Wang N, et al. Perioperative systemic lidocaine for postoperative analgesia and recovery after abdominal surgery: a meta-analysis of randomized controlled trials. *Dis Colon Rectum.* 2012;55:1183–1194.
48. Kwon YS, Kim JB, Jung HJ, et al. Treatment for postoperative wound pain in gynecologic laparoscopic surgery: topical lidocaine patches. *J Laparoendosc Adv Surg Tech.* 2012;22:668–673.
49. Marret CR, Bonnet F. Effects of acetaminophen on morphine side-effects and consumption after major surgery: meta-analysis of randomized controlled trials. *Br J Anaesth.* 2005;94:505–513.
50. Miranda HF, Puig MM, Prieto JC, Pinardi G. Synergism between paracetamol and non-steroidal anti-inflamatory drugs in experimental acute pain. *Pain.* 2006;121:22–28.
51. Horlocker TT, Wedel DJ, Rowlingson JC, et al. Regional anesthesia in the patient receiving antithrombotic or thrombolytic therapy: American Society of Regional Anesthesia and Pain Medicine evidence-based guidelines (third edition). *Reg Anesth Pain Med.* 2010;35:64–101.
52. Krane EJ, Dalens BJ, Murat I, et al. The safety of epidurals placed during general anesthesia. *Reg Anesth Pain Med.* 1998;23:433–438.
53. Levy BF, Tilney HS, Dowson HM, et al. A systematic review of postoperative analgesia following laparoscopic colorectal surgery. *Br J Surg.* 2011;98:1068–1078.
54. Lapmahapaisan S, Tantemsapya N, Aroonpruksakul N, Maisat W, Suraseranivongse S. Efficacy of surgical transversus abdominis plane block for postoperative pain relief following abdominal surgery in pediatric patients. *Paediatr Anaesth.* 2015;25(6):614–620.
55. El-Morsy GZ, El-Deeb A, El-Desouky T, Elsharkawy AA, Elgamal MA. Can thoracic paravertebral block replace thoracic epidural block in pediatric cardiac surgery? A randomized blinded study. *Ann Card Anaesth.* 2012;15(4):259–263.
56. Wu Y, Liu F, Tang H, et al. The analgesic efficacy of subcostal transversus abdominis plane block compared with thoracic epidural analgesia and intravenous opioid analgesia after radical gastrectomy. *Anesth Analg.* 2013;117:507–513.
57. Sahin L, Sahin M, Gul R, Saricicek V, Isikay N. Ultrasound-guided transversus abdominis plane block in children: a randomised comparison with wound infiltration. *Eur J Anaesthesiol.* 2013;30:409–414.
58. Long JB, Birmingham PK, De Oliveira GS Jr, et al. Transversus abdominis plane block in children: a multicenter safety analysis of 1994 cases from the PRAN (Pediatric Regional Anesthesia Network) database. *Anesth Analg.* 2014;119:395–399.
59. Khan RS, Ahmed K, Blakeway E, et al. Catastrophizing: a predictive factor for postoperative pain. *Am J Surg.* 2011;201(1):122–131.
60. Riddle L, Keefe FJ, Nay WT, et al. Pain coping skills training for patients with elevated pain catastrophizing who are scheduled for knee arthroplasty: a quasi-experimental study. *Arch Phys Med Rehabil.* 2011;92:859–865.
61. Guirguis MN, Abd-Elsayed AA, Girgis G, Soliman LM. Ultrasound-guided transversus abdominis plane catheter for chronic abdominal pain. *Pain Pract.* 2013;13(3):235–238.
62. Macrae WA. Chronic pain after surgery. *Br J Anaesth.* 2001;87:88–98.
63. Kehlet H, Jensen TS, Woolf CJ. Persistent postsurgical pain: risk factors and prevention. *Lancet.* 2006;367(9522):1618–1625.
64. Nikolajsen L, Brix L. Chronic pain after surgery in children. *Curr Opin Anaesthesiol.* 2014;27:507–512.
65. Page MG, Stinson J, Campbell F, et al. Identification of pain-related psychological risk factors for the development and maintenance of pediatric chronic postsurgical pain. *J Pain Res.* 2013;6:167–180.
66. Walker SM. Biological and neurodevelopmental implications of neonatal pain. *Clin Perinatol.* 2013;40:471–491.
67. Wilkins KL, McGrath PJ, Finley GA, et al. Phantom limb sensations and phantom limb pain in child and adolescent amputees. *Pain.* 1998;78:7–12.
68. Blichfeldt-Eckhardt MR, Ording H, Andersen C, et al. Early visceral pain predicts chronic pain after laparoscopic cholecystectomy. *Pain.* 2014;155(11):2400–2407.
69. Keller SM, Carp NZ, Levy MN, Rosen SM. Chronic post thoracotomy pain. *J Cardiovasc Surg (Torino).* 1994;35(6)(suppl 1):161–164.
70. Brandsborg B, Nikolajsen L, Hansen CT, Kehlet H, Jensen TS. Risk factors for chronic pain after hysterectomy: a nationwide questionnaire and database study. *Anesthesiology.* 2007;106:1003–1012.
71. Capape S, Mora E, Mintegui S, et al. Prolonged sedation and airway complications after administration of an inadvertent ketamine overdose in emergency department. *Eur J Emerg Med.* 2008;15:92–94.
72. Horton JD, Dezee KJ, Ahnfeldt EP, Wagner M. Abdominal wall endometriosis: a surgeon's perspective and review of 445 cases. *Am J Surg.* 2008;196(2):207–212.
73. Takeuchi K, Smale S, Premchand P, et al. Prevalence and mechanism of non-steroidal anti-inflammatory drug-induced clinical relapse in patients with inflammatory bowel disease. *Clin Gastroenterol Hepatol.* 2006;4:196–202.

REVIEW QUESTIONS

1. During exploratory laparotomy for ileostomy reversal, a 30-kg, 10-year-old child with Crohn's disease receives a low-dose ketamine infusion with the goal of reducing postoperative pain. Accidentally, a dose of 1,000 mg of ketamine is administered over a period of 50 minutes. Which of the following is most likely to occur in the recovery period, 2 hours later?

A. Nausea
B. Chest pain
C. Dry mouth
D. Apnea

2. A 13-year-old girl has a 4-month history of periumbilical pain, accompanied by nausea, that does not respond to codeine and acetaminophen. The pain started suddenly 3 weeks after an open appendectomy and prevents her from going to school. On physical examination, the Carnett's sign is positive. Which of the following is most likely to be true about her pain?

A. It is improved by defecation.
B. It is worse when resting supine.
C. It is worse when sneezing.
D. It is worse during menstruation.

3. A 15-year-old girl has recurrent abdominal pain circumscribed to a small area at the border of the right rectus muscle. Previously, on two separate occasions, she had complete resolution of pain that lasted a month after trigger-point injection with bupivacaine. Her last injection was 6 weeks ago. In addition to pain, now she has frequent episodes of diarrhea. What is the best next step in management?

A. Repeat trigger-point injection with bupivacaine
B. Trigger-point injection with bupivacaine and betamethasone
C. A referral to a clinical psychologist to improve her coping skills
D. A stool guaiac test

ANSWERS

1. A. Ketamine can cause adverse effects, such as excessive sedation, hallucinations, delirium, excessive salivation, clonus, hypertonicity, nausea, vomiting, transient diplopia, nystagmus, rash, elevation of intracranial and intraocular pressures, and cardiovascular stimulation (tachycardia and hypertension). Answer B is incorrect; in a young patient without cardiac problems, ketamine-induced tachycardia and hypertension are unlikely to cause chest pain. Answer C is not correct because ketamine causes hypersalivation, not dry mouth. Answer D is not correct because apnea and respiratory depression are likely to occur at the time of ketamine peak concentration and not hours after administration. The excessive sedation induced by a ketamine overdose may cause airway obstruction.[71]

2. C. The pain experienced by this patient is likely caused by ACNES. The pain associated with ACNES is positional: it is least in the supine position (therefore answer B is not correct) and it is worse when sitting or lying on the affected side. Pain is aggravated by activities that tense the abdominal muscles, such as walking, stretching, sneezing (so answer C is correct), or laughing. Answer A is not correct because pain relieved with defecation is a characteristic of irritable bowel syndrome and not ACNES. Answer D is not correct because pain associated with menses suggests endometriosis. In abdominal wall endometriosis, the pain may be cyclic, with menses, or continuous.[72]

3. D. Although abdominal pain may have the same etiology (entrapment of the anterior cutaneous nerve between the abdominal muscles), the new onset of diarrhea is concerning, and the patient should undergo evaluation for an organic source of pain, such as Crohn's disease. Answers A, B, and C are not correct because repeating the trigger-point injection and referring the patient to a psychologist should be considered only after other causes of pain have been ruled out.

QUESTIONS AND ANSWERS

This chapter has accompanying questions and answers that are available to subscribers as part of the Oxford eLearning platform. To access the questions, follow the link below, or go to http://oxfordmedicine.com/painmanagementreview

20.

CHRONIC PELVIC PAIN

Rahul Rastogi, Saima Kamal, and Shuchita Garg

STEM CASE AND KEY QUESTIONS

A 49-year-old female with a remote history of vaginal prolapse underwent a mesh implant 3 years previously. One year after surgery, she started to have vaginal pain and dyspareunia. She was started on Lyrica 50 mg twice a day. She continued to have moderate to severe vaginal pain and dyspareunia, and was later started on oxycodone/acetaminophen 5/325 mg orally every 6 hours as needed. Two years ago she underwent a second surgery for mesh removal. She reported no benefit after the second surgery and her pain was unchanged. By this time, she was titrated up to pregabalin 100 mg twice a day and oxycodone/acetaminophen 10/325 mg orally every 4 hours as needed. She was diagnosed with chronic pelvic pain syndrome (CPPS) and was referred to an academic pain management clinic for consultation and further management. Now, her pain is in the perineal area, radiates to the medial aspect of her thigh, rectum, and hypogastric area. She describes the pain as constant, sharp, burning, with intensity of 8–9/10 on VAS. The pain is aggravated by urination, defecation, sexual intercourse, and prolonged sitting, and the patient reports no specific alleviating factors. On exam she has tenderness over the medial aspect of her thigh, vulva, and rectal area and exquisite tenderness to palpation of bilateral ischial spines. On vaginal exam, she is tender to palpation of the vaginal walls and has significant spasm of pelvic floor muscles. She complains the pain gives her difficulty in falling and staying asleep. Her past medical history is significant for hypertension and diabetes. She had to quit her job as a secretary since it entailed prolonged sitting, which was intolerable for her.

WHAT IS THE DIFFERENCE BETWEEN CHRONIC PELVIC PAIN (CPP) AND CPPS?

CPP is defined as nonmalignant pain below the umbilicus that has persisted for more than 6 months and is associated with a specific identifiable pathology, like infection, endometriosis, and pudendal neuralgia. CPPS is not associated with any identifiable pathology; the symptoms are related to multiple organ systems, such as gastrointestinal, genitourinary, and musculoskeletal dysfunction. It has many negative psychosocial connotations and often the patients have a history of physical or sexual abuse.

WHAT IS THE DIFFERENTIAL DIAGNOSIS OF CPP FOR THIS PATIENT?

Upon examining the patient, you reach the conclusion that the most likely differential diagnoses are adhesions, pudendal neuralgia, pelvic floor muscle spasm/dysfunction, vulvodynia, endometriosis, and pelvic inflammatory disease.

HOW WILL YOU EVALUATE AND TREAT THIS PATIENT?

In view of her history of surgery, adhesions seem to be the most likely cause of CPPS in this patient. Ultrasound of the abdomen/pelvis and/or CT pelvis could be considered but might not be very helpful as a diagnostic tool. They could be helpful to rule out any mass or space-occupying lesion causing the patient's symptoms.

A thorough discussion should be initiated with the patient, including discussion of the importance of a multidisciplinary approach, and understanding and setting up realistic patient expectations while a treatment plan is clearly laid out. Focused pelvic floor physical therapy should be started. Trigger-point injections can be performed in the pelvic floor muscles to potentially decrease the muscle spasm. Botulinum toxin injection into pelvic floor muscles and the perineal area under ultrasound guidance can help as well. Tricyclic antidepressants (TCA), such as nortriptyline 10 mg at bedtime, could be added for pain-related insomnia, along with the continuation of pregabalin in view of the neuropathic component. One should discuss the possible side effects of long-term opioid therapy for chronic nonmalignant pain and advise the patient to limit her use of opioids to treatment of severe episodes of pain only.

The patient returns for a follow-up visit 4 weeks after her first visit, and she reports mild to moderate improvement in her sleep pattern and mild to moderate improvement in her pain from pelvic floor exercises and botulinum injection therapy. Her exam findings are unchanged from her prior visit.

WHAT WILL BE THE NEXT STEP IN MANAGING THIS PATIENT?

The importance of a multidisciplinary approach to pain management should be reiterated to the patient and clear goals of care should be revisited and discussed with her.

Pudendal nerve block under fluoroscopic guidance for diagnostic and prognostic purposes could be considered at this point. Continued pelvic floor muscle exercises on a regular basis should be recommended. Increases in the doses of nortriptyline to 25 mg at bedtime and pregabalin to 150 mg twice a day should be advised. A referral should be made to a pain psychologist for cognitive-behavioral therapy.

HOW WOULD YOU INTERPRET THE RESULTS OF THE PUDENDAL NERVE BLOCK AT THE PATIENT'S NEXT FOLLOW-UP APPOINTMENT AFTER 6 WEEKS?

If the patient reports moderate to significant improvement in her pain after the pudendal nerve block, it would indicate that the diagnostic pudendal nerve block was positive for pudendal nerve involvement. She could be counseled about further interventions that could improve functionality. Regardless of the benefit from the intervention, she should continue to perform pelvic floor exercises. During episodes of extreme pain she should utilize the coping skills she learned in cognitive-behavioral therapy, such as stress management, sleep hygiene, and deep breathing and relaxation techniques. Meanwhile, neuropathic medications should be continued.

The patient wants to know if there is an intervention that can provide long-term pain relief, as she wants to go back to work.

WHAT OTHER INTERVENTIONS CAN WE OFFER HER?

The option of pulsed radiofrequency, a neuroablative technique that provides analgesia without destruction of neural tissue, could be considered. The intermittent pulses allow heat to dissipate, thus preserving the pudendal nerve from destruction. This intervention has the potential to helping the patient for 3 to 6 months. The option of sacral stimulation could be considered as an alternative, if pulsed radiofrequency treatment of the pudendal nerve fails to provide adequate relief.

WHY IS THE MULTIDISCIPLINARY APPROACH TO PAIN MANAGEMENT IMPORTANT IN THIS PATIENT POPULATION?

CPP is a complex medical condition because of its inconsistent natural history, uncertain etiology, and associated psychosocial implications. It is refractory to various forms of treatment and results in a great deal of frustration not only for the patient but for the treating physician as well. The best results are achieved through a multidisciplinary approach, where a combination of interventions, together with medications, physical therapy, and coping techniques, have a higher likelihood of success.

DISCUSSION

CPP is a chronic or persistent pain perceived in structures related to the pelvis in either men or women. The pain can be located in the pelvis, the anterior abdominal wall (at or below the umbilicus), low back, or buttocks and is severe enough to cause functional disability and to motivate the patient to seek medical care. Pelvic pain arises from the visceral or somatic system and encompasses structures innervated by spinal segments at T10 and below.

When persistent pelvic pain is associated with a specific disease or pathology, it is CPP; if it is not associated with a specific disease or pathology, it is CPPS. CPPS is often associated with negative cognitive, behavioral, sexual, or emotional consequences, as well as symptoms suggestive of lower urinary tract, sexual, bowel, pelvic floor, and/or gynecologic dysfunction, without obvious inflammation or other specific pathology explaining the symptoms.[1,2]

EPIDEMIOLOGY OF PELVIC PAIN

Given a lack of consensus on the definition, CPP often remains underdiagnosed.[1] Epidemiologic studies have reported that the prevalence of CPP in women ranges from 5.7% to 26.6%,[3] and in men it ranges from 2.7% to 13.8%.[4,5]

In the United Kingdom, the annual prevalence of CPP in primary care settings is estimated to be 3.8% in women 15 to 73 years old, which is higher than the prevalence of migraine (2.1%), and is similar to that of asthma (3.7%) and back pain (4.1%).[6] Lifetime incidence of CPP is as high as 33%, with less than 1% of patients being seen by a pain specialist; instead, patients are likely to receive treatment from a gynecologist, primary care physician, urologist, or gastroenterologist.[7]

CPP in women accounts for 10% of referrals to gynecologists, 40% of all gynecologic diagnostic laparoscopies, and 12% of total hysterectomies.[8]

CPP creates a significant socioeconomic burden through direct health care costs, work absenteeism, infertility, and a decreased mother-wife role in the family. Estimated direct annual costs of health care for CPP in the United States are close to $880 million, and costs can exceed $2 billion when indirect costs are included, such as time off from work.[3]

ETIOLOGY OF PELVIC PAIN

The etiology of pelvic pain is usually multifactorial, involving somatic, visceral, or neurogenic components. There is considerable overlap with coexisting conditions, such as endometriosis, chronic pelvic inflammatory disease, irritable bowel syndrome, interstitial cystitis, and urethral syndrome.[9] About 30% to 50% of patients with CPP are classified as having "CPP without obvious pathology." About 25% of patients continue to have unresolved pelvic pain after hysterectomy for pelvic pain relief.[10] Among patients who undergo exploratory laparoscopy, one-third are diagnosed with endometriosis, one-third are diagnosed with adhesions, and one-third have no identifiable pathology.[11] CPP is associated with a high rate of psychologic comorbidities; more than 50% of patients have a history of physical or sexual abuse.[12]

Although CPP mostly affects women, men can also have CPP. Common causes of CPP in men are chronic (nonbacterial) prostatitis, chronic orchialgia, and prostatodynia.[13]

TYPES OF CPP

CPP can be classified by location, phenotype, system involved, and symptom distribution. Classification of pelvic pain is challenging because > 50% of the time there is more than one disease process and system involved. The authors have developed an axis-based approach that involves hierarchical classification in a stepwise manner,[1,14] as illustrated in Figure 20.1.

NERVE SUPPLY TO PELVIS

Thoracolumbar and sacral spinal segments converge in peripheral neuronal plexuses and innervate pelvic structures. Somatic fibers arise from T12-S5, while visceral fibers arise from T10-S5. Autonomic supply is mainly from hypogastric plexuses, while the pudendal nerve (S2-S4) is the primary somatic nerve for the pelvis. Thoracolumbar afferent visceral fibers not only supply urogenital structures but also supply the distal ileum, sigmoid colon, and rectum (Figure 20.2).

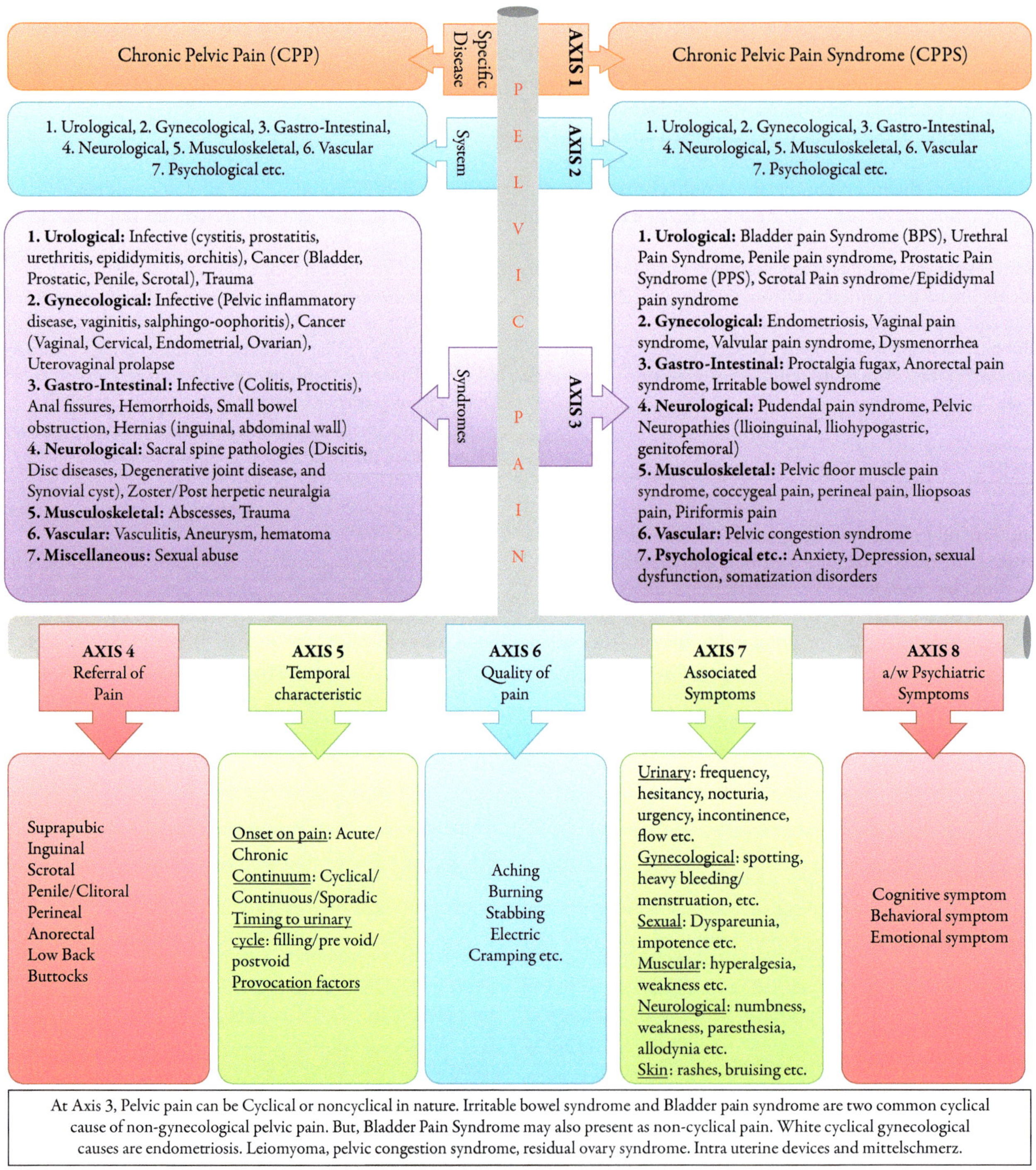

Hierarchical Classification of Pelvic Pain

Figure 20.1. Hierarchical classification of pelvic pain.

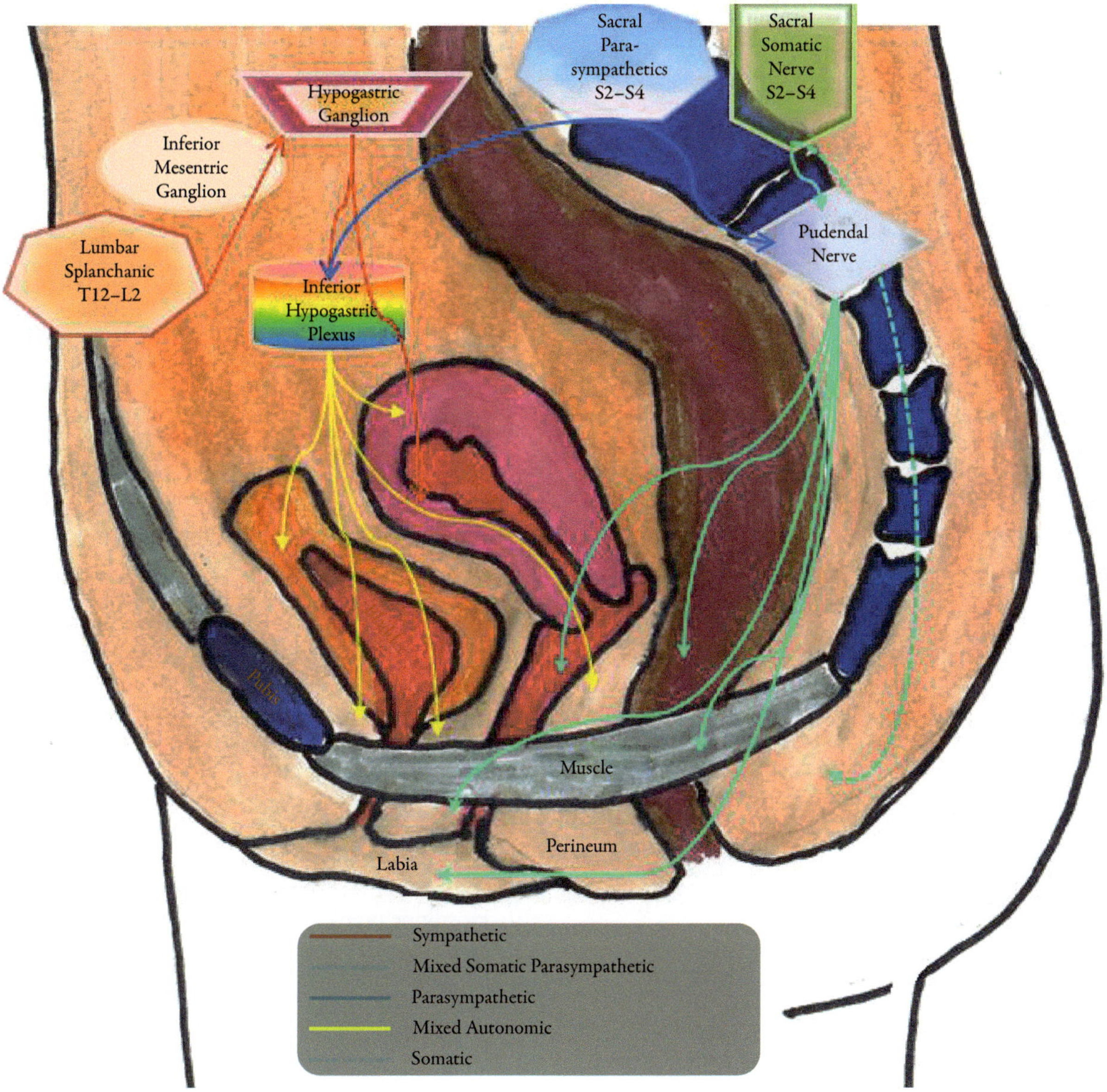

Figure 20.2. Nerve supply of pelvis.

PATHOPHYSIOLOGY

The pathophysiology of pelvic pain is poorly understood, and several theories have been postulated to explain its underlying mechanisms.[15]

- Peripheral injury and inflammation cause release of inflammatory mediators that cause nociceptive stimulation and sensitization.
- Visceral cross-sensitization: As a result of transmission of noxious stimuli from affected pelvic structures to adjacent normal structures, functional changes arise in normal pelvic structures. There are two possible explanations for this:
  - One neuronal cell body can branch in several axons to supply several targets, leading to antidromic stimulation and release of neuropeptides (cGRP and substance P) in adjacent pelvic organs, which ultimately results in hyperalgesia, i.e., neurogenic inflammation.
  - Temporal summation and convergence of sensory input within the spinal cord results in viscero-visceral convergence.
- Release of proinflammatory mediators and the presence of neurogenic inflammation result in persistent peripheral hyperalgesia, i.e., peripheral sensitization.
- NMDA and AMPA receptor activation at the spinal cord level results in facilitation of noxious stimuli in the CNS, causing allodynia, i.e., central sensitization.
- Modulation of pain signals at the dorsal horn via descending inhibitory cortical pathways plays a major role in perception and persistence of pelvic pain.

DIAGNOSIS OF CPP/CPPS

All patients with CPP should have a thorough history, physical examination, and appropriate workup to aid in developing a differential diagnosis.

History

A detailed history is necessary for complete evaluation and effective management of this complex condition. A complete history should include, location, character, radiation/distribution, aggravating/alleviating factors, associated symptoms, relation with menstrual cycle and urinary or bowel movements, and responsiveness to prior treatment modalities. In addition, careful documentation of psychosocial factors, including sexual history, is very important. A written pelvic pain questionnaire (available online from the International Pelvic Pain Society, www.pelvicpain.org) may be completed in privacy prior to the in-person consultation.

Physical Examination

A detailed physical exam can greatly help in narrowing down the differential diagnosis. It should include examination of the relevant musculoskeletal system, neurologic exam, and the exam of the lower abdominopelvic area, i.e., thoracolumbar spine, sacral spine, pelvic girdle, lower abdominal area, pelvic floor musculature, suprapubic/inguinal region for hernia or neuropathy, external genitalia, and rectovaginal area. Rectovaginal exam should be performed to assess pelvic floor muscle function/spasm, pelvic entrapment neuropathy, coccygeal pain, and pelvic masses.

Diagnostic Workup

Diagnostic testing for CPPS is of limited use. Blood and urine tests can be performed to rule out infective etiology. Ultrasonography can be helpful in evaluation of a pelvic mass. In cases of severe persistent pain and unclear etiology, diagnostic laparoscopy can be performed to assess for an organic source of pain. Differential nerve blocks can be performed to diagnose specific neurologic involvement.

MANAGEMENT OF CPP/CPPS

In view of the complex interplay of multiple symptoms, different etiologic factors, and involvement of different organ systems, a multidisciplinary approach to management of CPP offers the most promise. The overall goal is to improve quality of life while optimizing functionality. In CPPS, where there is no identifiable cause, management involves a holistic approach to pain management, addressing behavioral, psychosocial, sexual, and spiritual components (Figure 20.3).

The patient should be referred to a specialist to rule out any possible end-organ disease/etiology. If an end-organ etiology is found, it should be addressed with disease- specific treatments directed by a specialist while the patient receives an analgesic regimen prescribed by a pain medicine specialist. The specific treatments are summarized in Table 20.1.[14]

The following modalities are usually used in management of pain in CPP/CPPS:

- Pharmacotherapy: CPPS is multimechanistic, thus pain adjuvants are helpful in its management.
  - Analgesics (e.g., acetaminophen, NSAIDs) are the first-line agents in cases of unknown origin with mixed symptoms. However, they are not very effective for CPPS associated with endometriosis.[16]
  - Antidepressants, such as tricyclic antidepressants (TCAs; amitriptyline, nortriptyline, imipramine) and serotonin norepinephrine reuptake inhibitors (SNRIs; venlafaxine, duloxetine), provide relief for the neuropathic component of CPPS.[14] SSRIs seem to be more effective if there is an underlying mood disorder. Duloxetine has shown better efficacy for urogenital symptoms.
  - Anticonvulsants (e.g., gabapentin, pregabalin) have shown good results in managing neuropathic pain and are well tolerated.[17] Concurrent use of gabapentin and amitriptyline has shown better efficacy than either of these medications alone in patients with CPP.[18]
  - Opioids have a limited role secondary to their long-term side effect profile but can be used after other options have been exhausted. With opioid use, practitioners should use opioid risk stratification/assessment tools and follow opioid prescribing guidelines for chronic pain published by the CDC.[19]
  - Hormone preparations have been suggested for pain associated with endometriosis[17]; however, their role in nonspecific CPPS remains unclear and limited. Medroxyprogesterone acetate has been shown to reduce pain associated with pelvic congestion syndrome.
- Interventional Therapies: Interventional therapies usually have a limited role in management of CPPS but, in some select cases, they can aid in diagnosis and prognosis while providing therapeutic benefit.
  - Local anesthetic injections alone are utilized for diagnosis of nerve entrapments (i.e., pudendal nerve, ilioinguinal nerve, genitofemoral nerve). Their prognostic role helps in planning more-invasive and longer-lasting treatment modalities, such as nerve release surgery, radiofrequency ablation, or botulinum toxin injections. Addition of steroids to local anesthetics can be used for therapeutic purposes.
  - Superior hypogastric nerve block and ganglion impar block (Figure 20.4 and Figure 20.5) have shown some benefit in visceral pelvic pain, but strong evidence is lacking for their role in the management of nonmalignant CPPS. Side effects, such as colonic dysmotility and sexual dysfunction, are possible; therefore, before considering these interventions, a thorough assessment of possible risks versus benefits and alternative treatment options should be made

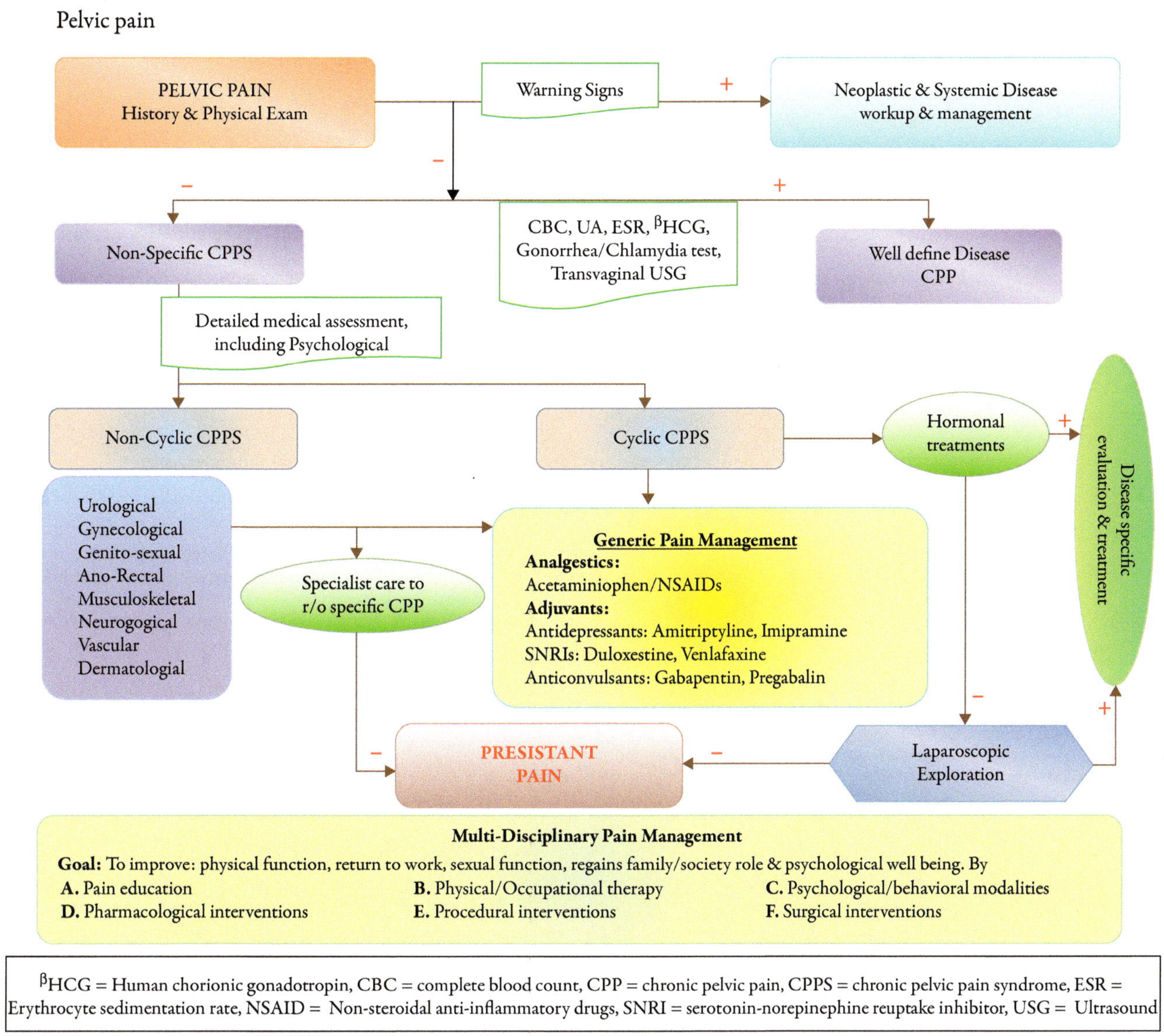

Figure 20.3. Management algorithm for chronic pelvic pain.

and discussed with the patient. If blockade is used, a combination of local anesthetic and steroids, and not neurolytic agents, should be used for nonmalignant CPP.

- Trigger-point injections in the abdominal wall and sacral, perineal, and vaginal areas have been suggested to provide some pain relief. Anecdotal evidence exists for benefit from acupuncture.
- Spinal cord stimulation and sacral neuromodulation through implanted electrodes can provide relief in carefully selected patients with CPPS.[20,21]
- Surgical modalities should be reserved for severe functional limitations, because surgical outcome for pain relief is extremely poor.

- Psychotherapy: CPPS, like any chronic pain condition, is associated with emotional, cognitive, behavioral, sexual, and social problems. Thus, psychotherapy plays a vital role in multidisciplinary pain management. Understanding the patient's personality and prior life experiences is of utmost importance in understanding the patient's current psychologic state; therefore, an early, comprehensive, psychologic assessment is valuable for effective management of CPPS. A pain psychologist helps patients to develop positive thoughts and healthy coping strategies, while progressively challenging and eliminating negative behaviors.[22]

  There is good evidence supporting the role of group cognitive-behavioral therapy or combined psychology and physical therapy (somato-cognitive group therapy) in chronic pain. Disease-specific group therapy may be even more beneficial for the participants.[23] There is considerable variability among CPPS patients; therefore, incorporating individualized therapy into a CPPS group behavioral program can be more effective.[22,24]

- Physical therapy: CPPS is commonly associated with myofascial triggers, and a thorough transvaginal exam of the pelvic musculature identifies specific myofascial

Table 20.1. COMMON TREATMENTS FOR SPECIFIC DISEASES

SYSTEM	SPECIFIC DISEASES	FIRST-LINE TREATMENTS	LATER TREATMENTS
Urologic	Bladder pain syndrome	Conservative treatment, patient education, general pain management, pelvic floor relaxation	Intravesical therapies, cystoscopy with hydrodistension, neuromodulation, cystectomy
	Prostatic pain syndrome	Antibiotics, quercetin, conservative treatment, general pain management	Alpha-blockers, anticholinergics, finasteride, phytotherapy, pentosan, trigger-point injections, neuromodulation, prostatectomy
	Scrotal pain syndrome	General pain management, nerve blocks, antibiotics	Surgical treatments (i.e., orchiectomy, epididymectomy, microsurgical denervation of spermatic cord)
Gynecologic	Endometriosis	Hormonal treatments, general pain management, physical therapy	Hysterectomy, lysis of adhesions, ablation/resection of endometriosis, uterosacral nerve ablation
Anorectal	Proctalgia fugax	Patient education, sublingual nifedipine or nitroglycerin, benzodiazepines, botulinum toxin injection	Internal anal sphincterectomy
	Anorectal pain	Abscess drainage, diltiazem or nitroglycerin ointment	Controlled anal dilatation, fissurectomy, sphincterectomy, sacral neuromodulation
Neurologic	Neuralgias	General pain management, nerve blocks	Radiofrequency ablation, neuromodulation, nerve release surgery
Musculoskeletal	Pelvic floor dysfunction	Biofeedback, pelvic floor exercises, general pain management	Pelvic dilatation, transvaginal stretching
Vascular	Pelvic congestion syndrome	General pain management	Embolization of varices or supplying vessels

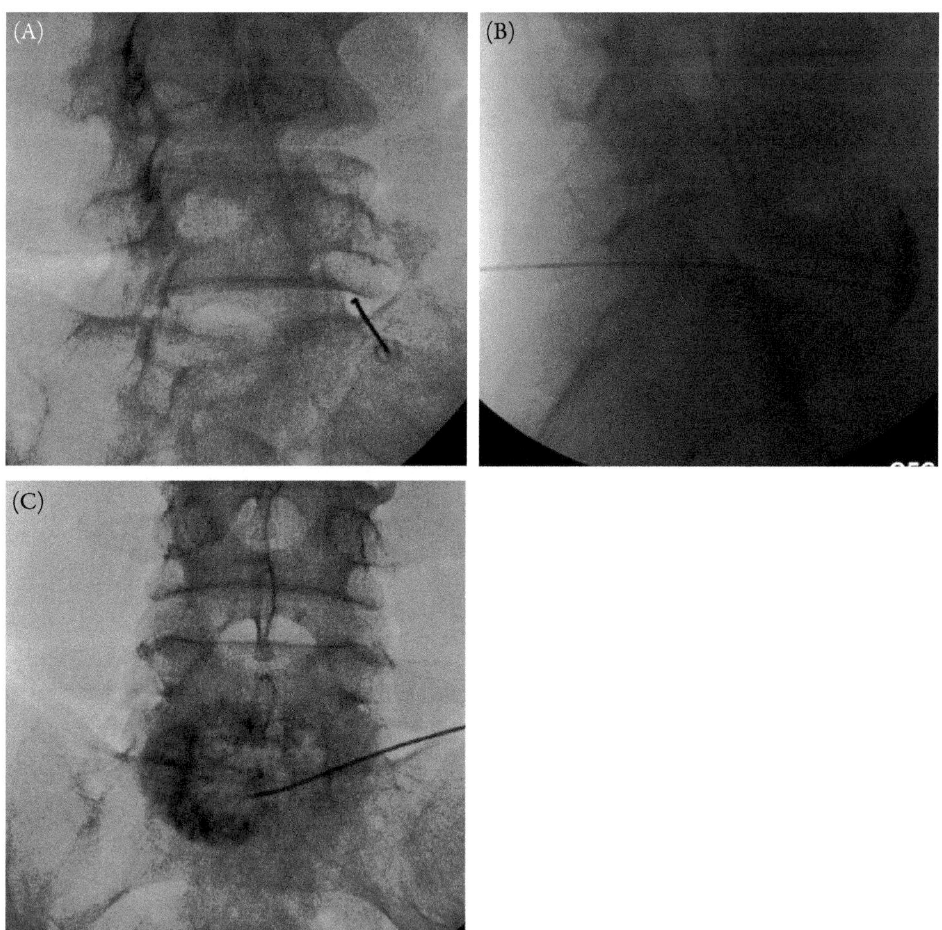

Figure 20.4. Superior hypogastric nerve block, transdiscal approach. (A) shows initial needle entry in oblique fluoroscopic view. (B) and (C) show final needle placement in lateral (B) and posteroanterior (C) with excellent spread of dye and medication. Image courtesy of University of Chicago Library.

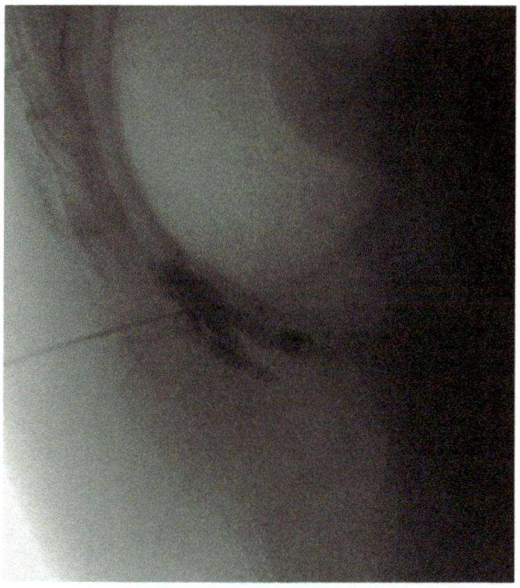

Figure 20.5. Ganglion impar. Lateral fluroscopic view shows needle placement through the sacrococcygeal membrane and excellent spread of dye around ganglion impar. Image courtesy of University of Chicago Library.

trigger points. Pelvic floor physical therapies, including the transvaginal approach, are very helpful in reducing musculoskeletal pain and increasing mobility in CPPS.[25]

CONCLUSION

- Chronic nonmalignant pelvic pain is a common, complex medical condition with multifactorial etiology and multisymptom presentation that is often associated with psychosocial factors. It affects both men and women and has socioeconomic consequences if not optimally treated.
- CPP/CPPS management continues to be a frustration for patients and a challenge for health care professionals.
- Available therapeutic options are still considered experimental due to lack of strong clinical evidence. More research is needed to find out efficacious modalities for management of CPP/CPPS.
- Given its complex nature, the diagnosis and management of CPP can be delayed secondary to lack of knowledge among primary care physicians. It is prudent to increase awareness of this debilitating condition among primary care practitioners, so that the patients are referred to appropriate specialists in a timely manner.
- Management of CPP/CPPS starts by having a detailed discussion with the patient regarding goals of management. Physicians need to be judicious with their choice of investigations and interventions, to minimize associated risks and costs. Unfortunately, it is emotionally traumatic for the patients to realize the complexity of the condition and the lack of definite cure.
- A psychologist can help early in identifying the complex interplay of psychologic comorbidities. As with any other chronic pain condition, optimal results are seen with a multidisciplinary approach to its management while setting up realistic expectations for both physician and patient.

REFERENCES

1. Fall M, Baranowski AP, Elneil S, et al. EAU guidelines on chronic pelvic pain. *Eur Urol.* 2010;57(1):35–48.
2. Wesselmann U, Czakanski PP. Pelvic pain: a chronic visceral pain syndrome. *Curr Pain Headache Rep.* 2001;5(1):13–19.
3. Ahangari A. Prevalence of chronic pelvic pain among women: an updated review. *Pain Physician.*2014;17(2):E141–E147.
4. Bartoletti R, Cai T, Mondaini N, et al. Prevalence, incidence estimation, risk factors and characterization of chronic prostatitis/chronic pelvic pain syndrome in urological hospital outpatients in Italy: results of a multicenter case-control observational study. *J Urol.* 2007;178(6):2411–2415; discussion 2415.
5. Nickel JC, Downey J, Hunter D, Clark J. Prevalence of prostatitis-like symptoms in a population based study using the National Institutes of Health chronic prostatitis symptom index. *J Urol.* 2001;165(3):842–845.
6. Zondervan K, Barlow DH. Epidemiology of chronic pelvic pain. *Baillieres Best Pract Res Clin Obstet Gynaecol.* 2000;14(3):403–414.
7. Brookoff D. Genitourinary syndromes: interstitial cystitis, chronic prostatitis, pelvic floor dysfunction and related disorders. In: Smith HS, ed. *Current Therapy in Pain.* Philadelphia: Saunders-Elsevier; 2009:205–215.
8. Reiter RC. A profile of women with chronic pelvic pain. *Clin Obstet Gynecol.* 1990;33(1):130–136.
9. Zondervan KT, Yudkin PL, Vessey MP, et al. Chronic pelvic pain in the community—symptoms, investigations, and diagnoses. *Am J Obstet Gynecol.* 2001;184(6):1149–1155.
10. Stovall TG, Ling FW, Crawford DA. Hysterectomy for chronic pelvic pain of presumed uterine etiology. *Obstet Gynecol.* 1990;75(4):676–679.
11. Stout AL, Steege JF, Dodson WC, Hughes CL. Relationship of laparoscopic findings to self-report of pelvic pain. *Am J Obstet Gynecol.* 1991;164(1 Pt 1):73–79.
12. Walling MK, Reiter RC, O'Hara MW, Milburn AK, Lilly G, Vincent SD. Abuse history and chronic pain in women: I. Prevalences of sexual abuse and physical abuse. *Obstet Gynecol.* 1994;84(2):193–199.
13. Barbalias GA, Nikiforidis G, Liatsikos EN. Alpha-blockers for the treatment of chronic prostatitis in combination with antibiotics. *J Urol.* 1998;159(3):883–887.
14. Engeler D, Baranowski AP, Borovicka J, et al. Guidelines on chronic pelvic pain. European Association of Urology. http://uroweb.org/wp-content/uploads/EAU-Guidelines-Chronic-Pelvic-Pain-2015.pdf
15. Origoni M, Leone Roberti Maggiore U, Salvatore S, Candiani M. Neurobiological mechanisms of pelvic pain. *Biomed Res Int.* 2014;903848.
16. Allen C, Hopewell S, Prentice A, Gregory D. Nonsteroidal anti-inflammatory drugs for pain in women with endometriosis. *Cochrane Database Syst Rev.* 2009; 2:CD004753.
17. Cheong YC, Smotra G, Williams AC. Non-surgical interventions for the management of chronic pelvic pain. *Cochrane Database Syst Rev.* 2014;3:CD008797.
18. Sator-Katzenschlager SM, Scharbert G, Kress HG, et al. Chronic pelvic pain treated with gabapentin and amitriptyline: a randomized controlled pilot study. *Wien Klin Wochenschr.* 2005;117(21-22):761–768.
19. Dowell D, Haegerich TM, Chou R. CDC guideline for prescribing opioids for chronic pain—United States, 2016. *JAMA.* 2016;315(15):1624–1645.
20. Kapural L, Narouze SN, Janicki TI, Mekhail N. Spinal cord stimulation is an effective treatment for the chronic intractable visceral pelvic pain. *Pain Med.* 2006;7(5):440–443.

21. Sokal P, Zielinski P, Harat M. Sacral roots stimulation in chronic pelvic pain. *Neurol Neurochir Pol.* 2015;49(5):307–312.
22. Baranowski AP. Chronic pelvic pain. *Best Pract Res Clin Gastroenterol.* 2009;23(4):593–610.
23. Haugstad TS, Haugstad GK, Kirste UM, Kirschner R, Hakonsen E. Somatocognitive therapy for chronic pelvic pain. *Tidsskr Nor Laegefo ren.*2012;132(3):272–273.
24. Albert H. Psychosomatic group treatment helps women with chronic pelvic pain. *J Psychosom Obstet Gynaecol.* 1999;20(4):216–225.
25. Bedaiwy MA, Patterson B, Mahajan S. Prevalence of myofascial chronic pelvic pain and the effectiveness of pelvic floor physical therapy. *J Reprod Med.* 2013;58(11-12):504–510.
26. Speer LM, Mushkbar S, Erbele T. Chronic pelvic pain in women. *Am Fam Physician.* 2016;93(5):380–387.
27. Stacy J, Frawley H, Powell G, Goucke R, Pavy T. Persistent pelvic pain: rising to the challenge. *Aust N Z J Obstet Gynaecol.* 2012;52(6):502–507.

REVIEW QUESTIONS

1. Which of the following is not true for CPP?

   A. It is associated with significant burden on the health care system and costs.
   B. It affects quality of life and causes emotional suffering.
   C. Physical pain symptom burden is significantly higher than psychologic symptoms.
   D. It is a challenge for treating physicians.

2. CPPS is differentiated from CPP by

   A. Presence of persistent pain in the pelvic area for more than 3 months.
   B. There is no definitive etiology or pathology.
   C. Presence of negative cognitive, behavioral, and emotional consequences.
   D. Symptoms are suggestive of multisystem involvement.

3. The prevalence of CPP

   A. Is not associated with irritable bowel syndrome.
   B. Is higher in men than women.
   C. Is significantly lower than that for asthma.
   D. Is higher than the prevalence of migraines.

ANSWERS

1. C. CPP is defined as nonmalignant pain in lower abdominal-pelvic structures that has persisted for more than 6 months. CPP is associated with a high rate of psychologic comorbidities and > 50% of patients have a history of physical or sexual abuse. CPP creates a significant socioeconomic burden through direct health care costs, work absenteeism, infertility, and a decreased mother-wife role in the family. Estimated direct annual costs of health care for CPP in the United States are close to $880 million, and costs can exceed $2 billion when indirect costs, including time off work, are included.[1,9,12]

2. B. CPPS is defined as nonmalignant pain in lower abdominal-pelvic structures that has persisted for more than 6 months with no definite etiology.[2]

3. D. Epidemiologic studies have reported that the prevalence of CPP among women ranges from 5.7% to 26.6%,[3] and in men it ranges from 2.7% to 13.8%.[4,5] In the United Kingdom, the annual prevalence of CPP in primary care settings is estimated to be 3.8% in women 15 to 73 years old, which is higher than the prevalence of migraine (2.1%), and is similar to that of asthma (3.7%) and back pain (4.1%).[6]

QUESTIONS AND ANSWERS

This chapter has accompanying questions and answers that are available to subscribers as part of the Oxford eLearning platform. To access the questions, follow the link below, or go to ✔ http://oxfordmedicine.com/painmanagementreview

21.

TESTICULAR PAIN

Andrew J. McNeil, Ajay Antony, and Marc O. Maybauer

STEM CASE AND KEY QUESTIONS

A 57-year-old male presents to the outpatient clinic with chronic left-sided pain from the left scrotum and testicle radiating to his upper left inguinal hernia scar. The patient rates the pain on average as 7/10 on the Visual Analog Scale (VAS) and 9/10 at its worst. The pain is described as a shooting, burning pain that is aggravated by movement and bending. The pain started about 5 years earlier, shortly after his inguinal hernia repair. He states he has seen general surgery and was "cleared." The patient states warm compresses have helped in the past, but now the pain is unremitting and even oral medications (percocet, baclofen, and ibuprofen) that he had received from his primary care provider have not helped. The rest of the patient's review of systems exam is unremarkable.

The patient's past medical history is significant for hypertension, diabetes that is diet controlled, and obesity (BMI 31). His past surgical history is significant for cryptorchidism surgery at age 1 year, indirect inguinal hernia repair approximately 5 years previously, prostate biopsy for elevated PSA that showed benign prostatic hyperplasia (BPH) 7 years ago, and vasectomy 6 years ago. The patient is divorced and has had five partners in the last month. He states he usually uses protection in the form of a condom. He has a history of one DUI 8 years ago and admits to significant alcohol intake in the past. He denies illicit drug use or current alcohol use, but admits to smoking. He has no known drug allergies and takes only lisinopril to assist with blood pressure control.

In clinic today the patient's blood pressure is 155/62, heart rate is 89, temperature is 37°C, height is 172 cm, and his weight is 95 kg. Physical exam is significant for left testicular tenderness to palpation; not noted are edema, erythema, or color changes. A well-healed left inguinal hernia scar is noted. There is limited lumbar extension due to pain in the left groin and extending into the left testicle; otherwise, all other findings are within normal limits (WNL). The patient does not have any labs or imaging with him and states he remembers his primary care physician mentioning that all his labs were WNL except his HbA_{1c} was slightly elevated.

WHAT TYPE OF PAIN IS THIS PATENT DESCRIBING?

Based on his history, the patient's pain seems to be neuropathic; however, with the pain's being exacerbated by palpation and the patient's myofascial restriction in the area, he is probably suffering from some myofascial pain as well.

WHAT IS THE DEFINITION OF CHRONIC ORCHIALGIA? WHAT IS THE DIFFERENTIAL DIAGNOSIS FOR THIS PATIENT'S PAIN?

Chronic orchialgia is defined as pain in the testicle(s) that has been present for more than 3 months, is intermittent or constant in nature, and significantly interferes with daily activities.[1] Many have expanded the definition to include chronic scrotal pain, and the structures included to encompass the epididymis, spermatic cord, testicle, and supporting structures.

With the patient's history of elevated PSA and cryptorchidism, malignancy should be investigated. The differential diagnosis should also include postvasectomy pain and postinguinal hernia pain. Furthermore, the patient could have chronic epididymitis or a sexually transmitted infection (STI).

WHAT TESTS WOULD YOU WANT TO ORDER?

Given the patient's sexual history, STI screening would be warranted. A urinalysis and CBC would also aid in ruling out infectious causes. A repeat PSA would also give more information about his prostate and the potential for malignancy. An ultrasound would be warranted for an abnormal physical exam or urinalysis. Finally, CT or MRI would only be warranted if suspicion of malignancy was high (MRI) or if an evaluation of an implantable device was needed (CT).

WHAT TYPES OF MEDICATIONS ARE USEFUL IN TREATING HIS PAIN PATTERN?

NSAIDs, antidepressants, or gabapentinoids would all be reasonable choices for suspected neuropathic and myofascial pain. NSAIDs can help with nociceptive pain, while many of the other agents mentioned help with neuropathic pain. Antibiotics may be used if infection is suspected. Goals of therapy would be adequate efficacy, limiting potentially harmful side effect profiles, and choosing drugs that work on concurrent comorbidities, such as a serotonin–norepinephrine reuptake inhibitor (SNRI) for pain in the setting of depression.

WHAT TYPES OF TREATMENT MODALITIES SHOULD BE CONSIDERED FIRST, ONCE MALIGNANCY AND INFECTION ARE RULED OUT?

Conservative modalities are key to the successful treatment of this patient's ongoing pain. Although further interventions may be needed, the patient should be counseled on the benefits of smoking cessation, weight loss, and warm/cold packs applied to painful area. Further, physical therapy with focus on pelvic floor physiotherapy, biofeedback, and transcutaneous electrical nerve stimulation (TENS) have been shown to be effective. The patient may also benefit from pain psychology with a focus on cognitive-behavioral therapy (CBT).

WHAT OTHER INTERVENTIONS COULD BE TRIED?

Invasive interventions may include spermatic cord block, ilioinguinal/genitofemoral nerve block, or obturator nerve block. Pulsed radiofrequency (pRF) lesioning may be attempted at any of these peripheral nerves for longer-term pain relief. Peripheral nerve stimulation may be attempted as well. Microsurgical decompression of the spermatic cord can be considered if short-term relief obtained from diagnostic block of the spermatic cord with local anesthetic is successful but short lived. Salvage orchiectomy is considered a last resort.

WOULD SPINAL CORD STIMULATION (SCS) BE AN OPTION?

Yes, SCS should be considered for intractable pain of the trunk and limb when conservative treatment fails. Options for lead placement would be at the level of the conus medullaris (L1-L2) or at the sacral nerve root level (S2-S4).

WHAT OTHER TREATMENT MODALITIES MAY BE EMPLOYED TO ASSIST WITH PAIN CONTROL?

Nutritional modifications, acupuncture, meditation, CBT, and herbal supplements could be considered as adjunct treatment modalities.

DISCUSSION

DEFINITION, INCIDENCE, AND ETIOLOGY

Orchialgia, testicular pain, can be a complex, debilitating, and frustrating condition for patients and providers. When the pain has been present for 3 months or more, the condition is generally thought to cross from acute to chronic.[1–5] This arbitrary duration is undoubtedly not a true fixed point, but rather a process. Primary care, emergency medicine, surgical subspecialties, and chronic pain medicine specialists are just a few of the medical specialties that will encounter orchialgia.[5]

Orchialgia can present with bilateral or unilateral pain, can be constant or intermittent, and often interferes with the patient's daily activity.[1,4] Although the strict definition is pain in the testes, it is often useful and necessary to consider other vital structures in the area that may be causing referred pain and/or direct pain to the testes. Thus, this chapter highlights the etiology, diagnosis, and treatment options relevant to not only the testes but also the inguinal region, spermatic cord, and vas deferens, as well as the scrotum and supporting tissues. Therefore, from this point forward we define the aforementioned structures as scrotal content, as Levine does.[1] It has been estimated that scrotal content pain affects 100,000 men annually in the United States.[6]

Davis et al.[4] found that over 50% of patients with chronic scrotal content pain have no known/identifiable organic cause, and thus the pain was classified as idiopathic. The patient may seek out multiple providers and be shuffled from subspecialty to subspecialty in an effort to find a "single silver bullet" treatment option that simply does not exist. Patients often become frustrated and disheartened as they are placed on various medications and undergo procedures that may or may not provide the desired pain relief. The exact mechanism of their pain may not be fully understood and can be complex to manage. The "silver bullet" is often not a single intervention/surgery or medication but rather a process that involves a combination of treatment modalities.

When the etiology is known, it may be helpful and often will lead to a more directed and standardized treatment regimen. However, even with optimal treatment, a patient who has progressed from the acute phase to a more chronic phase may develop a refractory pain pattern. Box 21.1 lists possible etiologies of chronic scrotal content pain.

Box 21.1. **ETIOLOGIES OF SCROTAL CONTENT PAIN**

- Infection (e.g., epididymitis, UTI)
- Orchitis/epididymo-orchitis
- Torsion
- Cancer
- Cyst
- Obstruction
- Varicocele
- Spermatocele
- Trauma
- Iatrogenic (postsurgical: inguinal hernia repair, vasectomy)
- Referred pain (radiculitis, urethral stricture, IBS, prostatitis, nephrolithiasis)
- Psychologic (e.g., stress)
- Idiopathic

ANATOMY AND PATHOPHYSIOLOGY

Scrotal content pain can have somatic, visceral, and/or neuropathic components. The testes receive autonomic parasympathetic innervation from the ganglia of T10-T12 and the epididymis/vas deferens from T12-L1. Additionally, afferent and efferent fibers have been found to come from the pelvic plexus as well as the sacral parasympathetic nerves.[2] They receive somatic branches from the genitofemoral and ilioinguinal nerves. The sensory input is complex, from ilioinguinal, iliohypogastric, and genitofemoral nerves.[1,2] L1-L2 also provides the afferent limb of the cremasteric reflex, its presence or absence being a useful tool for the evaluation of acute testicular pain, and the posterior scrotum is innervated by branches of the pudendal nerve, S1-S3.[2] Pain is ultimately processed in the brain but is transmitted via the myelinated A-delta fibers and unmyelinated C fibers through the intraspinal nerves to the dorsal horn. From there it ascends the spinothalamic tract to the brain. Acute pain often involves specialized nociceptors that initially are stimulated by noxious stimuli and trigger the above cascade.

Both the acute and chronic pain mechanisms are not fully understood. However, active research is being done in both. One theory of how a pain pattern transforms from acute to chronic is through "central wind-up" or "hard wiring." Woolf and Salter[7] suggested that the initial insult triggers a pathologic process of the central nervous system rather than reaction to a stimulating noxious event. This leads to central modulation and a decreased threshold for developing an action potential. Ultimately, this leads to spontaneous firing and the previously mentioned central wind-up or hard wiring.[1]

Further, another theory suggests that individuals may be predisposed to development of chronic pain through a "double-hit" process. The theory suggests that a patient with an underlying subacute process, such as inflammation or infection, or a genetic process, already has nerve degeneration, a process called Wallerian degeneration,[1,5] and nerve hypersensitivity. If the patient is then exposed to a second insult in the area, such as surgery or trauma, he has an increased propensity to develop chronic pain.

EVALUATION

As with most things in the health care arena, a comprehensive history and physical are critical to the evaluation process. A clear history should be obtained focusing on the pain's nature and onset, inciting event, duration, location, character, radiation, aggravating factors, and alleviating factors. The average, best, and worst pain should be scaled using a formal metric, such as the VAS. Furthermore, the pain's effect on the patient's overall quality of life should be assessed using a validated scale, such as the Pain Impact Questionnaire (PIQ-6).[1] Identifying previously trialed interventions and medications, with duration of trial, any noted side effects, and response/relief of pain, should be fully undertaken by the provider. Additionally, the medications the patient is currently taking for pain, as well as for his general health, should be investigated.

The physical exam should focus on assessment of the scrotal content pain and identifying if the pain is reproducible with manipulation. Specifically, the clinician should evaluate for hernias, testicular irregularity/masses, cysts, and prior surgical scars. Other possible causes of pain should be ruled out, such as low back pain, ureteral stones, and infection. The patient should be evaluated in the standing, sitting, and lying positions.

TESTING/IMAGING

Testing should be focused, with the assistance of the findings from the history and physical. In general, patients suffering from chronic scrotal content pain should at a minimum be evaluated with a urinalysis. Additional serologic/urine testing for STIs or subacute scrotal content infections may be warranted depending on the history and physical findings.

Imaging is a critical evaluation and the simplest form can be achieved by ultrasound. The ultrasound can be of the testes specifically or an abdominal ultrasound if the patient presents with signs and symptoms concerning for a pelvic or abdominal etiology for the scrotal content pain. Ultrasound of the testes is described as the most reliable imaging for intrascrotal lesions of a nonimplantable nature.[2,9] It is suggested that scrotal ultrasound need not be performed in a patient with scrotal content pain if the urinanalysis and physical exam are normal.[2,5,10]

Advanced imaging, such as CT and MRI, may assist with diagnosis of referred pain generators, such as urolithiasis, radiculitis, and abdominal disorders. MRI may assist in the diagnosis of nonpalpable testicular masses when ultrasound has difficulty discriminating.[2]

DIRECTED TREATMENT OPTIONS FOR DIAGNOSED ETIOLOGIES

If the patient is found to have an acute process, he should be treated with appropriate therapy. If no acute findings are identified, then it is paramount to exclude any possible neoplasm. As noted, the use of routine testicular ultrasound in patients with chronic scrotal content pain but normal urinalysis and physical exam has fallen out of favor. However, the reassurance to the patient and physician that a testicular ultrasound provides, the limited risk to the patient, and the low financial burden to the system may justify obtaining one.[3]

For restriction to flow in the urinary tract, specifically due to prostate hypertrophy, it has been suggested that alpha-blockers are first-line therapy.[2] For obstructive etiologies that can be surgically removed, a surgical consult should be strongly considered.[11]

Antibiotics play a role in the treatment process if infection is a concern. Commonly, epididymitis, orchitis, or prostatitis requires combination therapy with doxycycline and a fluoroquinolone.[2,8] Levofloxacin is considered first-line therapy for chronic bacterial prostatitis because it has enhanced prostate penetration.[8] In patients at risk for, or found to have, an STI, the treatment should be directed per guidelines.[5] For bacterial urinary tract infections, the common causative organism *Escherichia coli* should be targeted with a course of either ciprofloxacin or levofloxacin for 10 days.[5]

Postsurgical chronic scrotal content pain has been estimated to be present in approximately one-third of postvasectomy patients, but only approximately 50% require medical intervention.[12] Often the pain is relieved with a simple procedure to eliminate any obstruction of the epididymis by nodules or granulomas. If scrotal content pain is found to be due to a referred pain generator, such as radicular, vascular, or gastrointestinal origin, then referral to the appropriate specialist is appropriate.[2]

CONSERVATIVE TREATMENT OPTIONS

It is vital to develop a good rapport with the patient immediately. It is important to inform him that there probably will not be a single silver bullet that will alleviate all of his pain. Additionally, there will be further testing and questions that need to be asked. It is important to document every interaction with the patient in a clear and concise form, because the patient may seek financial compensation.[1,2]

The base of the treatment model should be focused on conservative therapy and an understanding that the process will take time. It is imperative that the patient be counseled on smoking cessation and weight loss if either is indicated by findings in the history or physical exam. Further, regular exercise and a good home stretching exercise program will ensure that the patient does not slip into a generalized deconditioned state that will worsen other pain generators and feed the scrotal content pain.[13] There has been success with various physical therapy modalities, such as manual therapy, to improve posture, musculoskeletal anomalies, and soft tissue restrictions.[14] Biofeedback using electromyography and verbal cues that teach the patient relaxation techniques has been shown to be a successful treatment option.[15,16] There has been reported success with the use of TENS, and a trial of 1 to 3 months has been recommend as safe and effective.[3,17,18] Successful treatment of refractory idiopathic scrotal content pain must focus on optimizing the patient holistically in an effort to augment his overall pain control. To that end, the use of physical therapy for low back pain and sacroiliac/hip pain must be implemented as well.

The effect of chronic scrotal content pain on the psyche is vital to assess and to treat as well. Often there is a large component of depression, anxiety, and comorbid psychiatric disorders; therefore, referral to psychiatric subspecialties for assistance is critical.[2,5] The development of improved coping skills and overall CBT have been shown to be effective and thus referral to a specialized psychologist will likely assist in improving the patient's quality of life.[16,19]

ANALGESIC AND ADJUNCTIVE PHARMACOLOGIC TREATMENT OPTIONS

The analgesic pharmacologic options to treat idiopathic scrotal pain should follow the World Health Organization's established stepwise approach (see Table 21.1). Many recommend that the initial therapy start with a 1-month trial of NSAIDs and the stepwise approach to analgesia, coupled with empiric antibiotics.[3–5] If the pain is not alleviated by the initial non-opioid plus adjunctive therapy, the therapy may progress to a weak opioid, such as codeine, combined with the step 1 treatment. If the patient still does not receive optimal relief, therapy may escalate to step 3, which includes opioids plus step 1 drugs. Caution should be used, because there is a high prevalence (approximately 27%) of chemical dependency in the genital pain population according to a study of 48 patients.[5] In addition, long-term opioid use for chronic pain should be generally discouraged.

Table 21.1. **WORLD HEALTH ORGANIZATION STEPWISE ANALGESIC APPROACH**

WHO STEPWISE ANALGESIC APPROACH, STARTING AT STEP 1 AND ADVANCING TO EACH SUBSEQUENT STEP IF PAIN PERSISTS	
Step 1	Non-opioids (aspirin or acetaminophen) + step 1 + adjunctive
Step 2	Weak opioids (e.g., codeine) + step 1 + adjunctive
Step 3	Strong opioids (e.g., morphine) + step 1 + adjunctive

Modified from Kumar P, Mehta V, Nargund VH. Clinical management of chronic testicular pain. *Urol Int.* 2010;84:125–131.

Adjunctive therapy with low-dose antidepressants, such as tricyclic antidepressants (TCAs), has been shown to assist with pain control as well.[3,18] Commonly, a trial of amitriptyline or nortriptyline has been shown to be effective.[3,5,20] The patient should start out on a low dose at bedtime and should be monitored for side effects, such as sedation and disorientation. Furthermore, TCAs should not be tried if the patient has a contraindication to TCAs, such as recent MI, prolonged QT, and subsequent monoamine oxidase inhibitor (MAOI) use.[21] Other antidepressants, such as selective serotonin reuptake inhibitors (SSRIs), SNRIs, and MAOIs, play a role in the holistic treatment of the chronic pain patient.[18] MAOIs should be used with caution because they can precipitate a hypertensive crisis with ingestion of tyramine-rich foods, such as wine and cheese. Additionally, they interact with many other medications and predispose the patient to serotonin syndrome.[21]

Other adjuncts, such as gabapentin, a central calcium channel modulator/anticonvulsant, have been shown to provide good relief for neuropathic pain. Again, the dose should be started low and slowly titrated while monitoring for side effects and renal function.[1,20] If gabapentin is not tolerated, the patient may benefit from a trial of pregabalin.

INTERVENTIONAL TREATMENT OPTIONS

A selective nerve block may be indicated to assist with the diagnosis as well as possible therapeutic relief of scrotal content pain. A spermatic cord block can be performed using a mixture of 1% lidocaine and 0.25% marcaine plus dexamethasone. This mixture is injected into the perivasal tissues and then medial and lateral to the external inguinal ring (to block the ilioinguinal nerve and the genitofemoral nerve, respectively).[5] Relief of pain has been shown to help predict which patients will obtain relief from microsurgical denervation of the spermatic cord.[22] An obturator block can be performed to assist with the diagnosis of possible obturator entrapment syndrome, which can lead to referred pain to the scrotum. Furthermore, if the pain appears to be more posterior scrotal content in nature, an S3 nerve block may assist with diagnosis and treatment of this pain as well. One case series by Cohen and Foster showed promise for possible pRF to the ilioinguinal, iliohypogastric, and genitofemoral nerves for the treatment of chronic scrotal content pain. Three patients received pRF and reported continued relief at 6 months after the procedure.[23] Additionally, pRF of ilioinguinal nerves has shown promise in case reports of pain after inguinal herniotomy for up to 9 months; however, robust evidence in the form of randomized controlled trials or even case series is lacking.[24]

Sympathetic block, such as a superior hypogastric block, can be used for both diagnostic and therapeutic purposes. It can also be used as a bridge to manage pain until more conservative therapy can be optimized, such as physical therapy. Sympathetic block also has been found to be effective when combined with a ganglion impar block.[25]

Peripheral nerve stimulation with field stimulation has been successfully performed using an ultrasound- and fluoroscopy-guided technique. Placement of the ilioinguinal nerve lead using ultrasound was followed by final placement of both leads under fluoroscopy (respectively). SCS is based on the gate-control theory of pain proposed in 1965 by Melzack and Wall.[26] In 2012, Kapural et al. showed that SCS was an effective therapy for pelvic pain.[27] It is reasonable to consider SCS a possible treatment modality for chronic scrotal content pain, for assistance in treating not only referred pain generators but also direct generators based on anatomic location. However, at this time, there are no robust data to support this practice. Finally, there has been some promising efficacy with transrectal pelvic plexus blockade for chronic scrotal content pain.[2]

SURGICAL TREATMENT OPTIONS

Epididymectomy may be considered if the pain is restricted to the epididymis. This procedure has been reported to have good results for postvasectomy pain.[28] Additionally, vasectomy reversal has provided pain relief to approximately 69% to 84% of patients suffering from postvasectomy pain syndrome, according to Myers et al.[29]

Microdenervation of the spermatic cord (MDSC) was first performed in 1978 and has become more common if conservative therapy fails.[30] A successful selection measure for this procedure is relief of pain by spermatic cord block.[1,30] Other surgical procedures include varicocelectomy, robotic-assisted microsurgical vasoepididymostomy, and microablation of the spermatic cord. Salvage intervention includes orchiectomy.[5]

ALTERNATIVE TREATMENT OPTIONS

Acupuncture has been used successfully as an alternative to treat chronic pain generators. Strong evidence-based data is limited; however, smaller case series have been done that show promise for this treatment option. The successful treatment of chronic orchialgia was achieved using electroacupuncture combined with conventional amitriptyline. In 2011, Zhong et al.[31] successfully treated 56 individuals with electroacupuncture at sites Shenshu (BL 23), Ciliao (BL 32), Sanyinjiao (SP 6), and Taichong (LR 3).[1] The combined amitriptyline and electroacupuncture group received superior pain control over a control group that received only amitriptyline. The study was limited in size and follow-up; however, it did show promise of a low-risk treatment option.

CONCLUSION

- Chronic orchialgia affects nearly 100,000 individuals in the United States each year.
- Orchialgia is defined as chronic if it exceeds 3 months in duration.
- While the definition of orchialgia is pain originating from the testes, the evaluation of pain in the male genitalia requires consideration of pain generators involving the entire scrotal content.
- Scrotal content pain can have somatic, visceral, and/or neuropathic components and can be complex and difficult to diagnose.
- As many patients with chronic orchialgia have primary or secondary psychiatric comorbidity, antidepressants with analgesic properties may play a significant role in treatment.
- A high rate of chemical dependence is seen in patients with chronic orchialgia, requiring clinicians to be mindful of prescribing habits and to consider alternative therapies.
- Diagnostic and therapeutic injections, pRF lesioning, and neuromodulation strategies have been employed for the treatment of chronic orchialgia.
- Surgical treatment options include MDSC, epididymectomy, varicocelectomy, robotic-assisted microsurgical vasoepididymostomy, microablation of the spermatic cord, and orchiectomy.

REFERENCES

1. Levine L. Chronic orchialgia: evaluation and discussion of treatment options. *Ther Adv Urol.* 2010;2(5-6):209–214.
2. Kumar P, Mehta V, Nargund VH. Clinical management of chronic testicular pain. *Urol Int.* 2010;84(2):125–131.
3. Bhardwa JM, Kumar P, Nargund V. The aetiology, pathophysiology and management of chronic orchialgia. *BJU Int.* 2003;92(4):491.
4. Davis BE, Noble MJ, Weigel JW, Foret JD, Mebust WK. Analysis and management of chronic testicular pain. *J Urol.* 1990;143(5):936–939.
5. Brahmbhatt JV, Gudeloglu A, Parekattil SJ. Chronic orchialgia: workup and management. In: Jacob BP, Chen DC, Ramshaw B, Towfigh S (eds.), *The SAGES Manual of Groin Pain.* New York, NY: Springer International Publishing; 2016:343–361.
6. Tojuola B, Layman J, Kartal I, Gudelogul A, Brahmbhatt J, Parekattil S. Chronic orchialgia: review of treatments old and new. *Indian J Urol.* 2016;32:21–26.
7. Woolf CJ, Salter MW. Neuronal plasticity: increasing the gain in pain. *Science.* 2000;288:1765–1768.
8. Naber KG. Management of bacterial prostatitis: what's new? *BJU Int.* 2008;101: 7–10.
9. Lau MM, Taylor PM, Payne SR. The indications for scrotal ultrasound. *Br J Radiol.* 1999;72:833–837.
10. Van Haarst EP, Van Andel G, Rijcken TH, Schlatmann TJ, Taconis WK. Value of diagnostic ultrasound in patients with chronic scrotal pain and normal findings on clinical examination. *Urology.* 1999;54:1068–1072.

11. Gary CL, Powell CR, Amling CL. Outcomes for surgical management of orchialgia in patients with identifiable intrascrotal lesions. *Eur Urol.* 2001;39:455–459.
12. McMahon AJ, Buckley J, Taylor A, Lloyd SN, Deane RF, Kirk D. Chronic testicular pain following vasectomy. *Br J Urol.* 1992;69:188–191.
13. Rosenbaum TY, Owens A. The role of pelvic floor physical therapy in the treatment of pelvic and genital pain-related sexual dysfunction. *J Sex Med.* 2008;5:513–523.
14. Anderson WD, Sawyer T, Chan C. Sexual dysfunction in men with chronic prostatitis/chronic pelvic pain syndrome: improvement after trigger point release. Paradoxical relaxation training. *J Urol.* 2006;176:1534–1549.
15. Cornel EB, van Haarst EP, Schaarsberg RW, Geels J. The effect of biofeedback physical therapy in men with chronic pelvic pain syndrome type III. *Eur Urol.* 2005;47:607–611.
16. Clemens JQ, Nadler RB, Schaeffer AJ, Belani J, Albaugh J, Bushman W. Biofeedback, pelvic floor re-education, and bladder training for male chronic pelvic pain syndrome. *Urology.* 2000;56:951–955.
17. Fitzwater JB, Kuehl TJ, Schreir JJ. Electrical stimulation in the treatment of pelvic pain due to levator ani spasm. *J Reprod Med.* 2003;48:573–577.
18. Costabile RA, Hahn M, McLeod DG. Chronic orchialgia in the pain prone patient: the clinical perspective. *J Urol.* 1991;146:1571–1574.
19. McCracken LM, Dennis CT. Behavioral and cognitive-behavioral treatment for chronic pain. *Spine.* 2002;27:2564–2573.
20. Sinclair AM, Miller B, Lee LK. Chronic orchialgia: consider gabapentin or nortriptyline before considering surgery. *Int J Urol.* 2007;14:622–625.
21. Dharmshaktu P, Tayal V, Kalra BS. Efficacy of antidepressants as analgesics: a review. *J Clin Pharmacol.* 2012;6–17.
22. Benson JS, Abern MR, Larsen S, Levine LA. Does a positive response to spermatic cord block predict response to microdenervation of the spermatic cord for chronic scrotal content pain? *J Sex Med.* 2013;10:876–882.
23. Cohen SP, Foster A. Pulsed radiofrequency as a treatment for groin pain and orchialgia. *Urology.* 2003;61:645xxi–645xxiii.
24. Werner MU, Bischoff JM, Rathmell JP, Kehlet H. Pulsed radiofrequency in the treatment of persistent pain after inguinal herniotomy: a systematic review. *Reg Anesth Pain Med.* 2012;3:340–343.
25. Ahmed DG, Mohamed MF, Mohamed SA. Superior hypogastric plexus combined with ganglion impar neurolytic blocks for pelvic and/or perineal cancer pain relief. *Pain Physician.* 2015;1:E49–E56.
26. Melzack R, Wall PD. Pain mechanisms: a new theory. *Science.* 1965;150:971–979.
27. Kapural L, Janicky T, Narouze S, Mekhail N. Spinal cord stimulation is an effective treatment for the severe pelvic visceral pain. *Pain Med.* 2006;7:440–443.
28. Hori S, Sengupta A, Shukla CJ, Ingall E, McLoughlin J. Long-term outcome of epididymectomy for the management of chronic epididymal pain. *J Urol.* 1996;182:1407–1412.
29. Myers SA, Mershon CE, Fuchs EF. Vasectomy reversal for the treatment of the post-vasectomy pain syndrome. *J Urol.* 1997;157:518–520.
30. Levine LA, Matkov TG. Microsurgical denervation of the spermatic cord as primary surgical treatment of chronic orchialgia. *J Urol.* 2001;165:1927–1930.
31. Zhong LJ, Wang J, Ding XH. Therapeutic effects of electroacupuncture on chronic orchialgia. *Zhongguo Zhen Jiu.* 2011;1:40–42.

REVIEW QUESTIONS

1. A 16-year-old boy presents to the emergency department with sudden-onset severe testicular pain. The right testicle is high-riding and there is an extremely weak cremasteric reflex. What is the best diagnostic tool if physical exam is unable to confirm the diagnosis?

A. Ultrasound
B. X-ray
C. MRI
D. CT

2. What nerve roots provide innervation for the afferent limb of the cremasteric reflex?

A. L3-L4
B. L5-S1
C. S2-S4
D. L1-L2

3. A 65-year-old male is prescribed amitriptyline for chronic testicular pain that causes poor sleep. Which of the following is a contraindication to this drug?

A. History of short QT interval
B. Recent MI
C. History of insomnia
D. History of masseter spasm

ANSWERS

1. A. After a thorough history and physical exam, ultrasound is the quickest and most sensitive diagnostic tool to evaluate for testicular emergencies. The case describes acute testicular torsion, which can be confirmed with ultrasound after an abnormal physical exam. MRI or CT (answers C and D) may assist with urolithiasis, radiculitis, or abdominal pathology. X-ray (answer B) would be best for evaluating bony structures.[3,5]

2. D. The presence or absence of the cremasteric reflex can be useful in evaluating acute testicular pain. It is absent with testicular torsion or damage to the ilioinguinal nerve. Its afferent limb is L1-L2.[2]

3. B. Amitriptyline is a TCA often used for the treatment of chronic pain with a neuropathic component. A common side effect is sleepiness, which makes it a logical choice for a patient with poor sleep. Contraindications include recent MI, long QT syndrome, concurrent administration of MAOI, and prior hypersensitivity to TCA.[21] Amitriptyline can aid in the treatment of insomnia. Long QT interval and TCA administration can cause torsade de pointes, not short QT intervals. A history of masseter spasm (answer D) is concerning for malignant hyperthermia, a hypermetabolic response to inhalational anesthetics.

QUESTIONS AND ANSWERS

This chapter has accompanying questions and answers that are available to subscribers as part of the Oxford eLearning platform. To access the questions, follow the link below, or go to
✔ http://oxfordmedicine.com/painmanagementreview

22.

CHRONIC BACK PAIN IN THE ELDERLY: SPINAL STENOSIS

Nebojsa Nick Knezevic, Benjamin Cantu, Ivana Knezevic, and Kenneth D. Candido

STEM CASE AND KEY QUESTIONS

A 64-year-old woman with history of diabetes and hypertension presents to the pain management center with a primary complaint of low back pain. Back pain has been a chronic issue for her for almost 10 years and is unrelated to any particular injury. She has been having difficulty standing up from a sitting position and with standing for more than 10 minutes. When she complained for the first time to her primary care physician (PCP), she was prescribed a course of physical therapy, which provided some temporary relief. Her pain began gradually, building up to a 8/10 rating on a numeric pain rating scale, and she was started on an NSAID (ibuprofen up to 1600 mg/day) and a generic muscle relaxant. Since the symptoms were not completely resolved with that regimen, gabapentin 600 mg three times a day was also prescribed by her PCP and this step provided some pain relief that persisted for several months. However, the patient's pain had gotten worse in the last month and she was referred to our center as the patient complained that she is she was unable to complete daily household chores. The patient was reporting a numeric pain score of 9/10, characterized as burning pain and which was accompanied by "pins and needles" radiating from the lower back to the buttocks, more on the left than right, with occasional numbness in that area. Pain was aggravated by walking or prolonged sitting or standing and was relieved by lying with a pillow under the most painful area. Patient was a smoker of approximately 7 cigarettes/day for the past 30 years. She denied having any extremity weakness or any urinary bladder issues and she did not have prior surgeries to address these issues. MRI showed diffuse and generalized lumbar spinal stenosis and spondylosis without overt nerve root or foraminal compression, except at L2-L3 where it was severe, and at L4-L5 where it was moderate, due to degenerative changes in the bony elements.

WHAT IS THE ETIOLOGY OF CHRONIC LOW BACK PAIN (CLBP) IN THE ELDERLY? WHAT SHOULD BE CONSIDERED IN THE DIFFERENTIAL DIAGNOSIS?

Because of the patient's age, > 60 years old, the suggested etiology for CLBP is predominantly spinal stenosis. An age-related change in intervertebral disk nutrient metabolism is often a cause of disk degeneration. Lack of nutrients along with progressive loss of interdiskal hydration is a reason for annular disruption leading to disk herniation and spinal canal encroachment, causing stenosis. The differential diagnosis should also include bony osteophyte formation, facet joint degeneration, or a hypertrophic ligmentum flavum, which are common sources of narrowing of the central canal and lateral recesses and lead to a trefoil type of deformity. A patient's long-term spondylitic changes contribute to disk degeneration and liberation of inflammatory mediators (histamine, lactate, bradykinin, calcitonin-gene related peptide, vasoactive intestinal peptide, substance P, phospholipase A_2) from neural structures that contribute to local and radicular pain.

IS MRI ALWAYS INDICATED IN THE DIAGNOSTIC PROCESS? ARE THERE ANY OTHER COST-EFFECTIVE BUT VALUABLE INVESTIGATIVE RESOURCES?

Thorough physical examination with extensive medical history acquisition should be the basis for making the CLBP diagnosis in the elderly and is still noted to be an essential tool when evaluating patients for the first time. Clinically based evidence suggests that MRI is the most appropriate imaging modality to use; however, it is considered expensive and the above-mentioned approach is strongly encouraged as the first-line strategy, especially in the elderly, who gradually develop CLBP symptoms.

WILL THIS PATIENT'S CLBP EVER DIMINISH? WHY HAVE THE APPLIED TREATMENT OPTIONS FAILED TO PROVIDE RELIEF?

Disk degeneration is a natural maturation process underlying aging. Pain symptoms may be kept under control by applying available treatment options while not addressing the underlying evolution of the degeneration and hence not providing even a modicum of resolution or cure. This patient's pain relief was moderately obtained by incorporating bed rest, manual therapeutic manipulation, and massage in the early stages of the pain symptom experience. However, pharmacologic therapy with an NSAID, followed (using the WHO stepwise approach) by opioid use (and also gabapentin) later, failed to provide a satisfactory level of pain relief with the same continuation of the patient's lifestyle (confounding factors included being diabetic and overweight) and gabapentin was predominantly effective for her neuropathic pain, not her nociceptive symptoms associated with anatomic spondylosis.

CAN MULTIPLE "PAIN KILLER" THERAPY IMPROVE THE PAIN EXPERIENCE WHILE CAUSING NO ADVERSE EFFECTS IN THE PATIENT?

With the patient's comorbidities (diabetes, high blood pressure), choosing an adequate opioid treatment should be undertaken with great caution. Combining multiple opioids often has a high risk of engendering side effects in older populations (such as constipation, urinary retention, mental confusion, drowsiness, risk of falls and fractures, and respiratory depression, especially with synergistic effects with other pharmaceuticals).

IS SURGERY INDICATED FOR THIS PATIENT? WHAT ARE THE OTHER TREATMENT OPTIONS IF SHE IS DEEMED NOT TO BE A SURGICAL CANDIDATE?

Before turning to surgery for the treatment of spinal stenosis due to severe spondylosis, especially in the elderly with underlying conditions like those noted in this patient, and in general, the following should be considered. It has been shown that surgery is associated with an exceedingly slow recovery process in the elderly. Other interventional treatments are available and could provide symptom control, at least transiently, including use of modalities such as epidural steroid injections, which can provide longer-term pain relief than many conventional medications. However, in this patient, steroid use had to be closely monitored, because repeated steroid injections could raise blood sugar levels and elevate blood pressure due to retention of sodium and water. If pain control is difficult to achieve and to sustain with an interventional approach, other noninvasive methods have to be utilized before accepting a decision to proceed with surgery.

DISCUSSION

EPIDEMIOLOGY OF CHRONIC BACK PAIN IN THE ELDERLY

CLBP is a common reason for frequent physician office visits by the elderly.[1] The prevalence of CLBP has been steadily increasing among the elderly as the population ages, with those more than 65 years old representing 12.3% of CLBP sufferers.[2] Although earlier data suggested that CLBP in the elderly was declining,[3] in a recent 7-year longitudinal cohort study, its prevalence was found to be increasing in this demographic group, specifically in those age 70 to 77.[4]

ETIOLOGY OF CLBP IN THE ELDERLY

Factors found to be predictors of CLBP were female sex, social isolation, hypertension, and joint pain.[5] A common contributor to chronic back pain in the elderly is degenerative spinal stenosis. It is estimated that relative and absolute stenosis have a prevalence of 47% and 19.4%, respectively, in people 60 to 69 years old.[4] Although the numbers correlate with observed stenosis on imaging and patients are not always symptomatic, there is evidence that absolute stenosis is associated with a threefold increased risk of developing low back pain.[4] Furthermore, spinal stenosis constitutes the most common reason for elderly patients with CLBP to undergo surgical intervention.[6]

PATHOPHYSIOLOGY OF CLBP

Various factors contribute to the pathophysiology of disk degeneration as we age, with an end result of development of CLBP. One of the primary components of the process is changes in the nutrient capacity of the intervertebral disk.[7,8] Endplate permeability decreases, causing a decline in the metabolic exchange of nutrients and oxygen between vertebral vessels and disks. The lack of nutrition to the disk, combined with the retention of damaged molecules, is believed to be the initial insult to the aging disk.[9]

Due to the increase in metabolic requirement and a reduction in elimination of metabolic waste products, pH decreases, leading to inactivation of cellular processes in the nucleus pulposus.[10,11] As time passes, fluid loss in disks brings vertebrae and adjacent facet joints closer together by decreasing the relative disk height. Compounded with repeated micromotion, continuous damage to the longitudinal ligaments and outermost annulus causes osteoblastosis within the vertebrae and thus bony osteophyte formation. Osteophytes and further disk height loss lead to a decline in the range of motion and an increase in nociception during spinal loading.[8–11]

Disruption to the annular layers of the disk is another key contributor in age-related disk injury.[11,12] Tears, such as peripheral rim lesions (involving the outermost annulus), circumferential tears (splitting between the two major layers of the annulus), and radial fissures (tears that spread outward from the nucleus), all represent mechanisms of injury to the disk.[7,10]

When nuclear material escapes the outer annulus and travels toward the central canal or lateral recesses, irritation of the surrounding structures increases. As further disk degeneration proceeds, the ligamentum flavum folds on its own, becoming more fibrotic and hypertrophic. The thickened ligamentum flavum constitutes another means of impingement on the thecal sac and other neural elements.[12]

Disk degeneration leading to disk herniation, osteophyte formation, facet degeneration, and hypertrophic ligamentum flavum all serve as potential sources to create narrowing of the central canal and lateral recesses, leading to degenerative spinal stenosis. Nerves then become compressed from mechanical obstruction and microvascular changes are created.[3] As these changes occur, inflammatory mediators are released from neural structures, aiding in central sensitization and release of nociceptive neuropeptides from dorsal root ganglia, contributing to local and radicular pain.[10,11]

DIAGNOSIS

When approaching patients with CLBP, clinicians should first rule out nondegenerative pathology. History and physical examination should be the initial approach to rule out underlying disease that would require prompt attention. Screening may be performed by asking a standard series of questions and by an adequate musculoskeletal and neurologic exam.[13]

Recently, a Delphi study, including 279 clinicians in multiple specialties from 29 different countries with a mean of 19 years in practice, aimed at creating standardized criteria for the diagnosis of lower back pain, specifically spinal stenosis. The task force found significance from the collected data when six questions were asked, which yielded 80% certainty in a diagnosis of spinal stenosis (Box 22.1).[14]

Studies for the clinical evaluation of spinal stenosis through physical exam have received less attention than diagnosis through imaging, but physical exam is still noted as a valuable tool for providers when evaluating patients for the first time.[15] Fritz et al.[15] conducted a study on 93 patients and a multivariate analysis and found significant correlations between lumbar spinal stenosis and the following clinical signs:

1. Age > 65
2. Abnormal Romberg test
3. Wide-based gait
4. Thigh pain following 30 sec of lumbar extension

Box 22.1. DELPHI STUDY STANDARDIZED QUESTIONS AND CO-RELATED CLINICAL SIGNS FOR LUMBAR SPINAL STENOSIS DIAGNOSIS

Standardized Criteria for Diagnosis of LBP

1. Does the patient have leg or buttock pain while walking?
2. Does the patient flex forward to relieve symptoms?
3. Does the patient feel relief when using a shopping cart or bicycle?
4. Does the patient have motor or sensory disturbance while walking?
5. Are the pulses in the foot present and symmetric?
6. Does the patient have lower extremity weakness?

Modified from Tomkins-Lane C, Melloh M, Lurie J, et al. Consensus on the clinical diagnosis of lumbar spinal stenosis: results of an International Delphi Study. *Spine (Phila Pa 1976)*. 2016;41(15):1239–1246.

When imaging is indicated for diagnosis and for guidance in determining appropriate treatment, clinically based evidence suggests that MRI is the most appropriate modality (Figure 22.1).

If MRI is unavailable or contraindicated, CT scanning with or without myelography is the next best imaging tool.[11] It should be noted that a clinician should use good judgment in evaluating candidates for immediate imaging. In a study analyzing rising health care costs in the elderly and use of imaging, it was found that more than half the patients had MRI performed without showing any "red flag" signs.[16]

CONSERVATIVE NONPHARMACOLOGIC TREATMENTS

Although there is not a consensus on the best approach for chronic back pain, conservative therapy is often initially suggested. Besides pharmacologic therapy, different nonpharmacologic treatment options, such as physical therapy, injections, electrical stimulation, manipulations, and cognitive approaches, could and should be considered.

Activity Modification

There has been no strong evidence to support bed rest for the treatment of degenerative spinal stenosis. Short periods of rest up to 2 days may be helpful in alleviating acute exacerbations of pain. Instruction should be given for avoiding activities that increase back extension, but encouragement to return to normal activities as soon as possible is beneficial.[17]

Manipulation and Acupuncture

Chiropractic manipulation, traction, and acupuncture are modalities gaining more popularity among patients with CLBP. Reviews of their efficacy for low back pain, however, have not been convincing.[18] In spinal stenosis specifically, manipulation has not been shown to improve symptoms with clinical significance.[18] Further investigation of this therapeutic method is warranted.

Short-lived benefits have been shown with acupuncture for CLBP compared to placebo, but not compared to sham acupuncture.[19] Prolonged symptom relief with acupuncture has not been proven. Thus, perhaps this modality is useful when used as an adjuvant with other treatment methods.[20]

Physical Therapy

Physical therapy and exercise are often prescribed for sufferers of back pain. Based on a review of the iterature on patients with spinal stenosis, limited evidence showed benefit from physical therapy as a single treatment approach. However, based on clinical experience, the North American Spine Society (NASS) does suggest a limited course of active physical therapy to determine the degree of therapeutic effect experienced.[18,21] Many exercise plans have been described for use in older adults. Since there is not strong evidence to prove that

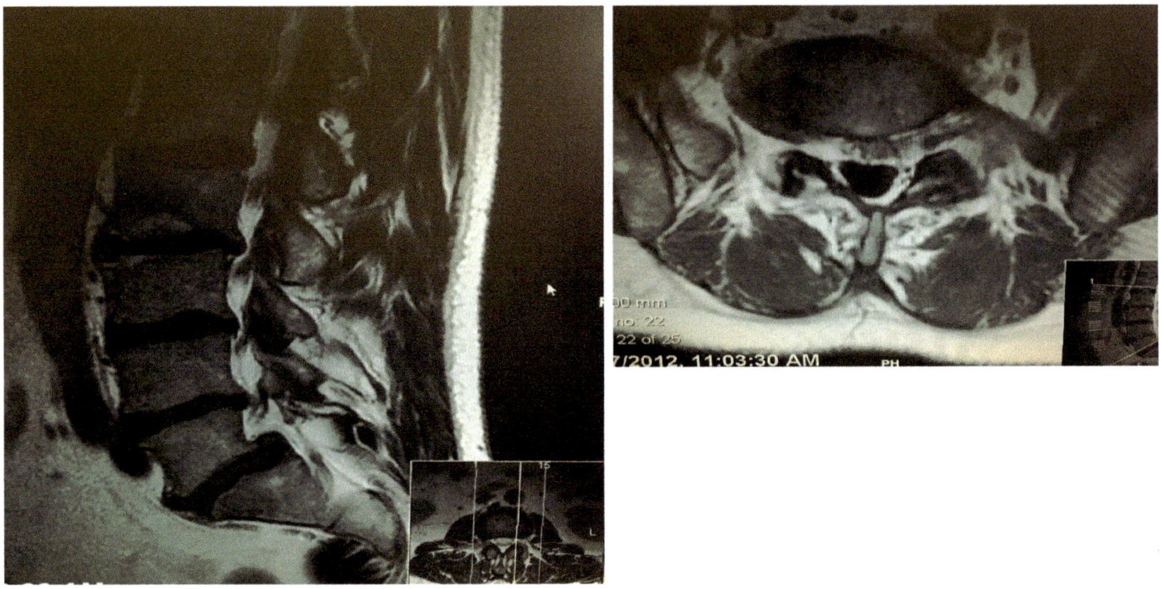

Figure 22.1. MRI images (sagittal and axial) from a patient who has degenerative disk changes and spinal stenosis.

one plan is better than another, patient preference is important to ensure compliance.[18,21]

TENS/PENS

There have been studies involving an older population and the use of transcutaneous and percutaneous electrical nerve stimulation (TENS and PENS, respectively).[22,23] Older patients were found to have improvements in resting pain, movement-evoked pain, and disability; however, they required a higher amplitude than younger cohorts to achieve similar results. This may reflect an important clinical characteristic that should be taken into account when dosing TENS in the older population.[22]

PHARMACOLOGIC TREATMENTS

NSAIDs/Acetaminophen

Evidence would suggest that a trial of acetaminophen is reasonable when analgesic therapy is initiated, due to its reasonable safety profile in the elderly, as long as the recommended daily dose is not exceeded.[24] NSAIDs are often employed for initial pharmacologic pain relief as well.[22] However, these drugs frequently produce side effects in the elderly; therefore, it is important to monitor patients closely for any gastrointestinal, renal, hepatic, or cardiovascular signs and symptoms. The lowest dose and shortest duration should be attempted, along with proton pump inhibitors prescribed to decrease adverse GI effects.[25,26]

Opioids

Opioids can be prescribed after failure of the NSAIDs or acetaminophen; however, caution is advised with chronic use due to the potential side effects in older adults, such as constipation, urinary retention, mental confusion, drowsiness, and increased risk of falls and fractures.[27,28] Evidence of long-term efficacy for pain control is minimal with these agents, and there is still not sufficient evidence to endorse their longer use for improving pain and function in patients.[18,27]

Muscle Relaxants

Muscle relaxants may be helpful in managing low back pain, but they are not indicated in spinal stenosis. They may be of some use with acute exacerbations of back spasm related to spinal stenosis, but their long-term use is not suggested.[29]

Antidepressants

Many clinical trials have supplied evidence supporting use of antidepressants in pain control. Efficacy has been proven in various disorders involving neuropathic pain; however, antidepressant use in the treatment of chronic back pain is less clear. Tricyclic antidepressants (TCAs) were one of the first groups of antidepressants shown to have some benefit with nonneuropathic pain. In placebo-controlled studies involving subjects with chronic back pain, nortriptyline showed analgesic effects in patients with no preexisting symptoms of depression.[30] However, it should be noted that, due to the adverse effects of TCAs, caution should be used in prescribing these medications to the elderly. Serotonin-norepinephrine reuptake inhibitors, such as duloxetine, have shown some benefit in treating nonneuropathic pain, with a better side effect profile than TCAs, but the studies conducted in older populations have had small sample sizes.[31,32] Data have shown duloxetine to be effective for low back pain when compared to placebo for CLBP without a radicular component.[33]

Anticonvulsants

Gabapentin and pregabalin have been well studied and have been shown to be effective for neuropathic pain syndromes;

however, new studies are pointing to their use in low back pain, particularly in spinal stenosis.[34,35] Gastroretentive gabapentin showed improvement in pain and increased sleep in elderly patients with spinal stenosis and a radiating component.[34] Pregabalin showed improvement in patients ages 65 and older with low back pain and pain in a lower limb when compared to opioids, which were effective in relieving low back pain without lower limb symptoms.[35]

INTERVENTIONAL TREATMENTS

When pharmacologic and physical therapies fail, epidural injections are often performed. The problematic nociceptive target is accessed using transforaminal (Figure 22.2), interlaminar (Figure 22.3), and caudal approaches, and glucocorticoids with added local anesthetic are usually injected into the epidural space. There have been many studies both validating and challenging the efficacy of these injections, particularly for spinal stenosis.[20,36,37] Studies have attempted to prove long-term benefits from epidural injections as well. In a randomized, double-blind, controlled trial involving 120 patients, subjects were given interlaminar epidural steroid injections for central spinal stenosis and were followed for 2 years.[38] Patients were randomized to receive either steroid and local anesthetic or local anesthetic alone. Results of the study showed significant improvement in both groups. Patients in the "success category" showed symptomatic improvement at 2 years, with an average of five to six procedures within that time frame, confirming the importance of patient selection in successful outcomes for these treatments.[38]

In a recent systematic review of 52 randomized clinical trials, with either placebo or active control groups, the authors analyzed the efficacy of epidural injections for significant pain control in patients with spinal stenosis. Conclusions from the review found that there is level 2 evidence supporting the long-term efficacy of interlaminar and caudal epidural injections performed with either local anesthetic alone or anesthetic and steroids.[36] There was also a significant benefit (level 3) to transforaminal approaches for short-term relief.[36]

We should note that epidural steroid injections have been shown to increase blood glucose levels systemically by greater than 100-fold in patients with diabetes compared to preinjection baseline levels.[39] Therefore, it is important to monitor these individuals, especially among the elderly with degenerative spinal disease, in whom diabetes is a common problem.[39]

SURGICAL TREATMENTS

There are many surgical techniques available for patients who become candidates for surgery. Previous reviews of clinical studies have revealed success rates varying between 26% and 100%.[40] Decompressive laminectomy is the most common procedure employed currently. However, in a randomized trial with a concurrent cohort study involving 13 surgical centers with 654 participants, there was no difference in long-term benefits at the 8-year follow-up between those who underwent decompressive laminectomy and nonoperated patients.[41]

Evidence suggests new options, such as minimally invasive techniques, are viable in correctly selected candidates. Although higher repeated surgery rates were reported compared to laminectomy, the associated risks of removal and replacement are substantially lower than with the open procedure of a laminectomy.[42,43] Furthermore, the overall rate of improvement of symptoms for up to 2 years makes this a valuable procedure for candidates not requiring immediate surgical decompression due to severe spinal stenosis.

NEUROMODULATION

Spinal cord stimulation (SCS) is used to treat recalcitrant pain poorly responsive or nonrespondive to less-invasive treatment modalities. It is also used for the treatment of recurrent or

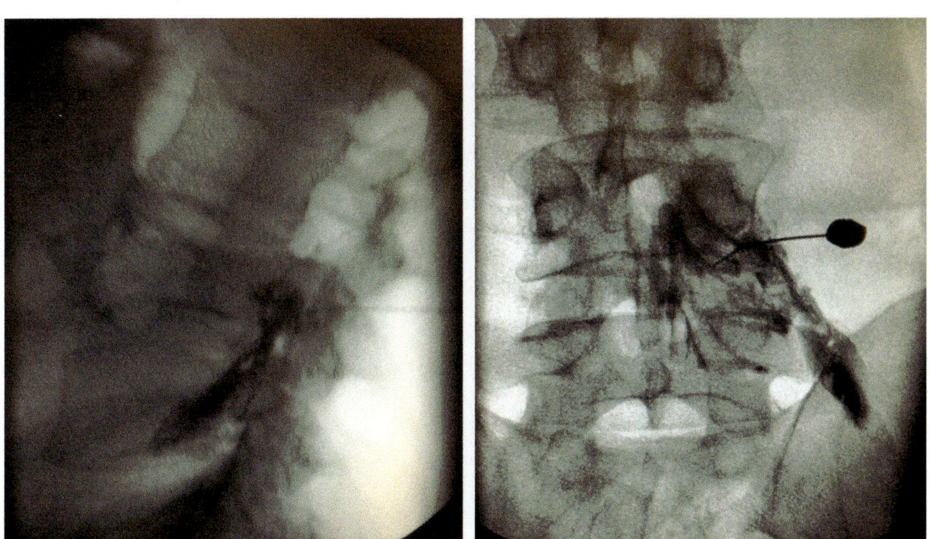

Figure 22.2. Transforaminal epidural steroid injection at L4-L5 level, fluoroscopic images (lateral and AP views).

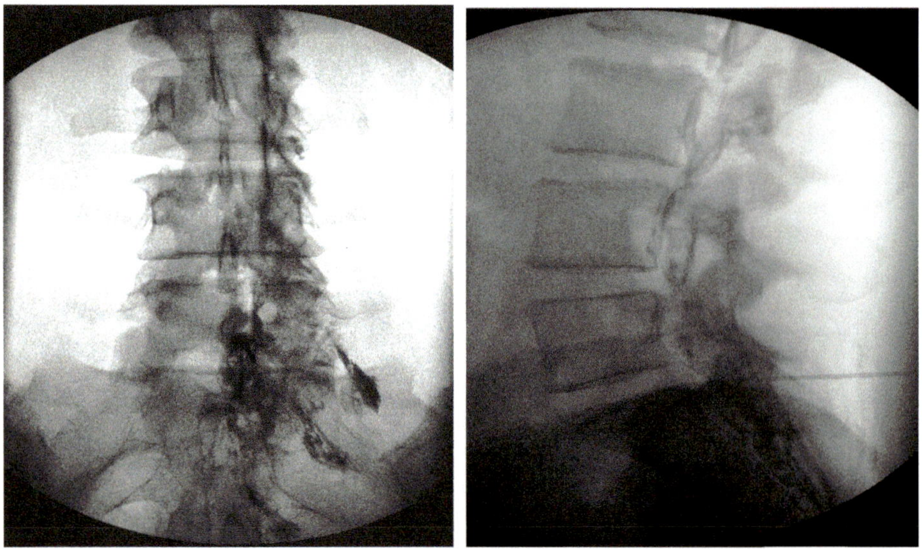

Figure 22.3. Interlaminar epidural steroid injection at L5-S1 level using parasagittal approach, fluoroscopic images (AP and lateral views).

persistent back pain after spinal surgery known as "failed back surgery syndrome" or "postlaminectomy syndrome." The procedure entails placement of either a surgical paddle or percutaneous leads connected to a power source into the epidural space at a spinal level corresponding to a dermatome covering the painful area (Figure 22.4).[44]

Many patients have been successfully treated over the years, as exemplified in the published literature.[45–48] Newer technology (high-frequency or HFS), using a nonparesthesia, anatomic approach to CLBP and radicular lower extremity pain, has recently become available.

INTRATHECAL DRUG DELIVERY SYSTEMS (IDDS)

Intrathecal drug delivery is used to provide an alternate mode of administration of narcotics to patients with chronic noncancer pain. It might especially benefit those on long-term opioid therapy who derive insufficient pain relief despite frequent administration or dose escalation of the opioid medication. With IDDS, the continuous supply of a given medication dose around the clock allows for stable pain control while eliminating peaks and troughs associated with the oral opioid use.[49]

CONCLUSIONS

- CLBP is a common reason for frequent physician office visits among the elderly.
- Disk degeneration and spinal stenosis are the primary reasons for CLBP in the elderly.
- Detailed medical history and physical examination are important to rule out underlying diseases that would require prompt attention medically and surgically.

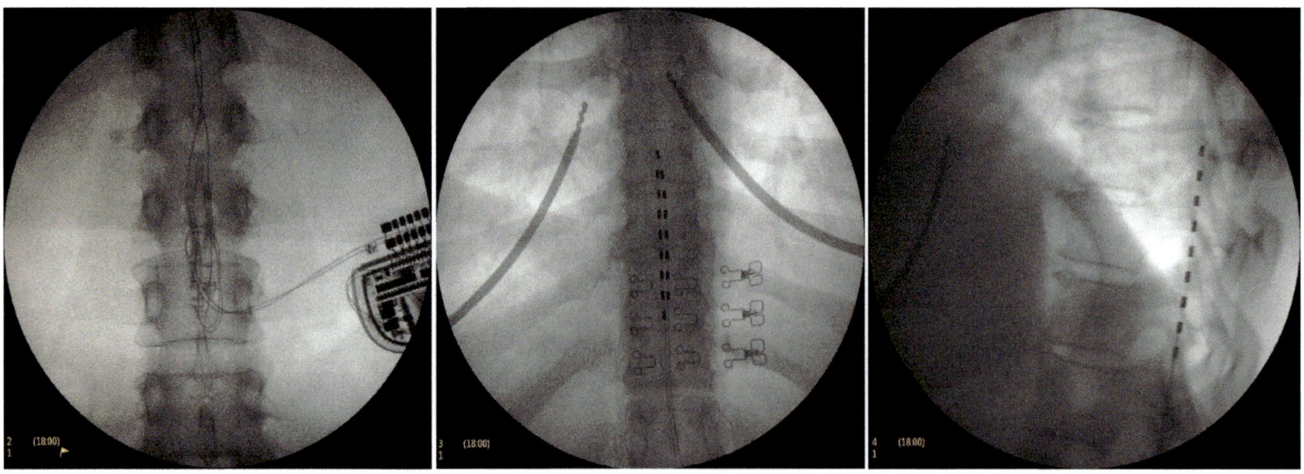

Figure 22.4. X-ray images showing the spinal cord stimulator (leads placed at T7 level, and implantable pulse generator, IPG) implanted in a patient with spinal stenosis.

- MRI in elderly patients is frequently overutilized and uneconomical.
- Treatment options include conservative treatments, pharmacologic agents, physical therapy, electrical stimulation, manipulations, and interventional procedures with epidural injection of steroids and/or local anesthetics.
- In most cases, a combination of conservative and interventional procedures provides pain relief and avoids surgical options, which are a concern due to multiple comorbidities in older patients.

REFERENCES

1. Deyo RA, Mirza SK, Martin BI. Back pain prevalence and visit rates: estimates from U.S. national surveys, 2002. *Spine (Phila Pa 1976)*. 2006;31(23):2724–2727.
2. Freburger JK, Holmes GM, Agans RP, et al. The rising prevalence of chronic low back pain. *Arch Intern Med*. 2009;169(3):251–258.
3. Lavsky-Shulan M, Wallace RB, Kohout FJ, et al. Prevalence and functional correlates of low back pain in the elderly: the Iowa 65+ Rural Health Study. *J Am Geriatr Soc*. 1985;33(1):23–28.
4. Kalichman L, Cole R, Kim DH, et al. Spinal stenosis prevalence and association with symptoms: the Framingham Study. *Spine J*. 2009;9(7):545–550.
5. Jacobs JM, Hammerman-Rozenberg C, Cohen A, et al. Chronic back pain among the elderly: prevalence, associations, and predictors. *Spine (Phila Pa 1976)*. 2006;31(7):E203–E207.
6. Deyo RA, Mirza SK, Martin BI, et al. Trends, major medical complications, and charges associated with surgery for lumbar spinal stenosis in older adults. *JAMA*. 2010;303(13):1259–1265.
7. Adams MA, Roughley PJ. What is intervertebral disc degeneration, and what causes it? *Spine (Phila Pa 1976)*. 2006;31(18):2151–2161.
8. Buckwalter JA. Aging and degeneration of the human intervertebral disc. *Spine (Phila Pa 1976)*. 1995;20(11):1307–1314.
9. Beattie PF. Current understanding of lumbar intervertebral disc degeneration: a review with emphasis upon etiology, pathophysiology, and lumbar magnetic resonance imaging findings. *J Orthop Sports Phys Ther*. 2008;38(6):329–340.
10. Videman T, Nurminen M. The occurrence of anular tears and their relation to lifetime back pain history: a cadaveric study using barium sulfate discography. *Spine (Phila Pa 1976)*. 2004;29(23):2668–2676.
11. Abe Y, Akeda K, An HS, et al. Proinflammatory cytokines stimulate the expression of nerve growth factor by human intervertebral disc cells. *Spine (Phila Pa 1976)*. 2007;32(6):635–642.
12. Freemont AJ, Watkins A, Le Maitre C, et al. Current understanding of cellular and molecular events in intervertebral disc degeneration: implications for therapy. *J Pathol*. 2002;196(4):374–379.
13. American Geriatrics Society Panel on Pharmacological Management of Persistent Pain in Older Persons. Pharmacological management of persistent pain in older persons. *J Am Geriatr Soc*. 2009;57(8):1331–1346.
14. Tomkins-Lane C, Melloh M, Lurie J, et al. Consensus on the clinical diagnosis of lumbar spinal stenosis: results of an International Delphi Study. *Spine (Phila Pa 1976)*. 2016;41(15):1239–1246.
15. Fritz JM, Delitto A, Welch WC, et al. Lumbar spinal stenosis: a review of current concepts in evaluation, management, and outcome measurements. *Arch Phys Med Rehabil*. 1998;79(6):700–708.
16. Weiner DK, Kim YS, Bonino P, et al. Low back pain in older adults: are we utilizing healthcare resources wisely? *Pain Med*. 2006;7(2):143–150.
17. Coomes EN. A comparison between epidural anaesthesia and bed rest in sciatica. *Br Med J*. 1961;1(5218):20–24.
18. Mayer TG. The North American Spine Society focuses on multidisciplinary spine care. *Spine J*. 2001;1(1):1–4.
19. Leibing E, et al. Acupuncture treatment of chronic low-back pain—a randomized, blinded, placebo-controlled trial with 9-month follow-up. *Pain*. 2002;96(1-2):189–196.
20. Atlas SJ. Epidural steroid injections are not effective for patients with lumbar spinal stenosis. *Evid Based Med*. 2015;20(1):16.
21. Rundell SD, Gellhorn AC, Comstock BA, et al. Clinical outcomes of early and later physical therapist services for older adults with back pain. *Spine J*. 2015;15(8):1744–1755.
22. Simon CB, Riley JL III, Fillingim RB, et al. Age group comparisons of TENS response among individuals with chronic axial low back pain. *J Pain*. 2015;16(12):1268–1279.
23. Weiner DK, Perera S, Rudy TE, et al. Efficacy of percutaneous electrical nerve stimulation and therapeutic exercise for older adults with chronic low back pain: a randomized controlled trial. *Pain*. 2008;140(2):344–357.
24. Atlas SJ, Keller RB, Wu YA, Deyo RA, Singer DE. Long-term outcomes of surgical and nonsurgical management of lumbar spinal stenosis: 8 to 10 year results from the Maine Lumbar Spine Study. *Spine (Phila Pa 1976)*. 2005;30(8):936–943.
25. Abdulla A, Adams N, Bone M, et al. Guidance on the management of pain in older people. *Age Ageing*. 2013;42(suppl 1):i1–i57.
26. Savigny P, Watson P, Underwood M. Early management of persistent non-specific low back pain: summary of NICE guidance. *BMJ*. 2009;338:b1805.
27. Chaparro LE, Furlan AD, Deshpande A, et al. Opioids compared with placebo or other treatments for chronic low back pain: an update of the Cochrane Review. *Spine (Phila Pa 1976)*. 2014;39(7):556–563.
28. Miller M, Stürmer T, Azrael D, Levin R, Solomon DH. Opioid analgesics and the risk of fractures in older adults with arthritis. *J Am Geriatr Soc*. 2011;59(3):430–438.
29. Deyo RA. Drug therapy for back pain. Which drugs help which patients? *Spine (Phila Pa 1976)*. 1996;21(24):2840–2849; discussion 2849–2850.
30. Atkinson JH, Slater MA, Willias RA, et al. A placebo-controlled randomized clinical trial of nortriptyline for chronic low back pain. *Pain*. 1998;76(3):287–296.
31. Mancini M, Gianni W, Rossi A, et al. Duloxetine in the management of elderly patients with major depressive disorder: an analysis of published data. *Expert Opin Pharmacother*. 2009;10(5):847–860.
32. Raskin J, Wiltse CG, Siegal A, et al. Efficacy of duloxetine on cognition, depression, and pain in elderly patients with major depressive disorder: an 8-week, double-blind, placebo-controlled trial. *Am J Psychiatry*. 2007;164(6):900–909.
33. Smith HS, Smith EJ, Smith BR. Duloxetine in the management of chronic musculoskeletal pain. *Ther Clin Risk Manag*. 2012;8:267–277.
34. Yaksi A, Ozgonenel L, Ozgonenel B. The efficiency of gabapentin therapy in patients with lumbar spinal stenosis. *Spine (Phila Pa 1976)*. 2007;32(9):939–942.
35. Sakai Y, Sakai Y, Ito K, et al. Pharmacological management of chronic low back pain in older patients: a randomized controlled trial of the effect of pregabalin and opioid administration. *Eur Spine J*. 2015;24(6):1309–1317.
36. Kepler C. Epidural injections with glucocorticoid and lidocaine for spinal stenosis did not confer additional benefit compared with lidocaine alone. *J Bone Joint Surg Am*. 2015;97(4):342.
37. Manchikanti L, Kaye AD, Manchikani L, et al. Efficacy of epidural injections in the treatment of lumbar central spinal stenosis: a systematic review. *Anesth Pain Med*. 2015;5(1):e23139.
38. Manchikanti L, Cash KA, McManus CD, et al. A randomized, double-blind controlled trial of lumbar interlaminar epidural injections in central spinal stenosis: 2-year follow-up. *Pain Physician*. 2015;18(1):79–92.
39. Even JL, Crosby CG, Song Y, et al. Effects of epidural steroid injections on blood glucose levels in patients with diabetes mellitus. *Spine (Phila Pa 1976)*. 2012;37(1):E46–E50.

40. Turner JA, Ersek M, Herron L, et al. Surgery for lumbar spinal stenosis. Attempted meta-analysis of the literature. *Spine (Phila Pa 1976)*. 1992;17(1):1–8.
41. Kaloostian P, Gokaslan Z. Surgical versus non-surgical management of lumbar spinal stenosis. *Curr Rehabil Phys Med Rep*. 2013;1:169–173.
42. Lauryssen C, Jackson RJ, Baron JM, et al. Stand-alone interspinous spacer versus decompressive laminectomy for treatment of lumbar spinal stenosis. *Expert Rev Med Devices*. 2015;12(6):763–769.
43. Wu AM, Zhou Y, Li Q-L, et al. Interspinous spacer versus traditional decompressive surgery for lumbar spinal stenosis: a systematic review and meta-analysis. *PLoS One*. 2014;9(5):e97142.
44. Linderoth B, Foreman RD. Physiology of spinal cord stimulation: review and update. *Neuromodulation*. 1999;2(3):150–164.
45. Burchiel KJ, Anderson VC, Brown FD, et al. Prospective, multicenter study of spinal cord stimulation for relief of chronic back and extremity pain. *Spine (Phila Pa 1976)*. 1996;21(23):2786–2794.
46. Turner JA, Loeser JD, Bell KG. Spinal cord stimulation for chronic low back pain: a systematic literature synthesis. *Neurosurgery*. 1995;37(6):1088–1095; discussion 1095–1096.
47. Taylor RS, Van Buyten JP, Buchser E. Spinal cord stimulation for chronic back and leg pain and failed back surgery syndrome: a systematic review and analysis of prognostic factors. *Spine (Phila Pa 1976)*. 2005;30(1):152–160.
48. North RB, Ewend MD, Lawton MT, et al. Failed back surgery syndrome: 5-year follow-up after spinal cord stimulator implantation. *Neurosurgery*. 1991;28(5):692–699.
49. Caraway D, Walker V, Becker L, et al. Successful discontinuation of systemic opioids after implantation of an intrathecal drug delivery system. *Neuromodulation*. 2015;18(6):508–515; discussion 515–516.

REVIEW QUESTIONS

1. A 63-year-old male with history of osteoporosis slipped on the ice and landed on his buttocks. He complains of persistent pain in the middle of his lower back. On physical exam, he reports severe midline tenderness to palpation. The most likely etiology is:

A. Sacroiliac joint pain
B. Spinal stenosis
C. Vertebral compression fracture
D. Posterior disk bulge

2. A 58-year-old female with a history of hypertension presents in clinic; she has complaints of lower back pain when completing household chores, cooking, or when bending for vacuuming or twisting at the waist, and she has needed to hire a homemaker. She has no bowel or bladder complaints. On the exam she has full strength and normal sensation and reflexes, as well as a negative straight leg test. What is the confirmatory diagnostic imaging test best suited for her condition?

A. MRI of the spine
B. Plain radiographs of the lumbar spine
C. CT
D. X-ray

3. An 82-year-old male presents with more than a 3-year history of moderate to severe low back pain radiating in the right buttock after walking. Pain is relieved after lying down and while resting in the bed despite a regular NSAID regimen. The patient does not have night sweats, chills, or fever. What is the next step in the patient's pain management?

A. Physical therapy
B. Hip and pelvis radiographs
C. Plain radiographs of the lumbar spine
D. Epidural steroid injections

ANSWERS

1. C. A history of osteoporosis and the presence of midline tenderness to palpation make vertebral compression fracture (VCF) the most probable diagnosis. While sacroiliac joint (SIJ) pain is a common complaint, the patient would have tenderness at the SIJs on physical exam, and a FABER (flexion, abduction, external rotation) test would be positive (A is incorrect). Answer B is incorrect, because spinal stenosis is characterized by lower back pain radiating down to the posterior thighs and is increased with extension of the spine. None of these is present in this patient. Similarly, D is not correct because a herniated disk would most likely lead to radiating pain, sometimes all the way to the toes. It is aggravated by forward flexion and actions that increase intra-abdominal pressure, such as coughing, sneezing, and defecation.

2. A. MRI has become a standard diagnostic imaging study in accurate visualization of the spinal bony structures and their relations to the surrounding soft tissue indicating any annular tears, edema, or nerve compression. All the other options have limited use, especially as an initial diagnostic measure, but may be utilized later as a confirmatory follow-up of the initiated treatment. However, whatever imaging studies are performed, the results have to be correlated with clinical presentation and physical exam results.

3. A. Corticosteroids can result in reduced bone density, increased risk of bone fracture, and immunosuppression. Hence, they are to be avoided as the initial approach to pain management in spinal stenosis, particularly in elderly patients, because epidural injections of a local anesthetic are not definitively proven to enhance pain reduction in patients with lumbar spinal stenosis. Their use should be considered after a documented failure of more conservative measures and then only if the patient is deemed not to be a reasonable candidate for surgery or neuromodulation.

QUESTIONS AND ANSWERS

This chapter has accompanying questions and answers that are available to subscribers as part of the Oxford eLearning platform. To access the questions, follow the link below, or go to http://oxfordmedicine.com/painmanagementreview.

23.

CHRONIC LOW BACK PAIN IN A YOUNG PATIENT

Nebojsa Nick Knezevic, Teresa M. Kusper, and Kenneth D. Candido

STEM CASE AND KEY QUESTIONS

A 25-year-old male athlete presented to a pain clinic with a chief complaint of pain in the lumbar area radiating into the left buttock and left leg, exacerbated by lifting and twisting while reaching overhead. The pain started a few months ago after he slipped on a field during a sandlot football game. Upon presentation, the patient rated his pain as 9/10 on a numeric pain rating scale. He had been using topical creams and cooling patches, which provided only minimal relief. Three days before evaluation, the pain had worsened when the patient lifted his sports bag after football practice. Physical examination was remarkable for limited flexion during Adam's forward bend test, as well as the straight leg raising (SLR) test being positive for back pain on the left at 40°. Neurologic exam showed no deficits. His primary care physician ordered an MRI, which confirmed presence of an intervertebral disk herniation at the L4-L5 level and referred him for additional interventions.

HOW IS LOW BACK PAIN (LBP) DEFINED AND CATEGORIZED BASED ON SYMPTOM DURATION? BECAUSE THE PATIENT IS EAGER TO RETURN TO HIS USUAL ACTIVITIES INVOLVING COMPETITIVE SPORTS, HOW WOULD YOU EXPLAIN TO HIM THE CONDITION HE IS SUFFERING FROM?

In discussing his problem with the patient, you inform him that he suffers from LBP, a condition that is defined as pain, spasm, stiffness, or tension localized below the costal margin and above the inferior gluteal folds, and which can emanate from various structures of the lumbar or sacral spine. Certain characteristics of the pain can offer a clue to an underlying pathology and can aid in selecting an effective treatment strategy. Acute pain occurs suddenly and lasts < 4 weeks. Subacute pain ranges from 4 to 12 weeks and has a propensity to transform into longstanding back pain. Chronic low back pain (CLBP) is defined as pain that persists for more than 3 months from its onset. It can be constant and unrelenting, or it may consist of multiple recurrent episodes separated in time. Management varies based on the chronicity of the pain. Most frequently, the pain is nonspecific, without an underlying pathology, and tends to improve within a few weeks with conservative management. At other times, the pain can be triggered by structural abnormalities, or by other serious pathologies requiring approaches that are more aggressive.

WHAT ARE THE MOST COMMON ETIOLOGIES OF CLBP? WHAT IS THE MOST LIKELY DIAGNOSIS IN THIS PATIENT? WHICH INFORMATION PROVIDED ALLOWS NARROWING DOWN THE DIFFERENTIAL DIAGNOSIS?

The differential diagnosis of CLBP includes three broad categories of causes: mechanical, nonmechanical, and visceral. Mechanical causes include discogenic pain, strains and sprains, disk herniations, spondylosis, facet arthropathy, spondylolisthesis, spondylolysis, foraminal or spinal stenosis, fractures, and congenital derangements, such as kyphosis, scoliosis, and spina bifida. Nonmechanical causes encompass inflammatory arthritic conditions, infections, neoplastic disease, Scheuermann disease (osteochondrosis), and Paget's disease. The final category is pain referred from visceral structures: gastrointestinal, renal, pelvic, and vascular sources. In this patient, the presence of an identifiable inciting event permits ruling out nonmechanical and visceral causes of the back pain. Additionally, restriction of forward flexion on physical exam and presence of positive diagnostic maneuvers (SLR test) point to a mechanical etiology, most likely disk herniation causing nerve root impingement.

IS IMMEDIATE IMAGING INDICATED IN PATIENTS WITH CLBP? IS IT NECESSARY FOR THIS PATIENT?

In a majority of cases, imaging is not required for patients with acute LBP. Immediate MRI or CT is indicated for patients with neurologic deficits or for those exhibiting symptoms consistent with spinal cord compression, including cauda equina syndrome (LBP, radiculopathy, saddle anesthesia, urinary retention, atonic anal sphincter, decreased or absent reflexes) or conus medullaris syndrome (symptoms similar to cauda equina, except more likely bilateral, normal/increased anal tone, and preserved bulbocavernosus reflex). Imaging is also indicated for patients presenting with signs of spinal infection or vertebral compression fracture, and for individuals with night sweats, unintentional weight loss, or nocturnal back pain, because these symptoms frequently herald a neoplastic process. This patient could be diagnosed clinically based on his presentation and physical exam. An appropriate plan of management can be instituted in his case without the necessity of obtaining diagnostic imaging.

DESCRIBE THE SIGNIFICANCE OF THE SLR TEST. WHAT OTHER MANEUVERS CAN BE USED TO AID IN DIAGNOSING A HERNIATED INTERVERTEBRAL DISK?

The SLR test is performed to evaluate for sciatic nerve stretch and compression. The patient lies supine, and the physician places one hand under the heel of the extremity to be tested, and the other hand on the anterior aspect of the knee in order to keep the leg in the extended position. The examiner then lifts the leg while flexing the hip. Patients commonly report pain during this maneuver, which most often is due to hamstring tightness rather than compression of the sciatic nerve. In order to avoid false-positive results, the physician should lower the leg just enough for the pain to go away and then she or he should dorsiflex the foot. This maneuver is called Braggard's test; pain radiating down the leg results from sciatic nerve pulling upon dorsiflexion and the test is very sensitive and positive for sciatic nerve compression. Nerve root tension between 30° and 70° of hip flexion is considered a positive finding (normal hip flexion is 70° to 80°).

WHAT TREATMENT APPROACH WOULD MOST BENEFIT THIS PATIENT?

Initially, conservative treatment, consisting of nonsteroidal anti-inflammatory drugs (NSAIDs) for mild to moderate pain, should be undertaken, in accordance with the World Health Organization (WHO) stepwise approach to pain management. Opioid analgesics are not usually recommended as a first-line option; however, they can be prescribed in cases of severe pain. Bed rest is not recommended, whereas physical therapy with a focus on spinal stabilization, flexibility, and strengthening exercises can be of great value. This patient had tried topical analgesics and cooling patches without much success. He may be started on a trial of oral medication and physical therapy, and he can then be re-evaluated in 1 month. If no improvement is noted, he might be a candidate for an epidural steroid injection.

DISCUSSION

EPIDEMIOLOGY AND RISK FACTORS IN YOUNGER PATIENTS

Prevalence of CLBP in pediatric patients ranges between 20% and 46% worldwide, and increases during childhood, reaching an adult level around the age of 18.[1] A number of anthropometric factors appear to be implicated in the emergence of chronic back pain in the pediatric population. Growth process, daily habits affecting posture and body mechanics, school-related and extracurricular activities, and traumatic events can all incite back pain in the pediatric population. A critical time of growth between 11 and 14 years of age predicts the onset of LBP before the age of 22.[2] The literature shows that a significant portion of spinal ailments stem from participation in athletic activities. Back pain has been reported in 50% to 80% of older adolescent athletes participating in wrestling, gymnastics, soccer, and tennis.[3] Kurgansky et al. supplied detailed epidemiologic data that shed light on the top diagnoses and etiologies of CLBP and/or radiculopathy in a young population referred for epidural steroid injections (Table 23.1).[4]

Although the vast majority of the spinal problems are acquired, juvenile degenerative disease appears to be the underlying culprit in a small portion of the pediatric population.[5] It also appears that disk disease correlates with recurrences of LBP in young people at an older age.[6]

The prevalence of CLBP in the young adult population varies with age (Table 23.2),[5,7–15] but according to the literature might range between 4% and 47.7%.[16,17]

Discogenic LBP is more common in younger patients, while CLBP due to zygapophyseal and sacroiliac joints predominates in older adults.[9] However, the sacroiliac joint (SIJ) is a well-recognized source of CLBP in younger patients. The pain emanating from the SIJ can be precipitated by traumatic events or it can be triggered by sports-related injuries as part of complex sprains.[12] Vining et al. reviewed radiographic images of 247 individuals suffering from CLBP and provided specific information regarding the most common etiology for the chronic back pain as well as within-age-group comparison of the prevalence for the specific etiology.[15] The study reveals that degenerative disk disease and degenerative spondylolisthesis are more prevalent in individuals more than 40 years old.[15] As evidenced by the reports discussed, age-related, work-related, and traumatic events constitute the vast majority of the causes for LBP in young adults.

DIAGNOSIS

Workup of any back pain complaint should commence with a detailed inquiry about the patient's medical history, with a primary focus on the circumstances surrounding the onset of the symptoms. Special attention must be given to sitting and ambulation habits, posture, and existence of confounding comorbidities. Presence or absence of specific associated symptoms will influence the choice of the diagnostic and therapeutic modalities. Any suspicious symptoms indicative of an infectious, malignant, or neurologic process require prompt diagnostic workup and appropriate medical or surgical intervention. Detailed evaluation with physical exam concentrating on the assessment of posture, gait, weight bearing, and contours of the spinal curvatures, palpation and percussion of the musculoskeletal components, and body mechanics may elicit critical findings sufficient for accurate diagnosis and appropriate treatment. Generally, pediatric patients warrant earlier

Table 23.1. **CHARACTERISTICS OF PATIENTS* 9 TO 20 YEARS OLD WITH CLBP AND/OR RADICULOPATHY REFERRED FOR EPIDURAL STEROID INJECTIONS**

ETIOLOGY OF PAIN	REFERRING DIAGNOSIS	SPORTS INVOLVED IN THE PAIN

• Traumatic events (22%)
• Sports-related injuries (68.8%)
• Motor vehicle accidents (10.4)
• Falls not related to sports (8.3%)
	• Disk herniation alone (60.7%)
	• Disk herniation in combination with other spinal diagnosis (31.9%)
	• Spinal diagnoses (with or without disk herniation):
	  • Spondylolysis (11.4%)
	  • Scoliosis (10.5%)
	  • Facet joint pain (10.0%)
	  • Spondylolisthesis (8.3%)
	  • Transitional vertebra (7.0%)
	  • Spinal canal stenosis (3.9%)
	  • Schmorl's nodes (3.1%)
	  • Sacroiliac joint pain (3.1%)
	  • Spina bifida (2.6%)
	  • Spinal cord tethering (1.3%)
	  • Arachnoiditis (1.3%)
		• Basketball (23.0%)
		• Baseball or softball (16.8%)
		• Soccer (16.2%)
		• Lacrosse (10.6%)
		• Football (9.9%)
		• Dance (7.5%)
		• Cheerleading (7.5%)
		• Track and field (7.5%)
		• Field hockey (6.8%)
		• Swimming (6.2%)
		• Volleyball (6.2%)

*N = 224; athletes = 161; median duration of symptoms = 9 months.

Modified from Kurgansky et al.[4]

imaging than the adults, after 3 weeks of persistent back pain in absence of any suspicious symptoms (Figure 23.1).[3]

TREATMENT

Nonpharmacologic Management

A number of psychologic and physical modalities can be utilized for the management of back pain and other pain syndromes. Physical therapy, osteopathic or chiropractic spinal manipulations, and acupuncture are frequently employed alone or in combination with other treatment options. Physical therapy is used to increase back and hip range of motion and core stability and to strengthen lumbar musculature, and it is one of the essential components of the multidisciplinary approach.[1] Osteopathic and chiropractic manipulative therapeutic options are still poorly understood, and limited insight is offered by a handful of available scientific studies.[18,19] Bronfort et al. showed that either supervised trunk exercise, home exercise, or chiropractic spinal manipulation in patients 18 to 65 years old with CLBP improved pain and reduced the patients' medication use after 12 weeks of therapy.[20] Acupuncture is widely employed to alleviate a variety of chronic pain syndromes, especially when used concomitantly with other forms of treatment.

Pharmacologic Management

NSAIDs are the cornerstone of the initial approach to pain management, and they are usually used before other treatment modalities are attempted. The effectiveness of nonselective NSAIDs in reducing pain intensity and disability due to chronic nonspecific LBP has been demonstrated by six out of 13 randomized controlled trials (RCTs) included in a Cochrane review.[21] Similarly, a beneficial response in terms of pain reduction and global improvement was described in various reports on selective COX-2 inhibitors in CLBP patients.[21,22] Celecoxib provided superior benefit to acetaminophen[23] and tramadol in RCTs.[24]

Although opioids are widely accepted medications for acute and chronic pain syndromes, their use is associated with questionable efficacy and dubious long-term outcomes in chronic back pain syndromes. Opioids are also associated with numerous adverse effects, the most notable being constipation (41%), nausea (32%), and somnolence (29%).[25] Moreover, given the inherent abuse, addiction, tolerance, and dependence potential, narcotics ought to be prescribed cautiously and only when benefits outweigh the risks and/or other treatment options have been exhausted.

Muscle relaxants are prescribed to treat a number of painful musculoskeletal disorders, including back pain, neck pain, fibromyalgia, and myofascial pain syndrome. The goal of such treatment is to ameliorate pain by diminishing muscle spasticity. Antispasmodics accounted for 18.5% of all prescriptions written for back pain in 2000, with cyclobenzaprine, carisoprodol, and methocarbamol being the most commonly used.[26] Strong evidence exists in support of short-term use of nonbenzodiazepine and benzodiazepine muscle relaxants for nonspecific LBP.[27–29] Cyclobenzaprine is the most widely investigated muscle relaxant, and its efficacy for LBP has been demonstrated by several independent studies; however, the majority of the studies pertain to acute LBP.[29–31]

Antiepileptic drugs include a broad group of agents, such as phenytoin, valproic acid, carbamazepine, topiramate, lamotrigine, tiagabine, pregabalin, and gabapentin. Pregabalin has been extensively studied and has shown that can alleviate neuropathic pain in chronic lumbosacral radiculopathy.[32,33] According to the available evidence, no differences in effectiveness have been found between pregabalin and opioids[34] and pregabalin and amitriptyline.[35]

Antidepressants are used as adjunctive pharmacologic agents, and they are thought to reduce the experience of pain

Table 23.2. PREVALENCE AND ETIOLOGY OF CHRONIC BACK PAIN BY AGE GROUP

ETIOLOGY	AGE (YEARS)	PREVALENCE (%)	PARTICIPANTS	STUDY
Facet arthrosis	1. 18–30 2. 31–40 3. 41–50 4. 51–60 5. 61–70	1. 28 2. 18 3. 28 4. 44 5. 21	303 patients with chronic nonspecific (not radicular) lumbar back pain of > 6 months, ages 18–90 years	Retrospective analysis[10]
1. Disk bulge 2. Disk herniation 3. Disk degeneration 4. Modic change 5. Facet osteoarthritis 6. Central canal stenosis 7. Anterolisthesis 8. Retrolisthesis 9. Lumbar interspinous bursitis (Baastrup disease)	7–89 (mean age 44)	1. 64.9 2. 39.9 3. 50.6 4. 27.8 5. 53.1 6. 9.3 7. 14.7 8. 5.9 9. 8.2	539 consecutive patients (51% males, 49% females undergoing lumbar MRI for lumbago or sciatica)	Retrospective analysis[13]
Axial spondyloarthritis	20–45 (mean age 36.3)	24	364 primary care patients (57% women, 43% men) with CLBP; median duration of 9.0 years	Cross-sectional study[14]
1. Discogenic pain 2. Sacroiliac joint pain 3. Facet joint pain	Mean age 42.5	1. 56.6 2. 26 3. 19	27 patients (78% women) with CLBP due to motor vehicle collisions; mean duration of symptoms 24 months	Chart review[8]
1. Disk degeneration 2. Isthmic spondylolisthesis 3. Degenerative spondylolisthesis 4. Lumbosacral transitional segments	21–65 (mean age 44.8)	1. 49 2. 5 3. 18 4. 14	247 patients with CLBP > 12 weeks; 91% participants with CLBP > 12 months	Retrospective study[15]
Sacroiliac joint syndrome due to: 1. Traumatic event (motor vehicle collision, falls onto the buttocks, postpartum, football, pelvic fracture) 2. Cumulative injury (lifting, running) 3. Idiopathic	30–76 (mean age 48.2)	1. 44 2. 21 3. 35	54 patients (59.3% women, 40.7% men) with low back or buttock pain diagnosed with sacroiliac joint syndrome; syndrome duration averaging 20.6 months	Retrospective descriptive cohort study[12]
1. Intervertebral disk 2. Lumbar facet joints 3. Sacroiliac joints 4. Vertebral fracture 5. Pelvic fracture 6. Baastrup disease 7. Fusion hardware	Mean age: 1. 43.7 2. 59.6 3. 61.4 4. 79.0 5. 71.3 6. 75.3 7. 59.6	1. 41.8 2. 30.6 3. 18.2 4. 2.9 5. 1.8 6. 1.8 7. 2.9	156 patients with CLBP; mean duration 12 months	Chart review[9]
Discogenic pain	Median age 36.7	39	92 consecutive patients (61 men and 31 women) with CLBP who underwent discography; median duration of pain 18.5 months	Cross-sectional study[7]
1. Facet joint pain 2. Discogenic pain 3. Sacroiliac pain	Mean age 47.5 (107 patients < 65 years old)	1. 40 2. 26 3. 2	120 randomly selected patients (79 women, 41 men) with CLBP; mean duration 9.1 years	Prospective randomized study[11]
Degenerative disk disease	< 21 (mean age 17.1)	76 patients	1,877 patients with CLBP	Retrospective chart review[5]

Table created using references 5 and 7 to 15 as scholarly sources.

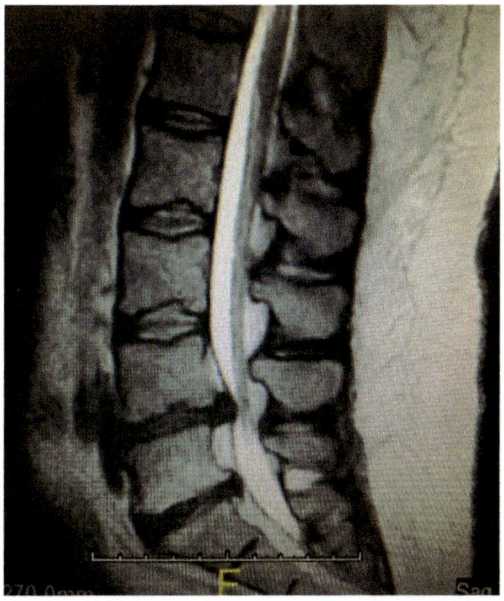

Figure 23.1. MRI of lumbar disk herniation at L4-L5 and L5-S1 levels.

by modulation of the descending pain inhibitory pathways. By treating insomnia and depressive symptoms, the drugs alter perception of pain, but these benefits must be weighed against possible adverse effects, such as constipation, drowsiness, dry mouth, and dizziness.[36] Tricyclic antidepressants show great promise in alleviating pain syndromes, especially pain with neuropathic components. Success in relieving chronic back and leg pain was demonstrated by separate investigators.[35,37] Favorable treatment outcomes in patients with CLBP on serotonin-norepinephrine reuptake inhibitor (SNRI) therapy were found in two separate RCTs.[38,39] However, an analysis of 15 studies comparing duloxetine to other medications (NSAIDs, COX-2 inhibitors, opioids, SSRIs) shows comparable efficacy between duloxetine and the other pharmacologic agents used in CLBP.[40]

Interventional Pain Management

Epidural steroid injections (ESI) are the most commonly utilized interventional modality for a broad range of clinical diagnoses (Figure 23.2).

Increased use of ESI is illustrated in different reports.[41,42] Sciatica, radiculopathy, and herniated disk account for 41% of the injections, while axial LBP accounts for 36%, and spinal stenosis for 23%.[41] The proposed mechanism of action of the steroid injection is the reduction of inflammation around the nerve roots caused by the chemicals liberated from the diseased intervertebral disks and leaking nucleus pulposus material.[43] Additionally, steroids appear to have antinociceptive[44] and swelling-reducing properties.[45] The injections are most often recommended to patients with radicular pain, dermatomal pain distribution, and neurologic symptoms of 1 to 12 months' duration.[46] The literature shows conflicting evidence for, and discordant conclusions about, the effectiveness of interlaminar, transforaminal, and caudal epidural steroid injections. Three different approaches to epidural injection are available in clinical practice: steroid with sodium chloride solution, steroid with local anesthetic, or local anesthetic alone. A recent comparative systematic review and meta-analysis assessing the efficacy of interlaminar, transforaminal, and caudal ESI for LBP due to lumbar radiculopathy and spinal stenosis evaluated 39 different trials with a cumulative total of 4,794 patients.[47] The review demonstrated significant efficacy of injections consisting of lidocaine alone or steroid combined with lidocaine solution in reducing pain and improving function in patients with CLBP.[47]

The procedures included in facet joint interventions category include intra-articular steroid injections, medial branch blocks, and radiofrequency ablation of medial branches (Figure 23.3). These techniques are indicated for treatment of facet arthropathy or facet joint syndrome. They can be used in young adults or the pediatric population in the presence of axial CLBP incurred during sports and with a clinical picture consistent with facet joint sprain. In the older adult population, utilization of facet joint injections in Medicare beneficiaries between 2000 and 2012 increased by 11% per year for lumbosacral injections and by 15% for cervicothoracic injections.[48] Manchikanti et al. performed a systematic review of 21 RCTs examining the effectiveness of facet joint injections and found level 2 evidence for lumbar facet injections and level 3 evidence for lumbosacral facet injections.[49]

Therapeutic sacroiliac joint (SIJ) interventions include intra-articular steroid injection, periarticular application of local anesthetic and steroid, and pulsed or cooled radiofrequency neurotomy. A systematic review of 11 studies with a total number of patients ranging from 20 to 155 was conducted to assess the effectiveness of these interventions.[50] The results indicate fair evidence of effectiveness for the cooled radiofrequency ablation procedure, and limited evidence for intra-articular and periarticular injections and pulsed RFA interventions.[50]

In younger adults in whom a conservative regimen fail to improve pain in suspected sports-related sprains, intra-articular or periarticular injections may offer short-term pain relief, sometimes enough for patients to enroll in physical therapy and stretching exercises essential for long-term relief.

Trigger-point injections are used to relieve myofascial pain by injecting a medication or combination of different agents, such as local anesthetic and steroid, local anesthetic with steroid and opioid, or botulinum toxin A into several separate points in specific muscles or muscle groups. Trigger points can also be treated with the dry needling technique.

Surgical Interventions

Surgery is usually reserved for cases of protracted back pain not responding to conservative treatments or for LBP accompanied by evidence of bowel and/or bladder dysfunction, cauda equina syndrome, or worsening neurologic deficits. The choice of a specific surgical approach depends on the pathology contributing to LBP. Lumbar spine fusion is recommended for patients with intractable LBP due to degenerative disk disease who fail nonoperative management, although the available literature indicates long-term benefit is largely questionable.[51,52] Open diskectomy and

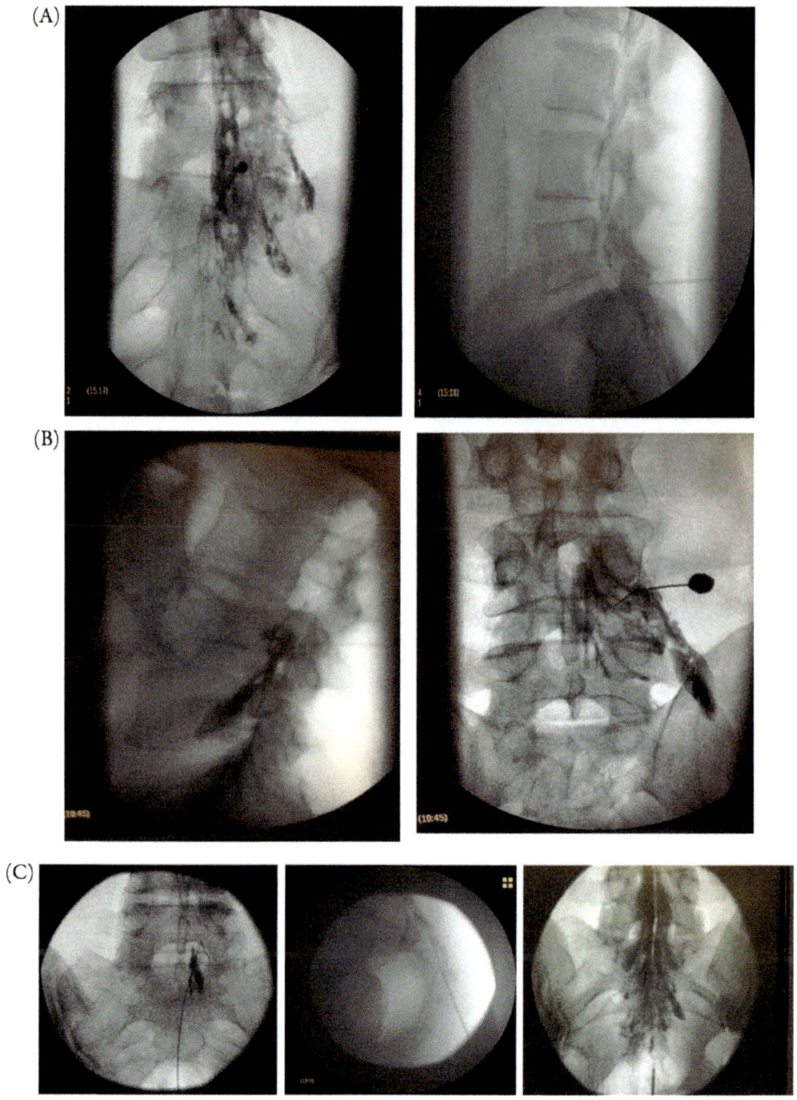

Figure 23.2. X-ray fluoroscopic images of (A) Interlaminar epidural steroid injections (IL- LESI) parasagittal approach, (B) Transforaminal epidural steroid injections (TF-ESI), and (C) Caudal epidural steroid injections.

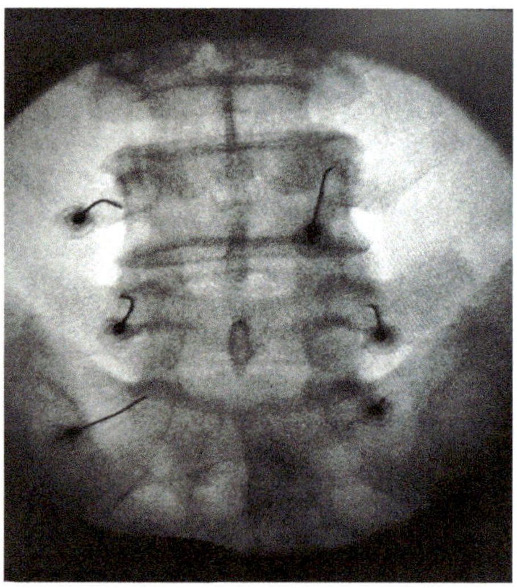

Figure 23.3. Radiographic image of lumbar medial branch block of L3-L4, L4-L5, and L5-sacral ala.

microdiskectomy are utilized for herniated disk with radicular extremity pain.[53,54]

CONCLUSIONS

- CLBP is a common complaint across different age groups.
- Etiology varies among pediatric, adolescent, and adult patients.
- Patient history is a critical element of the assessment.
- Not all back pain requires imaging, but imaging should not be postponed in cases with suspected neurologic damage, infection, or metastatic disease.
- Treatment options include nonpharmacologic management, conservative treatment with medications, interventional techniques and surgical interventions.

REFERENCES

1. Landry BW, Fisher PR, Driwscoll SW, et al. Managing chronic pain in children and adolescents: a clinical review. *PMR.* 2015;7(11 suppl):S295–S315.
2. Poussa MS, Heliovaara MM, Seitsamo JT, et al. Anthropometric measurements and growth as predictors of low-back pain: a cohort study of children followed up from the age of 11 to 22 years. *Eur Spine J.* 2005;14(6):595–598.
3. Waicus KM, Smith BW. Back injuries in the pediatric athlete. *Curr Sports Med Rep.* 2002;1(1):52–58.
4. Kurgansky KE, Rodriguez ST, Kralj MS, et al. Epidural steroid injections for radiculopathy and/or back pain in children and adolescents: a retrospective cohort study with a prospective follow-up. *Reg Anesth Pain Med.* 2016;41(1):86–92.
5. Dimar JR II, Glassman SD, Carreon LY. Juvenile degenerative disc disease: a report of 76 cases identified by magnetic resonance imaging. *Spine J.* 2007;7(3):332–337.
6. Salminen JJ, Erkintalo MO, Pentii J, et al. Recurrent low back pain and early disc degeneration in the young. *Spine (Phila Pa 1976).* 1999;24(13):1316–1321.
7. Schwarzer AC, April CN, Derby R, et al. The prevalence and clinical features of internal disc disruption in patients with chronic low back pain. *Spine (Phila Pa 1976).* 1995;20(17):1878–1883.
8. DePalma M, Ketchum J, Saullo T, et al. Structural etiology of chronic low back pain due to motor vehicle collision. *Pain Med.* 2011;12(11):1622–1627.
9. DePalma MJ, Ketchum JM, Saullo T. What is the source of chronic low back pain and does age play a role? *Pain Med.* 2011;12(2):224–233.
10. Manchikanti L, Manchikanti KN, Cash KA, et al. Age-related prevalence of facet-joint involvement in chronic neck and low back pain. *Pain Physician.* 2008;11(1):67–75.
11. Manchikanti L, Singh V, Pampati V, et al. Evaluation of the relative contributions of various structures in chronic low back pain. *Pain Physician.* 2001;4(4):308–316.
12. Chou LH, Slipman CW, Bhagia SM, et al. Inciting events initiating injection-proven sacroiliac joint syndrome. *Pain Med.* 2004;5(1):26–32.
13. Maes R, Morrison WB, Parker L, Schweitzer ME, Carrino JA. Lumbar interspinous bursitis (Baastrup disease) in a symptomatic population. *Spine (Phila Pa 1976).* 2008;33(7):E211–E215.
14. Van Hoeven L, Luime J, Han H, Vergouwe Y, Weel A. Identifying axial spondyloarthritis in Dutch primary care patients, ages 20–45 years, with chronic low back pain. *Arthritis Care Res.* 2014;66(3):446–453.
15. Vining RD, Potocki E, McLean I, et al. Prevalence of radiographic findings in individuals with chronic low back pain screened for a randomized controlled trial: secondary analysis and clinical implications. *J Manipulative Physiol Ther.* 2014;37(9):678–687.
16. Mallen C, Peat G, Thomas E, et al. Severely disabling chronic pain in young adults: prevalence from a population-based postal survey in North Staffordshire. *BMC Musculoskelet Disord.* 2005;6:42.
17. Campbell P, Forster NE, Thomas E, et al. Prognostic indicators of low back pain in primary care: five-year prospective study. *J Pain.* 2013;14(8):873–883.
18. Licciardone JC, Gatchel RJ, Aryal S. Recovery from chronic low back pain after osteopathic manipulative treatment: a randomized controlled trial. *J Am Osteopath Assoc.* 2016;116(3):144–155.
19. Licciardone JC, Gatchel RJ, Aryal S. Targeting patient subgroups with chronic low back pain for osteopathic manipulative treatment: responder analyses from a randomized controlled trial. *J Am Osteopath Assoc.* 2016;116(3):156–168.
20. Bronfort G, Maiers MJ, Evans RI, et al. Supervised exercise, spinal manipulation, and home exercise for chronic low back pain: a randomized clinical trial. *Spine J.* 2011;11(7):585–598.
21. Enthoven WT, Roelofs PD, Deyo RA, et al. Non-steroidal anti-inflammatory drugs for chronic low back pain. *Cochrane Database Syst Rev.* 2016;2:CD012087.
22. Chung JW, Zeng Y, Wong TK. Drug therapy for the treatment of chronic nonspecific low back pain: systematic review and meta-analysis. *Pain Physician.* 2013;16(6):E685–E704.
23. Bedaiwi MK, Sari I, Wallis D, et al. Clinical efficacy of Celecoxib compared to acetaminophen in chronic nonspecific low back pain: results of a randomized controlled trial. *Arthritis Care Res.* 2016;68(6):845–852.
24. O'Donnell JB, Ekman, EF, Spalding WM, et al. The effectiveness of a weak opioid medication versus a cyclo-oxygenase-2 (COX-2) selective non-steroidal anti-inflammatory drug in treating flare-up of chronic low-back pain: results from two randomized, double-blind, 6-week studies. *J Int Med Res.* 2009;37(6):1789–1802.
25. Kalso E, Edwards JE, Moore RA, et al. Opioids in chronic non-cancer pain: systematic review of efficacy and safety. *Pain.* 2004;112(3):372–380.
26. Luo X, Pietrobon R, Curtis LH, et al. Prescription of nonsteroidal anti-inflammatory drugs and muscle relaxants for back pain in the United States. *Spine (Phila Pa 1976).* 2004;29(23):E531–E537.
27. van Tulder MW, Touray T, Furlan AD, et al. Muscle relaxants for nonspecific low back pain: a systematic review within the framework of the Cochrane collaboration. *Spine (Phila Pa 1976).* 2003;28(17):1978–1992.
28. Chou R, Peterson K, Helfand M. Comparative efficacy and safety of skeletal muscle relaxants for spasticity and musculoskeletal conditions: a systematic review. *J Pain Symptom Manag.* 2004;28(2):140–175.
29. Toth PP, Urtis J. Commonly used muscle relaxant therapies for acute low back pain: a review of carisoprodol, cyclobenzaprine hydrochloride, and metaxalone. *Clin Ther.* 2004;26(9):1355–1367.
30. Browning R, Jackson JL, O'Malley PG. Cyclobenzaprine and back pain: a meta-analysis. *Arch Intern Med.* 2001;161(13):1613–1620.
31. Brown BR Jr, Womble J. Cyclobenzaprine in intractable pain syndromes with muscle spasm. *JAMA.* 1978;240(11):1151–1152.
32. Baron R, Freynhagen R, Tolle TR, et al. The efficacy and safety of pregabalin in the treatment of neuropathic pain associated with chronic lumbosacral radiculopathy. *Pain.* 2010;150(3):420–427.
33. Saldana MT, Navarro A, Perez C, et al. Patient-reported outcomes in subjects with painful lumbar or cervical radiculopathy treated with pregabalin: evidence from medical practice in primary care settings. *Rheumatol Int.* 2010;30(8):1005–1015.
34. Sakai Y, Ito K, Hida T, et al. Pharmacological management of chronic low back pain in older patients: a randomized controlled trial of the effect of pregabalin and opioid administration. *Eur Spine J.* 2015;24(6):1309–1317.
35. Kalita J, Kohat AK, Misra UK, et al. An open labeled randomized controlled trial of pregabalin versus amitriptyline in chronic low backache. *J Neurol Sci.* 2014;342(1-2):127–132.
36. Salerno SM, Browning R, Jackson JL. The effect of antidepressant treatment on chronic back pain: a meta-analysis. *Arch Intern Med.* 2002;162(1):19–24.
37. Orbai AM, Meyerhoff JO. The effectiveness of tricyclic antidepressants on lumbar spinal stenosis. *Bull NYU Hosp Joint Dis.* 2010;68(1):22–24.
38. Skljarevski V, Zhang S, Desaiah D, et al. Duloxetine versus placebo in patients with chronic low back pain: a 12-week, fixed-dose, randomized, double-blind trial. *J Pain.* 2010;11(12):1282–1290.
39. Skljarevski V, Liu P, Zhang S, et al. Efficacy and safety of duloxetine in patients with chronic low back pain who used versus did not use concomitant nonsteroidal anti-inflammatory drugs or acetaminophen: a post hoc pooled analysis of 2 randomized, placebo-controlled trials. *Pain Res Treat.* 2012;2012:296710.
40. Cawston H, Davie A, Paget MA, et al. Efficacy of duloxetine versus alternative oral therapies: an indirect comparison of randomised clinical trials in chronic low back pain. *Eur Spine J.* 2013;22(9):1996–2009.
41. Friedly J, Chan L, Deyo R. Increases in lumbosacral injections in the Medicare population: 1994 to 2001. *Spine (Phila Pa 1976).* 2007;32(16):1754–1760.

42. Manchikanti L, Pampati V, Falco FJ, et al. Assessment of the growth of epidural injections in the Medicare population from 2000 to 2011. *Pain Physician.* 2013;16(4):E349–E364.
43. Bogduk N. Epidural steroids. *Spine (Phila Pa 1976).* 1995;20(7):845–848.
44. Johansson A, Hao J, Sjolund B. Local corticosteroid application blocks transmission in normal nociceptive C-fibres. *Acta Anaesthesiol Scand.* 1990;34(5):335–338.
45. Byrod G, Otani K, Brisby H, et al. Methylprednisolone reduces the early vascular permeability increase in spinal nerve roots induced by epidural nucleus pulposus application. *J Orthop Res.* 2000;18(6):983–987.
46. Fanciullo GJ, Hanscom B, Seville K, et al. An observational study of the frequency and pattern of use of epidural steroid injection in 25,479 patients with spinal and radicular pain. *Reg Anesth Pain Med.* 2001;26(1):5–11.
47. Manchikanti L, Knezevic NN, Boswell MV, et al. epidural injections for lumbar radiculopathy and spinal stenosis: a comparative systematic review and meta-analysis. *Pain Physician.* 2016;19(3):E365–E410.
48. Beckworth WJ, Jiang M, Hemingway J, et al. Facet injection trends in the Medicare population and the impact of bundling codes. *Spine J.* 2016;16(9):1037–1041.
49. Manchikanti L, Kaye AD, Boswell MV, et al. A systematic review and best evidence synthesis of the effectiveness of therapeutic facet joint interventions in managing chronic spinal pain. *Pain Physician.* 2015;18(4):E535–E582.
50. Hansen H, Manchikanti L, Simopoulos TT, et al. A systematic evaluation of the therapeutic effectiveness of sacroiliac joint interventions. *Pain Physician.* 2012;15(3):E247–E278.
51. Mannion AF, Brox JI, Fairbank JC. Comparison of spinal fusion and nonoperative treatment in patients with chronic low back pain: long-term follow-up of three randomized controlled trials. *Spine J.* 2013;13(11):1438–1448.
52. Froholdt A, Reikeraas O, Holm I, et al. No difference in 9-year outcome in CLBP patients randomized to lumbar fusion versus cognitive intervention and exercises. *Eur Spine J.* 2012;21(12): 2531–2538.
53. Veresciagina K, Spakauskas B, Ambrozaitis KV. Clinical outcomes of patients with lumbar disc herniation, selected for one-level open-discectomy and microdiscectomy. *Eur Spine J.* 2010;19(9):1450–1458.
54. Dewing CB, Provencher MT, Riffenburgh RH, et al. The outcomes of lumbar microdiscectomy in a young, active population: correlation by herniation type and level. *Spine (Phila Pa 1976).* 2008;33(1):33–38.
55. Chou R, Qaseem A, Owens DK, et al. Diagnostic imaging for low back pain: advice for high-value health care from the American College of Physicians. *Ann Intern Med.* 2011;154(3):181–189.
56. Bogduk N, Holmes S. Controlled zygapophysial joint blocks: the travesty of cost-effectiveness. *Pain Med.* 2000;1(1):24–34.
57. Cohen SP, Williams KA, Kurihara C, et al. Multicenter, randomized, comparative cost-effectiveness study comparing 0, 1, and 2 diagnostic medial branch (facet joint nerve) block treatment paradigms before lumbar facet radiofrequency denervation. *Anesthesiology.* 2010;113(2):395–405.
58. Kaspiris A, Grivas TB, Zafiropoulou C, et al. Nonspecific low back pain during childhood: a retrospective epidemiological study of risk factors. *J Clin Rheumatol.* 2010;16(2);55–60.

REVIEW QUESTIONS

Box 23.1. **PATIENT INFORMATION**

A 17-year-old athletic male presents to the clinic with a sudden onset of sharp LBP, which started 5 days earlier after he jumped up and twisted his back trying to throw a pass during a basketball game. The patient denies radicular leg pain, paresthesias, weakness in his lower extremities, and urinary and fecal incontinence. Bilateral paraspinal spasm and tenderness are noted on physical exam; otherwise, the examination is unremarkable. X-ray of the lumbar spine is unremarkable.

1. Refer to the patient in Box 23.1. Which of the following is the most likely diagnosis?

   A. Spondylolisthesis
   B. Acute lumbar strain
   C. Acute lumbar intervertebral disk herniation
   D. Spondylolysis

2. Refer to the patient in Box 23.1. Which of the following approaches would be indicated as an initial treatment for this patient?

   A. Bed rest for 1 week
   B. Ibuprofen and light physical activity
   C. Initiate cyclobenzaprine
   D. Trigger-point injections

3. Refer to the patient in Box 23.1. If the patient had decreased sensation on the medial aspect of the lower leg, absent patellar reflex, and impaired motor strength of knee extensors, what would be the most likely diagnosis?

   A. Herniated disk at L4-L5
   B. Compression of the lateral femoral cutaneous nerve
   C. Anterior spondylolisthesis of L5 on S1
   D. Tight piriform muscle

ANSWERS

1. B. An acute lumbar sprain causes LBP provoked by a strenuous activity, and that is usually well localized and without any neurologic deficits. Spondylolisthesis is a forward slippage of one vertebra in relation to the one below. Spondylolysis is a defect in the pars interarticularis of the neural arch, which appears as a collar around the neck of a Scottie dog on an oblique radiograph. Both would be evident

on radiographic imaging, which is negative in this patient, therefore Answers A and D are incorrect. Answer C is incorrect because herniated lumbar disk will often present as radiating pain associated with paresthesia and/or weakness, which are absent in this patient.

2. B. Ibuprofen and light physical therapy are the best initial approach to treatment of acute LBP.[20,21] Bed rest is not recommended. (Answer A is incorrect.) Answer C is incorrect because cyclobenzaprine might provide benefit for acute back pain with spasms,[29–31] but it is not a first-line option. Trigger-point injections are indicated for myofascial pain persisting despite conservative management. They would not be the initial step in the management of this patient. (Answer D is incorrect.)

3. A. Clinical evaluation and physical examination can significantly aid in establishing a positive diagnosis. However, in the pediatric population, imaging studies need to ordered after 3 weeks of persistent LBP.[3] When radicular symptoms occur in addition to LBP, clinical diagnosis is the main tool for establishing the diagnosis and designing treatment. Compression of the L4 nerve roots would manifest as sensory loss along the medial lower leg, weakness of the knee extensors, and diminished patellar tendon reflex. Compression of the lateral femoral cutaneous nerve (known as meralgia paresthetica) results in pain and paresthesias along the lateral aspect of the thigh. (Answer B is incorrect.) Spondylolisthesis of L5 on S1 may compress the L5 nerve root, which would result in sensory loss over the lateral calf, dorsum of the foot, and web space between the first and second toes. Also, there would be weakness of the knee flexors and not the extensors. (Answer C is incorrect.) Piriform muscle tightness can compress the sciatic nerve and trigger sciatic neuropathy, which is characterized by impairment of knee flexion and sensory loss below the knee except for the medial aspect of the lower leg. (Answer D is incorrect.)

QUESTIONS AND ANSWERS

This chapter has accompanying questions and answers that are available to subscribers as part of the Oxford eLearning platform. To access the questions, follow the link below, or go to ✔ http://oxfordmedicine.com/painmanagementreview

24.

POSTLAMINECTOMY SYNDROME

Kenneth D. Candido, Tatiana Tverdohleb, and Nebojsa Nick Knezevic

STEM CASE AND KEY QUESTIONS

A 56-year-old male with a history of chronic low back pain (CLBP) presented to the clinic with persistent pain after decompression L4-L5 laminectomy performed 3 months earlier. Before laminectomy, the patient complained of low back pain (LBP) with right-sided radicular symptoms for 4 years. His imaging studies revealed a 5-mm centrally bulging intervertebral disk at L4-L5, hypertrophy of the facet joints, and hypertrophied ligamentum flavum at the L4–L5 level, which caused a trefoil deformity and narrowing of the spinal canal with bilateral L4-L5 nerve root impingement at the neuroforamina.

The patient failed conservative therapy that consisted of use of pain medications from different therapeutic classes (oxycodone 5 mg q8h, naproxen 500 mg q12h, pregabalin 225 mg q24h, duloxetine 40 mg q24h). Also, he did not respond to physical therapy measures, and two epidural steroid injections provided short-term pain relief (VAS score at baseline was 8/10 and went down to 6/10 after the injections, for 2 weeks each time). After these measures failed to produce sustainable pain relief, the patient agreed to proceed with spinal surgery. As stated, his LBP persisted after spinal surgery with no change (VAS score remained 8/10).

WHAT IS POSTLAMINECTOMY SYNDROME AND WHAT SHOULD BE CONSIDERED IN THE DIFFERENTIAL DIAGNOSIS? HOW WOULD YOU EXPLAIN TO THE PATIENT THE FACT THAT HIS PAIN PERSISTED AFTER THE SURGERY?

Postlaminectomy syndrome (PLS) is defined as persistent or recurrent LBP after otherwise anatomically successful lumbar spine surgery. In this case, the patient reported persistent LBP following decompression laminectomy spine surgery with minimal to no change in the pain intensity. His physical examination revealed increased stiffness of the low back paraspinal muscles and midline lumbar pain with positive radicular symptoms. The spinal radiography did not detect any bone spurs or bone misalignments, any thecal sac abnormalities, or any other non-back-related pathologies, essentially showing successful anatomic spine decompression. In the absence of any anatomic pathology and in the presence of continued 8/10 pain, similar to the patient's presurgical value, the patient was diagnosed with PLS.

WHAT IS THE NEXT STEP IN PLS MANAGEMENT? HOW WOULD YOU EXPLAIN THE NEXT TREATMENT STEPS TO THE PATIENT?

Currently there are no published, established, and accepted guidelines for the management of PLS. Therefore, after excluding other factors in the potential etiology of LBP (i.e., surgical complications, such as inflammation, epidural edema, and red flags like abdominal aortic aneurysm rupture, neoplasm, infection), treatment can be started with pharmacologic therapy and with a physical rehabilitation program. Also, diagnostic and therapeutic interventions, such as medial branch blocks and nerve root blocks, can help distinguish the source of the pain and provide pain relief at the same time. The patient in this case had undergone pharmacologic therapy (oxycodone 5 mg q8h, naproxen 500 mg q12h, pregabalin 225 mg q24h, duloxetine 40 mg q24h) in combination with epidural steroid injections and lumbar medial branch blocks after surgery with minimal pain improvement (VAS score reduced from 8/10 to 6/10).

IS ADDITIONAL REVISION SURGICAL MANAGEMENT APPROPRIATE FOR THE PATIENT?

After pharmacologic and interventional management failed to improve the patient's pain and functionality, and a reoperation process was excluded due to the patient's refusal to consider that option, the clinicians decided to proceed with a spinal cord stimulation (SCS) trial. The patient reported outstanding relief of his pain and improved functionality (> 75% pain relief, reduction in medication consumption by 50%, improved tolerance for ambulation and sitting). After a 1-week trial, SCS was discontinued and 4 additional weeks were allowed to pass to permit wound healing, then a permanent spinal cord stimulator (SCS) with two leads was implanted, with more than 90% improvement in the patient's pain. At the 1-year follow-up, the patient had the same level of pain (1/10) and he had returned to work and to his social activities and hobbies with few restrictions concerning the SCS, which had been reprogrammed twice during that period.

WHAT SHOULD HAVE BEEN DONE FOR THE PATIENT TO PREVENT PLS?

In order to prevent PLS, we need to consider the risk factors that are manageable before, during, and after decompressive laminectomy. One of the most common preoperative risk factors is miscommunication and/or misinterpretation of the surgery goals by the patient, which can lead to higher procedural expectations than are commensurate with reality. In particular, surgeons may overstate the success rates and minimize the failure rates of these types of procedures, whether intentionally or unintentionally. In the case presented here, is still unclear what risk factors might have contributed to the persistence of the pain.

It is strongly recommended that the surgeon prevent and recognize the risk factors at every stage, including pre-, intra-, and postoperative risk factors.

DISCUSSION

Postlaminectomy syndrome (PLS) is commonly referred to as failed back surgery syndrome (FBSS), rebound radicular syndrome, postoperative persistent syndrome, or post-lumbar-surgery syndrome and is defined as persistent or recurrent back pain after otherwise anatomically successful lumbar spine surgery (Figure 24.1).[1–7] The definition implies that persistent or recurrent chronic back pain is a result of a functional failure of the back to respond to the intervention, as opposed to an anatomic failure of surgery.[4]

The incidence of pain detected after back surgery is in the range of 5% to 74.6%, and the need for reoperation varies from 13.4% to 35%.[8–11] The frequency of FBSS in the general population is estimated to range from 20 to 2,000 per 100,000 people.[12] In 1997, in the United States, the number of spine surgeries reached 317,000; 5 years later, in 2002, there was drastic increase to over one million spinal procedures performed.[13–17]

ETIOLOGY AND PATHOGENESIS

Risk Factors for PLS

Preoperative risk factors include:

- Selection of an inappropriate candidate for surgery based on imaging results with poor clinical correlation[18]
- Selection of patients with nonsurgical causes of radiculopathy and neuropathy (i.e., those caused by infections, metabolic abnormalities, vasculitis)[11]

Intraoperative risk factors include:

- Operation on the wrong level due to segmentation defects without eliminating the pain generator[18,19]
- Incomplete decompression can lead to persistent pain

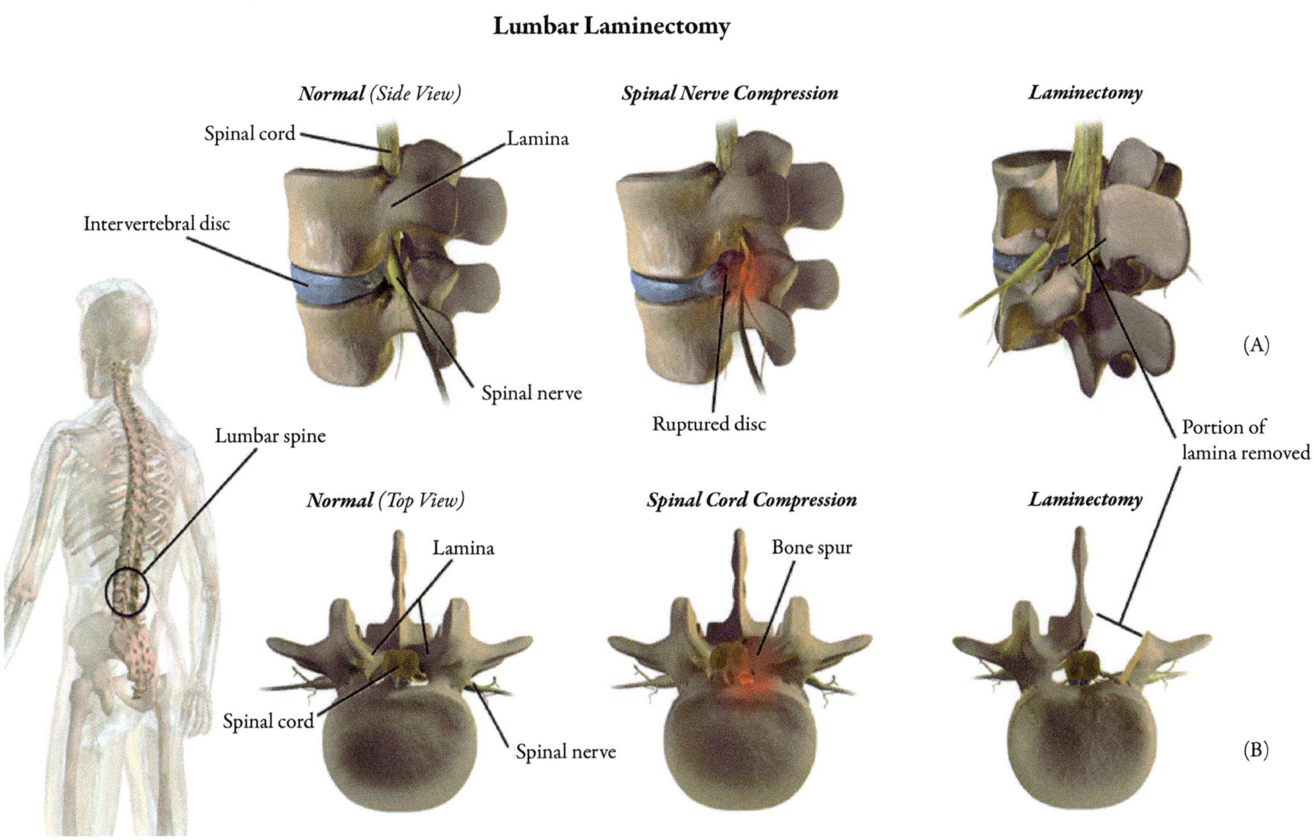

Figure 24.1. Lumbar laminectomy. (A) Sagittal view. (B) Axial view. SOURCE: https://commomns.wikimedia.org/wiki/File:LumbarLaminectomy.png. Author Bruce Blaus. (The image is licensed under Creative Commons Attribution-Share Alike 4.0 International license.)

- Presence of disk fragments in the neural foramina, spinal stenosis, extraforaminal disk herniation, nerve kinking by the adjacent pedicle[18,19]
- Excessive and aggressive retraction[18,19]
- Pars articularis fracture during decompression
- Inability to accomplish the surgery goals (decompression for foraminal stenosis due to ligamentous hypertrophy can lead to destabilization of the segment and persistent pain)[18]

Postoperative risk factors include:

- Hematoma, infection
- Epidural fibrosis, which can lead to decreased vascular supply to the nerve roots and decreased cerebrospinal fluid circulation and nutrition of the nerve roots (Figure 24.2)
- Arachnoiditis, which can result in axial and lower limb pain (arachnoiditis can be assessed with MRI)[18]
- Normal anatomic architecture disruption and altered biomechanics[18,20]
- Loss of disk height after discectomy may result in compression and pain
- Recurrence of disk herniation at the site of operation due to uneven load distribution[18,21]
- Myofascial pain

Epidural fibrosis is almost inevitable after back surgery that involves manipulation of the epidural space. A laminectomy involves peeling off the ligamentum flavum that is adherent to it; as nature abhors a vacuum, the void created by the peeling off results in the obligatory production of an epidural scar. Epidural fibrosis can contribute to postoperative persistent pain in 20% to 36% of cases.[18,22–28] It can compress the nerve roots and may cause pain on back movement as well as impede CSF circulation and nutrition and can subsequently lead to nerve root hypersensitivity.[29–31]

Muscle manipulation during spinal surgery is an expected part of the process that can result in muscle injury and trauma, including the formation of lactic acidosis and nonfunctional skeletal muscle metabolites, and in association with other factors can lead to persistent back pain after surgery.[32] Muscle trophicity can be affected by repeated surgeries, leading to progressive instability of the spine.[33] Further tension and biomechanical overloading of the muscle and tendons can induce severe muscle pain. Theoretically, the pain is believed to be related to the chemical mediators that are produced in overused and traumatized muscles and which increase the impulse activity of nociceptors.[32]

Inflammation within the functional unit can cause muscle spasm in order to prevent more muscle movement that would lead to more pain. The pain from muscle spasm is also attributed to contraction under ischemic conditions.[32,34]

Glycogen storage depletion and mononeuronal firing can lead to muscular fatigue and subsequent impairment of the neuromusculoskeletal function of the paravertebral muscles, with episodes of acute LBP further worsening the FBSS.[34–36]

Every spine surgery has the capacity to change the weight distribution among the structures of the spine; therefore, spinal instability can occur due to altered biomechanics after surgery.

Laminectomy can lead to facet joint incompetence with resultant axial pain. The decompression procedure can destabilize the joint, resulting in instability and pain (Table 24.1).[37]

DIAGNOSIS OF PLS

Patient History

Diagnosis of PLS starts with detailed evaluation of the patient history, which provides valuable information about the etiology

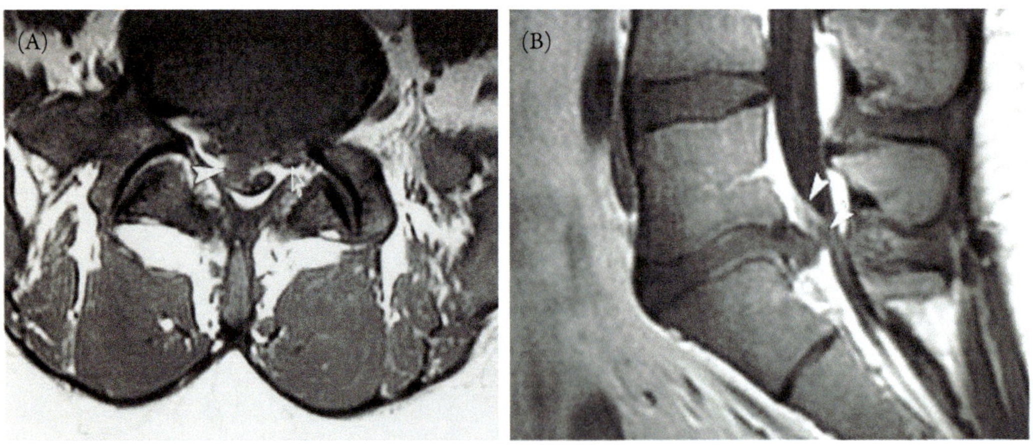

Figure 24.2. Patient with symptoms of recurrent low back pain after laminectomy. (A) Contrast-enhanced T1-weighted MRI at L5-S1 level: focal paracentral protrusion with ventral thecal sac effacement and invasion of the neural foramen. (B) Left-sided nerve root displacement with postoperative fibrosis displaced by the herniation. Reproduced with permission from *J Chiropr Med.* 2012; 11(4):249–253.

Table 24.1. **BACK PAIN GENERATORS AND CONDITIONS THAT LEAD TO DECOMPENSATION OF THE PRIMARY PROCESS AFTER SPINAL SURGERY**

TYPICAL BACK PAIN GENERATORS	ATYPICAL BACK PAIN GENERATORS
• Recurrent disk herniation • Peridural scarring • Nerve root compressed by scarring • Deformity of the dural sac • Herniation of the adjacent disk • Spinal instability • Facetectomy • Pseudomeningocele • Arachnoid cysts • Arachnoiditis • Foraminal restenosis	• Spondylolisthesis • Spinal stenosis • Scoliosis and spine deformity • Iliolumbar syndrome • Piriformis syndrome • Sacroiliac disease • Sacralization of the transverse process • Spinal infections • Tumor

Modified from References 32, 38, and 39.

of the pain, psychologic and social aspects of the patient's coping with the pain, and the previous treatment modalities and investigations. When asking the patient to describe the pain, it is important to compare preoperative and postoperative symptomatology. It needs to be clarified whether the pain has recurred or is persistent and whether it has the same location or a new location. In all cases of LBP, red flags should be identified to differentiate the pain from fractures, neoplasms, infections, or possible rupture of, or leakage from, an abdominal aneurysm.[40]

Psychosocial factors, which include the patient's emotional profile, work environment, and social relations and interaction, play a significant role in the postoperative pain response. The Roland-Morris Questionnaire evaluates mild to moderate functional disability, the Oswestry Scale tests severe disability as well as social aspects, and the Dallas Pain Questionnaire assesses four aspects of daily living: daily activities (leisure, work), anxiety, depression, and social interaction.[41–45]

Physical Exam

The purpose of the physical examination is to rule out serious pathology or a serious complication from the spinal surgery and to localize the source of the pain.

General examination helps in evaluating the posture, gate, and patient functionality.

Examination of the spine allows the examiner to determine the stability of the spine in the frontal and sagittal planes, stiffness, abdominopelvic muscle strength, and pain, which can be focal or global (following a nerve root distribution). Range of motion testing helps determine whether the patient has back pain or radicular pain. Additionally, palpation can reveal vertebral or paravertebral trigger points, surgical scars, indentations, and step-offs.[18,46]

Motor control can be assessed with two easy screening tests. Balance is examined from the hands and knees position with opposite arm and leg extension. The second test requires the patient to maintain a stable prone plank position from a modified push-up position where the patient starts prone and elevates to the elbows and balls of the feet.[11]

Examination of the sacroiliac joint (SIJ) should be performed with a combination of SIJ pain provocation tests, in order to exclude the SIJ as a source of pain in PLS.[47–49]

Clinical Investigations

Imaging is an important component of patient assessment that helps to establish a diagnosis, to determine a definitive treatment, and to arrive at a prognosis.

Plain radiographs can evaluate the surgical site, bone misalignment, and degenerative changes, and spondylolisthesis can be detected on flexion-extension views.[50] When evaluating a radiographic film, it is important to distinguish findings specific to FBSS from expected postoperative normal findings, for example, herniation of the thecal sac through a new laminectomy defect, which can produce a mass effect and which is considered normal if it decreases over the next 30 to 60 days.[18,19,21] Postoperative fibrosis, inflammation, and epidural edema can mimic recurrent disk herniation seen on a noncontrast MRI, while inflammation can be distinguished from recurrent disk herniation on contrast administration with T1 imaging.[18,21] The severity of postoperative fibrosis and adhesions within the epidural space correlates with recurrent radicular and activity-related pain. Due to this unfortunate finding, studies have established grading systems for evaluation and prediction of epidural fibrosis.[23,51–55]

Electrodiagnostic study is particularly helpful when there is a need to differentiate causes of neuropathic pain.[40]

Interventional Diagnostic Procedures

Lumbar medial branch blocks under fluoroscopic guidance are diagnostic for zygapophysial joint pain.[56,57] According to the International Association for the Study of Pain (IASP), controlled diagnostic blocks have identified 15% to 45% of patients with facet joints as their source of pain and 16% of patients with recurrent back pain from the facet joints after spinal surgery.[58–61]

SIJ Blocks

It is estimated that 2% of patients with FBBS suffer from pain caused by the SIJ.[62–64] Apart from positive provocation tests, SIJ block is still required to make a more accurate diagnosis.[65]

Selective Nerve Root Block

Transforaminal injection of local anesthetic and steroid under imaging guidance can be performed mainly for radicular pain and can identify the source of pain. The response to the injection helps determine whether surgery will have a positive impact on pain related to a herniated disk.[66–68]

Provocative Lumbar Discography

Nowadays, provocative lumbar disography is considered a diagnostic aid that has to be correlated with clinical findings.

Its usefulness was questioned due to the presence of pain after intradiscal injection in 40% of an asymptomatic (volunteer) patient population as well as the presence of a high rate of injection-induced pain in a population with psychologic disorders.[69]

TREATMENT OF PLS

A review of treatment options for CLBP revealed utilization of more than 60 pharmaceutical products, 20 different injection therapies, and 32 different manual therapy approaches.[70] However, the treatment of FBSS is far more challenging and often requires drastic therapies to manage pain and improve patients' functional status.

CONSERVATIVE TREATMENTS

Pharmacotherapy

The American Pain Society and Cochrane reviews have published clinical practice guidelines for CLBP management (Box 24.1) but no review of PLS management was found.[18,71,72] There is a lack of studies on therapeutic management of PLS. Most studies retrospectively review case reports, and well-designed studies show the inferiority of pharmacologic management alone.[3] Often non-opioid medications are insufficient in these settings and use of opioids in managing PLS is becoming controversial, especially when instrumented lumbar fusion was performed; therefore, these patients are maintained on multiple medications from different classes or receive additional interventional therapy. However, some studies showed improvement in pain scores using pharmaceutical therapy with different combinations of drugs and interventional therapy.[73,74] In 2010, Zencirci et al. conducted a randomized, controlled study of 42 patients with FBSS. Group one was administered epidural methylprednisolone plus oral naproxen, tizanidine, vitamin B and C complex (N = 21) and group two was administered oral gabapentin plus the group 1 treatment regimen. Pain was assessed by Visual Analog Scale (VAS) at 1, 3, and 6 months. Both group 1 and group 2 showed statistically significant changes in their VAS scores (for group 1, VAS was 77 at baseline and 56 at 6 months; for group 2, VAS was 80.5 at baseline, and 20.2 at 6 months; $p <$ 0.001).[73] Teixeira et al. conducted a prospective open-label case series on 56 patients with FBSS.[74] The investigators combined pharmacologic, interventional, and physical therapy (amitriptyline, chlorpromazine, naproxen, acetaminophen, codeine phosphate plus kinesiotherapy and muscle stretching with 1% lidocaine injection, if myofascial pain was present). At the final follow-up, the baseline VAS score decreased from 72 to 47 (p = 0.01).[74]

Box 24.1. PHARMACOLOGIC MANAGEMENT OF CHRONIC LOW BACK PAIN

- Nonsteroidal anti-inflammatory drugs or acetaminophen
- Cyclooxygenase-2 (COX-2) inhibitors
- Muscle relaxants (baclofen, tizanidine)
- Antidepressants (tricyclic antidepressants, selective serotonin reuptake inhibitors, and serotonin-norepinephrine reuptake inhibitors)
- Gabapentinoids
- Tramadol
- Opioids

Modified from Reference 11.

INVASIVE INTERVENTIONAL TECHNIQUES

Interventional techniques should be used in conjunction with pharmacologic therapy to improve functionality and decrease the intensity of pain. As discussed earlier, some procedures serve as both diagnostic and therapeutic methods.

When medial branch blocks had a positive response with induction of 80% pain relief, radiofrequency neurotomy was found to produce sustained analgesia. After appropriate diagnostic criteria and technique, 60% of patients had 90% pain reduction at 6 months' follow-up and 87% of patients had more than 60% pain reduction at 12 months.[75,76]

Caudal epidural steroid injections are used to improve radicular pain and were demonstrated to have a moderate effect for long-term relief in chronic lumbar radicular pain associated with PLS.[77] In some cases, a catheter placed through the sacral hiatus allows deposit of medication closer to the pain generator (Figure 24.3).

Epidural steroid injections have proved to be effective in instances of documented epidural fibrosis, disk disruption and herniation, and spinal stenosis, thus addressing several pathologic changes associated with PLS.[78] Furthermore, the normal anatomic architecture of the back structures is disrupted in patients after back surgery, where fibrosis and stenosis are commonly encountered; this makes it more challenging to accurately inject steroids into the epidural space and often increases the chance of dural puncture. Therefore, the procedure has to be performed under fluoroscopic guidance to maximize the chance of successful outcome.[79] The transforaminal approach is sometimes preferred to the interlaminar one due to significant risk for dural puncture and technical difficulties. Given the distorted anatomy, digital subtraction fluoroscopy may assist the proceduralist in identifying vascular uptake and avoiding possible complications (Figure 24.4).

Epidural fibrosis is commonly the cause of pain in patients with FBSS (36% of cases).[22,27] Its presence impedes the passage of the epidural medications to areas of interest. Heavner et al. and Manchikanti et al. demonstrated that epidural adhesiolysis with or without hypertonic saline neurolysis effectively treated the FBSS.[80,81] It is recommended that percutaneous adhesiolysis be reserved for FBSS patients who experience radicular pain and who have failed conservative and epidural injection treatments.

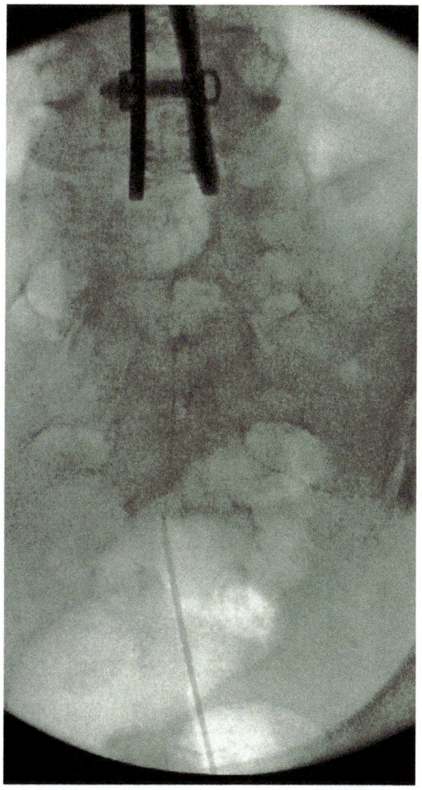

Figure 24.3. Caudal epidural steroid injection using a 21 G styleted catheter through an 18 G epidural needle placed in the sacral hiatus in a patient with PLS. Courtesy of Magdalena Anitescu, MD.

SURGICAL MANAGEMENT

SCS

After pharmaceutical and interventional management have failed, SCS trial followed by implantation is used for refractory PLS. The proposed mechanism of action is thought to be via the gate-control theory of pain and modulation of neurotransmitters in the dorsal horn.[82] North et al. conducted a study that compared patient satisfaction after SCS implantation or repeat back surgery; the authors concluded that the SCS group had a more favorable outcome than reoperation.[83] The PROCESS trial compared conventional medical management (CMM) with SCS in patients with FBSS. The primary outcome was pain relief of more than 50% at 6, 12, and 24 months. In the SCS group, 48% of patients reached the primary outcome goal, compared to only 9% in the CMM group ($p < 0.001$). However, a patient was eligible for permanent implantation of SCS only if the SCS screening trial was successful (Figure 24.5).[84]

Intrathecal Pumps

On literature review, no published RCTs on intrathecal infusion device systems for noncancer chronic pain were found; however, several observational studies had assessed the efficacy of the intrathecal pump in patients with FBSS.[18,85–87] It

(A)

(B)

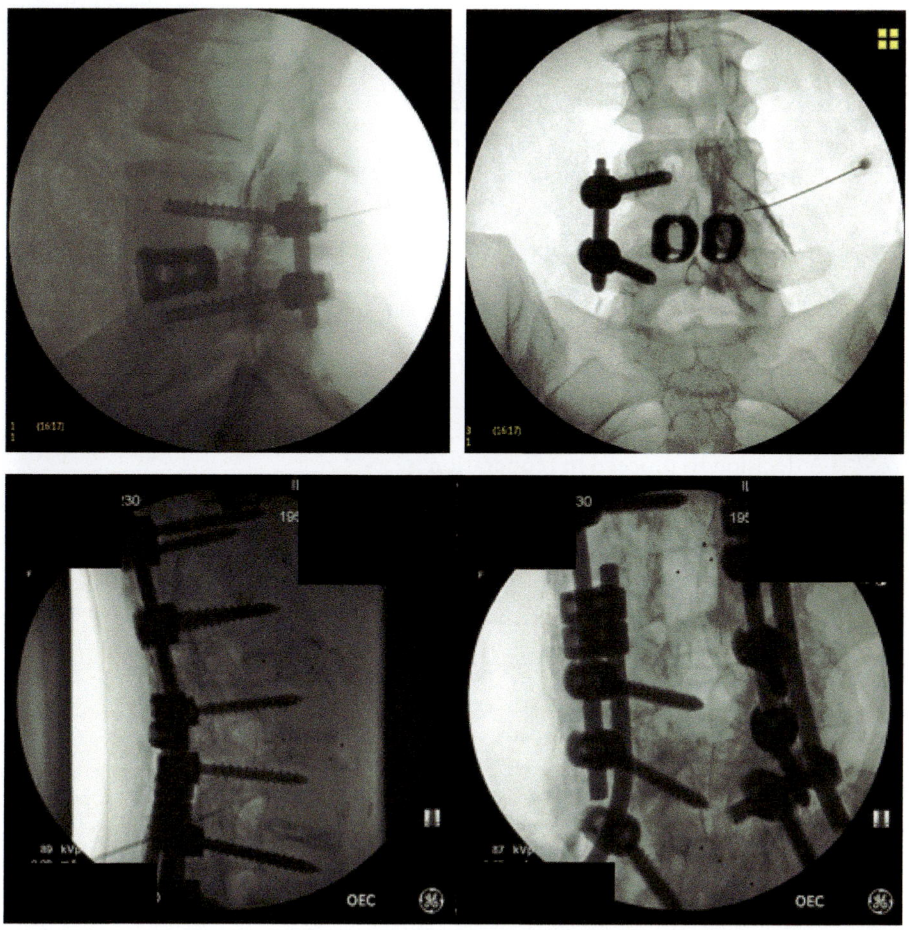

Figure 24.4. Epidural steroid injections in patients with lumbar spine instrumentation. (A) Transforaminal epidural steroid injection in a patient with FBBS. (B) Laminectomy surgery with spine fusion. Presence of hardware dramatically affects the precision of epidural steroid injection.

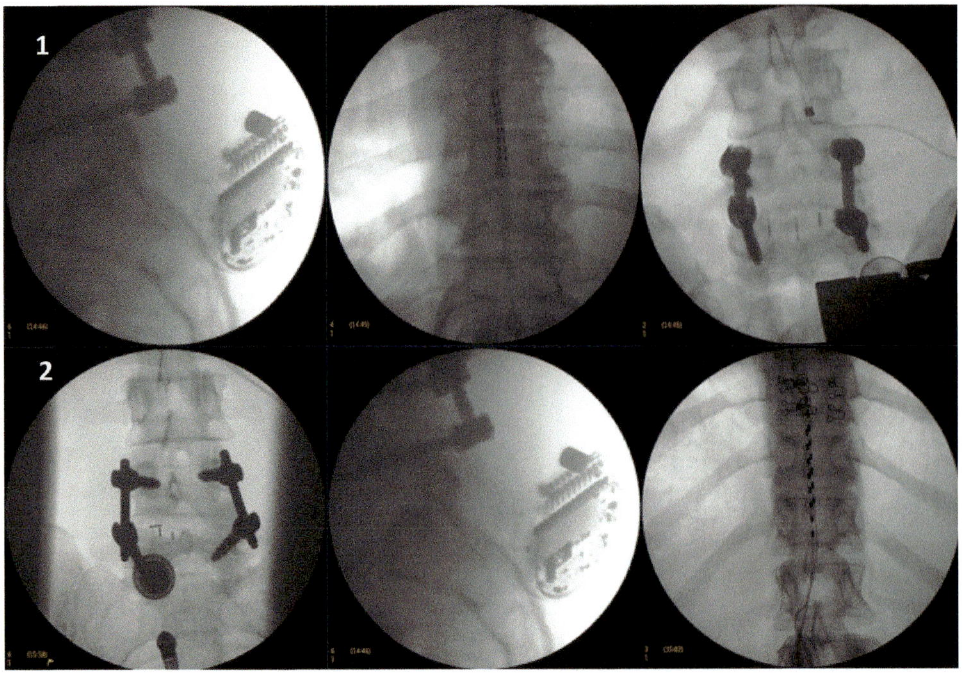

Figure 24.5. Two patients with postlaminectomy syndrome treated with spinal cord stimulation.

was found that effective pain reduction was experienced by 67.4% of patients at 6 months, while the mean pain reduction was 64%.[85,86] However, drug side effects with the device are not uncommon, with the nost prevalent being nausea and vomiting (33%), urinary retention (24%), and pruritus (26%).[88] Currently, with the existing evidence, intrathecal infusion devices can be recommended to patients who failed other treatment options (Figure 24.6). It is important for the patient to respond to orally administered opioid; otherwise, no effect from the intrathecal pump is expected due to opioid tolerance. Furthermore, patients have to undergo a psychologic evaluation prior to intrathecal pump implantation as well.[18]

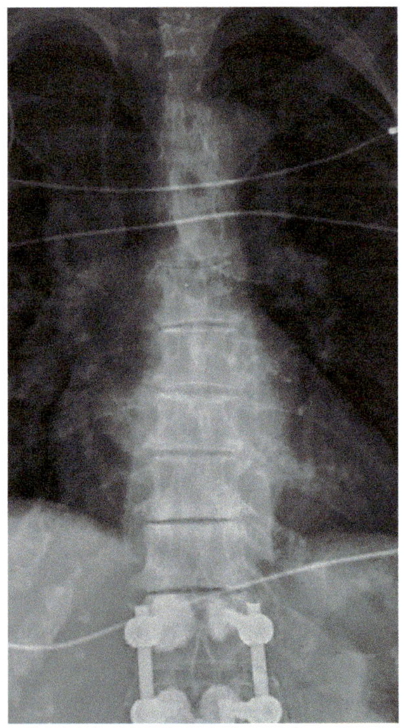

Figure 24.6. Intrathecal pump placement in a patient with postlaminectomy syndrome in which oral medications were associated with significant and intolerable side effects. The catheter is seen at the T8 level. There was significant scar tissue from the T12-S1 spinal fusion with cement enhancement at T12 and L1. A previous trial of spinal cord stimulation was unsuccessful in alleviating pain in this patient. After pump placement, pain was significantly reduced from 9/10 to 1/10 on the VAS, with improved function, appetite, and mood. (Photo courtesy of Magdalena Anitescu, MD.)

Reoperation

The rate of reoperation success in this category of patients proved to be very low, and with each additional procedure, it declines even more.[89–91] A decision to proceed to reoperation should involve a consultation with an expert surgeon who possesses experience with this group of patients. The lack of large randomized trials to guide clinicians to the best evidence-based decision is an indicator that proceeding with reoperation can be accomplished only in those instances where neurologic deficit is amenable to surgery.[92]

Physical Therapy and Rehabilitation Procedures

Miller et al. conducted a prospective study comparing the influence of interdisciplinary management (IDM) in patients with

FBSS and in non-FBSS patients with chronic back pain.[93] IDM included psychologic evaluation, physical therapy, cognitive-behavioral therapy (CBT), relaxation, biofeedback, stress management, and coping strategies, all of which were tailored to each patient on a case by case basis. Patients from the FBSS group showed significant improvement with physical therapy; however, no difference between groups was detected.[93]

There are three types of rehabilitation programs for patients with CLBP and patients with FBSS: exercise programs, back to school approaches, and spine functional restoration programs, which are being extensively developed. The spine functional restoration program consists of global muscle reinforcement and social, psychologic, kinesiophobia, and pain management aspects.[41] However, successful results depend on patients' motivation and active involvement during the program and after. The goal of the rehabilitation program is to increase the rate of return to work of such patients, which revealed results as high as 65% to 72%.[94]

CBT

CBT consists of teaching skills of relaxation, behavioral activation (such as goal setting and pacing strategies), change of perception (such as visual imagery), desensitization, and hypnosis.[41] CBT is beneficial for CLBP patients; however, the effectiveness of such therapy has not been studied in patients with FBSS.

CONCLUSIONS

- PLS is commonly referred to as FBSS and is defined as persistent or recurrent back pain after otherwise anatomically successful lumbar spine surgery.
- The incidence of pain detected after back surgery varies in the range of 5% to 74.6%.
- Epidural fibrosis can contribute to postoperative persistent pain in 20% to 36% of cases.
- Postoperative fibrosis, inflammation, and epidural edema can mimic recurrent disk herniation on a noncontrast MRI study; inflammation can be distinguished from recurrent disk herniation on contrast administration with T1 imaging.
- According to the IASP, controlled diagnostic blocks have identified 16% of patients with recurrent back pain from the facet joints after spine surgery.
- Non-opioid medications are often insufficient and opioids for PLS have become controversial.
- North et al. concluded that SCS had a more favorable outcome than reoperation in patients with FBSS.

REFERENCES

1. Aldrete JA. Postlaminectomy syndrome. In: Waldman SD, ed. *Pain Management*. 1st ed. Philadelphia, PA: Saunders; 2006:818.
2. Krutsch JP, McCeney MH, Barolat G, et al. A case report of subcutaneous peripheral nerve stimulation for the treatment of axial back pain associated with postlaminectomy syndrome. *Neuromodulation.* 2008;11(2):112–115.
3. Desai MJ, Nava A, Rigoard P, et al. Optimal medical, rehabilitation and behavioral management in the setting of failed back surgery syndrome. *Neurochirurgie.* 2015;61(suppl 1):S66–S76.
4. Watson CP. Bonica's management of pain. *J Pain Symptom Manag.* 2010;40(2):315–319.
5. Shipton EA. Low back pain and the post-laminectomy pain syndrome. *South Afr Med J.* 1989;76:20–23.
6. Borg PAJ, Krijnen HJ. Hyaluronidase in the management of pain due to post-laminectomy scar tissue. *Pain.* 1994;58:273–276.
7. Rigoard P, Desai MJ, Taylor RS. Failed back surgery syndrome: what's in a name? A proposal to replace "FBSS" by "POPS." *Neurochirurgie.* 2015;61:S16–S21.
8. Hussain A, Erdek M. Interventional pain management for failed back surgery syndrome. *Pain Pract.* 2014;14:64–78.
9. Choi HS, Chi EH, Kim MR, et al. Demographic characteristics and medical service use of failed back surgery syndrome patients at an integrated treatment hospital focusing on complementary and alternative medicine: a retrospective review of electronic medical records. *Evid Based Complement Alternat Med.* 2014;2014.
10. Bodiu A. Diagnosis and operatory treatment of the patients with failed back surgery caused by herniated disk relapse. *J Med Life.* 2014;7:533–537.
11. Shapiro C. The failed back surgery syndrome: pitfalls surrounding evaluation and treatment. *Phys Med Rehabil Clin N Am.* 2014;25:319–340.
12. Weber H. Lumbar disc herniation. A controlled, prospective study with ten years of observation. *Spine.* 1983;8:131–140.
13. National Center for Health Statistics. National Hospital Discharge Survey. Washington, DC. Department of Health and Human Services, Center for Disease Control; 1997. Series 13, No. 144.
14. 2000 spinal surgery update. *Orthop Netw News.* 2000;11(4). Available at: http://www.orthopedicnetworknews.com.
15. Lieberman IH. Disc bulge bubble: Spine economics 101. *Spine J.* 2004;4:609–613.
16. Wenger DR. Spine surgery at a crossroads. Does economic growth threaten our professionalism? *Spine.* 2007;32:2158–2165.
17. Deyo RA, Mirza SK. Trends and variations in the use of spine surgery. *Clin Orthop Relat Res.* 2006;443:139–146.
18. Chan C, Peng P. Failed back surgery syndrome. Review article. *Pain Med.* 2011;12:577–606.
19. Grossman RG, Loftus CM. *Principles of Neurosurgery.* 2nd ed. Philadelphia, PA: Lippincott-Raven; 1999:422–430.
20. Kumar MN, Baklanov A, Chopin D. Correlation between sagittal plane changes and adjacent segmental degeneration following lumbar spine fusion. *Eur Spine J.* 2001;10:314–319.
21. Herrara HI, Moreno de la Presa R, Gutierrez RG, et al. Evaluacion de la columna lumbar postquirurgica [Evaluation of the postoperative lumbar spine]. *Radiologia.* 2013;55:12–23.
22. Fritsch EW, Heisel J, Rupp S. The failed back surgery syndrome—reasons, intraoperative findings, and long-terms results: a report of 182 operative treatments. *Spine.* 1996;21:626–633.
23. Ross JS, Robertson JT, Frederickson RC, et al. Association between peridural scar and recurrent radicular pain after lumbar discectomy: magnetic resonance evaluation. *Neurosurgery.* 1996;38:855–863.
24. Trescot AM, Chopra P, Abdi S, et al. Systematic review of effectiveness and complications of adhesiolysis in the management of chronic spinal pain: an update. *Pain Physician.* 2007;10:129–146.
25. Chopra P, Smith HS, Deer TR, et al. Role of adhesiolysis in the management of chronic spinal pain: a systematic review of effectiveness and complications. *Pain Physician.* 2005;8:87–100.
26. Manchikanti L, Singh V. Epidural lysis of adhesions and myeloscopy. *Curr Pain Headache Rep.* 2002;6:427–435.
27. Kayaoglu CR, Calikoglu C, Binler S. Re-operation after lumbar disc surgery: results in 85 cases. *J Int Med Res.* 2003;31:318–323.

28. Maliszewski M, Tymowski M, Lelek P, et al. An attempt to use Gore-Tex surgical membrane in lumbar disc surgery. *Neurol Neurochir Pol.* 2004;38:271–277.
29. Coskun E, Suzer T, Topuz O, et al. Relationships between epidural fibrosis, pain, disability, and psychological factors after lumbar disc surgery. *Eur Spine J.* 2000; 9:218–3.
30. Jayson M. The role of vascular damage and fibrosis in the pathogenesis of nerve root damage. *Clin Orthop Relat Res.* 1992;279:40–48.
31. Rydevik BL. The effects of compression on the physiology of nerve roots. *J Manipulative Physiol Ther.* 1992;15:62–66.
32. Rigoard P, Blond S, David R, et al. Pathophysiological characterization of back pain generators in failed back surgery syndrome (part B). *Neurochirurgie.* 2015;61(suppl 1):S35–S44.
33. Lucas D, Bresler B. Stability of ligamentous spine. In: Report No.: Biomechanics Laboratory Report; 1961:40.
34. Bigland-Ritchie B, Cafarelli E, Vollestad NK. Fatigue of submaximal static contractions. *Acta Physiol Scand.* 1986;556(suppl):137–148.
35. Edwards RH. Human muscle function and fatigue. *Ciba Found Symp.* 1981;82:1–18.
36. Kukulka CG. Human skeletal muscle fatigue. *Dynamics of Human Biologic Tissues.* 1992.
37. Onesti ST. Failed back syndrome. *Neurologist.* 2004;10:259–264.
38. Aldrete JA. Failed back surgery syndrome. In: Waldman SD, ed. *Pain Management.* Philadelphia, PA: Elsevier/Saunders; 2007: 817–830.
39. Assaker R, Zairi F. Failed back surgery syndrome: to re-operate or not to re-operate? A retrospective review of patient selection and failures. *Neurochirurgie.* 2015;61(suppl 1):S77–S82.
40. Guyer RD, Paterson M, Ohnmeiss DD. Failed back surgery syndrome: diagnostic evaluation. *J Am Acad Orthop Surg.* 2006;14:534–543.
41. Durand G, Girodon J, Debiasis F. Medical management of failed back surgery syndrome in Europe: evaluation modalities and treatment proposals. *Neurochirurgie.* 2015;61:S57–S65.
42. Roland M, Morris R. A study of natural history of back pain. Part I: development of a reliable and sensitive measure of disability in low-back pain. *Spine.* 193;8(2):141–144.
43. Fairbank JC, Couper J, Davvies JB, et al. The Oswestry low back pain disability questionnaire. *Physiotherapy.* 1980;66:271–273.
44. Kopec JA, Esdaile JM, Abrahamowicz M, et al. The Quebec Back Pain Disability Scale. Measurement properties. *Spine.* 1995;20:341–352.
45. Lawlis GF, Cuencas R, Selby D, et al. The development of the Dallas Pain Questionnaire. An assessment of the impact of spinal pain on behavior. *Spine.* 1989;14:511–516.
46. Long DM. Failed back surgery syndrome. *Neurosurg Clin N Am.* 1991;2:117–125.
47. Young S, April C, Laslett M, et al. Correlation of clinical examination characteristics with three sources of low back pain. *Spine J.* 2007;16:1539–1550.
48. Hancock MJ, Maher CG, Latimer J, et al. Systematic reviews of tests to identify the disc, SIJ or facet joint as source of low back pain. *Eur Spine J.* 2007;16:1539–1550.
49. Laslett M, April CN, Mcdonald B, et al. Diagnosis of sacroiliac joint pain: validity of individual provocation tests and composites of tests. *Man Ther.* 2005;10:207–218.
50. Kizilkilic O, Yalchin O, Sen O, et al. The role of standing flexion-extension radiographs for spondylolisthesis following single level disc surgery. *Neurol Res.* 2007;29:540–543.
51. Bosscher HA, Heavner JE. Incidence and severity of epidural fibrosis after back surgery: an endoscopic study. *Pain Pract.* 2010;10:18–24.
52. Hurme M, Katevuo K, Nykvist F, et al. CT five years after myelographic diagnosis of lumbar disk herniation. *Acta Radiol.* 1991;32:286–289.
53. Wetzel FT, LaRocca H. The failed posterior lumbar interbody fusion. *Spine.* 1991;16:839–845.
54. Porchet F, Lombardi D, De Preux J, et al. Inhibition of epidural fibrosis with ADCON-L: Effect on clinical outcome one year following re-operation for recurrent lumbar radiculopathy. *Neurol Res.* 1999;21:S51–S60.
55. Ross JS, Obuchowski N, Modic MT. MR evaluation of epidural fibrosis: proposed grading system with intra- and inter- observer variability. *Neurol Res.* 1998;21:S23–S26.
56. Dreyfuss O, Scwarzer AC, Lau P, et al. Specificity of lumbar medial branch and L5 dorsal ramus blocks: a computed tomographic study. *Spine.* 1997;22:895–902.
57. Kaplan M, Dreyfuss P, Halbrook B, et al. The ability of the lumbar medial branch blocks to anesthetize the zygapophysial joint. *Spine.* 1998;23:1847–1852.
58. Schwarzer AC, Aprill CN, Derby R, et al. The relative contributions of the disc and zygapophyseal joint in chronic low back pain. *Spine.* 1994;19:801–806.
59. Manchikanti L, Boswell MV, Singh V, et al. Prevalence of facet joint pain in chronic spinal pain of cervical, thoracic, and lumbar regions. *MBC Musculoskelet Disord.* 2004;5:15–22.
60. Merskey H, Bogduk N. Classification of chronic pain. In: Boogduk N, Merskey H, eds. *Descriptions of Chronic Pain Syndromes and Definition of Pain Terms.* 2nd ed. Seattle, WA: IASP Press; 1994:180–181.
61. Manchikanti L, Manchukonda R, Pampati V, et al. Prevalence of facet joint pain in chronic low back pain in postsurgical patients by controlled comparative local anesthetic blocks. *Arch Phys Med Rehabil.* 2007;88:449–455.
62. Waguespack A, Schofferman J, Slosar P, et al. Etiology of long-term failures of lumbar spine surgery. *Pain Med.* 2002;3:18–22.
63. Slipman CW, Shin CH, Patel RK, et al. Etiology of failed back surgery syndrome. *Pain Med.* 2002;3:200–214.
64. Burton CV, Kirkbaldy-Willis WH, Yong-Hing K, et al. Causes of failure of surgery on lumbar spine. *Clin Orthop Relat Res.* 1981;157:191–199.
65. Hancock MJ, Maher CG, Latimer J, et al. Correlation of clinical examination characteristics with three sources of low back pain. *Eur Spine J.* 2007;16:1539–1550.
66. Vad VB, Bhat AL, Lutz GE, at al. Transforaminal epidural steroid injections in lumbosacral radiculopathy. *Spine.* 2002;27:11–16.
67. Bogduk N, Aprill C, Derby R. Selective nerve root blocks. In: Wilson DJ, ed. *Interventional Radiology of Musculoskeletal System.* London: Edward Arnold; 1995:121–132.
68. Eckel TS, Bartynski WS. Epidural steroid injections and selective nerve root blocks. *Tech Vasc Interv Radiol.* 2009;12:11–21.
69. Carragee EJ, Tanner CM, et al. Provocative discography inpatients after limited lumbar discectomy: A controlled, randomized study of pain response in symptomatic and asymptomatic subjects. *Spine.* 2000;25:3065–3071.
70. Haldeman S, Dagenais S. A supermarket approach to the evidence-informed management of chronic low back pain. *Spine J.* 2008;8:1–7.
71. Chou R, Huffman LH. Medications for acute and chronic low back pain: a review of the evidence for an American Pain Society/American College of Physicians Clinical Practice Guideline. *Ann Intern Med.* 2007;147:505–514.
72. Noble M, Treadwell JR, Tregear SJ, et al. Long-term opioid management for chronic noncancer pain. *Cochrane Database Syst Rev.* 2010;CD006605.
73. Zencirci B. Analgesic efficacy of oral gabapentin added to standard epidural corticosteroids in patients with failed back surgery. *Clin Pharmacol.* 2010;2:207–211.
74. Teixeira MJ, Yeng LT, Garcia OG, et al. Failed back surgery pain syndrome: therapeutic approach descriptive study in 56 patients. *Rev Assoc Med Bras.* 2011;7:286–291.
75. Dreyfuss P, Halbrock B, Pauza K, et al. Efficacy and validity of radiofrequency neurotomy for chronic lumbar zygapophysial joint pain. *Spine.* 2000;25:1270–1277.
76. Manchikanti L, Pampati S, Cash KA. Making sense of the accuracy of diagnostic lumbar facet joint nerve blocks: An assessment of the

implications of 50% relief, 80% relief, single block, or controlled diagnostic blocks. *Pain Physician.* 2010;13:133–143.
77. Abdi S, Datta S, Trescot AM, et al. Epidural steroids in the management of chronic spinal pain: a systematic review. *Pain Physician.* 2007;10:185–212.
78. Manchikanti L, Singh V, Cash KA, et al. Preliminary results of a randomized, equivalence trial of fluoroscopic caudal epidural injections in managing chronic low back pain: Part 3—Post surgery syndrome. *Pain Physician.* 2008;11:817–831.
79. Manchikanti L, Cash KA, Pampati V, et al. Evaluation of fluoroscopically guided caudal epidural injections. *Pain Physician.* 2004;7:81–92.
80. Heavner JE, Racz GB, Raj P. Percutaneous epidural neuroplasty. Prospective evaluation of 0.9% NaCl versus 10% NaCl with or without hyaluronidase. *Reg Anesth Pain Med.* 1999;24:202–207.
81. Manchikanti L, Rivera J, Pampati V, et al. One day lumbar epidural adhesiolysis and hypertonic saline neurolysis in treatment of chronic low back pain: a randomized double blind trial. *Pain Physician.* 2004;7:177–186.
82. Oakley JC, Prager JP. Spinal cord stimulation: mechanisms of action. *Spine (Phila Pa 1976).* 2002;27(22):2574–2583.
83. North RB, Kidd DA, Farrokh F, et al. Spinal cord stimulation versus repeated spine surgery for chronic pain: a randomized controlled trial. *Neurosurgery.* 2005; 56:98–106.
84. Kumar K, Taylor RS, Jacques L, et al. Spinal cord stimulation versus conventional medical management for neuropathic pain: A multicenter randomized controlled trial in patients with failed back surgery syndrome. *Pain.* 2007;132:179–188.
85. Winkelmuller M, Winkelmuller W. Long term effects of continuous intrathecal opioid treatment on chronic pain of nonmalignant etiology. *J Neurosurg.* 1996;85:458–467.
86. Roberts LJ, Finch PM, Goucke CR, et al. Outcome of intrathecal opioids in chronic non-cancer pain. *Eur J Pain.* 2001;5:353–361.
87. Deer TR, Caraway DL, Kim CK, et al. Clinical experience with intrathecal bupivacaine in combination with opioid for the treatment of chronic pain related to failed back surgery syndrome and metastatic cancer pain of the spine. *Spine J.* 2002;2:274–278.
88. Turner JA, Sears JM, Loeser JD. Programmable intrathecal opioid delivery systems for chronic non-cancer pain: a systematic review of effectiveness and complications. *Clin J Pain.* 2007;23:180–195.
89. North RB, Campbell JN, James CS, et al. Failed back surgery syndrome: 5-year follow-up in 102 patients undergoing repeated operation. *Neurosurgery.* 1991;28:685–690.
90. Kim SS, Michelson CB. Revision surgery for failed back surgery syndrome. *Spine.* 1992;17:957–960.
91. Waddell G, Kummel EG, Lotto WN, et al. Failed lumbar disc surgery and repeat surgery following industrial injuries. *J Bone Joint Surg Am.* 1979;61:201–207.
92. Deyo RA. Back surgery—Who needs it? *N Engl J Med.* 2007; 356:2239–2243.
93. Miller B, Gatchel RJ, Lou L, et al. Interdisciplinary treatment of failed back surgery syndrome (FBSS): a comparison of FBSS and non-FBSS patients. *Pain Pract.* 2005;5:190–202.
94. Poulain C, Kerneis S, Rozenberg S, et al. Long-term return to work after a functional restoration program for chronic low-back pain patients: a prospective study. *Eur Spine J.* 2010;19:1153–1161.

REVIEW QUESTIONS

1. A 62-year-old male comes to the pain clinic with recurrent LBP. The patient underwent right-sided L5-S1 lumbar laminectomy surgery about 3 months earlier. Currently he describes his pain as 8 out of 10 on the VAS, localized to the lumbar right side and shooting down his right leg. What is the next step in management?

A. CT of the lumbar spine
B. Prescribe an opioid medication
C. Epidural steroid injection
D. Perform physical exam followed by plain radiography of the lumbar spine

2. A 45-year-old male with a history of CLBP and failed conservative and interventional therapy decided to undergo low back surgery. The surgeon explained the risks and benefits, addressed the patient's expectations in terms of pain relief after surgery, and conducted a complete patient evaluation along with extensive imaging studies. Postoperatively, at the follow-up visit, the patient still complained of LBP. What are the most likely contributing postoperative risk factors for persistent pain in this patient?

A. Doctor–patient miscommunication
B. Inappropriate selection of the surgical candidate
C. Intraoperative misdiagnosis
D. Epidural fibrosis

3. A 51-year-old female who underwent spine surgery has been complaining of recurrent radicular pain. The surgeon completed a physical exam and ordered a plain radiograph that was inconclusive. The surgeon highly suspects nerve root entrapment. What is the next step in management?

A. Prescribe pain medication.
B. Conduct an electrophysiologic study.
C. Order MRI.
D. Perform an epidural steroid injection.

ANSWERS

1. D. The patient in this case most likely has recurrent LBP due to PLS; however, a very detailed history and physical exam are required to exclude red flag symptoms. Plain radiographs can evaluate the surgical site, bony misalignment, and degenerative changes, and spondylolisthesis can be detected on flexion-extension views.[50] Answers A, B, and C can follow after a complete history and physical evaluation have been performed and a plain radiograph has excluded spinal instability.

2. D. Epidural fibrosis is almost inevitable after back surgery that involves manipulation of the epidural space. Epidural fibrosis can contribute to postoperative persistent pain in 20% to 36% of cases. It can compress the nerve roots and may cause pain on back movement as well as impede CSF circulation and nutrition, which can subsequently lead to nerve root hypersensitivity. Answers A and B are preoperative risk factors and from the described case, the doctor addressed all of the

patient's concerns and the patient was considered an appropriate candidate for surgery since he failed all of the available therapies except surgery. Answer C is an intraoperative risk factor.

3. C. MRI provides useful information about the cause of symptoms. It can differentiate between scar tissue (postoperative epidural fibrosis) and recurrent or residual disk herniation. Nerve root enhancement after gadolinium injection on a postoperative MRI correlates with recurrent or residual symptoms. Answer A is not correct because an extensive examination and investigation have to be performed to find out the cause of the pain and proceed with appropriate treatment. Answer B, electrophysiologic study, is useful when a neuropathic component to the pain is present or suspected. Answer D, epidural steroid injection, is not appropriate at this time.

QUESTIONS AND ANSWERS

This chapter has accompanying questions and answers that are available to subscribers as part of the Oxford eLearning platform. To access the questions, follow the link below, or go to http://oxfordmedicine.com/painmanagementreview

25.

COCCYGODYNIA

Anna Woodbury and Vinita Singh

STEM CASE AND KEY QUESTIONS

A 56-year-old male presents with pain on sitting. The pain began after a skiing accident 3 years previously. He has tried heat, ice, massage and over-the-counter medication (ibuprofen, acetaminophen) without significant relief of pain. He localizes the pain to his tailbone area and describes it as stabbing, aching, and throbbing. The pain sometimes radiates into his groin and hips. He denies weakness, numbness, incontinence, or any red flag signs, though he does report worsening pain with bowel movements. He is unable to sit on hard benches for long periods of time. The pain has severely affected his quality of life, as he is a very spiritual person and he can no longer sit through church services. He has also become increasingly depressed due to the effect of pain on his quality of life.

WHAT DEFINES COCCYGODYNIA? WHAT IS THE PATHOPHYSIOLOGY OF COCCYGODYNIA? WHAT SHOULD BE CONSIDERED IN THE DIFFERENTIAL DIAGNOSIS OF COCCYGODYNIA?

Physical exam reveals extreme tenderness over the tailbone area as well as tenderness of bilateral posterior sacroiliac spines and pain in the groin upon flexion, abduction, and external rotation of the hips. Manipulation of the coccyx results in reproduction of his usual pain and demonstrates hypomobility of the sacrococcygeal joint. No cysts or other lesions are palpable on rectal exam, and there are no visible lesions on inspection of the area.

WHEN IS ADDITIONAL IMAGING NECESSARY? WHAT TYPE OF IMAGING SHOULD BE OBTAINED?

X-ray imaging of the patient's lumbar spine, hips, and pelvis reveals an old tailbone fracture as well as moderate degenerative disease in the sacroiliac joints. Review of systems is negative for fever or unexplained weight loss. However, the patient reports worsening depression despite using fluoxetine. During an assessment of his depressive symptoms, the patient reveals that he was also the victim of sexual abuse as a child, and wonders if this may contribute to the pain. This has prevented him from engaging in some types of massage that he has read are helpful in coccygodynia.

WHAT NONINVASIVE THERAPIES ARE RECOMMENDED FOR THE TREATMENT OF COCCYGODYNIA?

After a discussion with his psychiatrist regarding his pain and depression, a decision is made to transition him from fluoxetine to duloxetine in order to better manage both his pain and depression. Though ibuprofen has not been of benefit, he is willing to try another nonsteroidal anti-inflammatory drug (NSAID), so you prescribe meloxicam. You also encourage him to pursue intrarectal massage with a licensed physical therapist certified in this technique.

WHAT INTERVENTIONS ARE AVAILABLE FOR THE TREATMENT OF COCCYGODYNIA?

He reports that his depression has improved on duloxetine 30 mg taken twice daily, but he has seen only mild benefit in terms of pain relief with this and the meloxicam. He went to one massage session, but could not tolerate the therapy. He still rates his pain as severe, and cannot sit for long periods of time. He has purchased a coccyx seat cushion, but is still unable to sit even with this prosthetic. He has tried acupuncture, and states he experiences some benefit, but only for 2 to 3 days, and then the pain returns. Chiropractor treatments have been helpful for his low back and groin pain, but not for the pain in his tailbone. He asks if there is any type of injection available to treat his type of pain. You inject a small amount of local anesthetic and steroid directly into the point of maximum tenderness over his tailbone. Within minutes, the patient is thrilled. He reports 100% pain relief. However, he calls your clinic multiple times overnight and the next day stating that the pain has returned and is worse than before.

IS OPIOID MEDICATION APPROPRIATE FOR THE TREATMENT OF COCCYGODYNIA?

The patient visited an urgent care clinic over the weekend and has been taking hydrocodone, with some relief of the pain, but he acknowledges that the narcotic is worsening his depressive symptoms. He states that he would like to avoid further pills if possible, and continues to ask if there is anything you can do interventionally to provide long-term pain relief. After discussing the risks, benefits, and alternatives of various therapies available, the patient consents to proceed with a ganglion impar block. He again receives tremendous but short-lived relief with the block. He states that he wants a more permanent solution and is willing to undergo any risks in order to achieve pain relief.

WHAT LONG-TERM SOLUTIONS ARE AVAILABLE FOR THIS PATIENT'S PAIN? IF SURGERY IS AVAILABLE, AT WHAT POINT WOULD YOU RECOMMEND IT?

After further discussion of all potential options and their risks and benefits, the patient wishes to proceed with ganglion impar neurolysis, which you perform under fluoroscopic guidance. The patient experiences > 75% relief of his tailbone-related pain. He reports ongoing analgesia at his 3-month follow-up visit, and he is extremely grateful for your care.

DISCUSSION

Coccygodynia or coccydynia is a rare, painful condition localized in the region of the coccyx. The coccyx has several important anatomic functions:

1. It serves as an insertion site for multiple muscles, ligaments, and tendons.
2. Along with the ischial tuberosities, it provides weight-bearing support to a person in the seated position.
3. It provides positional support to the anus.[1]

ETIOLOGY AND PATHOGENESIS

The most common cause of coccygodynia is trauma; it can happen after falling on the buttocks, repetitive microtrauma, or after childbirth.[2] Microtrauma can occur from prolonged sitting on a hard, narrow, or uncomfortable surface, such as a bike seat, especially in obese individuals. In the absence of any inciting event, other causes, such as infections and tumor, should be excluded. Neoplasms and infections should always be ruled out. Coccygodynia can also represent referred pain from the lumbar spine, pelvic floor muscles, or visceral structures (the rectum, the sigmoid, and the urogenital system). The S4, S5, and coccygeal nerves are sensory nerves that are commonly involved in the development of coccygodynia. Coccygodynia can also be associated with nonorganic causes, such as somatization disorder. Obesity and female gender are associated with increased risk of developing coccygodynia. Women are reported to be five times more likely to develop coccygodynia than men.[1]

CLINICAL PRESENTATION

Pain from coccygodynia is located in the tailbone and is typically worse with prolonged sitting, leaning back while seated, prolonged standing, and rising from a seated position. Pain may also be present with sexual intercourse or defecation.[1] A history of trauma to the buttocks is helpful, but it is not always present in coccygodynia due to the variety of causes for tailbone pain.

PHYSICAL EXAMINATION

Inspection of the surrounding skin and soft tissue may reveal evidence of pilonidal cysts or fistulas. External palpation or rectal examination should be done to rule out presence of bone spicules, local swelling, or coccygeal masses. There is often tenderness over the site when coccygodynia is the result of direct trauma or an abnormality of the sacrococcygeal joint itself. However, as expected, there is no tenderness to palpation over the coccyx when pain is radicular or referred. This can help in distinguishing the root cause of a patient's coccygeal pain. In performing a rectal exam for coccygeal pain, the coccyx should be grasped between the forefinger and thumb. Manipulation often elicits pain. It may also reveal hypermobility or hypomobility of the sacrococcygeal joint.[3] Normal range of motion is generally thought to be 0° to 22°, although some studies report that less than 13° is considered abnormal.[3,4]

DIAGNOSIS

Diagnosis is primarily clinical, based on history and physical exam. Imaging studies, including lateral sacral radiographs, dynamic radiographs, and MRI, can help examine the shape of the coccyx and diagnose sacrococcygeal joint hypermobility or hypomobility.

1. Radiographs can identify fractures, hypermobility, luxation, subluxation, hypomobility, ossification, and osteolytic lesions caused by tumors or infectious processes, all thought to be potential mechanistic contributors to coccygodynia. A dynamic series includes standing and sitting X-rays. Lateral view in this series can measure coccygeal mobility. Maigne and Tamalet have suggested that mobility of more than 25° (hypermobility) and luxation of more than 25% (subluxation) should be considered abnormal. The mean mobility (flexion or extension) of the coccyx in patients without coccygodynia has been found to be 9.3° ± 5.7° (range from 0° to 22°; Figure 25.1).[4]

2. MRI can be used for better visualization of the shape of the coccyx, especially the tip, and also to rule out dorsal bursitis, cysts, tumors (Figure 25.2), or neural lesions.[5]

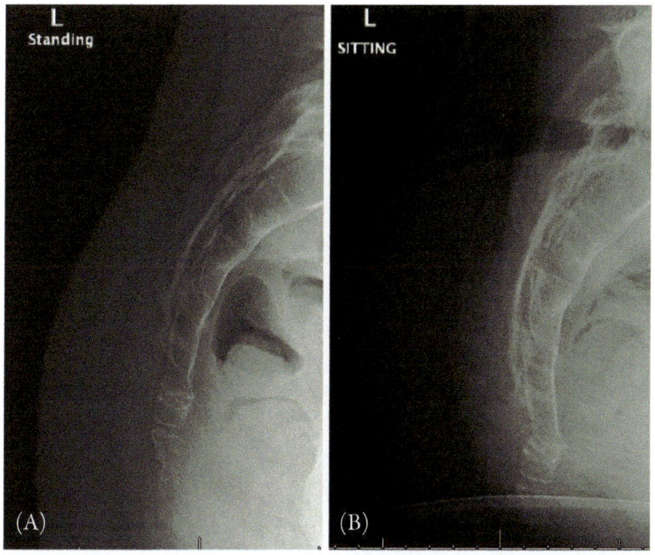

Figure 25.1. Radiographic image of sacrum, standing (A) and sitting (B) in a patient with significant chronic coccygodynia after a motor vehicle accident. Courtesy of University of Chicago Image Library.

3. Isotope bone scans of the sacrococcygeal area may assist in the detection of occult fractures prior to radiographic visualization.

TREATMENTS

Conservative Treatments

Conservative treatment is successful in 90% of cases, and many cases resolve without medical treatment.[6] Treatment options include NSAIDs, hot baths, membrane-shaped cushions, intrarectal massage and manipulation, local injections, ganglion impar blocks, radiofrequency thermocoagulation, and psychotherapy. For patients who do not respond to these interventions, coccygectomy is often recommended.[5,7] Relatively simple measures are sufficient in most cases. Over-the-counter modified wedge-shaped cushions (coccygeal cushions) can relieve the pressure on the coccyx while the patient is seated.[1] Poor sitting posture should be corrected. Heat or cold application to the site may be considered. NSAIDs are the most common analgesic prescribed. Opioids generally are not recommended and should be reserved for severe pain, such as from an acute injury that is not responsive to other measures.

Invasive Techniques

In cases where coccygodynia is a result of lower lumbosacral radicular pain (for example, coccygodynia as a result of Tarlov cysts), caudal epidural steroid injections can be used in treatment (Figure 25.3).[8]

The ganglion impar (ganglion of Walther) may also be targeted for treatment. It is one of the lowest portions of the sympathetic trunk, and is located in the pelvis, midline and anterior to the sacrococcygeal junction. Ganglion impar block (Figure 25.4) can be helpful in refractory cases of coccygeal pain and pelvic pain and is often used for pain associated with neoplasms. It can be followed by neurolysis if a local anesthetic block of the ganglion impar is successful.[9] Ganglion impar radiofrequency ablation and pulsed radiofrequency ablation have been used for chronic coccygeal pain to achieve long-term relief as well[10,11] (Figure 25.4). In select cases, coccygodinia can be accompanied by perineal and low pelvic pain; in those situations a diagnostic pudendal nerve block may differentiate between pudendal neuralgia and pain originating from the coccyx or from the perineal viscerae (Figure 25.5).

There has also been a case report of spinal cord stimulation (SCS) used in the treatment of coccygodynia, although evidence for use of this technique in coccygodynia is limited and requires further research.[1] In severe, refractory cases of coccygodynia, coccygectomy with complete removal of the coccyx up to the sacrococcygeal junction can be performed

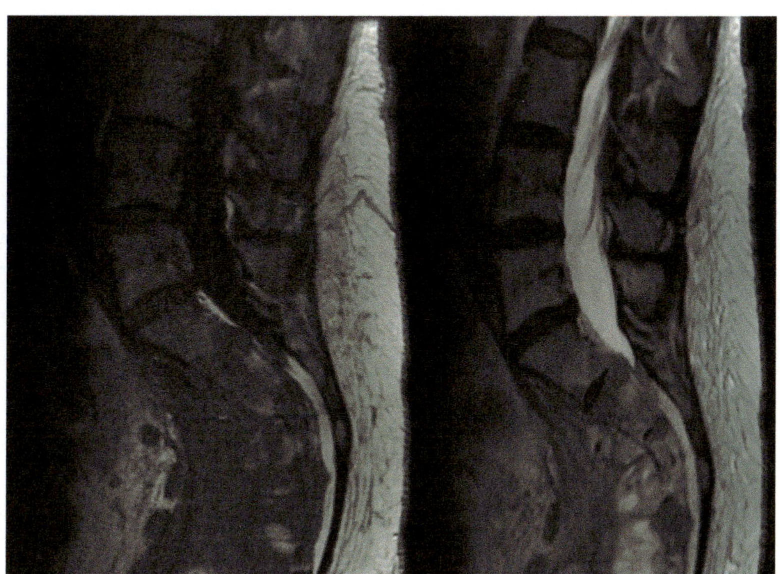

Figure 25.2. MRI revealing bony metastases to the sacrum. Courtesy of University of Chicago Image Library.

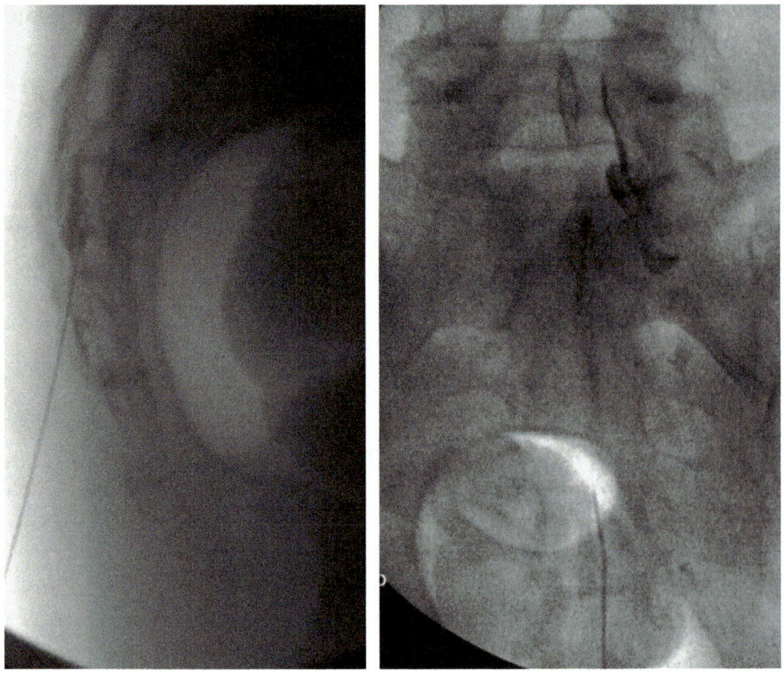

Figure 25.3. Caudal epidural steroid injection. In the lateral view, the needle (left) is fluoroscopically guided into the epidural space through the sacral membrane with the coccyx anterior (below) and the sacrum posterior (above). Appropriate epidural spread of contrast is noted. Courtesy of University of Chicago Image Library.

(Figure 25.6), although patients should be informed that complications, such as infection, phantom pain, and fistula, can occur.[7,12–14]

In a prospective study of coccygectomy for coccygodynia in 98 patients, significant improvement was noted 2 years postoperatively, with treatment failure primarily associated with higher levels of pain, opiate use, psychiatric illness, poor quality of life, and three or more medical comorbidities.[15] Local anesthetic injection to the tailbone with or without steroid can be diagnostic in identifying those who may benefit from this surgery and can be therapeutic in its own right.[15–17]

CONCLUSIONS

- Coccygodynia involves pain in the tailbone area that is aggravated by sitting on hard surfaces, leaning back while seated, rising from sitting to standing position, and prolonged standing.

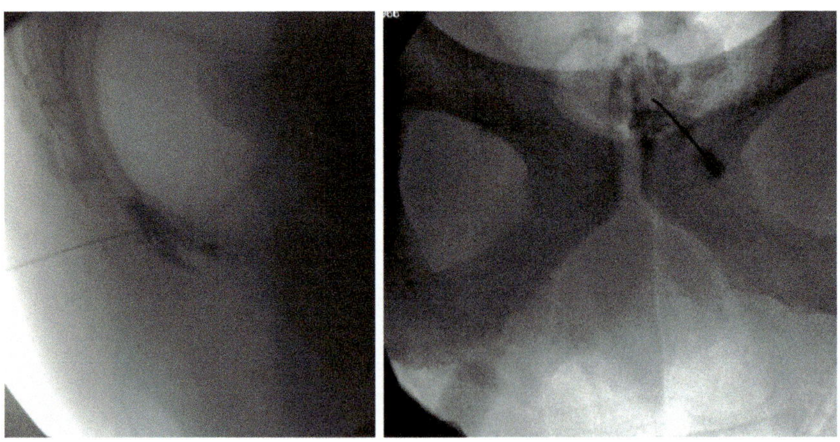

Figure 25.4. Ganglion impar injection. Fluoroscopy is done in the lateral view with the patient in the prone position. In the lateral view, the needle (below) is fluoroscopically guided through the sacrococcygeal ligament to lie approximately anterior (right) to the coccyx and posterior (left) to the rectum at the level of the ganglion impar. Appropriate spread of contrast is noted at this level. Courtesy of University of Chicago Image Library.

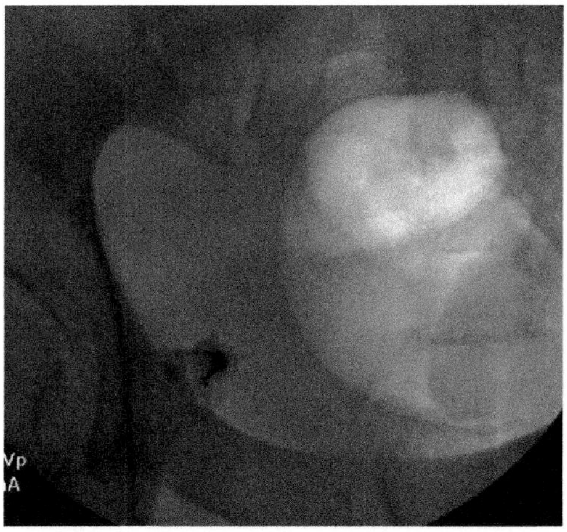

Figure 25.5. Pudendal nerve block. Fluoroscopic image of the needle placement and dye spread in a patient in prone position undergoing a left pudendal nerve block. after needle is touching the ischial spine, it is then advanced slightly medial to pass in close proximity to the pudendal nerve. Pudendal nerve blocks can also be performed in cases consistent with pudendal neuralgia.

- Coccygodynia is primarily a clinical diagnosis, although imaging can be helpful in establishing etiology and ruling out infectious or cancerous causes for coccygeal pain.
- Risks factors for coccygodynia include obesity and female gender.
- Conservative treatments are successful in 90% of cases.
- Minimally invasive interventional pain procedures include local anesthetic injection, ganglion impar blockade, and neurolytic procedures.
- Coccygectomy is recommended for definitive surgical treatment in refractory coccygodynia.

REFERENCES

1. Lirette LS, Tolba R, Eissa H. Coccydynia: an overview of the anatomy, etiology, and treatment of coccyx pain. *Ochsner J.* 2014;14(1):84–87.
2. Patijn J, Hayek S, Mekhail N, Van Zundert J, van Kleef M. 14. Coccygodynia. *Pain Pract.* 2010;10:554–559.
3. Maigne JY, Doursounian L, Chatellier G. Causes and mechanisms of common coccydynia: role of body mass index and coccygeal trauma. *Spine (Phila Pa 1976).* 2000;25(23):3072–3079.
4. Maigne JY, Guedj S, Straus C. Idiopathic coccygodynia. Lateral roentgenograms in the sitting position and coccygeal discography. *Spine.* 1994;19:930–934.
5. De Andres JCS. Coccygodynia: a proposal for an algorithm for treatment. *J Pain.* 2003;4:257–266.
6. Thiele G. Coccygodynia: cause and treatment. *Dis Colon Rectum.* 1963;6:422–436.
7. Trollegaard AA, Hellberg S. Coccygectomy: an effective treatment option for chronic coccydynia: retrospective results in 41 consecutive patients. *J Bone Joint Surg Br.* 2010;242–245.
8. Foye PM, Buttaci CJ, Stitik TP, Yonclas PP. Successful injection for coccyx pain. *Am J Phys Med Rehabil.* 2006;85:783–784. doi:10.1097/01.phm.0000233174.86070.63.
9. Bogduk N. Ganglion impar blocks for coccydynia: a case series prerequisite for efficacy trial. *Pain Med.* 2015;16:1245. doi:10.1111/pme.12838.
10. Toshniwal GR, Dureja GP, Prashanth SM. Transsacrococcygeal approach to ganglion impar block for management of chronic perineal pain: a prospective observational study. *Pain Physician.* 2007;10:661–666.
11. Foye PM. Ganglion impar pulsed radiofrequency for coccyx pain. *J Pain Symptom Manag.* 2011;41:e11–e12, author reply e12. doi:10.1016/j.jpainsymman.2010.12.003.
12. Perkins R, Schofferman J, Reynolds J. Coccygectomy for severe refractory sacrococcygeal joint pain. *J Spinal Disord Tech.* 2003;16:100–103.
13. Behrbalk E, Uri O, Maxwell-Armstrong C, Quraishi NA. Diagnosis and treatment of a rectal-cutaneous fistula: a rare complication of coccygectomy. *Eur Spine J.* 2016;25:1920–1922. doi:10.1007/s00586-014-3579-1.

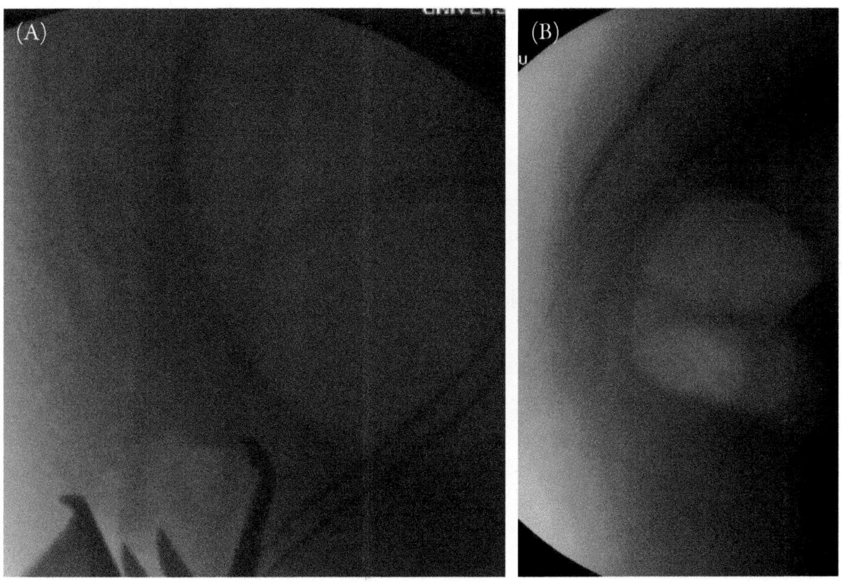

Figure 25.6. Coccygectomy. Coccyx is surgical removed under direct vision and using fluoroscopic guidance; patient with coccygectomy can still benefit from caudal epidural steroid injections if surgery is unsuccessful. Spinal cord stimulator can be used in refractory chronic pain not responsive to more conservative measures. The images show intraoperative fluoroscopic image of coccygectomy (A) as well as a caudal epidural steroid injection, lateral view, in the same patient several months after the surgery (B) also showing absence of the coccyx.

14. Patel A, Reeves C, Devang P. Poster 387. Phantom pain from coccygectomy treated with chemical neurolysis. *PM R.* 2016;8:S287. doi:10.1016/j.pmrj.2016.07.314.
15. Hanley EN, Ode G, Jackson BJ III, Seymour R. Coccygectomy for patients with chronic coccydynia: a prospective, observational study of 98 patients. *Bone Joint J.* 2016;98-B:526–533. doi:10.1302/0301-620X.98B4.36641.
16. Mitra R, Cheung L, Perry P. Efficacy of fluoroscopically guided steroid injections in the management of coccydynia. *Pain Physician.* 2007;10:775–778.
17. Nathan ST, Fisher BE, Roberts CS. Coccydynia: a review of pathoanatomy, aetiology, treatment and outcome. *J Bone Joint Surg Br.* 2010;92:1622–1627. doi:10.1302/0301-620X.92B12.25486.

REVIEW QUESTIONS

1. A 65-year-old woman with a history of depression presents with new-onset tailbone pain that has been worsening over the last month. She denies any history of trauma or falls. She has no children. She does not ride a bike or participate in any other repetitive activities that may affect the coccyx. X-ray is negative for fracture or significant degenerative disease. She is tender to palpation over the coccyx, and some local swelling is noted on rectal exam. She has lost 20 pounds over the last 2 weeks without attempting to diet or exercise. She does note that she has had decreased appetite and occasional night sweats. What is the most appropriate next step in management?

   A. Repeat X-ray
   B. Obtain MRI
   C. Refer her to a psychologist
   D. Perform a ganglion impar block

2. A 26-year-old woman presents to your office with new-onset coccygeal pain after falling on her buttocks. She is extremely distressed. In tears, she asks, "Will this ever get better?" You reply:

   A. Yes. Most cases of coccygodynia resolve on their own or with conservative therapy.
   B. Yes. However, you will most likely need surgery for the pain to resolve.
   C. No. It is most likely cancer, and you will need intense chemoradiation therapy.
   D. No. Most cases of coccygodynia are chronic and progressive.

3. A 70-year-old man presents with a 3-month history of coccygodynia. He has a history of prostate cancer in remission. You obtain a MRI that shows a bulging L3-4 disk, facet hypertrophy with foraminal stenosis at the right L5, Tarlov cysts, and no evidence of cancer recurrence. The most likely cause of his coccygodynia is:

   A. L3-L4 disk bulge
   B. Facet hypertrophy
   C. Tarlov cysts
   D. Neural tumor

ANSWERS

1. B. This is idiopathic coccygodynia. However, given its time course, in combination with weight loss, decreased appetite, night sweats, and local swelling, an MRI would be appropriate to evaluate for infection or neoplasm prior to proceeding with any injection.[5] Answer A is incorrect, as repeat X-ray may delay diagnosis. Answer C is incorrect, since, although the patient has a history of depression, a psychosomatic basis for her coccygodynia is a diagnosis of exclusion—neoplasm and infection must be ruled out first. Answer D is incorrect because an appropriate diagnosis should be made and imaging obtained before proceeding with an invasive procedure. An injection at this time has the potential to spread a treatable infection or neoplasm.

2. A. Most cases of coccygodynia resolve on their own or with conservative therapy. Answers B and C are incorrect because coccygectomy is rarely necessary, and cancer is not a common cause of coccygodynia. Answer D is incorrect in the setting of acute-onset coccygeal pain.[5]

3. C. Tarlov cysts are CSF-filled bulges of the meninges located in the sacral area (S1-S5) and can cause coccygodynia. While radicular symptoms can lead to coccygodynia, the other answers are less likely in this scenario. Answer D is unlikely, since a neural tumor would have been seen on MRI if present.

QUESTIONS AND ANSWERS

This chapter has accompanying questions and answers that are available to subscribers as part of the Oxford eLearning platform. To access the questions, follow the link below, or go to http://oxfordmedicine.com/painmanagementreview

26.

HEAD AND NECK CANCER PAIN

Esther Caballero-Manrique and Carlos A. Pino

STEM CASE AND KEY QUESTIONS

A 58-year-old male with a 60-pack/year smoking history and remote history of alcohol abuse presents to his primary care doctor with a neck "bump" that has been present for the last 4 weeks. Upon questioning, the patient also reports pain in his ears and hoarseness that started months ago. The day before his office visit, he had an episode of hemoptysis, and this is what prompted him to come to the doctor.

Physical exam by his physician reveals a rock-hard, fixed mass on the right aspect of his neck. A CT is obtained, and it reveals a subglottic mass in the larynx highly suspicious for carcinoma. The mass extends to the vocal cords but does not appear to lead to vocal cord fixation. Fine-needle aspiration biopsy of the mass is performed, confirming diagnosis of squamous cell carcinoma.

The patient meets with an oncologist and is scheduled for radiation therapy. In addition, he is started on scheduled ibuprofen and acetaminophen for odynophagia.

WHAT IS THE DIFFERENTIAL DIAGNOSIS FOR ODYNOPHAGIA? WHAT ARE THE WORLD HEALTH ORGANIZATION (WHO) GUIDELINES FOR A STEPWISE MEDICATION APPROACH TO CANCER PAIN?

The patient's pain is improved with ibuprofen and acetaminophen, but he is now constantly anxious after learning his diagnosis. He is started on lorazepam as needed. He is scheduled for radiation therapy, which is expected to be curative. On day 10 of radiation treatment, he complains to his radiology team of pain in his tongue and mouth and an inability to eat acidic foods. Examination reveals erythema in the oral cavity and two ulcers on the base of the tongue; the patient is diagnosed with stage II mucositis.

HOW IS MUCOSITIS GRADED? HOW IS IT TREATED?

The patient is started on bicarbonate rinses every 3 hours; however, he continues to have odynophagia. He goes to his dentist for a cleaning, as advised by his oncologist. He is switched to a mixture of viscous lidocaine, sodium bicarbonate, and diphenhydramine to swish and discard six times a day. He continues treatment as scheduled, but his mucositis continues to worsen; he is offered oxycodone for pain control but, because his brother was addicted to narcotics and eventually died from an overdose, the patient would like to avoid opioids if possible. A physical exam reveals extensive mucosal erythema in the oropharynx, with three ulcers on the inferior aspect of the tongue. The patient is unable to swallow liquids and is hospitalized for IV hydration; his radiation treatment is put on hold. He is started on gabapentin 300 mg nightly, which is increased gradually to 900 mg three times a day. He is also started on topical doxepin every 4 hours. After 2 weeks, he is finally able to sip fluids. He is restarted on radiation treatment while continuing his new pain regimen and although he continues to have extensive oral erythema and ulcers, his pain is improved with the doxepin and the other pain medications. He is discharged home, and he is able to complete his radiation treatment.

Two months after discharge, however, the patient's primary care physician notes the patient has lost 10 kg. Upon questioning, the patient describes difficulty swallowing food. He is started on a grade 2 dysphagia diet (pureed or soft foods and liquids); his dysphagia is attributed to his radiation treatment. He continues to lose weight, and his oncologist brings up the possibility of a feeding tube. The patient begins sobbing and tells his oncologist that it is becoming increasingly hard to cope with his disease. A feeding tube seems to be an extreme measure and he sees it as an end-of-life procedure.

WHAT ARE THE ADJUVANTS RECOMMENDED BY WHO FOR CANCER PAIN? WHY ARE ADJUVANTS AND DEPRESSION TREATMENT PARTICULARLY IMPORTANT IN HNC PATIENTS?

The patient is started on sertraline and psychotherapy. A feeding tube is inserted to supplement his oral intake. He does well for over a year, but 14 months after the end of his treatment, a visit to his oncologist reveals new hoarseness, ear pain, and facial numbness. A PET scan is performed, and it reveals recurrence of the tumor, with lymph node metastasis.

When the tumor board meets later that week, it is decided that the best course will be chemotherapy and surgical excision of the tumor via neck dissection, with lymph node resection.

The patient undergoes curative surgery, which unfortunately included partial sacrifice of the superficial cervical plexus (although the accessory nerve was preserved). He recovers well, but develops pain in his right neck and shoulder.

WHAT CAUSES NECK AND SHOULDER PAIN AFTER NECK DISSECTION? HOW CAN THIS PAIN BE TREATED?

The patient undergoes subcutaneous botulinum toxin A injection in the neck, which improves his pain; however, he develops significant weakness of the neck musculature, which makes it difficult for him to hold his head up.

WHAT ARE THE SIDE EFFECTS OF BOTULINUM TOXIN INJECTIONS? WHAT DOSE OF BOTULINUM TOXIN WOULD YOU USE IN THIS CASE?

The patient's weakness improves over the next few months. His shoulder pain is moderately controlled with periodic injections with local anesthetic and steroids, and his ear pain is relieved with gabapentin. Unfortunately, he is readmitted for aspiration pneumonia 8 months after surgery. The patient had changed his code status after surgery to "do not intubate" and "do not resuscitate" due in part to the burden of his disease on his daily life. He dies peacefully in the hospital.

DISCUSSION

Every year, more than 48,000 patients are diagnosed with head and neck cancer (HNC) in the United States.[1] HNC is defined as cancer arising from the nasal cavity, sinuses, lips, mouth, salivary glands, throat, or larynx. The primary risk factors for HNC are tobacco use, alcohol consumption, human papillomavirus (HPV) infection, and Epstein-Barr virus (EBV) infection. Curative treatment modalities vary; they range from radical neck dissection, which is physically deforming, to definitive chemotherapy or radiotherapy, or transoral robotic therapy, and selective (rather than radical) neck dissection for staging. Some patients also need postoperative chemotherapy and radiation therapy. Mortality and morbidity are significant in HNC, where even the treatments may be toxic. After HNC treatment, 5-year mortality rates may reach nearly 20%; common causes are second cancers that arise from therapy, advanced age, cardiopulmonary disease, sepsis, organ failure, pulmonary embolism, vascular disease, or surgical complications.[2]

Pain in HNC results from mucosal injury, invasion by tumor with resultant inflammation or ischemia, necrosis, infection of bone, and nerve compression or irritation. Up to 85% of patients report pain at diagnosis. The rich innervation of the orofacial region, coupled with the constant motion of the head and neck with oral intake and speech, are contributing factors to significant pain in HNC.[3] Furthermore, cancer treatment itself can be a source of severe pain, with mucositis and osteoradionecrosis being the most severe and difficult to treat complications. It is particularly important to address pain in HNC patients because head and neck pain affects crucial aspects of patients' lives, including the ability to speak, to eat, to swallow oral medicines, and even to produce facial expressions, and any difficulty can compound the affective aspect of pain.[4]

In the past, HNC was most often associated with heavy smoking and/or drinking, but the demographic has changed to younger (with average age in the 50s) white males, many of them without significant history of smoking or alcohol abuse. This is due in part to HPV, which is estimated to be the cause of 70% of HNC.[5]

Pain in HNC patients can lead to hospitalization, feeding tube insertion, and even interruption of treatment due to severe adverse events (especially due to radiotherapy), with resultant decrease in survivorship. Odynophagia, or pain upon swallowing, can be caused by inflammation, infection, or malignancy. In older patients with risk factors for HNC (smoking, alcohol abuse), odynophagia should raise suspicion of malignancy. This is especially true if other signs of malignancy exist, such as hemoptysis, blood in the oral cavity, or weight loss.

The WHO guidelines for cancer pain relief were developed with the goal of improving cancer pain treatment worldwide. An international group of experts published the guidelines in 1986.[6] The guidelines consist of a systematic approach to cancer pain to be adapted to the individual patient. The first step is anticancer treatment, along with symptomatic treatment, including medications and nonpharmacologic (Box 26.1) modalities.

The WHO guidelines further described the stepwise approach for medications to be used for pain control. In patients with mild pain, non-opioid drugs (NSAIDs and acetaminophen) are to be used. In patients with moderately severe pain, if non-opioids do not provide adequate relief when given on a scheduled basis, a weak opioid (codeine in the 1986 guidelines) can be prescribed to be used along with the non-opioids discussed. For patients with severe pain, the guidelines recommend morphine (a "strong opioid"). At each step, the guidelines suggest using adjuvants, more so in the setting of nerve injury. The guidelines of 1986 suggest corticosteroids, anticonvulsants, neuroleptic drugs, antidepressants, and anxiolytics, depending on the patient.

Other recommendations are titration of dose to effect, use of oral over intravenous dosage forms when possible, aggressive

Box 26.1. **NONPHARMACOLOGIC THERAPIES FOR THE MANAGEMENT OF PAIN IN HNC**

Conservative Therapies

Cervical collar
Physical therapy
Massage therapy
Transcutaneous electrical nerve stimulation (TENS)
Acupuncture
Biofeedback
Cognitive-behavioral therapy (CBT)

Box 26.2. INTERVENTIONAL PAIN THERAPIES FOR THE MANAGEMENT OF HNC

Trigger-point injections (TPI)
Botulinum A toxin injections
Peripheral nerve blocks
  Maxillary nerve
  Mandibular nerve
  Glossopharyngeal nerve
Sphenopalatine ganglion block
Stellate ganglion block
Trigeminal ganglion block
Intrathecal infusion

treatment of insomnia, systematic treatment of side effects, and close monitoring of the patient's symptoms, as medication side effects or new pain from disease progression may surface. Some experts have suggested an additional step in the WHO ladder consisting mainly of interventional procedures to treat cancer pain.[7] A list of interventional procedures that may help manage pain in patients with HNC is given in Box 26.2.

Figure 26.1 shows fluoroscopic images of a sphenopalatine block performed in a patient with tongue cancer.

The challenges posed in treatment of HNC pain are many, including inadequate knowledge of pain physiology and management by providers as well as fear of opioid addiction. Recently, the focus has shifted toward pain prevention with NSAIDs, opioids, and antiepileptic drugs.[8] Prevention may in turn decrease the dosage of opioids needed to control pain. In patients undergoing chemotherapy, NSAIDs and acetaminophen should be used with caution, as their antipyretic properties can mask fevers. Patients being treated for HNC with chemotherapy are at increased risk of infection due to the immunosuppressive effects of chemotherapy. The risk is compounded by physiologic changes induced by the disease process or the treatment. For instance, aspiration pneumonia is prevalent in this patient population due to large amounts of thick saliva produced by the salivary glands that are subject of inflammation and injury; in addition, radiation leads to increase risk of aspiration.[5]

PAIN MECHANISMS

Acute pain in HNC patients can be caused by the disease process (i.e., tumor leading to local inflammation, periosteal pressure, nerve invasion and compression, vascular damage, and muscle spasms), or by therapy (be it chemotherapy, radiotherapy, or surgery).

Chronic pain in HNC can be caused by disease progression or by complications of therapy, including mucosal infection, mucosal atrophy, neuropathy, dental caries, temporomandibular disorders, necrosis of the bone or of the mucosa, and postherpetic neuralgia.

Inflammation

Inflammation can be caused either by the tumor or by therapy (radiation, chemotherapy, or surgery). Reactive oxygen species (ROS) are released in response to tumor spread and inflammation in HNC. ROS in turn cause endothelial damage and increase vascular permeability, along with releasing nitric oxide (NO), which has been associated with neuropathic pain. Inflammatory cytokines also induce tumor necrosis factor (TNF) release, which is associated with neuropathic pain and is a key mediator in mucositis. COX-2 is upregulated in HNC,

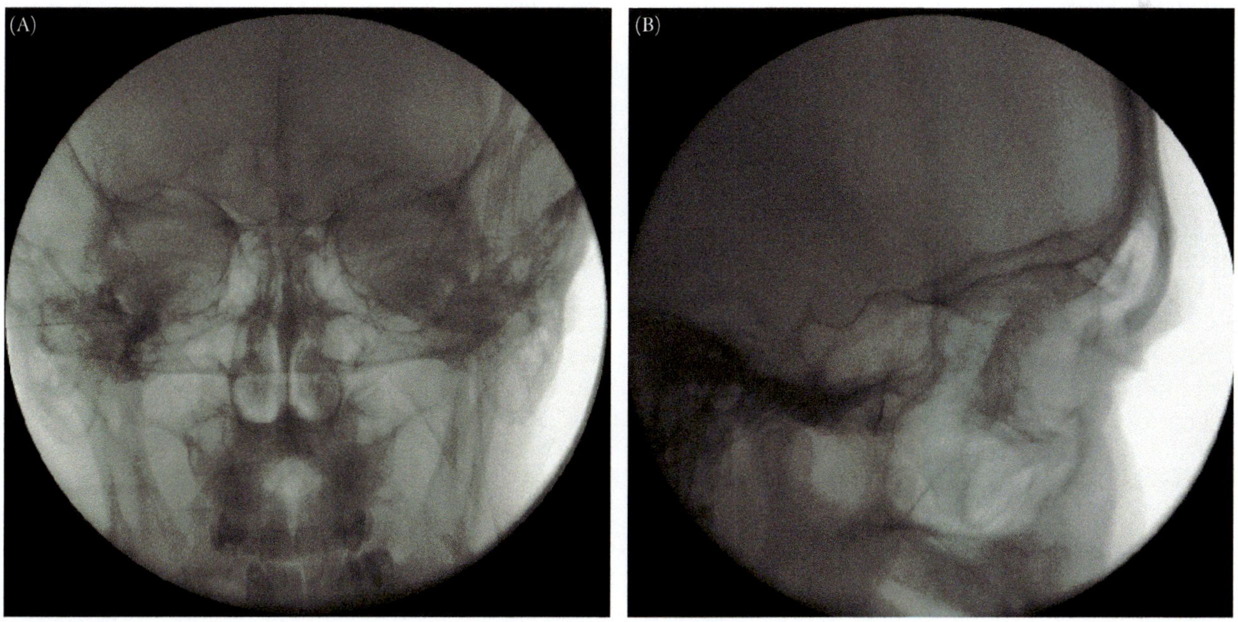

Figure 26.1. (A and B) Fluoroscopic images of sphenopalatine block performed on a patient with tongue cancer. The sphenopalatine ganglion is in the pterygopalatine fossa, which is adjacent to the middle turbinate. The needle is seen toward middle turbinate, with contrast injection showing that injection is not intravascular or intranasal.

leading to high levels of prostaglandins, which can lead to sensitization of C-type fiber afferents (thus affecting nociception) and Aδ mechanoreceptors mediating hyperalgesia.

Neuropathic Pain

Neuropathic pain results from direct nerve injury via nerve compression or invasion by tumor, neurotoxicity due to chemotherapeutic agents, or nerve injury after surgery. Neuropathic pain is more common in HNC than in other cancers. Facial, ear, and shoulder neuropathic pain are all common among HNC patients, typically consisting of constant pain with acute exacerbations several times a day; other neuropathic sensations can also be present, such as hyperalgesia, allodynia, paresthesias, and dysesthesias.[9]

The most important excitatory neurotransmitter playing a central role in neuropathic pain transmission is glutamate, which activates *N*-methyl-D-aspartate (NMDA) receptors and by doing so increases central nervous system excitability.[10] At the level of the dorsal horn, this translates into increased efficiency of synapses between primary afferents and second-order neurons after injury.

The primary afferents release neurotransmitters leading to calcium influx and activation and deactivation of a number of receptors in the cell. Postsynaptic neurons have calcium channels made up of proteins that include the $\alpha 1$ pore-forming units and $\alpha 2$ modulatory units. The $\alpha 2\delta$ subunit is of particular interest because it regulates the activation and inactivation of the calcium channel; this unit is upregulated significantly in C nociceptor fibers after nerve injury and is thought to be a key player in injury-related hypersensitivity and allodynia.[11]

Chemotherapeutic agents can also lead to neuropathic pain; painful peripheral polyneuropathy is common with some agents and usually leads to a glove-and-stocking distribution of neuropathy, with sensory loss, paresthesia, dysesthesia, pain, and muscle weakness.

Oxaliplatin-induced neuropathy leads to allodynia and dysesthesia in the hands and feet as well as pharyngeal dysesthesia, with shortness of breath and swallowing difficulty, sensations provoked by cold drinks.

Neuropathic Pain Treatment

Gabapentin and pregabalin are thought to be antagonists at the $\alpha 2\delta$ subunit of presynaptic voltage-dependent calcium channels. Neuropathic pain relief has been documented with both of these agents in cancer patients.[12] Pain improvement can be fast (within 1 or 2 weeks of initiation of treatment) and often leads to improvement in sleep and quality of life. Pregabalin also has anxiolytic effects, so it can be advantageous in patients who suffer from anxiety. Both are well tolerated, with somnolence and dizziness being the most common side effects upon initiation (although typically they improves with time).

Tricyclic antidepressants (TCAs), such as amitriptyline and imipramine, and serotonin-norepinephrine reuptake inhibitors (SNRIs), such as duloxetine and venlafaxine, are also used in the treatment of neuropathic pain. TCAs have been shown to be effective in the treatment of neuropathic pain in several randomized controlled trials.[13] Their use in HNC patients, however, might be limited by side effects, as they can lead to orthostatic hypotension, particularly in the elderly. They also have anticholinergic side effects, including xerostomia (dry mouth), which might be particularly significant in this population of patients, as they often develop xerostomia from radiation. Initiation of TCA treatment should be done gradually, with an initial dose of 25 mg daily (or 10 mg in the elderly) increasing up to 50 to 150 mg daily.[9]

Of the SNRIs, duloxetine has been proven to improve chemotherapy-induced peripheral neuropathy.[9] SNRIs are well tolerated, although they also can lead to dry mouth. Duloxetine, however, should not be used in patients with hepatic dysfunction.

Opioids are also used for treatment of cancer neuropathic pain, alone or in combination with any of the adjuvant agents discussed. Cancer pain in HNC is complex, and typically a neuropathic component is present in conjunction with other nociceptive mechanisms that cause pain. Opioids can treat neuropathic pain as well as nociceptive pain and they are generally used according to the WHO stepwise recommendations.

Cannabinoids have been shown to improve neuropathic pain. For instance, dronabinol 5 to 10 mg is well tolerated and has been shown to relieve neuropathic pain.[14]

Capsaicin is a topical agent thought to act via the transient receptor potential vanilloid 1 (TRPV1), depleting substance P from primary afferent nociceptors. Capsaicin has been shown to achieve modest pain reductions in peripheral neuropathy.

Topical lidocaine, in the form of a patch, is useful for relieving cancer-related neuropathic pain and chemotherapy-related peripheral neuropathy in the hands or feet. Caution should be exercised in patients taking class I antiarrythmics. The patches are well tolerated, with skin irritation being the main side effect. A maximum of three 5% patches should be applied (for a maximum of 12 hours) per day.

In noncancer pain, greater pain relief is achieved by combining gabapentin/pregabalin and TCAs than with either agent alone.[9] The addition of an antiepileptic or an antidepressant to existing opioid analgesia has been shown to lead to modest pain improvement, but with an increase in somnolence, dizziness, confusion, and dry mouth.[15]

For pain management in patients with HNC, the optimal approach is multimodal treatment that combines nonpharmacologic, pharmacologic, and interventional therapies designed individually for every patient.

CENTRAL SENSITIZATION

Central sensitization results from inflammation and neuronal injury; it is induced with repeated, intense nociception and continues even in the absence of nociception. When calcium enters the cell after neurotransmitter release, the α-amino-3-hydroxy-5-methyl-4-isoxazolepropionic acid (AMPA) and NMDA receptors undergo conformational changes that lead to postsynaptic hyperexcitability. Nociceptive transmission is augmented, the response to glutamate is increased, leading to hypersensitivity, and inhibitory neurotransmitters (glycine and gamma-aminobutyric acid [GABA]) are decreased; this disinhibition makes the dorsal horn neurons more susceptible to activation, triggering and maintaining central sensitization. Multiple substances are associated with central sensitization (glutamate,

NMDA, AMPA, substance P, bradykinin, nitric oxide). It is thought that the elevation of intracellular calcium leads to the increased synaptic activity that is part of central sensitization. This results is augmented nociceptive output, increased pain sensitivity, and generation of pain with innocuous stimuli.[16]

In HNC, inflammation and direct nerve injury (by tumor, cytotoxic agents, radiation, or surgery) can alter the sensory fibers, leading to central sensitization.[17]

Central Sensitization Preemption

Several groups have studied antiepileptic drugs (gabapentin and pregabalin) to treat or preempt central sensitization.[5,18,19] These medications inhibit glutamate release and NMDA activity; they also increase other inhibitory processes, leading to decreased incidence of chronic pain.

SURGICAL PAIN

HNC patients usually present with pain that may be worsened by surgery and typically improves with time. Shoulder and neck pain are typically associated with HNC surgery, due in part to trapezius or sternocleidomastoid muscle palsy after accessory nerve injury. Patients can also develop trapezius atrophy, shoulder girdle depression, limited shoulder abduction, and weakness. Neck and shoulder pain after neck dissection can be a significant cause of postoperative morbidity. Neuropathic pain can develop within the distribution of the superficial cervical plexus.

Subcutaneous botulinum toxin injections in the area of the cervical superficial plexus have been shown to decrease neuropathic pain after radical neck dissections.[20] Botulinum toxin A cleaves SNARE (soluble *N*-ethylmaleimide sensitive factor attachment protein receptor) proteins that are necessary for the docking of acetylcholine (ACh) vesicles to the presynaptic membrane. Interrupting the process of excessive ACh release may break a cycle of contracture, vessel compression, release of bradykinin, and acidosis and ultimately interrupt nociception. Other neurotransmitters have been postulated to play a role in this process, as SNARE proteins also block norepinephrine, epinephrine, substance P, and histamine. Botulinum toxin A has been found to inhibit central sensitization in studies that suggested that the toxin is transported by axons to the CNS in pathways that extend beyond ACh-dependent mechanisms.[21] Wittekindt and others studied the impact of the dose of botulinum toxin in neck and shoulder pain after neck dissection by injecting 10 mouse units/0.1 mL of saline (at 10 injection sites) or 20 mouse units/0.1 mL of saline at the same injection sites and found no difference in pain scale, although there was an improvement in quality of life in the lower-dose group.[20]

Complications of botulinum toxin injections are brachial plexopathy, polyneuritis, psoriasiform dermatitis, and muscle weakness.

MUCOSITIS

Painful mucositis is a common complication of HNC radiotherapy and chemotherapy, with severe mucositis developing in nearly 50% of patients by the fourth week of chemotherapy.[18] The process begins with an initiation phase, with damage to DNA and non-DNA structures triggered by chemotherapy and/or radiation therapy, followed by upregulation of messenger signals, leading to production of inflammatory cytokines. After this phase, signaling and amplification occur, where the inflammatory cytokines begin damaging tissues directly and lead to ulceration and inflammation, with loss of mucosal integrity. At this phase, the ulcers and inflammation are not just painful, but also lead to secondary bacterial colonization. Mucositis tends to be self-limited and healing begins once the provoking factor is removed.[22]

Treatment of mucositis involves topical and systemic analgesia. Topical analgesia is best delivered with a mixture of viscous lidocaine and a cleansing and a coating agent (typically referred to as "miracle mouthwash"). One example is a mixture of viscous lidocaine, sodium bicarbonate, and diphenhydramine that the patient swishes and discards several times a day. Topical application of morphine can also be used, but most commercial preparations contain ethanol and glycerin, which are contraindicated in the setting of mucositis. Topical doxepin can also be used, which has been shown to provide analgesia of up to 4 hours, and this relief is present even when mucositis progresses in severity.[23] Doxepin's mechanism of action is not fully understood, but it is thought that doxepin suppresses pain stimulation in cutaneous nociceptors due to sodium channel blockade and modulation of NMDA receptors.[24] Figure 26.2 shows a patient with mild mucositis with erythema and ulcers. Typically, patients can still swallow at this point. Figure 26.3 shows a patient with severe mucositis (extensive erythema and intolerable pain). At this stage, patients cannot tolerate swallowing liquids or solids.

If these measures fail, patients can be treated with oral, parenteral, or transdermal opioids. Studies have shown that gabapentin can prevent synapse remodeling in the setting of injury and decreased transmission of neuropathic pain impulses along with decrease excitatory synapse activity.[5] In particular, Bar Ad et al.[18] studied the effect of an escalating dose of gabapentin 2 weeks prior to HNC radiation treatment and found that although 80% of patients developed mucositis, only 35% required opioids during the last weeks of treatment.

OSTEORADIONECROSIS

This is considered the most devastating complication of radiation therapy in the head and neck area. It is defined as a radiation-induced ischemic necrosis of bone with associated soft tissue necrosis, occurring in the absence of primary or recurrent neoplasm. Although osteoradionecrosis can occur spontaneously, risk factors include location and tumor size, radiation dose, trauma (dental extractions), infection, and malnutrition. Oral cancers, particularly those of the tongue and floor of the mouth, are associated with a higher incidence of osteoradionecrosis,[25] and the mandible is more commonly affected than the maxilla.

Prevention of osteoradionecrosis is primarily achieved by attention to preradiation dental treatment; teeth do not inevitably need to be extracted. The majority of studies report

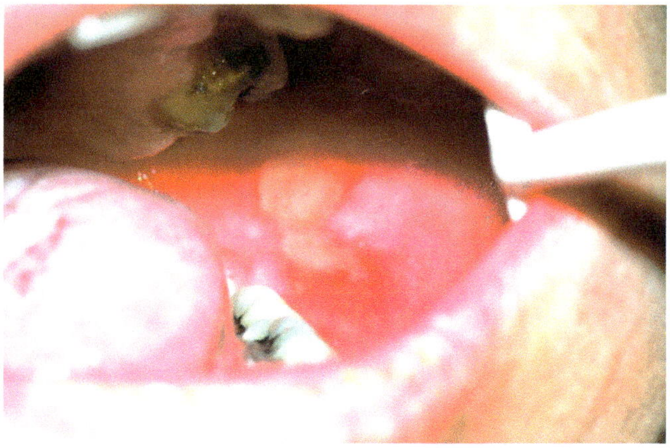

Figure 26.2. Oral mucositis in a patient who underwent radiation therapy for treatment of squamous cell cancer of the tongue. From Lalla RV, Sonis ST, Peterson DE. Management of oral mucositis in patients with cancer. *Dent Clin North Am*. 2008;52(1):61–viii.

a higher rate of osteoradionecrosis when extractions are performed after radiation therapy. Infection may be associated with osteoradionecrosis. Some lesions may be extensive enough that they will respond only to surgery and/or hyperbaric oxygen therapy.[26,27]

OVERVIEW

HNC pain is multifactorial, and it clearly has severe effects on quality of life, as patients' ability to eat, drink, kiss, talk, and move facial muscles is impacted by the disease, the treatments, and their complications.

Pain is typically present at the time of diagnosis due to tumor mass effect and inflammation, and there is usually a neuropathic pain component, either due to the cancer itself or due to radiation, chemotherapy, or surgery. This can lead to peripheral and central sensitization. In addition, mucositis is a complication of chemotherapy and radiation treatment and can become severe, affecting patients' ability to speak and to eat, and sometimes limiting the dose and duration of treatment. Management of pain for HNC is multimodal, with recent approaches aiming to preempt neuropathy and central sensitization with antiepileptics, such as gabapentin and pregabalin. Mucositis pain is treated using a stepwise protocol that includes basic oral care, rinses, topical anesthetics and coating agents, and systemic medications. Following neck dissection for HNC, patients usually experience disabling shoulder pain that can be treated with botulinum toxin injections or other interventional techniques.

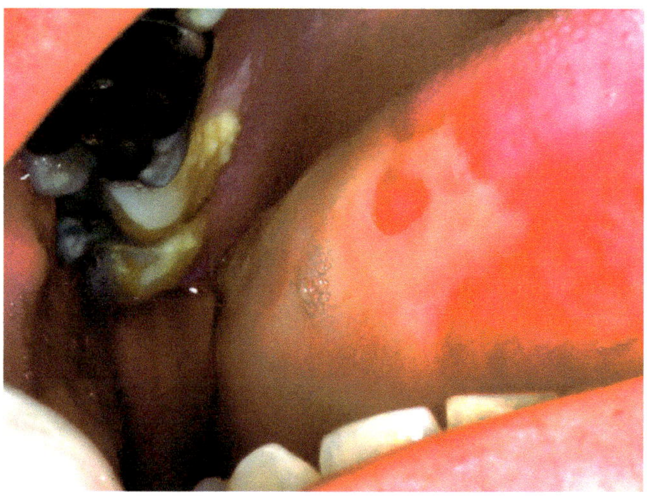

Figure 26.3. Severe mucositis, here involving the tongue. Severe ulcers usually lead to intolerable pain that prevents the patient from eating and drinking. From Lalla RV, Sonis ST, Peterson DE. Management of oral mucositis in patients who have cancer. *Dent Clin*. 2008;52(1):61–77.

CONCLUSIONS

- Head and neck cancer has significant effect on quality of life of those patients with major disability related to eating and talking.
- Pain in the HNC is present in all stages: diagnosis, immediate postsurgical and in survivors; in early stages is related to effects of cancer itself with inflammation and mass effect while in later stages related to sequelae of curative surgical procedures.
- Pain in HNC survivors follow a multimodal multidisciplinary approach with modulating agents, interventional procedures and physical therapy for optimal treatment of the residual refractory chronic pain.

REFERENCES

1. American Cancer Society. *Cancer Facts & Figures*. 2016. www.cancer.org.
2. Mell LK, Dignam JJ, Salama JK, et al. Predictors of competing mortality in advanced head and neck cancer. *J Clin Oncol*. 2010;28:15–20.
3. Epstein JB, Wilikie DJ, Fischer DJ, Kim Y, Villines D. Neuropathic and nociceptive pain in head and neck cancer patients receiving radiation therapy. *Head Neck Oncol*. 2009;1:1–26.
4. Epstein JB, Hong C, Logan RM, et al. A systematic review of orofacial pain in patients receiving cancer therapy. *Support Care Cancer*. 2010;18(8):1023–1031.
5. McMenamin EM, Grant M. Pain prevention using head and neck cancer as a model. *J Adv Pract Oncol*. 2015:6:44–48.
6. World Health Organization. *Cancer Pain Relief*. Geneva, Switzerland: World Health Organization; 1986.
7. Miguel R. Interventional treatment of cancer pain: the fourth step in the World Health Organization analgesic ladder? *Cancer Control*. 2000;7(2):149–156.
8. Paice JA, Ferrell B. The management of cancer pain. *CA-Cancer J Clin*. 2011:61:157–182.
9. Fallon MT. Neuropathic pain in cancer. *Br J Anaesth*. 2013;111:105–111.
10. Sah P, Hestrin S, Nicoll RA. Tonic activation of NMDA receptors by ambient glutamate enhances excitability of neurons. *Science*. 1989;246:815–818.
11. Basbaum A, Butista DM, Scherrer G, Julius D. Cellular and molecular mechanisms of pain. *Cell*. 2009;139:267–284.
12. Mishra S, Bhatnagar S, Goyal GN, Rana SP, Upadhya SP. A comparative efficacy of amitriptyline, gabapentin, and pregabalin in neuropathic cancer pain: a prospective randomized double-blind placebo-controlled study. *Am J Hospice Palliat Med*. 2012;29:177–182.

13. Finnerup NB, Sindrup AH, Jensen TS. The evidence for pharmacological treatment of neuropathic pain. *Pain.* 2010;150:573–581.
14. Finnerup NB, Otto M, McQuay HJ, Jensen TS, Sindrup SH. Algorithm for neuropathic pain treatment: an evidence based proposal. *Pain.* 2005;118:289–305.
15. Bennett MI. Effectiveness of antiepileptic or antidepressant drugs when added to opioids for cancer pain: systematic review. *Palliat Med.* 2011;25:553–559.
16. Latremoliere A, Woolf CJ. Central sensitization: a generator of pain hypersensitivity by central neural plasticity. *J Pain.* 2009;10:895–926.
17. Fishman SM, Ballantyne JC, Rathmell JP. *Bonica's Management of Pain.* Baltimore, MD: Lippincott, Williams & Wilkins; 2014.
18. Bar Ad V, Weinstein G, Dutta PR, Chalian A, Both S, Quon H. Gabapentin for treatment of the pain related to radiation-induced mucositis in patients with head and neck cancer treated with intensity modulated radiation therapy. *Head Neck.* 2010;116:173–177.
19. Clarke H, Bonin RP, Orser BA, Englesakis M, Wijeysundera DN, Katz J. The prevention of chronic postsurgical pain using gabapentin and pregabalin: a combined systematic review and meta analysis. *Anesth Analg.* 2012;115:428–442.
20. Wittekindt C, Liu WC, Preuss SF, Guntinas-Lichius O. Botulinum toxin A for neuropathic pain after neck dissection: a dose-finding study. *Laryngoscope.* 2006;116:1168–1171.
21. Benzon H, Rathmell JP, Wu CL, Turk DC, Argoff CE, Hurley RW. *Practical Management of Pain.* 5th ed. Mosby; 2013.
22. Epstein JB, Thariat J, Bensadoun RJ, et al. Oral complications of cancer and cancer therapy: from cancer treatment to survivorship. *Cancer J Clin.* 2012;62:62–68.
23. Epstein JB, Truelove EL, Oien H, Allison C, Le ND, Epstein MS. Oral topical doxepin rinse: analgesic effect in patients with oral mucosal pain due to cancer or cancer therapy. *Oral Oncol.* 2001;37:632–637.
24. Jayakrishnan R, Chang K, Ugurluer G, Miller R, Sio T. Doxepin for radiation therapy-induced mucositis pain in the treatment of oral cancers. *Oncol Rev.* 2015;9:290–299.
25. Curi MM, Dib LL. Osteoradionecrosis of the jaws: a retrospective study of the background factors and treatment in 104 cases. *J Oral Maxillofac Surg.* 1997;55:540–544.
26. Mounsey RA, Brown DH, O'Dwyer TP, Gullane PJ, Koch GH. Role of hyperbaric oxygen therapy in the management of mandibular osteoradionecrosis. *Laryngoscope.* 1993;54:605–608.
27. Chrcanovic BR, Reher P, Sousa AA, Harris M. Osteoradionecrosis of the jaw—a current overview—part 1. *J Oral Maxillofac Surg.* 2010;14(1):3–16

REVIEW QUESTIONS

1. What causes shoulder pain in surgically treated HNC?

   A. Trapezius or sternocleidomastoid muscle palsy after accessory nerve injury
   B. Tissue fibrosis
   C. Referred cervical pain
   D. Bursitis

2. What are the most common complications of botulinum toxin injections?

   A. Brachial plexopathy, polyneuritis, psoriasiform dermatitis, and muscle weakness
   B. Pain at the site of injection
   C. Hypersensitivity
   D. Rash

3. What were the goals of the WHO cancer pain relief guidelines of 1986?

   A. Improve survival
   B. Decrease complications of cancer treatment
   C. Decrease adverse events due to overdosing of opioids
   D. Improve cancer pain treatment worldwide

ANSWERS

1. A. Shoulder and neck pain are typically associated with HNC surgery, due in part to trapezius or sternocleidomastoid muscle palsy after accessory nerve injury. Patients also can develop trapezius atrophy, shoulder girdle depression, and limited shoulder abduction and weakness. Neck and shoulder pain after neck dissection can be a significant cause of postoperative morbidity. Neuropathic pain can develop within the distribution of the superficial cervical plexus.

2. A. Subcutaneous botulinum toxin injections in the area of the cervical superficial plexus have been shown to decrease neuropathic pain following radical neck dissections.[20] Botulinum toxin A cleaves SNARE proteins that are necessary for the docking of ACh vesicles to the presynaptic membrane; interrupting the process of excessive ACh release may break a cycle of contracture, vessel compression, release of bradykinin, and acidosis and ultimately interrupt nociception. Other neurotransmitters have been postulated to play a role in this process, because SNARE proteins also block norepinephrine, epinephrine, substance P, and histamine. Botulinum toxin A has been found to inhibit central sensitization in studies that suggested that the toxin is transported by axons to the CNS in pathways that extend beyond ACh-dependent mechanisms.[21] Wittekindt et al. studied the impact of the dose of botulinum toxin in neck and shoulder pain after neck dissection by injecting 10 mouse units/0.1 mL of saline (on 10 injection sites) or 20 mouse units/0.1 mL of saline on the same injection sites and found no difference in pain scale, although there was an improvement in quality of life in the lower-dose group.[20] Complications of botulinum toxin injections are brachial plexopathy, polyneuritis, psoriasiform dermatitis, and muscle weakness.

3. D. The WHO guidelines for cancer pain relief were developed with the goal of improving cancer pain treatment worldwide. In 1986, an international group of experts[6] published the guidelines, which consist of a systematic approach to cancer pain to be adapted to the individual patient.

QUESTIONS AND ANSWERS

This chapter has accompanying questions and answers that are available to subscribers as part of the Oxford eLearning platform. To access the questions, follow the link below, or go to ✔ http://oxfordmedicine.com/painmanagementreview

27.

MALIGNANT VISCERAL PAIN

James Wolf and Carlos A. Pino

STEM CASE AND KEY QUESTIONS

A 68-year-old man with history of hyperlipidemia, hypertension, and colonic polyps that were removed 10 years previously presents to his primary care physician for worsening constipation. He has also been more fatigued, and he thinks he has been "getting thinner" but has not weighed himself to investigate. Physical exam is notable for absent peritoneal signs and an irregular subcostal mass that descends with inspiration. No ascites, jaundice, or asterixis is noted. The patient has a heme-positive rectal exam and his hematocrit is 26%. He is referred to EGD and colonoscopy, which demonstrates an invasive adenocarcinoma. As part of a preoperative workup for metastasis, CT demonstrates a 6.5-cm mass in the left lobe of the liver.

WHAT ARE THE NEXT STEPS IN THE PATIENT'S TREATMENT? WHAT IS THE PATIENT'S PROGNOSIS? WHAT IS THE ROLE OF A PAIN SPECIALIST AT THIS POINT IN THE PATIENT'S CLINICAL COURSE?

The patient's CEA is found to be > 200, and endoscopic ultrasound-guided biopsy reveals positive mesenteric lymph nodes. The patient undergoes CT as well as hepatic ultrasound and a liver biopsy, which demonstrate metastatic colon adenocarcinoma. This represents an Astler-Coller class D malignancy, with median survival of 22 months.[1]

DESCRIBE THE TYPE OF PAIN YOU MIGHT EXPECT THIS PATIENT TO HAVE. WHAT PAIN-RELATED SYMPTOMS MIGHT HE HAVE NOW AND AS HIS DISEASE PROGRESSES? DO PATIENTS WITH DIFFERENT VISCERAL ORGANS AFFECTED HAVE SIMILAR PAIN?

The patient has poor response to 5-FU chemotherapy and declines surgery in favor of a palliative approach. His pain was initially managed adequately by his oncologist and primary care physician (PCP) with ibuprofen in addition to acetaminophen/oxycodone combination pills. Over the past month, however, he has had to increase his ibuprofen dose to the point where he has been having symptoms of gastritis. Acetaminophen/oxycodone was changed to separate acetaminophen tablets and PRN 10-mg oxycodone tablets in order to avoid toxic doses of acetaminophen.

WHAT IS THE PATHOPHYSIOLOGY UNDERLYING VISCERAL ABDOMINAL PAIN? DESCRIBE THE NEURONAL PATHWAYS THAT MEDIATE PAIN FROM THE VISCERA. WHAT OTHER PHARMACOLOGIC THERAPIES COULD YOU OFFER THIS PATIENT?

Over the subsequent 2 months, the patient's quality of life continues to decline, primarily due to advancing malignancy and uncontrolled pain. He receives limited benefit from increased doses of opioids, including methadone, transdermal fentanyl, and hydromorphone. His pain is still primarily visceral in location and quality but he also has severe constipation, nausea, fatigue, and sequelae of malnutrition. The patient has presented to the emergency department with an acute pain exacerbation and the palliative team consults you regarding an intrathecal pump.

WHAT ARE THE RISKS AND BENEFITS OF INTRATHECAL PUMPS? WOULD YOU CONSIDER OR NOT CONSIDER THIS MODALITY FOR THIS PATIENT? WHAT OTHER OPTIONS ARE AVAILABLE AT THIS POINT?

The patient undergoes neurolytic celiac plexus block, with drastic improvement in his pain. He has some persistent weakness of his right hip flexors and paresthesia in his right upper thigh, but his mobility and activity are severely limited at this point due to advanced disease. He and his family are extremely grateful to you. The patient's oncologist calls you 3 weeks later to tell you that the patient died peacefully.

WHAT ARE THE PRIMARY INDICATIONS FOR, AND CONTRAINDICATIONS TO, CELIAC PLEXUS BLOCK? HOW IS A CELIAC PLEXUS BLOCK PERFORMED? WHAT ARE THE MAJOR RISKS? WAS CELIAC PLEXUS BLOCK AN APPROPRIATE INTERVENTION FOR THIS PATIENT?

Discussion

In evaluating an intra-abdominal mass, imaging studies, blood tests for serum tumor markers, and tissue pathology are all employed, with the primary goals of determining the exact cell type and whether the tumor is primary or metastatic, and of defining its extent and invasiveness. Primary cancers can metastasize to solid visceral organs like the liver as well as to body cavities, such as the peritoneum, by hematologic or lymphatic mechanisms, as well as by direct extension. Patients with visceral metastasis do not often have a good prognosis, although certain tumor types can be curatively resected. Planning chemotherapy or radiation in order to render certain tumors more amenable to surgery must be coordinated by oncologists and surgeons. Recent evidence suggests that targeting primary tumors that have already metastasized for surgical resection may be of limited utility, and systemic therapy in these patients may yield better outcomes.[2]

Early in a patient's diagnosis and disease course, pain may not be a major issue. As prognosis becomes clearer, though, the patient as well as the treating physicians may have questions and concerns about pain that could arise due to chemotherapy, radiation, surgery, or advancing disease. Pain specialists should be able to confidently offer reassurance to patients and their families as well as pragmatism about the different modalities that can treat the pain and their efficacy.

Type and location of visceral cancer pain depend in large part on the structure affected. In this patient, afferents from the liver capsule, blood vessels, and biliary tract could all be responsible for transmitting painful stimuli, but hepatic metastasis typically causes pain when the tumor stretches the liver capsule. Intrahepatic metastasis often causes pain in the right subcostal region or right side of the back, and referred sites include the right neck, shoulder, and scapula. Quality of pain is often described as dull ache or abdominal pressure worsened by movement and deep inspiration. Anorexia and nausea are common. Hepatocellular carcinoma is uniquely associated with nontraumatic rupture, causing sudden and severe abdominal pain.[3]

Pancreatic cancer typically produces severe abdominal pain that radiates to the back and is often resistant to standard pharmacologic analgesic therapies. Blockage of the common bile duct can result in obstructive jaundice symptoms, such as icterus and pruritus. Injury to deep somatic structures of the posterior abdominal wall and involvement of the celiac plexus lead to a midline retroperitoneal syndrome manifested as a boring pain in the epigastric region that is worse in the supine position and sometimes improved by leaning forward.[3]

Intestinal obstruction, radiation enteritis, and pain due to intraperitoneal chemotherapy are common presentations not necessarily contingent on the type of malignancy diagnosed. Radiation enteritis presents as cramping, along with nausea or diarrhea, in about 50% of patients undergoing pelvic or abdominal radiotherapy, but it usually does not last long after treatments are completed. Intraperitoneal chemotherapy can cause chemical serositis, which may be experienced as pain or bloating.[3] As opposed to intestinal obstruction due to an acute process, such as a volvulus, chronic intestinal obstruction from an intra-abdominal malignancy may be caused by the tumor itself, autonomic neuropathy, or ileus. Pain from the intestinal obstruction can be either constant or colicky, and it is often accompanied by poor motility, manifested as vomiting or constipation.

VISCERAL PAIN

Visceral pain is experienced differently from somatic pain, in that patients often describe it as diffuse or vague, being more dull than sharp. Stronger emotional components are also observed with visceral pain, in addition to changes in autonomic outflow. One of the primary physiologic mechanisms for this difference is that, rather being innervated by only spinal nerves, visceral tissue is innervated by sets of nerves: either a combination of vagal and spinal nerves or a combination of sacral and spinal nerves (Figure 27.1).

Spinal visceral afferent fibers have their cell bodies in the dorsal root ganglia and terminate in laminae I and II of the dorsal horn of the spinal cord. Before reaching their terminals in the dorsal columns of the spinal cord, visceral nerves pass through the paravertebral ganglia, where they may travel rostrally or caudally through the sympathetic chain to enter the spinal cord at higher or lower spinal segments (Figure 27.2).

From here, the afferent fibers transmit noxious sensory stimuli to higher centers via the spinothalamic tract. Of note, postsynaptic second-order spinal visceral afferent fibers also synapse in the intermediolateral cell column and sacral parasympathetic nucleus, where they communicate with and influence sympathetic and parasympathetic efferent outflow to the viscera. Vagal visceral afferent fibers have cell bodies in the nodose ganglion and terminate in the nucleus tractus solitarii of the brainstem.[4] Vagal afferents form multiple connections with the hypothalamus, anterior cingulate cortex, and amygdala, which result in significant autonomic and emotional components of visceral pain.[5] Also, the perigenual cingulate gyrus, an area involved in processing of both pain and emotion, is a target of both spinal and vagal neuronal pathways.[6]

Visceral stimuli that cause perception of pain include traction on the mesentery, distension of hollow organs, contractions of muscle layers surrounding visceral organs, and chemical irritants.[7] Interestingly, cutting and burning of visceral structures do not seem to engender painful stimuli. A solid tumor itself can certainly cause obstruction, traction on the mesentery, and distension of hollow organs, leading

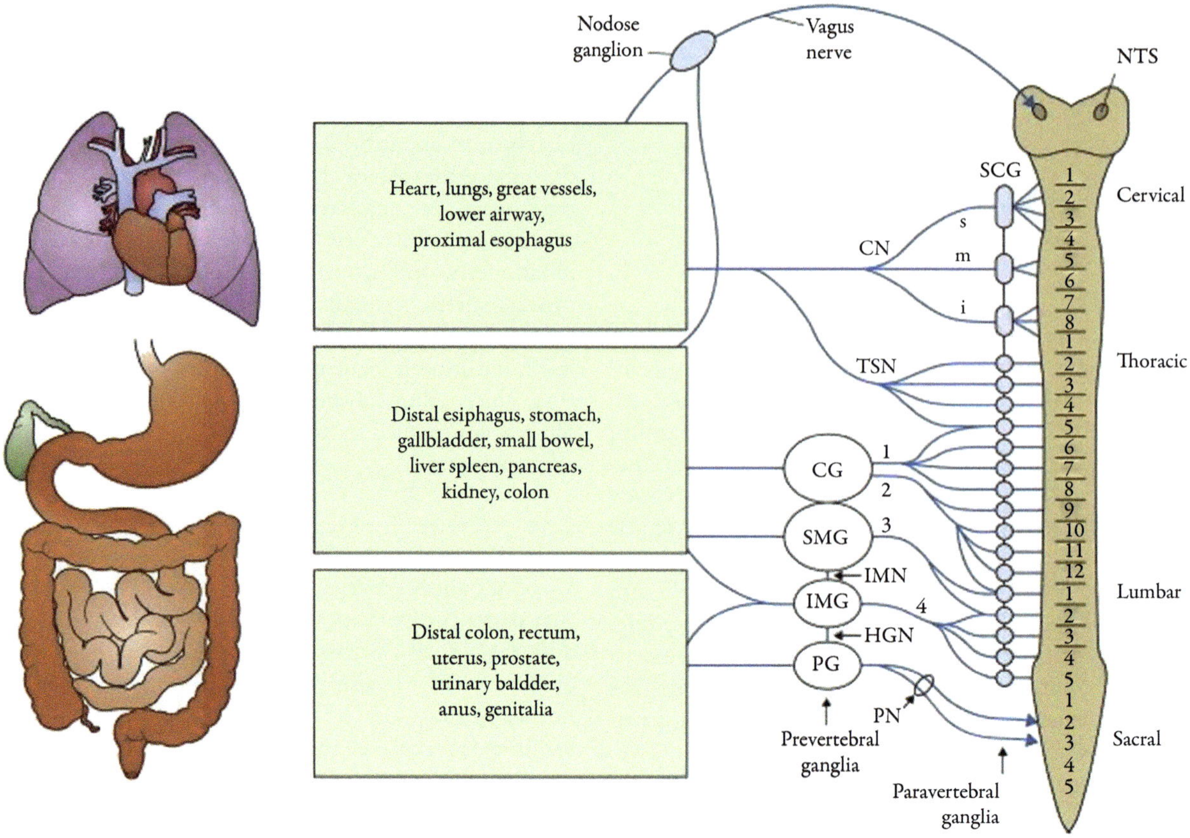

Figure 27.1. Visceral afferent nerves with cell bodies in the dorsal root ganglion innervate thoracic and abdominal viscera, terminating in the dorsal horn of the spinal cord. The vagus nerve, with cell bodies in the nodose ganglion, also innervates thoracic and abdominal viscera and has terminals in the nucleus tractus solitarii (labeled NTS in the figure). SCG, superior cervical ganglion; MCG, middle cervical ganglion; S, stellate ganglion; CG, celiac ganglion; SMG, superior mesenteric ganglion; IMG, inferior mesenteric ganglion; PG, pelvic ganglion; CN, cardiac nerves (s, m, i = superior, middle, inferior); TSN, thoracic splanchnic nerves (1, 2, 3, 4 = greater, lesser, least, lumbar); IMN, intermesenteric nerve; HGN, hypogastric nerve; PN, pelvic nerve. Reproduced with permission from Wall PD, McMahon SB, Koltzenburg M. *Wall and Melzack's Textbook of Pain*. 5th ed. Philadelphia, PA: Elsevier/Churchill Livingstone; 2006.

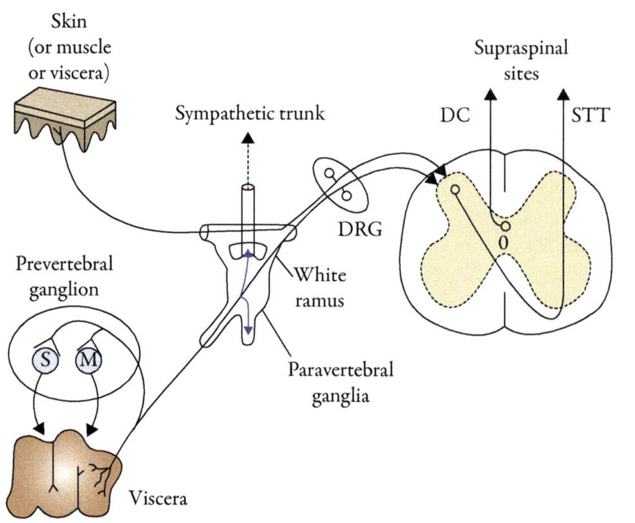

Figure 27.2. Spinal visceral afferent nerves with cell bodies in the dorsal root ganglion innervate thoracic and abdominal viscera, terminating in the dorsal column (DC) of the spinal cord. From here, visceral sensory information is transmitted rostrally in the contralateral spinothalamic tract (STT). Spinal visceral afferents may collateralize and terminate on secretory (S) or motor (M) neurons in the prevertebral ganglia and influence visceral secretions and motility. Reproduced with permission from Wall PD, McMahon SB, Koltzenburg M. *Wall and Melzack's Textbook of Pain*. 5th ed. Philadelphia, PA: Elsevier/Churchill Livingstone; 2006.

to stronger and more painful contractions of the smooth muscle layers. Furthermore, solid tumors can exert painful mechanical stress directly on a nerve. Of note, all of the aforementioned mechanisms can sensitize visceral afferent fibers by increasing their excitability via inflammatory mediators. This increased peripheral sensitization can lead to central sensitization, with the ultimate effect of a broader area of pain than might otherwise be expected based on the actual pathology.[7]

TREATMENT

An initial approach to treating malignant visceral pain should address the unique characteristics of visceral pain pathways discussed. Notably, the dual innervation of visceral structures by both spinal and vagal pathways may make certain visceral pain symptoms resistant to some regional block techniques. Furthermore, impaired visceral function, such as decreased gut motility seen with many analgesic medications, may actually worsen pain due to distended hollow organs or mesenteric traction.[8] Because metastatic and primary malignancies can cause pain through inflammatory, neuropathic, and mechanical mechanisms, at least attempting treatment with acetaminophen, steroids, nonsteroidal anti-inflammatory drugs (NSAIDs), and antineuropathic agents like antidepressants and anticonvulsants is reasonable, so long as no organ injury or dysfunction is present that precludes their use. In terms of less common drug therapies, serotonin antagonists, selective kappa opioid agonists, and anticholinergic agents have been explored as means for relieving visceral pain without impairing function, but evidence for significant benefit is scarce. Muscarinic cholinergic receptors are the primary mechanism of parasympathetically mediated visceral smooth muscle contraction, and two meta-analyses have shown that patients receiving drugs that block this mechanism experience improved pain.[9,10] Unfortunately, no single pharmacologic therapy is available at this time that shows efficacy at the level a clinician might expect of opioids for treating somatic pain. Because the non-opioid therapies alone may not offer acceptable efficacy for treating visceral pain, and because opioids can cause possibly painful functional impairment of visceral function, using non-opioid medications as adjuvant therapy to lower the required dose of opioid analgesics is a reasonable approach. *N*-methyl-D-aspartate (NMDA) receptor antagonists like ketamine are particularly useful in improving opioid analgesia and possibly sparing the opioid dose.[11]

In terms of procedural interventions, celiac plexus block, midline myelotomy, neuraxial catheter placement, and spinal cord stimulation are all options for patients with visceral pain. Because of their invasive nature and potential for serious side effects, these interventions are usually reserved for patients with end-stage disease. Neuraxial analgesia may be beneficial for patients with pain refractory to oral or parenteral medication or for those whose dosing requirements result in unacceptable adverse effects. Opioids, local anesthetics, and adjuvant drugs can be delivered to the epidural or intrathecal space either by an external pump or an implantable system. Clinicians must understand the resources available at the facility where the patient will be residing before placing either type of device. External infusion devices are more often used in end-of-life care, primarily because concerns regarding a patient's mobility are usually superseded by the aim of pain control and because dosages and boluses are easily titratable to a patient's pain level, which will be labile and progressive with advanced cancer. However, these devices require staff familiar with their programming and maintenance in order for them to be used safely and effectively. Permanent intrathecal pumps are more appropriate for non-palliative patients who are expected to have a chronic course of pain at a somewhat stable level.[12] Neuraxial procedures for palliative end-of-life care carry the same risks as those performed in the acute or perioperative setting. One important difference, though, is that indwelling epidural catheters convey a significant risk of infection that increases proportionally to how long they are in place.[13,14] The risk of infection in patients receiving epidural therapy via tunneled catheter for more than 70 days approaches 15%, whereas the incidence of infection extending to the epidural space is about 1%.[15] Because many of the infections are superficial and do not extend to the epidural space, they can often be managed without removal of the catheter.[13]

Less studied interventions for end-stage cancer pain of the viscera include spinal cord stimulation and midline myelotomy. A retrospective analysis of 70 patients receiving spinal cord stimulation for visceral pain showed that most had pain relief of 50%, with significantly decreased opioid use.[16] Surgical myelotomy is hypothesized to disrupt a ventromedial dorsal column pathway. Results have been promising, but few studies have been performed.

Conversely, celiac plexus block, specifically neurolytic celiac plexus block, has strong evidence supporting its utility in treating cancer pain. Important benefits of celiac plexus block are that it produces significant pain relief and even complete pain resolution, has a long duration of effect, and rarely causes severe complications. Ischia et al. found that, even with different techniques of celiac plexus block, 70% to 80% of patients had their pain completely resolved, and the pain relief lasted until death in 60% to 75% of patients.[17] Analgesic, nonneurolytic celiac plexus block can be attempted in benign conditions, such as chronic pancreatitis, and neurolytic celiac plexus block has been performed in select patient groups who have favorable response to analgesic celiac plexus block.

Anatomically, the celiac plexus is a collection of ganglia that vary significantly among individuals in terms of size, number, and precise location. Generally, the plexus is anterolateral to the aorta, surrounding the celiac artery roughly at the level of the first lumbar vertebra. Preganglionic fibers extend from the intermediolateral horn of levels T5-T12 of the spinal cord to exit along ventral roots of the spinal nerves and course through the white rami communicans into the sympathetic chain. Without synapsing there, the fibers pass through the sympathetic chain and ultimately reach the celiac ganglion as the greater splanchnic nerve (composed of fibers from T5-T10), lesser splanchnic nerve (composed of fibers from T10-T11), and least splanchnic nerve (composed of fibers from T11-T12). Postsynaptic fibers follow blood vessels to innervate the distal esophagus, stomach, duodenum, small intestine, ascending and proximal transverse colon, adrenal glands, pancreas, spleen, liver, and biliary system. Sensory afferent fibers travel this course without synapsing in the celiac ganglion; rather, they traverse it to their terminals in the dorsal horn of the spinal cord, as described.[3,4]

Multiple techniques exist for performing a celiac plexus block. Fluoroscopy, CT, and ultrasonography have been used to assist in needle guidance. Practitioners should consult an atlas and resources that describe the procedures in detail, but key points of common techniques are briefly described here. Deciding upon which approach and imaging technique to use mainly has to do with a practitioner's experience and the variability of anatomic structures and tumors that may negate or obligate certain needle trajectories.

The two-needle retrocrural technique is performed from the posterior approach. Two 20-G needles are inserted bilaterally and inferiorly to each transverse process of the L1 vertebra and then are advanced at an angle until the L1 vertebral body is contacted. "Walking off" the anterolateral aspect of the L1 vertebral body with the left-side needle and gradually advancing until aortic pulsations can be seen to move the needle itself should represent a needle tip position directly posterior to the aorta. The right-side needle is advanced beyond the anterolateral aspect of the L1 vertebral body to the anterolateral aspect of the aorta. Depending on the patient's anatomy and the ultimate position of the needle tips, injection here may actually yield a "splanchnic" block by interrupting the paired splanchnic nerves that arise from the sympathetic chain and then pass through the crura of the diaphragm before joining the celiac ganglion. Visceral afferent fibers that travel in the splanchnic nerves are the same as those that pass through the celiac plexus, so the ultimate results are the same.

Alternatively, using a single needle via the same entry point and trajectory with a unilateral approach is termed a single-needle periaortic technique. After the needle has been walked off the anterolateral aspect of the left-side L1 vertebral body, the clinician gradually advances the needle while observing for transmissions of the aortic pulse. The goal is to direct the needle slightly less medially and more anteriorly until the needle tip is anterior and lateral to the aorta. In this position, there is theoretically less risk of drug spreading to the spinal nerve roots. On fluoroscopic AP view, contrast should be noted slightly left of midline, and a later view should show a smooth, curvilinear shadow representing the preaortic space (see Figure 27.3).

A transaortic approach is also performed from a posterior position, but a smaller, 22-G needle with a more direct angle is used to reach the preaortic space by puncturing both the posterior and anterior walls of the aorta. After noting tactile changes in tissue density to indicate the walls of the aorta and aspiration of blood to identify the intravascular space, the clinician ultimately positions the needle tip in the preaortic space in the direct vicinity of the celiac plexus. AP fluoroscopic imaging should show contrast at the midline, with attention paid to make sure no contrast is in the peritoneal space.

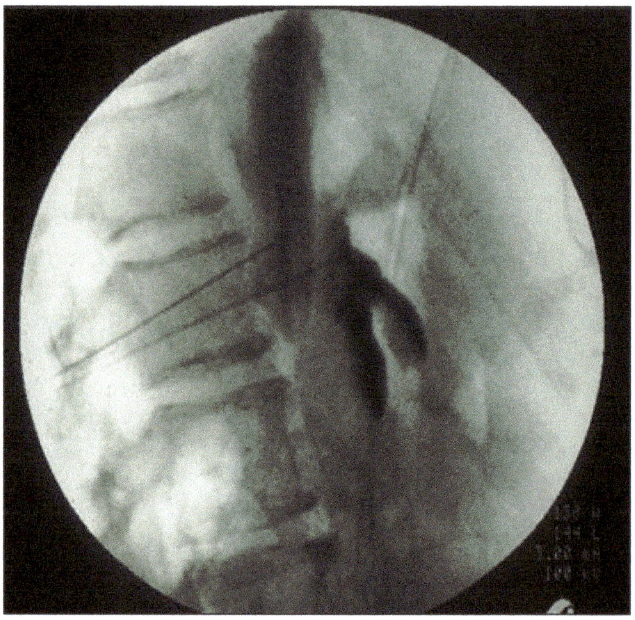

Figure 27.3. Celiac plexus block. Lateral view of retrocrural and anterocrural positions of the needle tip, with characteristic contrast distributions for each approach. Reproduced with permission from Benzon HT. *Practical Management of Pain*. 4th ed. Philadelphia, PA: Elsevier/Mosby; 2014.

In the above techniques, vigilant attention to needle aspiration is needed to identify any blood, CSF, or urine, because the kidney, aorta, and intrathecal space are all possible sites for unintended injections. Also, observation of a sensory or motor block with injection of a rapid-acting local anesthetic suggests that the needle tip is close enough to spinal nerve roots that any drug injected will affect them. Because alcohol, phenol, local anesthetic, or steroid can be injected depending on the indication and goal of the procedure, involvement of the spinal nerves could obviously be catastrophic if significant structures were exposed to a true neurolytic dose. Conversely, absence of a motor or sensory block in the lumbar dermatomes suggests that subsequent drug injected through the needles will not reach the spinal nerve roots.

Ultrasound-guided percutaneous celiac plexus block has the benefit of allowing the patient to be in the supine position. This makes it possible to administer the block at the bedside, with limited exposure to ionizing radiation. Using color Doppler to visualize the celiac trunk and mesenteric vessels, the practitioner injects local anesthetic or neurolytic agent between the structures.

Risks of celiac plexus block include hypotension (incidence about 38%), for which fluid bolus is often administered prophylactically before the blocking agent is administered. Due to the risk of vascular structure compromise, systemic anticoagulation or pathologic coagulopathy is a contraindication. Postblock diarrhea occurs in about 44% of patients, and this increased GI motility due to unopposed parasympathetic stimulation means that celiac plexus block should be avoided in patients with bowel obstruction. Epidural, subdural, subarachnoid, intrapleural, and intradiscal injections are all possible, as well as injury to spinal nerve roots, as discussed. Other uncommon adverse events include pneumothorax, trauma to kidneys and ureters, retroperitoneal hemorrhage, and spinal cord injury secondary to neurolytic spread to the anterior spinal artery.[18,19] Clinicians should keep in mind that noninterventional techniques like opioid therapy have substantial risks as well, and certain patients may benefit from having an efficacious procedure like celiac plexus block performed earlier in their disease course, as it may be associated with improved quality of life.[20]

CONCLUSIONS

- Visceral pain is experienced as dull and diffuse, with significant autonomic and emotional components because the viscera are innervated by a combination of either vagal and spinal nerves or sacral and spinal nerves. Spinal fibers synapse in the intermediolateral cell column, where they communicate with and influence sympathetic and parasympathetic efferent outflow to the viscera. Vagal afferents form multiple connections with the hypothalamus, anterior cingulate cortex, and amygdala that mediate emotional components of visceral pain.

- Visceral stimuli that cause perception of pain include traction on the mesentery, distension of hollow organs, contractions of muscle layers surrounding visceral organs, and chemical irritants. Cutting and burning of visceral structures do not seem to engender painful stimuli.
- Impaired visceral function (decreased gut motility) seen with many opioid analgesic medications may actually worsen pain due to distended hollow organs or mesenteric traction. Attempting multimodal treatments with acetaminophen, steroids, NSAIDs, NMDA antagonists, and antineuropathic agents like antidepressants and anticonvulsants is reasonable, but these non-opioid therapies alone or in combination may not offer acceptable efficacy for treating visceral pain. However, using non-opioid medications as adjuvant therapy to lower the required dose of opioid analgesics is a reasonable approach.
- Autonomic fibers originating from T5-T12 spinal levels travel through the white rami communicans and the sympathetic chain to enter the celiac plexus as the greater, lesser, and least splanchnic nerves. Visceral sensory afferent fibers travel with autonomic fibers through the celiac plexus without synapsing on their way to targets in the dorsal spinal cord.
- Celiac plexus block has strong evidence supporting its utility in treating cancer pain for significant periods of time, the technique being used sometimes being dictated by the anatomic location of the tumor. Hypotension and diarrhea are common but often short-lived side effects. Clinicians should keep in mind that, although rare catastrophic complications are possible with celiac plexus block, high-dose opioid therapy also has its own risks. Some clinical scenarios might warrant performing celiac plexus block earlier in a cancer patient's disease course rather than at the very end of life.

REFERENCES

1. Sternberg A, Sibirsky O, Cohen D, Blumenson LE, Petrelli NJ. Validation of a new classification system for curatively resected colorectal adenocarcinoma. *Cancer.* 1999;86(5):782–792.
2. Poultsides GA, Paty PB. Review: reassessing the need for primary tumor surgery in unresectable metastatic colorectal cancer: overview and perspective. *Ther Adv Med Oncol.* 2010;3(1):35–42.
3. Fishman SM, Ballantyne JC, Rathmell JP. *Bonica's Managment of Pain.* 4th ed. Baltimore, MD: Lippincott Williams & Wilkins; 2010.
4. Wall PD, McMahon SB, Koltzenburg M. *Wall and Melzack's Textbook of Pain.* 5th ed. Philadelphia, PA: Elsevier/Churchill Livingstone; 2006.
5. Zagon A. Does the vagus nerve mediate the sixth sense? *Trends Neurosci.* 2001;24(11):671–673.
6. Vogt BA. Pain and emotion interactions in subregions of the cingulate gyrus. *Nat Rev Neurosci.* 2005;6(7):533–544.
7. Mayer EA, Gebhart GF. Basic and clinical aspects of visceral hyperalgesia. *Gastroenterology.* 1994;107:271–293.
8. Benzon HT. *Practical Management of Pain.* 4th ed. Philadelphia, PA: Elsevier/Mosby; 2014.
9. Davenport K, Timoney AG, Keeley FX. Conventional and alternative methods for providing analgesia in renal colic. *BJU Int.* 2005;95(3):297–300.
10. Poynard T, Regimbeau C, Benhamou Y. Meta-analysis of smooth muscle relaxants in the treatment of irritable bowel syndrome. *Aliment Pharmacol Ther.* 2001;15(3):355–361.
11. Mercadante S, Arcuri E, Tirelli W, Casuccio A. Analgesic effect of intravenous ketamine in cancer patients on morphine therapy. *J Pain Symptom Manag.* 2000;20(4):246–252.
12. Farquhar-Smith P, Chapman S. Neuraxial (epidural and intrathecal) opioids for intractable pain. *Br J Pain.* 2012;6(1):25–35.
13. Rathmell JP, Lake T, Ramundo MB. Infectious risks of chronic pain treatments. *Reg Anesth Pain Med.* 2006;31(4):346–352.
14. Smitt PS, Tsafka A, Zande FT-VD, et al. Outcome and complications of epidural analgesia in patients with chronic cancer pain. *Cancer.* 1998;83(9):2015–2022.
15. Jong PCD, Kansen PJ. A comparison of epidural catheters with or without subcutaneous injection ports for treatment of cancer pain. *Anesth Analg.* 1994;78(1).
16. Kapural L, Deer T, Yakovlev A, et al. Technical aspects of spinal cord stimulation for managing chronic visceral abdominal pain: the results from the national survey. *Pain Med.* 2010;11(5):685–691.
17. Ischia S, Luzzani A, Ischia A, Faggion S. A new approach to the neurolytic block of the coeliac plexus: the transaortic technique. *Pain.* 1983;16(4):333–341.
18. Eisenberg E, Carr DB, Chalmers TC. Neurolytic celiac plexus block for treatment of cancer pain. *Anesth Analg.* 1995;80(2):290–295.
19. Conno FD, Caraceni A, Aldrighetti L, et al. Paraplegia following coeliac plexus block. *Pain.* 1993;55(3):383–385.
20. Oliveira RD, Reis MPD, Prado WA. The effects of early or late neurolytic sympathetic plexus block on the management of abdominal or pelvic cancer pain. *Pain.* 2004;110(1):400–408.

REVIEW QUESTIONS

1. The primary reason that visceral pain may be difficult to localize is:

   A. Poor representation of visceral afferents within nucleus tractus solitarii
   B. Convergence of visceral and somatic afferents on the same dorsal horn neurons
   C. Low threshold of visceral neuroreceptors
   D. Multiple concomitant causes of pain, including mechanical stretch, ischemia, inflammation, and neuropathy

2. Which of the following mechanisms play a role in visceral pain sensitization?

   A. Wind up of interneurons within dorsal horn and activation of silent primary afferents by inflammatory changes
   B. Wind up of interneurons within the dorsal horn, activation of silent primary afferents by inflammatory changes, and increased responsiveness of spinal neurons due to inflammatory changes
   C. Activation of silent primary afferents by inflammatory changes and increased responsiveness of spinal neurons due to inflammatory changes

D. Wind up of interneurons within the dorsal horn and increased responsiveness of spinal neurons due to inflammatory changes

3. Visceral receptors are located in all of the following except

A. Parenchyma
B. Mesentery
C. Mucosa
D. Smooth muscle

ANSWERS

1. B. There are multiple reasons for the diffuse and vague qualities of visceral pain, but its referral and localization to body wall structures is due to the convergence of visceral and somatic afferents on the same dorsal horn neurons. Vagal visceral afferent fibers terminate in the nucleus tractus solitarii, but visceral pain pathways have poor representation within the primary somatosensory cortex. Nevertheless, the majority of visceral afferents transmit information regarding motor or reflex functions, with few afferent neurons that are specialized for pain transmission.[3]

2. C. Repeated visceral stimuli increase the strength of reflex responses. Inflammation of visceral structures increases the magnitude of a response to a given mechanical stimulus and decreases the thresholds for the evocation of nociceptive responses. Some primary afferents are normally so nonreactive to most stimuli that they are essentially "silent" in nonpathologic states. In the context of an inflammatory tissue response, though, they become highly reactive to mechanical stimuli. Spinal neurons also change their responsiveness to visceral stimuli in the presence of inflammation, perhaps due to increased afferent activity, alteration of dorsal horn neurons, or altered modulation. Somatic central sensitization characterized by "wind up" of interneurons within the dorsal horn does not occur with visceral pain.[3]

3. A. Visceral receptors are located in mucosa, serosa, and muscle of hollow organs as well as visceral mesentery. They are not reported in the parenchyma of solid organs.[3]

QUESTIONS AND ANSWERS

This chapter has accompanying questions and answers that are available to subscribers as part of the Oxford eLearning platform. To access the questions, follow the link below, or go to ✔ http://oxfordmedicine.com/painmanagementreview

28.

POSTOPERATIVE ABDOMINAL WALL PAIN

Dan Dirzu, Ovidiu Palea, and Sarah Choxi

Abdominal pain accounts for almost 1.5% of office visits and nearly 5% of emergency department admissions each year in the United States.[1,2] In 35% to 51% of patients, no distinct physiologic, structural, or biochemical abnormality is identified.[3] In 2% to 3% of patients with chronic abdominal pain, the pain arises from the abdominal wall. The likelihood can be as high as 30% in patients with previously diagnosed chronic abdominal pain of no identifiable pathology.[4]

STEM CASE AND KEY QUESTIONS

A 28-year-old healthy female, who had a laparoscopic cholecystectomy 8 months earlier, suffers from severe pain in the right upper quadrant that began 6 months ago. Pain is exacerbated with postural changes. It is described as a constant pressure with an occasional superimposed burning sensation. Anti-inflammatories, opioid analgesics, topical ointments, and neuropathic medications have offered minimal relief. There is no change in the pattern of her pain after eating, urination, bowel movements, sexual activity, or menstruation. The patient has had a comprehensive workup: abdominal ultrasound, CT of the abdomen, barium radiography and endoscopy of the upper and lower digestive tract, endoscopic retrograde cholangiopancreatography, and diagnostic laparoscopy. Results were normal. On physical examination, point tenderness was elicited with palpation of the right upper quadrant of the abdomen in the area of a healed incision site from trocar placement during the laparoscopic cholecystectomy. The same pain was exacerbated when the patient was asked to lift her head and shoulders from the examination table to tense the abdominal muscles (positive Carnett's sign). The positive Carnett's sign suggests the source of the pain is the abdominal wall, as pain would lessen if the source were visceral.[5,6]

WHAT IS POSTOPERATIVE ABDOMINAL WALL PAIN?

Postoperative abdominal wall pain is chronic, unremitting pain unaffected by eating or bowel function but exacerbated by postural change. A localized, tender trigger point can be identified, although pain may radiate over a diffuse area of the abdomen.[7] A positive Carnett's sign favors an abdominal wall pain generator and not a visceral source.[5] The pain is likely from cutaneous nerve root or myofascial irritation.[7]

WHAT IS THE DIFFERENTIAL DIAGNOSIS FOR ABDOMINAL PAIN?

An organic cause for the pain should be excluded first. Organic causes vary from acute to chronic and from less serious to those requiring prompt medical attention. The location and pattern of pain, as well as its time course, are helpful in the diagnosis. Acute abdominal pain typically develops and resolves over hours or days; chronic abdominal pain may be intermittent or episodic and persist for weeks to months and occasionally years.

Nonorganic causes of abdominal pain include structural deformities, such as rectus sheath hematoma or incisional and other abdominal wall hernias. A thorough history is taken, with attention to particular warning signs (Box 28.1) to differentiate organic from nonorganic causes of abdominal pain (Box 28.2).

The history of surgery in the area of her current pain, with the finding of a positive Carnett's sign on physical examination in the absence of other intra-abdominal pathology, suggests that the patient has abdominal wall pain consistent with anterior cutaneous nerve entrapment syndrome (ACNES) in the area of trocar placement from the previous surgery.

ARE THE TREATMENTS DIFFERENT FOR ORGANIC AND NONORGANIC CAUSES OF PAIN? WHAT IS THE OPTIMAL TREATMENT PLAN FOR THE PATIENT?

Organic causes of pain necessitate a gastroenterology workup. Treatment for nonorganic causes depends on whether the pain is functional or structural. Functional abdominal pain is ongoing abdominal pain for which there is no identifiable biochemical, structural, or infectious cause. Both types of nonorganic pain may benefit from multimodal therapy: cognitive-behavioral therapy, biofeedback, and relaxation techniques in addition to pharmacotherapy and regional analgesia.[8] Abdominal wall pain may benefit from local anesthesia with steroids, neurolysis, neurectomy, or neurostimulation (Figure 28.1).[9]

Box 28.1. **SYMPTOMS OF ORGANIC CAUSES OF ABDOMINAL PAIN**

- unexplained weight loss
- fevers
- pain radiating to the back
- bilious emesis
- hematemesis
- hematochezia or melena
- diarrhea
- dysphagia
- arthritis
- anemia

The patient most likely has ACNES. An attempt to perform a rectus sheath block failed because the patient could not tolerate the placement of the ultrasound probe over the anterior rectus abdominis muscle due to exquisite tenderness. Subsequently, she was able to tolerate a transversus abdominis plane (TAP) block with local anesthetic and steroid for both diagnostic and therapeutic purposes.[5]

HOW IS A TAP BLOCK PERFORMED?

A high-frequency linear probe is placed lateral to the rectus sheath and all three layers of the abdominal muscles are visualized clearly (Figure 28.2).

A combination of triamcinolone 80 mg and 8 mL of 0.375% bupivacaine injected between the fascial layer of the internal oblique and transversus abdominis muscles using a 2-inch, 22-G echogenic needle and an in-plane approach (Figure 28.4) provided excellent pain relief, with patient's pain intensity decreasing from 7/10 to 2/10 on the Visual Analog Scale (VAS). After 1 week, a second injection was administered. After the second injection, the pain intensity on VAS decreased to 0/10. She remained symptom-free for 10 months until the pain returned.

Box 28.2. **COMMON FEATURES OF ABDOMINAL WALL PAIN**

- constant or fluctuating pain; not typically episodic
- postural pain
- pain unrelated to oral intake or bowel or bladder function
- abdominal tenderness unchanged or increased when abdominal wall muscles are tensed (Carnett's sign)
- discrete, tender trigger point that may or may not refer pain over a larger area
- trigger points along the lateral margins of the rectus abdominis muscles
- no findings of intra-abdominal process

ARE THERE OTHER TREATMENTS FOR LONGER, SUSTAINED RELIEF?

Sustained and often permanent pain relief can be achieved via chemical neurolysis or radiofrequency (RF) nerve ablation (Figure 28.3).[9,10] After the risks and benefits were explained to the patient, the pain physician performed a neurolytic TAP block under ultrasound guidance with 10 mL of 6% aqueous phenol. The patient tolerated the injection well and achieved complete pain relief without additional interventions.

DISCUSSION

INCIDENCE

Chronic abdominal wall pain is among the most common patient complaints seen by primary care doctors, surgeons, gastroenterologists, and pain physicians. The prevalence of chronic postsurgical pain after abdominal surgery ranges from 10% to 30%. Women, especially those 30 to 50 years old, are four times more likely to be affected than men.[11,12]

ETIOLOGY

The mechanism causing chronic postoperative abdominal pain is poorly understood. The pain is likely caused by inflammation, tissue and nerve damage, or alterations in central pain processing.[13] Surgical trauma rarely causes direct transection of nerve trunks. Injury is caused by stretching or impingement of nerves during tissue retraction or incision and during manipulation of skin, viscera, fascia, muscles, and joints.[14] Chronic postsurgical pain is likely a combination of nerve and tissue damage and alterations in central pain processing. Preoperative identification of susceptible patients and preventive strategies are a focus for protection against chronic postsurgical pain.[13] Among risk factors that have been identified for development of chronic postsurgical pain are young age, female sex, obesity, anxiety, depression, lack of optimism, stress, catastrophizing, low income, low self-rated health, lack of education, bariatric surgery, longer hospitalization, direct inguinal hernia, previous operation, bilateral repair, postoperative complications, remifentanil use during surgery, pain before surgery (both related and unrelated to surgical site), and time to return to work.[15–22] Protective

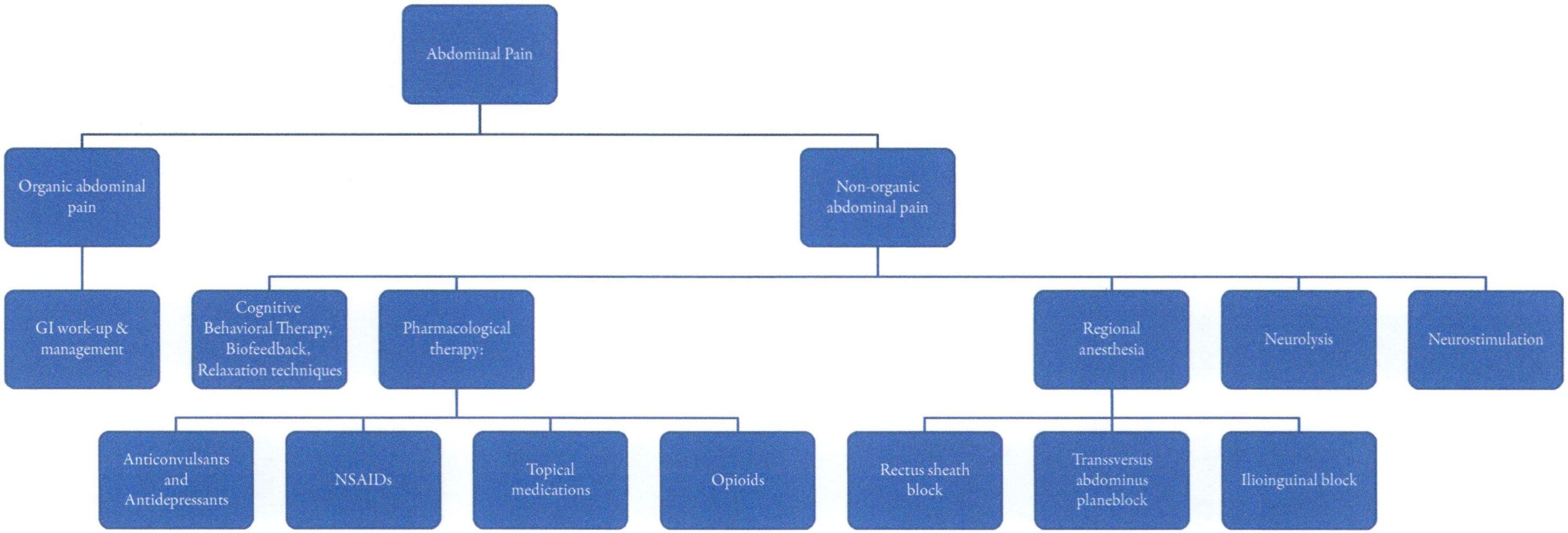

Figure 28.1. Abdominal pain management.

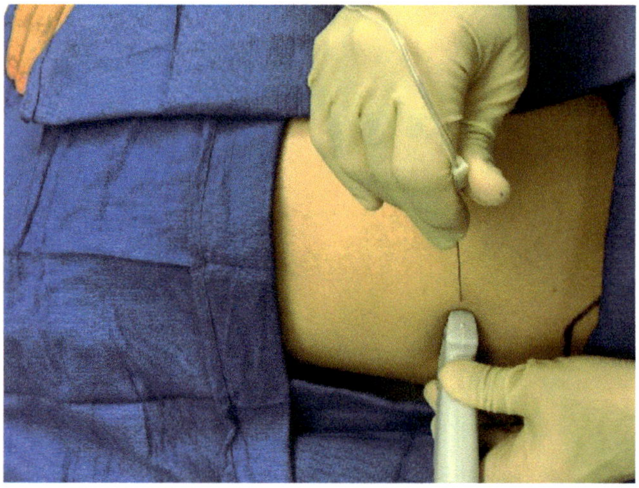

Figure 28.2. Ultrasound probe position for transversus abdominis plane block along lateral abdominal wall between the anterior superior iliac spine (purple line) and the lower costal margin. Needle position corresponds to in-plane technique.

factors against development of chronic postoperative pain are regional anesthesia, perioperative multimodal treatment of acute pain, preoperative use of gabapentin and *N*-methyl-D-aspartate (NMDA) receptor antagonists.[11,16,23,24]

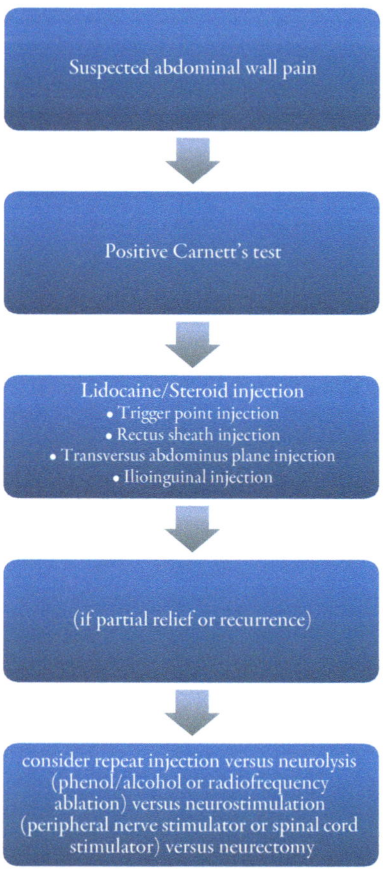

Figure 28.3. Diagnostic and therapeutic treatment algorithm for suspected chronic abdominal wall pain.

PATHOPHYSIOLOGY

Most data on chronic postsurgical pain are derived from research conducted in animals. In humans, some studies showed that elective neurectomy of selected segments of inguinal nerves is an effective technique for preventing chronic postherniorraphy pain.[25] Soft tissue trauma also generates chronic pain, but the result is not consistent with the extent of trauma. After even minor procedures, such as a hernia repair, there is a risk for chronic postoperative pain.[26,27] The duration of surgery appears to affect development of chronic pain postoperatively. Operations lasting longer than 3 hours have been associated with a greater risk than shorter procedures for development of chronic postsurgical pain. Patients who require longer operating times may have more extensive pathology, and more complex dissection that may predispose them to additional complications affecting the outcome of the operation.[28]

CLINICAL EXAMINATION AND DIAGNOSIS

The real challenge with chronic abdominal pain is to understand the etiology of the pain and to exclude potential organic causes, especially those requiring immediate attention and treatment (Table 28.1).

Incorrect diagnosis can lead to a cyclical pattern of unnecessary imaging, endoscopies, and diagnostic surgeries, which may worsen pain.[29] When possible, the clinician should clearly distinguish the pain source as abdominal wall pain or visceral pain. Carnett's test is a physical assessment of whether abdominal wall pain is unchanged or increased with raising the head and feet about 6 inches from the examination table while supine. This simple test is effective in differentiating abdominal wall pain from visceral pain. Precise localization of pain and a positive Carnett's sign are regarded as diagnostic for abdominal wall pain.[30] Targeted nerve blocks and trigger-point injections may also validate the diagnosis.[31] Pain reduction after local anesthetic injections close to abdominal wall nerves (i.e., in the transversus abdominis plane, ilioinguinal nerve, or iliohypogastric nerve) suggests abdominal wall pain, whereas pain reduction after sympathetic block points toward a visceral origin of the pain.

TREATMENT

Treatment options for abdominal wall pain include multimodal analgesic treatments using neuropathic pain medicine, muscle relaxants combined with interventional procedures such as local injection to the maximal point of tenderness, chemical neurolysis, pulsed RF ablation, and neurostimulation. In severe entrapment neuropathies, surgical release of the entrapped nerve can be used. Current treatment algorithms for chronic abdominal postsurgical pain are based mostly on case reports and extrapolation of data from other related conditions. Once there is strong suspicion of abdominal wall pain, the pain specialist may

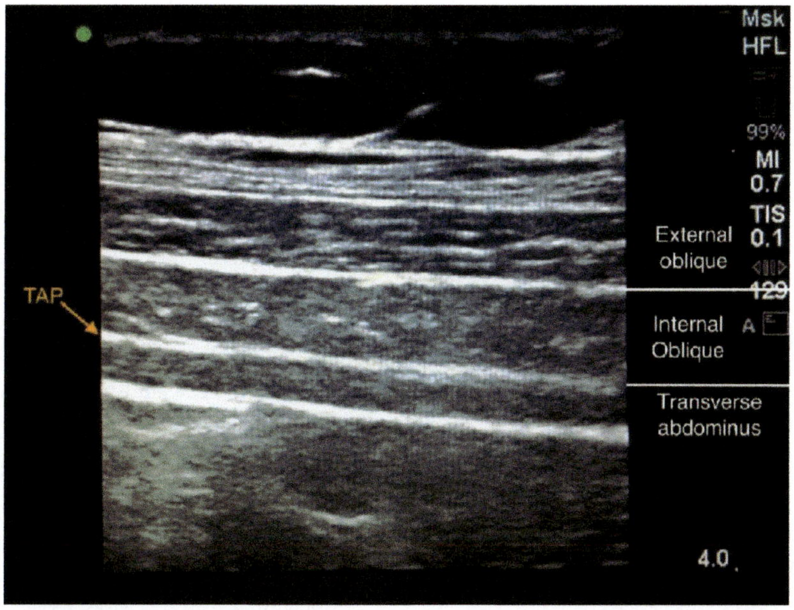

Figure 28.4. Ultrasound image showing external oblique, internal oblique, and transverse abdominis muscle layers and transversus abdominis plane (TAP).

perform a diagnostic and therapeutic block (nerve block or focal trigger point) with local anesthetic with or without steroid. The paucity of data, heterogeneity, and lack of control groups in the available literature preclude firm conclusions on the efficacy and safety of perineural steroids for chronic postsurgical pain.[32]

Many pharmacologic interventions have been explored for the prevention of chronic abdominal wall pain, including gabapentin, pregabalin, nonsteroidal anti-inflammatories, steroids, NMDA blockers, mexiletine, lidocaine, venlafaxine, and nitrous oxide.[33] Multimodal analgesia to achieve rapid relief is the primary goal of management. Anticonvulsants and antidepressants reduce sensitization and improve the endogenous pain-modulating system.[34] Gain in physical and social functioning is mandatory for continuation of therapy.[35,36] Pharmacologic treatment is only one element of a multidisciplinary approach.

If pharmacologic therapy yields no improvement or dose escalation causes intolerable side effects, minimally invasive therapies are considered. Chronic abdominal wall pain produced by nerve entrapment syndromes can be treated by ultrasound or fluoroscopically guided nerve blocks.[37] Chemical neurolysis with phenol and alcohol as well as pulsed RF ablation of the peripheral nerves or dorsal root ganglia (DRG) also have been effective for treating chronic abdominal wall pain refractory to nerve blocks.[38]

There have been many case reports of successful peripheral nerve stimulation for chronic abdominal wall pain.[39] Surgical neurectomy may be performed as a treatment of last resort in severe and debilitating cases. The patient should be made aware of the risk of deafferentation pain after these procedures, as pain may temporarily increase via a central sensitization phenomenon; in many cases, though, the condition is self-limited and tends to disappear with time.

CONCLUSIONS

- Chronic postoperative abdominal wall pain is poorly recognized.
- Pain arising from the abdominal wall can be diagnosed via a positive Carnett's sign (where the patient reports

Table 28.1. **ORGANIC CAUSES OF ACUTE AND CHRONIC ABDOMINAL PAIN**

ACUTE ABDOMINAL PAIN	CHRONIC ABDOMINAL PAIN
Abdominal aortic aneurysm	Angina
Appendicitis	Cancer
Cholangitis	Celiac disease
Cholecystitis	Crohn's disease
Cystitis	Endometriosis
Diabetic ketoacidosis	Gastritis
Diverticulitis	Hepatitis
Ectopic pregnancy	Hiatal hernia
Intussusception	Inguinal hernia
Myocardial infarction	Lead poisoning
Pancreatitis	Mittelschmerz
Pyelonephritis	Pelvic inflammatory disease
Ruptured spleen	Ulcerative colitis
Viral gastroenteritis	Hiatal hernia

increased pain with lifting the head from the examination table while supine).

- If nerve entrapment is suspected, nerve blocks can be performed with local anesthetics and steroids to decrease inflammation and alleviate pain. Physical therapy can complement the procedures. In severe cases, decompressive surgery may be employed.
- Refractory pain can be treated with minimally invasive techniques, such as chemical neurolysis, RF ablation, neurostimulation, and neurectomy.

REFERENCES

1. Woodwell DA, Cherry DK. National Ambulatory Medical Care Survey: 2002 summary. *Adv Data.* 2004;346:1–44.
2. Kamin RA, Nowicki TA, Courtney DS, Powers RD. Pearls and pitfalls in the emergency department evaluation of abdominal pain. *Emerg Med Clin North Am.* 2003;21(1):61–72.
3. Klinkman MS. Episodes of care for abdominal pain in a primary care practice. *Arch Fam Med.* 1996;5:279–285.
4. Koop H, Koprdova S, Schurmann C. Chronic abdominal wall pain: a poorly recognized clinical problem. *Dtsch Arztebl Int.* 2016;113.4:51–57.
5. Thomson H, Francis DM. Abdominal-wall tenderness: a useful sign in the acute abdomen. *Lancet.* 177;2(8047):1053–1054.
6. Thomson WH, Dawes RF, Carter SS. Abdominal wall tenderness: a useful sign in chronic abdominal pain. *Br J Surg.* 1991;78:223–225.
7. Suleiman S, Johnston DE. The abdominal wall: an overlooked source of pain. *Am Fam Physician.* 2001;64(3):431–439.
8. Benzon H, Srinivasa RN, Fishman SE, Liu S, Cohen SP. Chronic pain management in children and adolescents. *Essentials of Pain Medicine.* St. Louis, MO: Elsevier Health Sciences; 2014:403–408.
9. Mehta M, Ranger I. Persistent abdominal pain. Treatment by nerve block. *Anaesthesia.* 1971;26:330–333.
10. Hung JC, Azam N, Puttaniah V, Malhotra V, Gulati A. Neurolytic transversus abdominal plane block with alcohol for long-term malignancy-related pain control. *Pain Physician.* 2014;17(6):E755–E760.
11. McGarrity TJ, Peters DJ, Thompson C, McGarrity SJ. Outcome of patients with chronic abdominal pain referred to chronic pain clinic. *Am J Gastroenterol.* 2000; 95:1812–1816.
12. Costanza CD, Longstreth GF, Liu AL. Chronic abdominal wall pain: clinical features, health care costs, and longterm outcome. *Clin Gastroenterol Hepatol.* 2004;2:395–399.
13. van Rijckevorsel DC, de Vries M, Schreuder LT. Risk factors for chronic postsurgical abdominal and pelvic pain. *Pain Manag.* 2015;5:107–116.
14. Katz J, Seltzer Z. Transition from acute to chronic postsurgical pain: risk factors and protective factors. *Expert Rev Neurother.* 2009;9(5):723–744.
15. van den Berg AA, Ghatge S, Armendariz G, Cornelius D, Wang S. Responses to dural puncture during institution of combined spinal-epidural analgesia: a comparison of 27 gauge pencil-point and 27 gauge cutting-edge needles. *Anaesth Intens Care.* 2011;39(2):247–251.
16. Hallén M, Sevonius D, Westerdahl J, Gunnarsson U, Sandblom G. Risk factors for reoperation due to chronic groin postherniorrhaphy pain. *Hernia.* 2015;19(6):863–869.
17. Rashiq S, Dick BD. Post-surgical pain syndromes: A review for the non-pain specialist. *Can J Anaesth.* 2014;61(2):123–130.
18. Shipton E. Post-surgical neuropathic pain. *ANZ J Surg.* 2008;78(7):548–555.
19. Hinrichs-Rocker A, Schulz K, Järvinen I, Lefering R, Simanski C, Neugebauer EAM. Psychosocial predictors and correlates for chronic post-surgical pain (CPSP)—a systematic review. *Eur J Pain.* 2009;13(7):719–730.
20. Hoofwijk DM, Fiddelers AA, Peters ML, et al. Prevalence and predictive factors of chronic postsurgical pain and poor global recovery one year after outpatient surgery. *Clin J Pain.* 2015;31(12):1017–1025.
21. Chatel H, Madar Y, Leyder P, Bonneau C, Barrat C, Quilichini J. Prevalence and factors associated with persistent pain following body contouring surgery. *J Plast Reconstr Aesthet Surg.* 2016;69(5):700–705.
22. Sevonius D, Montgomery A, Smedberg S, Sandblom G. Chronic groin pain, discomfort and physical disability after recurrent groin hernia repair: impact of anterior and posterior mesh repair. *Hernia.* 2016;20(1):43–53.
23. Chaparro LE, Smith SA, Moore RA, Wiffen PJ, Giron I. Pharmacotherapy for the prevention of chronic pain after surgery in adults. *Cochrane Database Syst Rev.* 2013;7:CD008307
24. de Brito Cançado TO, Omais M, Ashmawi HA, Torres MLA. Chronic pain after cesarean section. Influence of anesthetic/surgical technique and postoperative analgesia. *Rev Bras Anestesiol.* 2012;62(6):762–774.
25. Nikolajsen L, Minella CE. Acute postoperative pain as a risk factor for chronic pain after surgery. *Eur J Pain.* 2009;3(2):29–32.
26. Montes A, Roca G, Sabate S, et al. Genetic and clinical factors associated with chronic postsurgical pain after hernia repair, hysterectomy, and thoracotomy: a two-year multicenter cohort study. *Anesthesiology.* 2015;122(5):1123–1141.
27. Zannoni M, Nisi P, Iaria M, Luzietti E, Sianesi M, Viani L. Wide nervous section to prevent post-operative inguinodynia after prosthetic hernia repair: a single center experience. *Hernia.* 2014;19(4):565–570.
28. Reddi D, Curran N. Chronic pain after surgery: pathophysiology, risk factors and prevention. *Postgrad Med J.* 2014;90:222–227.
29. Macrae WA. Chronic post-surgical pain: 10 years on. *Br J Anaesth.* 2008;101(1):77–86.
30. Greenbaum DS, Greenbaum RB, Joseph JG, Natale JE. Chronic abdominal wall pain, diagnostic validity and costs. *Digest Dis Sci.* 1994;39:1935–1941.
31. Baciarello M, Migliavacca G, Marchesini M, Valente A, Allegri M, Fanelli G. Transversus abdominis plane block for the diagnosis and treatment of chronic abdominal wall pain following surgery: a case series. *Pain Pract.* 2017. doi: 10.1111/papr.12570
32. Khan JS, Rai A, Sundara Rajan R, Jackson TD, Bhatia A. A scoping review of perineural steroids for the treatment of chronic postoperative inguinal pain. *Hernia.* 2016;20(3):367–376.
33. Radvansky BM, Shah K, Parikh A, Sifonios AN, Le V, Eloy JD. Role of ketamine in acute postoperative pain management: a narrative review. *Biomed Res Int.* 2015;2015:749837.
34. Streitberger K, Stüber F, Kipfer Buchli I, Stamer UM. Medikamentöse Schmerzbehandlung akuter und chronischer Abdominalschmerzen. *Ther Umschau.* 2011; 68(8):435–440. doi:10.1024/0040-5930/a000189.
35. Drossman DA. Severe and refractory chronic abdominal pain: treatment strategies. *Clin Gastroenterol Hepatol.* 2008;6:978–982.
36. Willimann P. Medikamentöse Schmerztherapie. *Ther Umschau.* 2011;68(9):512–516.
37. Boelens OB, Scheltinga MR, Houterman S, Roumen RM. Management of anterior cutaneous nerve entrapment syndrome in a cohort of 139 patients. *Ann Surg.* 2011;254(6):1054–1058.
38. Narouze S. Chronic abdominal wall pain: diagnosis and interventional treatment. In: Kapural L, ed. *Chronic Abdominal Pain.* New York, NY: Springer; 2015:189–194.
39. Pang D, Goroszeniuk T. Peripheral nerve stimulation for chronic abdominal pain. In: Kapural L, ed. *Chronic Abdominal Pain.* New York, NY: Springer; 2015:201–209.
40. Makharita M, Amr Y. Pulsed radiofrequency for chronic inguinal neuralgia. *Pain Physician.* 2015;18:E147–E155.

41. Skinner AV, Lauder GR. Rectus sheath block: successful use in the chronic pain management of pediatric abdominal wall pain. *Paediatr Anaesth.* 2007;17:1203–1211.
42. Akhnikh S, de Korte N, de Winter P. Anterior cutaneous nerve entrapment syndrome (ACNES): the forgotten diagnosis. *Eur J Pediatr.* 2014;173:445–449.

REVIEW QUESTIONS

1. Common causes of chronic abdominal pain in adults include

   A. Postherniorrhapy inguinal pain
   B. Diabetic ketoacidosis
   C. Abdominal aortic aneurysm
   D. Interstitial cystitis

2. A previously healthy 54-year-old male complains of acute abdominal pain, but there is no obvious cause for his pain. Medical conditions that should be investigated include all of the following conditions, except:

   A. Ventral hernia
   B. Postsurgical neuroma
   C. Rectus nerve entrapment
   D. Pyelonephritis

3. A 43-year-old man has had left groin pain for 6 months after an inguinal hernia repair. The patient describes the pain as stabbing pain radiating down to the left testicle. On examination, the patient has a well-healed incision and marked cutaneous allodynia and hyperalgesia. This patient most likely has

   A. Ilioinguinal neuralgia
   B. Mesh infection
   C. Recurrent hernia
   D. Incarcerated hernia

ANSWERS

1. A. The estimated prevalence of moderate to severe chronic pain after inguinal hernia repair is about 10% to 12%. Although abdominal aortic aneurysms, which are a manifestation of atherosclerosis, are found in adults, they usually do not cause abdominal pain. Diabetic ketoacidosis must be ruled out (in addition to myocardial infarction, pneumonia, pyelonephritis, and inflammatory bowel disease) as a cause of acute, not chronic, abdominal pain. Interstitial cystitis is a chronic condition resulting in bladder pressure and pelvic, not abdominal, pain.

2. D. The ventral hernia pain is episodic and disappears with postural changes. Postsurgical neuroma pain presents as localized tenderness over surgical scars several months after surgery. Rectus nerve entrapment occurs along the lateral edge of the rectus sheath, with worsening pain when the abdominal muscles are tensed. Chronic pain emanating from the abdominal wall is frequently unrecognized or confused with visceral pain. These conditions are diagnosed with a thorough history, physical examination, and imaging, such as CT. Pyelonephritis does not manifest with abdominal pain; it is associated with back pain.

3. A. Ilioinguinal neuralgia may develop after any surgery in the inguinal area that damages the ilioinguinal nerve. Pain may start immediately after the surgery or after a reasonable period of healing has passed. Wound infection, recurrent hernia, and mesh infection should be ruled out to avoid correctable causes of ilioinguinal pain. The pain is usually described as a sharp, electrical sensation or sometimes as a constant burning sensation in the groin area with occasional radiation into the testicles. Pain is exacerbated by light touch or rubbing by clothes. Treatment includes anticonvulsants and other adjuvant medications. If the pain persists, local anesthetic diagnostic and therapeutic block may be warranted. RF ablation, peripheral nerve stimulation, neurectomy, and repeat surgery should be reserved for resistant cases.

QUESTIONS AND ANSWERS

This chapter has accompanying questions and answers that are available to subscribers as part of the Oxford eLearning platform. To access the questions, follow the link below, or go to ✔ http://oxfordmedicine.com/painmanagementreview

29.

BACK PAIN: IT'S NOT ALWAYS ARTHRITIS

Tariq M. Malik

STEM CASE AND KEY QUESTIONS

A 45-year-old male has suffered from back pain for 4 weeks. He could not appreciate any inciting event. The pain has localized to his low back and does not radiate down his legs. Afebrile, he has not suffered any weight loss recently. He has continued working, even after he developed the back pain, but it is getting harder for him to complete his tasks at work. He has high blood pressure, does not have diabetes, and has no known drug allergies. His desk job makes it hard for him to sit through the whole day and work. The results of a neurologic examination by his primary care physician (PCP) are normal. At the patient's initial visit, the PCP recommended ibuprofen and 6 to 8 weeks of physical therapy to alleviate a suspected muscle spasm. However, 3 weeks later, the patient still complained of significant back pain, which was getting worse, and he complained that therapy was becoming more painful with each visit. He was referred to the pain clinic by his PCP for trigger-point injections. In the pain clinic, the history and physical examination are unremarkable except for a mild tenderness to deep percussion over the lumbar spine. The patient's gait is stable. The patient refuses trigger-point injection after a discussion of its risks and benefits. You recommend continued physical therapy for now and a return to clinic in 3 weeks.

THE PATIENT WANTS AN MRI BEFORE CONTINUING WITH PHYSICAL THERAPY. WHAT DO YOU SAY?

You explain that imaging studies are unnecessary in acute back pain in the absence of symptoms suggestive of cancer, infection, and nerve compression. Based on medical evidence, staying active and core strengthening exercises are recommended. You also make the patient aware that some insurance companies will not pay for imaging before physical therapy is completed. The patient returns to physical therapy and completes another week, but at the end of now the fifth week of back pain he calls the office in excruciating pain. He mentions that he has severe pain with every change of position and he cannot become comfortable at all; he has not slept for 3 days because of the pain.

WHAT IS THE NEXT STEP? WHAT WOULD YOU DO TO TREAT THE PATIENT? WOULD YOU ORDER IMAGING AT THIS POINT? WOULD YOU PRESCRIBE ANY MEDICATIONS?

You order an X-ray of the patient's lumbar spine; the results are unremarkable. The patient finally agrees to an epidural steroid injection that you suggest, thinking that he may have some degenerative changes in the facet joints and the disk. You prescribe a muscle relaxant along with ibuprofen for pain relief. You recommend an MRI before performing a back injection in view of his history of unrelenting back pain. The patient is unhappy because the process of getting approval for MRI from his insurance company may delay the epidural by a week or so.

HOW SHOULD YOU PROCEED? WOULD YOU PERFORM THE EPIDURAL STEROID INJECTION WITHOUT AN MRI? WOULD YOU PRESCRIBE AN OPIOID? WOULD YOU ADMIT THE PATIENT FOR PAIN CONTROL?

The patient has been taking NSAIDs (nonsteroidal anti-inflammatory drugs) for more than a month with no improvement in pain. He is in distress and anxious. Physical examination again reveals a tenderness to deep percussion over the lumbar spine. You emphasize the need for an MRI of the spine before any injection. He insists on an injection before the MRI and does not want to wait. Because you feel strongly about the indication for an MRI, while waiting for the radiology appointment and injection, you prescribe a methylprednisolone dose pack.

THE MRI SHOWS A LESION AT THE L4 BODY SUGGESTING MALIGNANCY. THE PATIENT IS REFERRED TO AN ONCOLOGIST FOR COMPLETE WORKUP. HE IS STILL IN PAIN AND WANTS TO KNOW WHAT TO DO

The oncologist admits the patient to the hospital for pain management and a workup of his tumor. The patient is given IV opioids, and you are asked to control the pain while the oncologic workup is in progress.

HOW DO YOU ALLEVIATE MALIGNANT SPINE PAIN?

Since MRI reveals extensive erosion of the body of the vertebra, you suggest surgical evaluation to treat any impending compression fracture and instability. After evaluating the patient, the neurosurgeon does not recommend surgery to treat pain in the absence of neurologic deficit at this time.

THE PATIENT'S PAIN IS NOT RESPONDING TO IV OPIOIDS AND STEROIDS. WOULD YOU SUGGEST AN INJECTION TO ALLEVIATE HIS PAIN?

MRI reveals no epidural spread of the tumor. He is not coagulopathic. You suggest kyphoplasty as the best option to quickly alleviate pain. You explain the procedure. The patient is agreeable. You order a lumbar CT to better delineate the spinal anatomy.

THE LUMBAR CT REVEALS NO MAJOR CLEFTS IN THE L4 BODY AND INTACT PEDICLES. YOU SCHEDULE THE PATIENT FOR AN L4 KYPHOPLASTY. THE PATIENT SAYS A RADIATION ONCOLOGIST TOLD HIM THAT PAIN CAN BE ALLEVIATED WITH RADIATION THERAPY. WHAT DO YOU SAY?

You agree with the radiation oncologist that radiation therapy is a good option. But you explain to the patient that the two options are complementary and not mutually exclusive. Pain relief from kyphoplasty is quicker than from radiation therapy. You explain that kyphoplasty will improve his pain so that he can get through radiation therapy, a multistep process that takes days to work.

THE PATIENT IS CONCERNED THAT A CEMENT LEAK FROM KYPHOPLASTY MAY CAUSE NERVE DAMAGE OR CARDIAC ARREST. HOW DO YOU ADDRESS HIS FEAR?

You explain that you plan to minimize the risk of cement leakage, which is already lower with kyphoplasty than with vertebroplasty for vertebral augmentation. You also plan radiofrequency (RF) ablation of the vertebral body tumor before injection of the cement, with the benefit of destroying the tumor and the vascularity of the tissue by a cautery effect.

The patient undergoes an uneventful L4 kyphoplasty with RF ablation of the vertebral bone metastases. He feels much better when ambulating. He undergoes simulation for radiation therapy and is discharged home after the first session to complete radiation therapy and chemotherapy as an outpatient.

DISCUSSION

In 2014, there were an estimated 1,665,540 new cancer cases diagnosed and 585,720 cancer deaths in the United States. Cancer is the second most common cause of death in the United States, accounting for nearly 1 of every 4 deaths. The 5-year survival of all patients with cancer at all sites has improved from 49% in 1975–1977 to 68% in 2003–2009.[1] After lung and liver, bone is the third most common location for metastatic cancer. About 60,000 new cases of spinal metastatic lesions are found each year, and 70% of all patients with metastasic cancer disease will develop spinal lesions, while 40% of all patients who die from cancer will have lesions in their spine.[2] The thoracic spine is most commonly affected by spinal metastasis, with the cervical spine being the least commonly affected. About 20,000 patients are treated for malignant spinal cord compressive symptoms annually.[3] Primary tumor of the spinal column is very uncommon; therefore, the vast majority of cancer in the spine comes from metastasis. The extensive network of interconnected valveless veins between Batson's venous plexus and the venous system of the prostate, breast, kidney, thyroid, and lung makes the spread of tumor (as well as infection) to the spine quite easy.[4] Breast cancer in women and prostate cancer in men are the most common cancers to spread to bone. Arterial embolization of tumor also may help seed metastases in the marrow of the vertebral bodies, but this route is a less frequent source of spread than the venous plexus.

Tumor in the spine causes pain, fracture, or compression of neuronal structures. Pain is multifactorial, persistent, and worse at night. It results from mechanical deformity, neuropathy from direct nerve irritation, and nociceptor activation from tissue destruction or inflammation causing swelling and tissue tension within the bone. A history of weight loss, night pain, previous tumor, or compression fracture in the absence of osteoporosis are clues that back pain may be of malignant origin. Uncovering malignant pathology requires a detailed history and physical examination. The primary goal of evaluation is to find out if the spinal lesion is a primary tumor or a metastatic lesion. The effort in treating a recently diagnosed vertebral body metastasis is directed toward finding the primary tumor, determining whether the spine is stable, and determining if the tumor has caused a fracture, cord compression, or other neural compromise. In general, the evaluation is done by the PCP or an oncologist.

Whenever a patient with back pain presents to a pain clinic, a proper evaluation is completed by the pain physician before a pain management plan is made. A detailed history, especially the presence of red flags, should be actively sought. The spine is palpated for any tender spots and careful neurologic examination is performed to elicit any sensory and motor deficits. If malignancy is suspected, then imaging is mandatory.

An X-ray of the spine is not very sensitive, and does not show bone destruction until 30% to 50% of bone is lost. Also it does not reveal subtle pathologic compression fractures.[5] Sensitivity of plain X-rays in detecting malignant lesions is around 40% to 50%. Lesions in the marrow up to 1 cm in size may not be visible; however, cortical lesions can be detected at much earlier stages. Simple spine radiographs are best used in evaluating bone pain in conjunction with a bone scan. The radiologic appearance of a tumor, when detectable, has been characterized as showing bone destruction, bone proliferation, and mineralization pattern, as well as the size and location of the tumor.[6]

A CT scan is more sensitive than plain radiography and can detect a lesion up to 6 months before it becomes visible on an X-ray. CT can show soft tissue invasion and bony lesions are better revealed than with X-rays. When MRI, CT, planar skeletal scintigraphy, and positron emission tomography (PET) were compared in a large-scale meta-analysis, CT had a sensitivity of 73% and a pooled specificity (per patient) of 95%.[7] On a per-patient basis, MRI was 91% sensitive and 95% specific. MRI is thus superior to both CT and planar skeletal scintigraphy and as good as PET-CT. Advantages of CT are that it is less susceptible to motion degradation, takes less time, and is better tolerated by claustrophobic patients.

MRI is better for evaluating marrow infiltration and soft tissue involvement and doesn't expose the patient to ionizing radiation, as CT does. Motion artifacts and metallic hardware (from previous spinal surgery), however, can degrade image quality. The presence of a pacemaker may make MRI impossible because not all pacemakers are MRI compatible. A number of advanced MRI sequences are available for various musculoskeletal malignancies; techniques such as chemical shift imaging, MRI spectroscopy, and diffusion-weighted imaging have been used in suspected cases of infiltrative tumors expanding beyond the bony structure of the spine. In several cases, MRI alone yields nonspecific results and differentiates a benign lesion from a malignant lesion less than 50% of the time.

Bone scans with technetium-99m (Tc-99m) methylene diphosphonate (MDP) are used to evaluate extent of disease and are more sensitive than X-ray in detecting tumors. A lesion must be metabolically active to be picked up by a bone scan. Radiographic correlation is still required to rule out nontumor pathology, such as inflammatory arthritis. SPECT (single-photon emission computed tomography) is even more sensitive than a Tc-99m bone scan; however, its cost limits its widespread use. In one study, the addition of SPECT to scintigraphy raised the negative predictive value of normal scintigraphic findings to 98%.[8]

As mentioned, imaging studies are essential in diagnosing vertebral bony metastases; a combination of radiologic techniques improves the sensitivity and specificity of the diagnosis and enables the clinician to better identify and treat the painful vertebrae.

The goal of therapy for metastatic lesions is palliative care for comfort, pain relief, and preservation of neurologic function. As majority of vertebral bone tumors are metastatic, and the prognosis depends on the primary tumor. When spinal metastases are encountered, life expectancy ranges from 6 months in lung cancer up to 18 months in prostate cancer. Prognosis also affects the plan for managing pain. Signs of nerve or cord compression, and any spinal instability, must be determined clinically and followed up with confirmatory radiologic studies. For symptoms of nerve or cord compression or mechanical instability, the treatment of choice is surgical intervention.[9] Radiation therapy is often added to surgical intervention in such instances. The intention is not to cure but to debulk as much tumor as possible, preserving or providing spinal stability with the least invasive procedure. Many interventions, however, are invasive, and debilitated patients have difficulty tolerating them.

When there is no nerve compression or spinal instability, or when comorbidities prevent a massive surgical intervention, the mainstay of treatment is radiation therapy, chemotherapy, or interventional pain procedures. Chemotherapy usually is reserved for chemosensitive tumors like neuroblastoma, Ewing's sarcoma, osteogenic sarcoma, germ cell tumors, and lymphoma. Chemotherapy can be a first-line treatment for cord compression from local epidural invasion by the tumor, especially lymphoma.[10] Pain relief from chemotherapy is slow and depends on tumor shrinkage, which normally takes weeks.

Radiation therapy is the first-line therapy for bony metastases and an adjuvant therapy after surgical resection and stabilization. Goals of radiation for bony metastases include stabilization of the tumor, relief of pressure on surrounding structures (e.g., neuronal tissue), and pain relief. Radiation therapy is urgently applied when a tumor has caused significant cortical destruction that threatens fracture and spinal instability, or tumor has eroded through bone, resulting in a soft tissue mass that is compressing nerves or spinal cord. Radiation also is indicated after surgical resection of a metastatic lesion with stabilization.[11] It improves pain significantly in more than 60% of cases, reducing opioid intake by patients. However, when used alone to treat cord compression, it is effective in 30% of cases, and its efficacy is highly dependent of the type of tumor.[12] Among the various tumors, multiple myeloma and lymphoma are generally radiosentive, responding well to radiation therapy; breast, lung, and prostate cancers are moderately sensitive. Renal cancer, melanoma, and gastrointestinal tract tumors are radioresistant. Yet there is no correlation between pain relief and histopathology. Pain relief occurs in steps and sometimes may take up to several weeks for the patient to achieve comfort. It is hypothesized that immediate pain relief comes from destruction of immune cells and reduced production of inflammatory chemicals or the neurolytic effect of radiation itself. Pain relief after 2 weeks comes from eradication of tumor cells. Radiation therapy is often dose-fractionated; a total of 30 Gy is given in 10 daily fractionated doses.[13] Meta-analyses of randomized trials have also shown equivalent outcomes with single- and multi-fraction regimens, and no difference in outcomes when compared to using biologic effective dose (BED).[14] The spine can be re-irradiated if there is inadequate pain relief after initial therapy, progression after initial therapy, or relapse. Radiation therapy is safe and effective with sufficient time between the two courses of treatment; however, a total limited dose is generally employed to prevent myelopathy.

The Mirels classification system (Table 29.1) is useful in predicting impending fracture and guiding the need for prophylactic pinning before radiotherapy, especially in long bones; it may be used as a guide for treating spinal metastases.[15]

Table 29.1. **MIRELS SCORING SYSTEM AND CLINICAL RECOMMENDATIONS**

SCORE	SITE OF LESION	SIZE OF LESION	NATURE OF LESION	PAIN
1	Upper limb	< ⅓ of cortex	Blastic	Mild
2	Lower Limb	⅓ to ⅔ of cortex	Mixed	Moderate
3	Trochanteric	> ⅓ of cortex	Lytic	Severe

SUMMED SCORE	CLINICAL RECOMMENDATION
< 7	Radiotherapy and observe
8	Clinical judgment
>9	Intervention

Adapted from Bagshaw HP, Tward JD. Current and emerging modalities. In: Randall RL, ed. *Metastatic Bone Disease.* New York, NY: Springer; 2016.

Several side effects and complications occur with radiation therapy; generally, benefit of the treatment outweighs risk, but patients may need to be aware that radiation of the spine can cause inflammation and swelling of the spinal cord, which may worsen an existing cord compression. Therefore, steroids are often given along with radiation treatment. Permanent myelopathy, especially when the maximal radiation dose is exceeded, can manifest from months to years after radiation treatment. Permanent damage is dose-dependent and is the dose-limiting factor when tumors are treated with radiation. Injury to the spinal cord occurs from damage to either oligodendrocytes or the vascular endothelium. Vascular damage leads to tissue necrosis; oligodendrocyte damage predominantly results in demyelination.

One of the most effective methods for prompt pain relief is vertebral augmentation therapy (VAT). Radiation therapy, although effective, can take up to 2 weeks to provide relief. VAT is done either with balloon tamponade to create a cavity before cement injection (kyphoplasty) or without creating a cavity with a balloon, by injecting more fluid cement in the fractured vertebral body (vertebroplasty). VAT provides pain relief by mechanical stabilization if there is a compression fracture. It is also considered preemptively if a tumor has eroded the bone and a compression fracture is impending. The VERTOS I, VERTOS II, CAFE, and FREE trials have shown clinically significant pain reduction after VAT when patients are selected appropriately.[16–19] There are several limitations to the procedure. First, VAT may not be effective when the lesion or tumor spreads into surrounding tissue, especially the epidural space, with signs of cord compression on MRI. Other than cord compression, systemic or local infection, complete erosion of the posterior body wall, and patient refusal are absolute contraindications. Relative contraindications include coagulopathy, complete collapse of vertebra, and short (days, hours) life expectancy. Anyone suffering from poor pain control with oral analgesics or opioids and who has a favorable anatomy is a good candidate for VAT. CT is better than MRI for evaluating the integrity of vertebral body walls and pedicles when planning for the procedure and can also offer information useful to the clinician in determining the technique used to access the vertebral body (basically if the procedure should be performed via a transpedicular or an extrapedicular method). Overall, vertebroplasty is as effective as kyphoplasty in metastatic vertebral compression fractures, although cement leaks outside the vertebral body are more common with vertebroplasty than with kyphoplasty.[20] VAT can be combined with radiation therapy to minimize local recurrence. Immediate analgesic effect of VAT is a big help to patients who otherwise may not be able to lie still for simulation session and for multiple radiation therapy sessions. VAT is also combined with other ablative therapies using RF or a cryoablation probe. The goal of either is to destroy both neural pain fibers and tumor cells by creating a 5- to 10-mm treatment margin beyond the tumor borders delineated during preoperative imaging. RF ablation uses a high-frequency alternating electrical current (200–1200 kHz) produced by an electrode, which produces heat by oscillation of ions. At temperature above 60°C, however, cell damage is irreversible. A temperature above 100°C chars and vaporizes tissues. Currently used RF devices for bone include OsteoCool RF Ablation System (Medtronic Inc., Minneapolis, MN) and DFINE STAR ablation (DFINE, Inc., San Jose, CA).

DFINE STAR has a unique tip deflection technology, facilitating directional guidance of the ablation tip.[21] It uses conventional RF ablation. Given the curved tip and steering capabilities, the procedure can be performed from one side (unipedicular) for navigation throughout the vertebral body (Figure 29.1).

After the STAR ablation instrument is placed within the center of the lesion, RF energy is delivered via the ablation electrode that is extended beyond the trocar. Two thermocouples within the ablation system monitor the temperature within the tumor in real time. There are two possible ablation areas, 3–2 cm and 2–1.5 cm, and they depend on the size of the tumor that is targeted as well as the location of the thermocouples (10–15 mm from the center of the ablation zone or 5–10 mm; Figure 29.2).

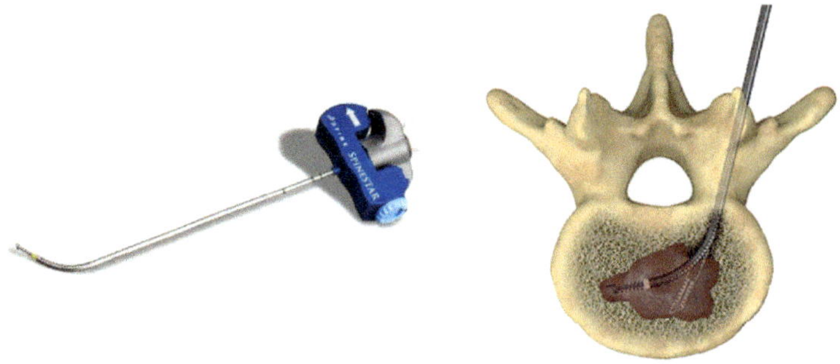

Figure 29.1. Cannula and radiofrequency probe. The curved probe allows a unipedicular approach to treat vertebral metastases. (Reprinted with permission from DFINE, Inc.)

After a maximum of 50°C is reached in the proximal thermocouple (the temperature at the most peripheral point of the ablation zone), the delivery of energy is discontinued, thus functioning as a safety mechanism. As with conventional RF ablation, some charring may occur, prompting removal of the probe and repositioning for maximal efficacy. Vertebral augmentation of the treated vertebra with vertebroplasty follows DFINE ablation for spinal stabilization.

The OsteoCool system uses water-cooled technology, employing two internally water-cooled bipolar probes that are heated to 70°C at the tip, with temperatures up to 90°C to 95°C in the center of the probe (Figure 29.3 and Figure 29.4).

With water-cooled technology, it is expected that the probes will not need to be repositioned during the procedure. Bilateral probe placement allows heat to extend synergistically into the tumor to create a spherical lesion, and the combination of the lesions created by each probe results in a significantly bigger lesion in the metastatic tumor, ensuring adequate destruction. Since the probes are continuously cooled, the temperature is constant around them and char formation is reduced. Since the RF lesion is significant, this technology is useful in tumors that involve the entire vertebral body, where an adequate placement ensures stabilization of the tumor. Specificity in heat lesioning time and intensity through the OsteoCool system depends on the probe size (7 mm, 10 mm, or 20 mm; Figure 29.5 and Figure 29.6).

The system is an upgrade of the Kyphon kit (Medtronic, Inc.) used in kyphoplasty. With OsteoCool, the drill has color markings corresponding to the final lesion. While the company recommends upgrading to a bigger size when using the

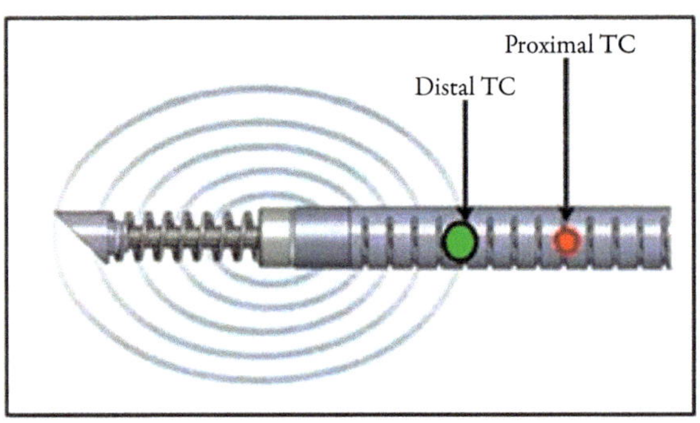

Figure 29.2. Radiofrequency ablation zone in DFINE STAR system. (Reprinted with permission from DFINE, Inc.)

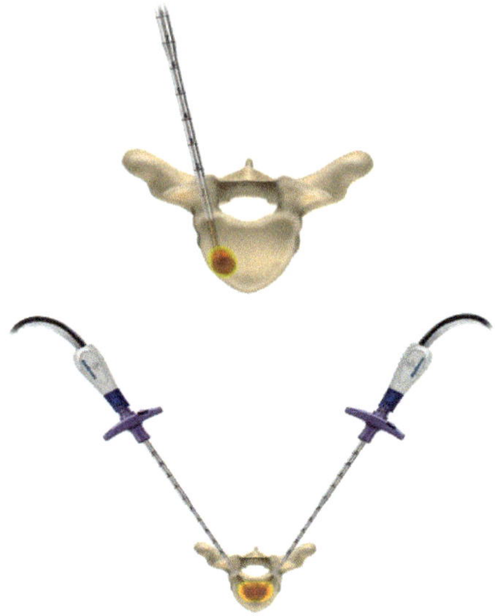

Figure 29.3. OsteoCool system.

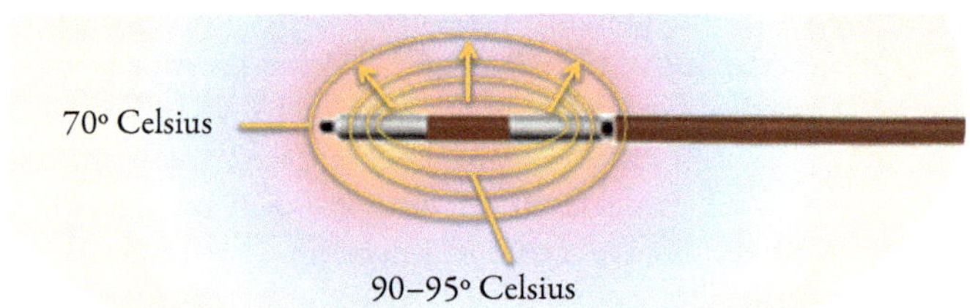

Figure 29.4. OsteoCool probe is temperature controlled, reaching 70°C at the tip and 90°C to 95°C within the lesion. (Reprinted with the permission of Medtronic, Inc.)

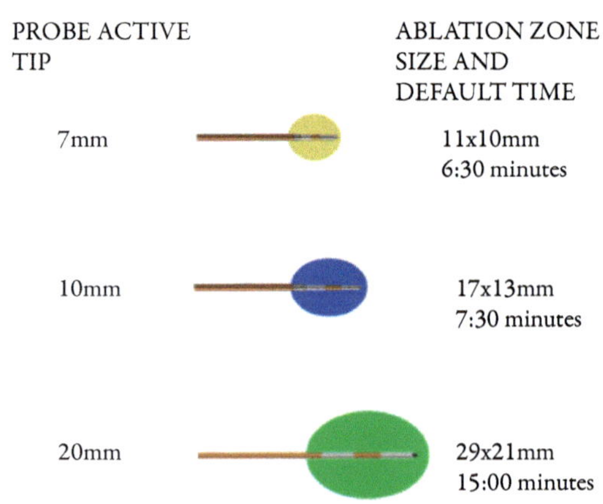

Figure 29.5. Disposable OsteoCool RF ablation probes. (Reprinted with the permission of Medtronic, Inc.)

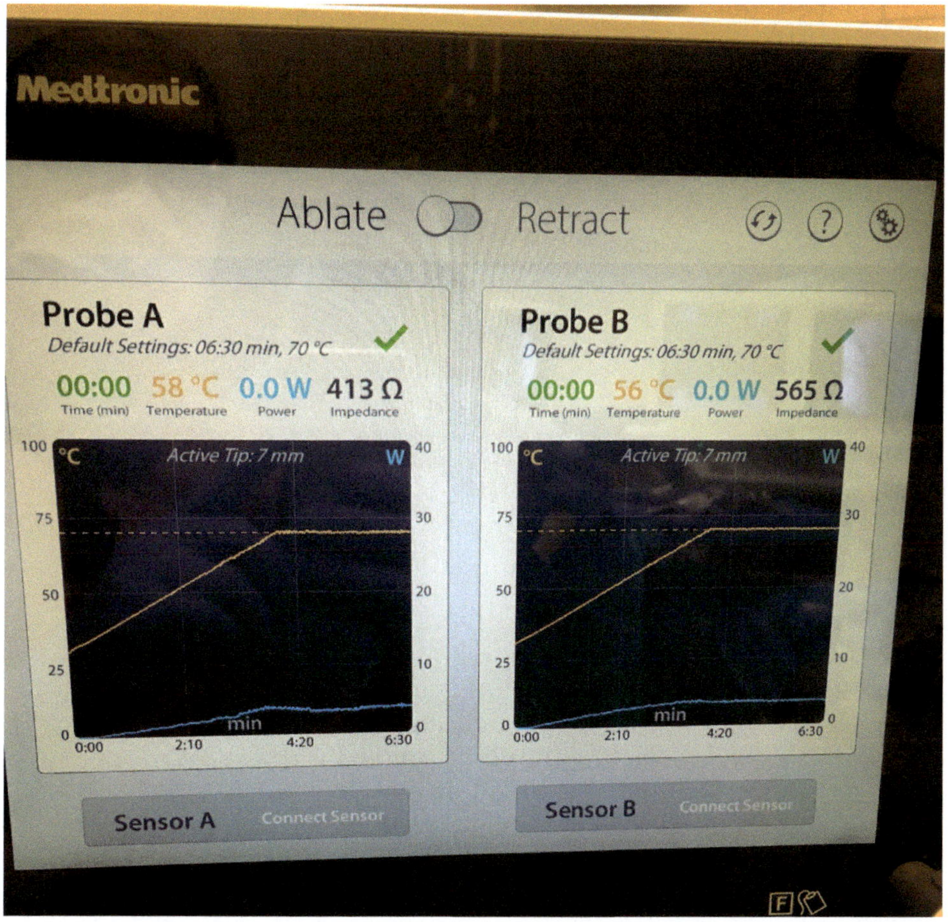

Figure 29.6. Heat record and application during RF lesioning; image taken at the end of lesioning with a 7-mm probe in the T7 vertebra. Image from the author's personal library.

color-coded drills, our clinical experience has usually been to downgrade to a smaller lesioning probe, especially if the tumor is close to the vertebral wall. The ablation process is recorded during the procedure, including measurement of the power and temperature during tumor heat treatment (Figure 29.7).

Following RF ablation, kyphoplasty is performed for stabilization of the vertebra (Figure 29.8).

OsteoCool and DFINE STAR are both bipolar devices. Ablation cycles vary between 6 min (7-mm probe of the OsteoCool system) and 15 min (DFINE), depending on the size, shape, location, and intrinsic characteristics of the tumor. A cauterizing effect, which reduces the risk of bleeding, is particularly advantageous when treating hypervascular tumors or coagulopathic patients. Despite the many precautions taken to prevent leakage of the cement into a vessel after ablation, uptake has been described, especially with vascular tumors in the middle of vertebrae, where normal vertebral plexuses are present (Figure 29.9 and Figure 29.10).

Cryoablation is another technology used to treat bone tumors. Therapy is based on the Joule-Thomson effect: rapidly expanding gas absorbs temperature from its surroundings. A temperature between −20°C and −40°C is necessary and should persist 1 cm beyond the tumor periphery.[22] One cycle consists of a freeze phase usually lasting 10 min followed by 8 min of thaw phase. Ablations frequently requires two freeze–thaw cycles. Some of the cryoprobes currently used for cryoablation are produced by Endocare (Healthtronics/Endocare Incorporated, Irvine, CA) and Galil Medical (Galil Medical, Arden Hills, MN). In cryoablation, intense cooling causes ice crystals to form within cells, disrupting cellular membranes and denaturing intracellular proteins, resulting

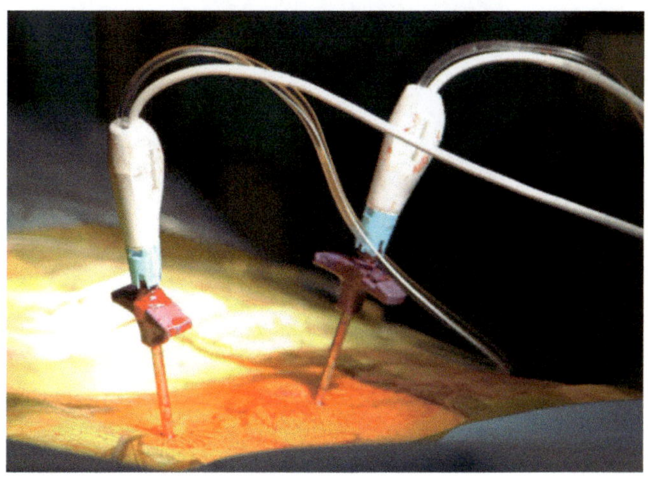

Figure 29.7. OsteoCool system with placed probes. Image from the author's personal library.

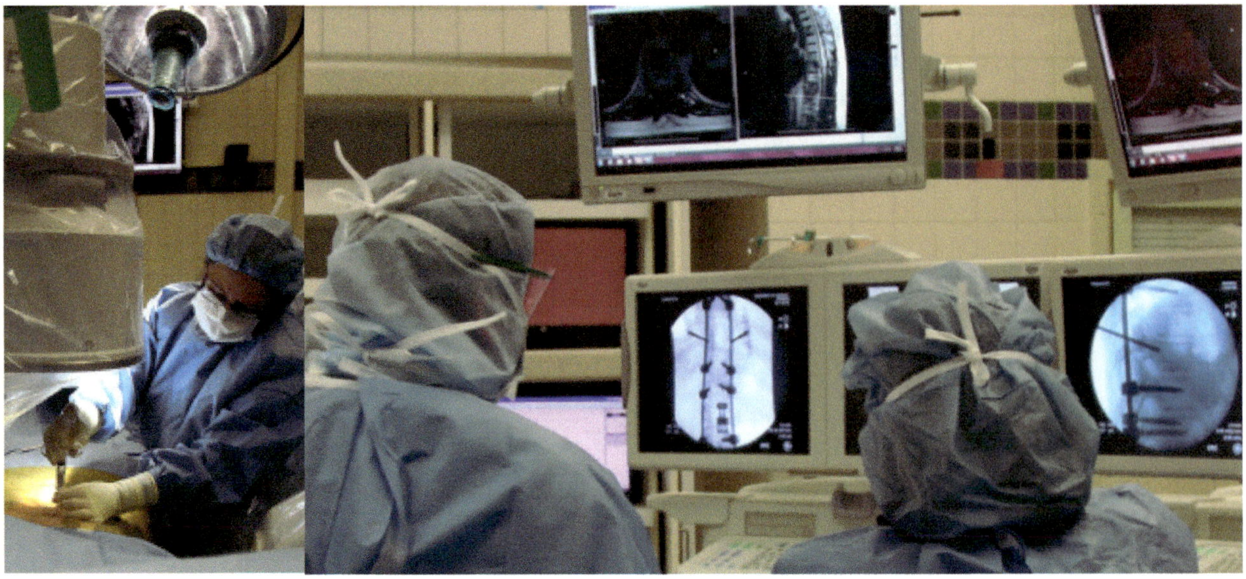

Figure 29.8. OsteoCool RF ablation followed by kyphoplasty. Image from the author's personal library.

in cell death. Cryoablation also produces ischemic injury by coagulating blood and interrupting blood flow to the tissue. Cryoablation uses smaller ablation probes, with probe size as small as 17 G (Galil Medical). Cryoablation also has the added benefit of a clearly visible ablation zone (ice ball) during the ablation, which can be seen on CT, MRI, or ultrasound. Ablated tissue is not cauterized, and bleeding from hypervascular tumors or in patients with underlying coagulopathy is not reduced. It takes longer to perform cryoablation than RF ablation, as each freeze–thaw cycle is about 18 to 20 min. It may take up to 1 hour to complete a procedure, depending on the size of the tumor and the number of freeze–thaw cycles needed. After ablation, the residual necrotic cavity is filled with cement to stabilize the bone cavity and to reduce the risk of future compression fracture.

Preemptive destruction of malignant tissue with ablative therapies potentially reduces the risk of local tumor displacement or extension into normal healthy tissues when it is followed by VAT. It also reduces the risk of cement leak, because injection into the low-pressure cavity created by ablation will keep cement inside the cavity instead of spilling into surrounding tissues. In one study, the odds ratio of cement leak was reduced to 0.262 (95% CI: 0.113 to 0.607; $P = 0.002$) after using RF ablation before injecting cement.[23] When necessary, cavity creation can be further facilitated after ablation by using balloon kyphoplasty. Combining these therapies should improve local tumor control and reduce pain by killing

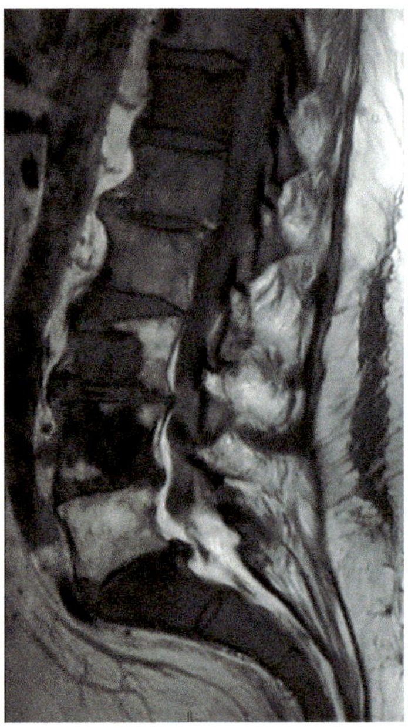

Figure 29.9. MRI showing multiple vertebral metastases. At the middle of L2 and L3, venous plexuses can be seen as white indentations in the vertebral body; cement caught in the plexuses can be taken up vascularly. Image from the library of the University of Chicago courtesy of Magdalena Anitescu.

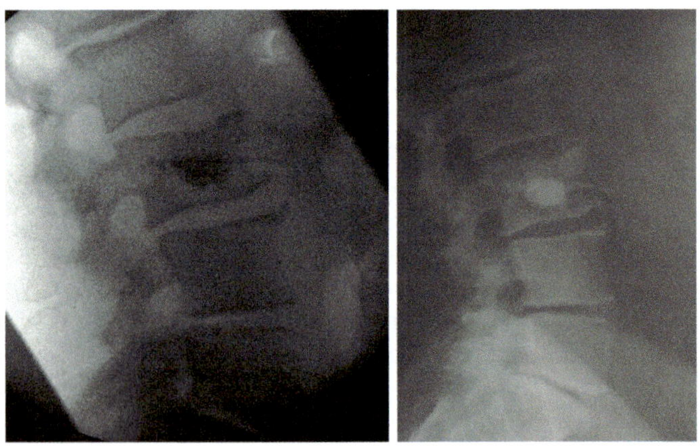

Figure 29.10. Same patient after L3 lesion OsteoCool RF ablation and subsequent kyphoplasty, showing asymptomatic cement leak and uptake of cement by venous plexuses. The first image was taken at the end of the kyphoplasty, in the operating room, and the second image was taken in the recovery room. Figure courtesy of Magdalena Anitescu.

resistant or residual tumor cells. In one study, pain control for malignant spinal lesions was more rapid and effective with combined RF ablation and radiation therapy than with standard radiation therapy.[24]

CONCLUSION

Traditionally, tumors have been treated with radiation, chemotherapy, and surgery. Now, interventional therapies have a larger role in malignancy-related conditions, especially when pain relief is the main objective. Interventional therapies are being used more and more when patients' comfort and spinal stabilization are desired. Vertebroplasty and kyphoplasty, along with RF ablation and cryoablation, are additional options for treating bone malignancy. Continued advances in the field of interventional pain management and image-guided procedures will offer cancer patients new treatments for pain relief until the day that a cure for cancer is found.

REFERENCES

1. American Cancer Society. *Cancer Facts & Figures*. Available at https://www.cancer.org/research/cancer-facts-statistics/all-cancer-facts-figures/cancer-facts-figures-2014.html
2. Posner JB. *Neurologic Complications of Cancer*. Philadelphia, PA: FA Davis; 2009.
3. Grant R, Papadopoulos SM, Greenberg HS. Metastatic epidural spinal cord compression. *Neurol Clin*. 1991;9(4):825.
4. Nathoo N, Caris EC, Weiner JA, Mendel E. History of vertebral venous plexus and the significant contribution of Breschet and Batson. *Neurosurgery*. 2011;69(5):1007–1014.
5. Salvo N, Christakis M, Rubenstein J, et al. The role of plain radiographs in management of bone metastases. *J Palliative Med*. 2009;12(2):195–198.
6. Lodwick GS. A probabilistic approach to the diagnosis of bone tumors. *Radiol Clin North Am*. 1965;3(3):487–497.
7. Yang HL, Liu T, Wang XM, Xu Y, Deng SM. Diagnosis of bone metastases: a meta-analysis comparing ^{18}FDG PET, CT, MRI and bone scintigraphy. *Eur Radiol*. 2011;21:2604–2617.
8. Chua S, Gnanasegaran G, Cook GJ. Miscellaneous cancers (lung, thyroid, renal cancer, myeloma, and neuroendocrine tumors): role of SPECT and PET in imaging bone metastases. *Semin Nucl Med*. 2009;39:416–430.
9. Laufer I, Rubin DG, Lis E, et al. The NOMS framework: approach to the treatment of spinal metastatic tumors. *Oncologist*. 2013;18(6):744–751.
10. Grubb MR, Currier BL, Pritchard DJ, et al. Primary Ewing's sarcoma of the spine. *Spine*. 1994;19:309–313.
11. Saarto T, James R, Tenhunen M, Kouri M. Palliative radiotherapy in the treatment of skeletal metastases. *Eur J Pain*. 2002;6(5):323–330.
12. Janjan NA. Radiation for bone metastases: conventional techniques and the role of systemic radiopharmaceuticals. *Cancer*. 1997;80:1628–1645.
13. Hartsell WF, Scott CB, Brunner DW, et al. Randomized trial of short- versus long-course radiotherapy for palliation of painful bone metastases. *J Nat Cancer Inst*. 2005;97(11):798–804.
14. Wu JS, Wong R, Johnson M, et al. Meta-analysis of dose-fractionation radiotherapy trials for the palliation of painful bone metastases. *Int J Radiat Oncol Biol Phys*. 2003;55(3):594–605.
15. Jawad MU, Scully SP. In brief: classifications in brief: Mirels' classification: metastatic disease in long bones and impending pathologic fracture. *Clin Orthop*. 2010;468(10):2825–2827.
16. Voormolen MH, Mali WP, Lohle PN, et al. Percutaneous vertebroplasty compared with optimal pain medication treatment: short-term clinical outcome of patients with subacute or chronic painful osteoporotic vertebral compression fractures. The VERTOS study. *AJNR Am J Neuroradiol*. 2007;28(3):555–560.
17. Wardlaw D, Cummings SR, Van Meirhaeghe J, et al. Efficacy and safety of balloon kyphoplasty compared with nonsurgical care for vertebral compression fracture (FREE): a randomised controlled trial. *Lancet*. 2009;373(9668):1016–1024.
18. Klazen CA, Lohle PN, de Vries J, et al. Vertebroplasty versus conservative treatment in acute osteoporotic vertebral compression fractures (VERTOS II): an open-label randomised trial. *Lancet*. 2010;376(9746):1085–1092.
19. Berenson J, Pflugmacher R, Jarzem P, et al. Balloon kyphoplasty versus non-surgical fracture management for treatment of painful vertebral body compression fractures in patients with cancer: a multicentre, randomised controlled trial. *Lancet Oncol*. 2011;12(3):225–235.
20. Burton AW, Mendoza T, Gebhardt R, et al. Vertebral compression fracture treatment with vertebroplasty and kyphoplasty: experience in 407 patients with 1,156 fractures in a tertiary cancer center. *Pain Med*. 2011;12(12):1750–1757.
21. Frodsham AE, Eisenmenger LB. Ablation and cement technologies. In: Randall RL, ed. *Metastatic Bone Disease*. New York, NY: Springer; 2016:203–219.
22. Beland M, Mayo-Smith W. Image-guided tumor ablation. In: Kaufman J, Lee M, eds. *Vascular and Interventional Radiology: The Requisites*. 2nd ed. Philadelphia, PA: Saunders (Elsevier); 2014.
23. David E, Kaduri S, Yee A, Chow E, et al. Initial single center experience: radiofrequency ablation assisted vertebroplasty and osteoplasty using a bipolar device in the palliation of bone metastases. *Ann Palliat Med*. 2017;
24. Di Staso M, Zugaro L, Gravina GL, et al. A feasibility study of percutaneous radiofrequency ablation followed by radiotherapy in the management of painful osteolytic bone metastases. *Eur Radiol*. 2011;21(9):2004–2010.

REVIEW QUESTIONS

1. With advancements in chemotherapy, the prevalence of metastatic bone disease is

   A. Decreasing
   B. Increasing
   C. Unchanged
   D. There is insufficient data

2. The most common complaint with a spinal malignant lesion is

   A. Weight loss
   B. Weakness
   C. Pain
   D. Cauda equina syndrome

3. In order of prevalence, the most common spinal level at which a metastatic tumor will be found is

   A. Cervical
   B. Lumbar
   C. Thoracic
   D. Sacral

ANSWERS

1. B. The prevalence of cancer is increasing. In 2014 it was estimated that 1.7 million new cancer cases were diagnosed, up from 1.3 million in 2013. With increasing prevalence and better therapeutic interventions, more people are living with cancer. Bones are vascular and are a prime target for metastatic seeding. Bone is the third most common site of tumor seeding after lung and liver.[1]

2. C. Pain is most likely complaint with a spinal malignant lesion.[2] Pain occurs from activation of nociceptors by the prostaglandins and other inflammatory mediators produced by immune cells. Mechanical deformity compression fracture and neuropathic nerve activation are also present. Cord compression or nerve root compression is present in less than 10% of cases.[3] While weight loss and weakness are commonly associated with cancer, they are nonspecific findings for spinal metastases.

3. C. The most common spinal level affected is thoracic, followed by lumbar and then cervical.[2,3]

QUESTIONS AND ANSWERS

This chapter has accompanying questions and answers that are available to subscribers as part of the Oxford eLearning platform. To access the questions, follow the link below, or go to http://oxfordmedicine.com/painmanagementreview.

30.

INTRATHECAL DRUG DELIVERY SYSTEMS

Deepti Agarwal, Ifeyinwa C. Ifeanyi, and Mercy A. Udoji

STEM CASE AND KEY QUESTIONS

A 35-year-old male is transferred to your hospital from an outside medical facility with complaints of severe abdominal pain, unintentional 30-lb (13.5-kg) weight loss, and subcostal chest pain that began 3 months earlier. His vital signs are within normal limits. His past medical history is notable for alcoholism (last drink 6 months ago), early-stage hepatic cirrhosis, tobacco abuse (one to two packs per day), and diabetes mellitus (type 1), well controlled with an insulin pump. An abdominal CT scan performed at the outside hospital was notable for a mass at the head of the pancreas, suspicious for adenocarcinoma, as well as nodules in the lung and liver, prompting transfer to your institution.

Before his transfer, the patient received intravenous (IV) fentanyl and hydromorphone, with minimal relief of his pain. He is scheduled for further workup and biopsy to determine a treatment plan. He is opioid naïve, but received hydrocodone and oxycodone with acetaminophen combination with some relief of pain. He currently rates his pain as 10/10 and is visibly uncomfortable, despite a recent dose of IV hydromorphone. You are consulted to help manage the patient's pain during his admission.

WHAT ARE YOUR THOUGHTS REGARDING THIS PATIENT'S PAIN MANAGEMENT AT THIS TIME? ARE YOU CONCERNED ABOUT OTHER FACTS IN HIS HISTORY? WHAT OTHER INFORMATION WOULD YOU LIKE TO GATHER FROM THE PATIENT OR HIS MEDICAL RECORDS?

Laboratory testing is notable for the following: alkaline phosphatase, 97 units/L; aspartate aminotransferase (AST), 879 units/L; alanine aminotransferase (ALT), 97 units/L; platelet count, 98,000; amylase, 352 units/L; lipase, 188 units/L. MRI-guided biopsy of his pancreatic and lung masses is completed successfully. The preliminary pathology report shows a moderately differentiated adenocarcinoma of the pancreas. Further imaging via PET scan is suspicious for metastases to the spine. The patient continues to complain of severe subcostal abdominal pain that "pierces" through his abdomen to his back and states that his current IV pain medicine regimen is not "touching" his pain for more than an hour at a time.

WHAT ARE THIS PATIENT'S OPTIONS FOR BETTER PAIN RELIEF? IS A MULTIMODAL ANALGESIA REGIMEN APPROPRIATE FOR THIS PATIENT? IF SO, WHAT AGENTS WOULD YOU USE?

A surgeon is consulted. The patient is not deemed a suitable candidate for surgical resection and palliative therapies are recommended due to multiple metastatic lesions. After prolonged discussion with the patient and his family, the decision is made that he will undergo radiation therapy for his vertebral metastatic disease and chemotherapy for his primary tumor.

Two months later, you are asked to see the patient again for worsening pain and metastatic spread of cancer to his colon, left lung, and pelvis. He continues to use oral medications but complains of inadequate analgesia and side effects (nausea, altered mental status, dizziness) that cause him not to want to take his medications. His severe pain has caused his chemotherapy to be delayed, placing the patient at increased risk for tumor spread, and reducing his life expectancy. The oncologist and patient would like to know if the patient is a candidate for an intrathecal drug delivery device (IDDD) at this time. They specifically ask about an intrathecal drug delivery (ITDD) system containing ziconotide.

WHAT DO YOU TELL THE PATIENT AND HIS ONCOLOGIST? WHAT ARE INDICATIONS FOR, AND CONTRAINDICATIONS TO, INTRATHECAL PUMP (ITP) PLACEMENT?

You bring the patient into the clinic for discussion of the risks and benefits of ITP placement. During your exam, you note that the patient appears emaciated (he has lost 40 pounds [18 kg] since his last visit 1 month ago). He reports lack of sleep and frequent awakenings due to pain. He also reports poor oral intake secondary to nausea from pain medications as well as persistent dizziness. He and his family would like him to have an ITP in an attempt to improve his quality of life and oral intake and perhaps allow the patient to better tolerate lifesaving chemotherapy. You consult with the oncologist and are informed that the patient's disease is very far advanced. His life expectancy is less than 3 months.

WHAT DO YOU TELL THE PATIENT ABOUT ITDD NOW? IS THIS PATIENT AN APPROPRIATE CANDIDATE FOR AN INTERNALIZED IDDD? WHAT ARE HIS OPTIONS FOR PAIN CONTROL GIVEN HIS LIMITED LIFE EXPECTANCY?

The patient undergoes placement of a percutaneous catheter with a subcutaneous access port for delivery of intrathecal medications. At this point, he is enrolled in hospice and has a nurse visiting his home three times a week to provide care for him and to refill his pump. During her latest visit, the patient complains of inadequate analgesia and increasing nausea and diarrhea.

ARE YOU CONCERNED? DOES THE IDDD NEED TO BE EXPLANTED? HOW DO YOU ADVISE THE HOSPICE NURSE TO PROCEED?

Discussion

As our understanding of chronic pain becomes more refined, we know that the diversity of patient background and of chronic pain conditions, mechanisms, and clinical manifestations contribute to a large population of patients who are unable to achieve adequate pain relief. Oral, transdermal, and parenteral drugs have long been effective analgesic agents; however, they require systemic administration. This can lead to inadequate pain control, systemic side effects, and tolerance, dependence, and addiction, with long-term use in escalating doses.[1] When patients are refractory to conventional medical management, ITDD may have certain advantages, including reduction in the amount of opioid needed, targeted drug delivery at the source of noxious input, and improved analgesia.

HISTORY OF INTRATHECAL ANALGESIA

The first documented spinal analgesic procedure (with cocaine) was performed by August Bier in 1898 for a series of lower extremity operations.[2] In spite of immense interest in the scientific study of intrathecal analgesia, it took another century, with the discovery of opiate receptors in the spinal cord, to uncover the scientific rationale for Bier's earlier work.[3,4] Following this, Fields and Basbaum described the descending pain inhibition system in the substantia gelatinosa.[5] Initially, use of intrathecal opioids was limited to obstetric patients and patients with intractable cancer pain.[6,7]

Over time, the efficacy and safety evidenced in succeeding studies established ITDD as an alternative therapy for other chronic pain states. The first implantable intrathecal opioid delivery device was introduced into clinical use in 1981 for the treatment of severe pain secondary to malignancy.[8] Originally, morphine was the gold standard for intraspinal analgesia, given its duration of action, understood mechanism of action, and ease of use. Alternative agents have been added to the selection for intraspinal therapy, such as hydromorphone, alpha-adrenergic agents, and baclofen, to help address other issues, such as neuropathic pain and spasticity.

PATIENT SELECTION

In order to optimize positive outcomes for ITDD, it is important to identify appropriate patients. When evaluating patients for ITDD, it is helpful to divide them into two broad categories: patients suffering from cancer pain due to a terminal illness, and patients with chronic nonmalignant pain (failed back surgery syndrome, postherpetic neuralgia, etc.).[9]

Patients suffering from cancer pain respond well to intrathecal opioids if they have been managed with oral opioids first. An IDDD should be considered if a patient continues to have pain despite opioid rotation and/or has intractable side effects (nausea, vomiting, sedation, etc.; see Box 30.1).

While reduced life expectancy is not a contraindication, one has to weigh the benefits and the risks (cost and ability to stabilize patients on an efficacious dose). The most recent consensus guidelines support ITDD in cancer patients regardless of expected survival.[10]

Patients experiencing chronic nonmalignant pain often have a more complicated clinical picture secondary to psychologic and behavioral factors that might influence their pain state. Factors to consider when selecting patients for implantation are listed in Box 30.2 and include:

- Failure of maximal medical therapy, which means ineffective analgesia with multiple oral and transdermal trials, physical therapy and rehabilitation, behavioral intervention (i.e., biofeedback), minimally invasive interventions (i.e., epidural and transforaminal injections), and alternative therapies (acupuncture).
- Favorable psychologic evaluation and realistic goals. The specifics are not defined,[12] but the purpose of the psychologic evaluation is to rule out any untreated

Box 30.1. **INDICATIONS FOR INTRATHECAL DRUG DELIVERY**

- Failure of oral medications to control the patient's pain
- Uncontrollable side effects from oral or IV administration
- Successful trial of intrathecal medications (trial not always performed for cancer patients)
- Life expectancy more than 3 months
- Favorable psychologic evaluation and lack of cognitive impairment
- Lack of absolute contraindications
- Clear source of pain

Box 30.2. **CONTRAINDICATIONS TO INTRATHECAL DRUG DELIVERY**

- Sepsis or systemic infection
- Thrombocytopenia or coagulopathy that is uncorrectable
- Local infection at proposed epidural or reservoir sites
- High CSF pressure
- Life expectancy < 3 months (for fully internalized system)

psychiatric illnesses, to define support systems available after the procedure, and to understand what psychological factors might influence the outcomes for a particular patient

- Medical contraindications ruled out.
- Favorable response to an intrathecal drug trial.

DEVICE SELECTION

When selecting which device to use, it is important to consider duration of expected use, need for dose titration, patient's general health, ambulatory status, and estimated life expectancy. The current available evidence does not indicate that bolus dosing results in better analgesia than continuous infusion. Many types of ITP are available on the market today and the choice of device to implant is influenced both by provider preference and by patient factors (see Box 30.3).

TRIAL

After patients have met appropriate selection criteria, the next step is an intraspinal drug trial. A trial not providing sufficient palliation (considered 50% improvement in pain and functional status), is considered a contraindication to implantation. During the trial, the chosen drug is infused through an indwelling catheter that is placed intrathecally or epidurally. It is recommended that the tip of the catheter be placed close to the dermatomal level responsible for the nociceptive impulse.

Box 30.3. **TYPES OF INTRATHECAL DRUG DELIVERY SYSTEMS**

- Percutaneous catheter used with external pump
- Percutaneous catheter with subcutaneous access port and external pump
- Implanted fixed rate ITP (InfusAID®, Codman 3000®)
- Implanted programmable ITP (Medtronic Synchromed®)

DRUG SELECTION

Medications used in implantable drug delivery systems include opioids, local anesthetics, adrenergic agonists, *N*-methyl-D-aspartate (NMDA) receptor agonists, and other experimental agents. Initially, opioids were used alone for intrathecal pharmacotherapy. With better knowledge of pain physiology, use of non-opioid adjuvants has been shown to be therapeutically advantageous in certain clinical situations (i.e., neuropathic pain).

Opioids

Intrathecal opioids act at μ-, δ-, and κ-receptors located in the substantia gelatinosa of the spinal cord dorsal horn, producing dose-dependent analgesia.[13,14] Opioid medications act pre- and postsynaptically by inhibiting neurotransmitter release from primary afferents via blockade of calcium channels and by opening G-protein-coupled complexes to cause efflux of potassium ions from the nerve cell.[15,16]

Morphine sulfate is considered the gold standard and is the only opioid the Food and Drug Administration (FDA) has approved for intrathecal delivery. Morphine has proven efficacy in cancer and noncancer pain.[17,18] Notable side effects of long-term intrathecal morphine delivery include: respiratory depression, pedal edema, hyperalgesia, catheter-tip granuloma, and hypothalamic-pituitary axis suppression. Hydromorphone is a highly potent semisynthetic hydrogenated ketone of morphine. The key advantage of using hydromorphone for intrathecal therapy is a better side effect profile (it is less hydrophilic, thus has a smaller area of spread) and improved analgesia in patients suffering from nociceptive pain.[19] Fentanyl and sufentanil are (less desirable) alternatives to morphine and hydromorphone. Their primary advantage is fewer systemic side effects and decreased risk of catheter-tip granuloma formation.[10]

Local Anesthetics

Local anesthetics are used as adjuvants for management of chronic neuropathic pain. Bupivacaine, the most commonly used, is an amide local anesthetic whose mechanism of action involves reversible binding to sodium channels to inhibit nerve impulse propagation. When used in conjunction with an opioid, such as morphine, it has proven synergistic analgesic effects in cancer and noncancer pain.[20,21,22]

Adrenergic Agonists

Agents in this class include clonidine and tizanidine. Adrenergic agonists act at receptor sites in the substantia gelatinosa, pre- and postsynaptic terminals of small primary afferents, indirectly reducing the release of substance P. Clonidine is the only adrenergic agonist FDA approved for intrathecal use. In general, these agents cause less respiratory depression than opioids do and have a role in control of neuropathic pain. The provider should be cautious with these agents because they may cause significant hypotension and transient sedation at higher doses.[23]

Calcium Channel Blockers

Ziconotide (also known as Prialt) is a highly selective N-type voltage-sensitive calcium channel antagonist derived from marine snail venom and is considered a first-line agent for refractory neuropathic pain. Despite its proven analgesic efficacy in patients with cancer, widespread use of this agent has been limited, due to its narrow therapeutic window and multiple side effects, including ataxia, hallucinations, nystagmus, urinary retention, and double vision.[24,25]

Gamma-Aminobutyric Acid (GABA) Agonists

Baclofen is a GABA-B agonist that is FDA approved for treatment of spasticity. It has a dual mechanism of action, causing decreased calcium conduction and excitatory amino acid release presynaptically, as well as increasing potassium conductance via neuronal hyperpolarization postsynaptically. Caution should be exercised when using this agent intrathecally because it has been associated with life-threatening withdrawal, manifesting as tachycardia, hallucinations, muscle rigidity, fever, blood pressure lability, and seizures. Pruritus is one of the earliest symptoms of baclofen withdrawal. Overdose of baclofen has been associated with respiratory depression, seizures, and death. Prompt treatment with IV physostigmine is recommended when overdose is suspected.[26]

Recommendations about which drug(s) to use and at what concentrations have been developed by the Polyanalgesic Consensus Conference, with the latest iteration published in 2012.[10,11] The recommendations include an algorithm for intrathecal management of nociceptive and neuropathic pain, with several drug recommendations and combinations based on the best available evidence (see Figure 30.1 and Figure 30.2 and Table 30.1).

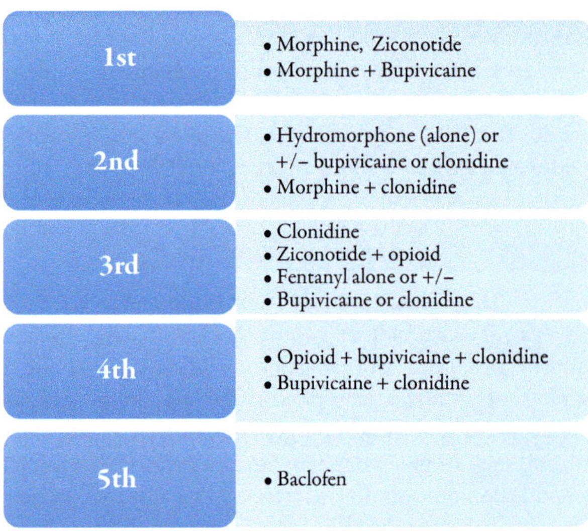

Figure 30.1. Algorithm for managing neuropathic pain with intrathecal medication.[11]

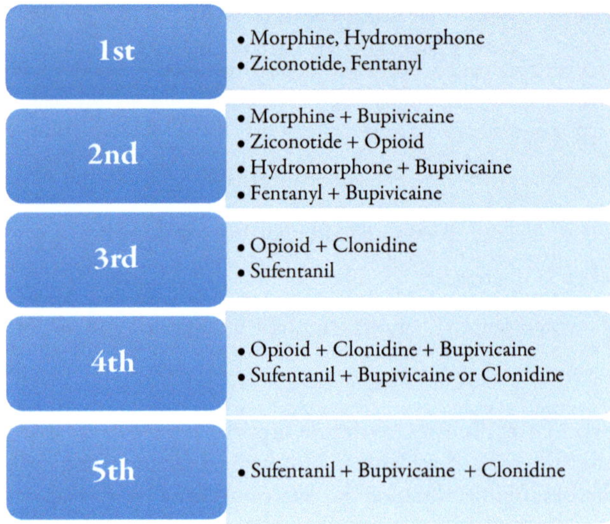

Figure 30.2. Algorithm for managing nociceptive pain with intrathecal medication[11].

COMPLICATIONS

Complications from the implantation of an ITP can be categorized into surgical, pharmacologic, mechanical, and patient-specific or medical (endocrine, infections) complications.[27] Box 30.4 lists helpful tips for preventing and managing complications.

Surgical

Intraoperative bleeding occurs for a number of reasons, most of which can be prevented with a thorough evaluation of the patient. Patients who are being anticoagulated or who use certain herbal supplements are not surgical candidates until appropriate precautions have been taken. The most up-to-date recommendations regarding perioperative management of anticoagulant medications are found in guidelines published by the American Society of Regional Anesthesia in 2015.[28]

Trauma to the periosteum or unexpected spinal tumor encountered during the procedure can increase the risk of bleeding into the epidural or intrathecal space. Significant and undetected bleeding may lead to hematoma, spinal cord compression, and resultant neurologic deterioration. Serial neurologic exams are necessary to recognize postoperative neurologic deficits. Worsening low back pain that is associated with motor weakness, sensory changes, and/or loss of bladder tone should warrant emergent imaging and neurosurgical consultation. Neurologic injury can result from the actual catheter placement, as well as from an inflammatory response that occurs at the catheter tip and is associated with drug delivery.[29] Although rare, the risk of damage to nerve roots during catheter insertion exists.

The risk of infection is common to all implanted devices, and prevention requires adherence to sterile techniques, appropriate antibiotic use, and recognition of new clinical symptoms (erythema, tenderness, swelling, drainage, fever, and leukocytosis). Operative infections are most often caused

Table 30.1. **RECOMMENDED STARTING DOSES FOR INTRATHECAL DRUG DELIVERY**[11]

DRUG	STARTING DOSE	FDA APPROVED	SPECIAL COMMENTS
Morphine	0.1–0.5 mg/day	Yes	Gold standard for intrathecal therapy, but with risk of hyperalgesia
Hydromorphone	0.02–0.5 mg/day	No	Fewer side effects, 5 times more potent than morphine
Fentanyl/Sufentanil	25–75/10–20 μg/day	No	Less risk of catheter-tip granuloma
Bupivacaine	1–4 mg/day	No	Good synergistic effects with opioids. Lidocaine, at high doses, can injure spinal roots.
Clonidine	40–100 μg/d	No	Alpha agonist, causes hypotension in high doses
Ziconotide	0.5–2.4 μg/d	Yes	Calcium channel antagonist, with small therapeutic window
Baclofen	25–100 μg trial bolus dose, depending on the patient	Yes	Rapid cessation can lead to life-threatening withdrawal symptoms

*Some information in this table is adapted from Deer TR, Prager J, Levy R et al. Polyanalgesic Consensus Conference 2012: Recommendations for the management of pain by intrathecal (intraspinal) drug delivery: report of an interdisciplinary expert panel. *Neuromodulation*. 2012; 15(5):436–466

by staphylococci with access through the skin, and thus use of a cephalosporin or vancomycin is generally effective.[30] If a patient is known to be methicillin-resistant *Staphylococcus aureus* positive, then treatment with vancomycin until the nasal swab is negative could help decrease risk of postoperative infections.

Box 30.4. **HELPFUL TIPS FOR PREVENTING AND MANAGING COMPLICATIONS**

- Neurologic history and exam should be documented prior to an intervention.
- Obtain preoperative CT or MRI to check for canal stenosis, arachnoiditis, or other intraspinal abnormalities that would make insertion of the catheter more difficult.
- Obtain imaging and document the catheter tip placement and position at implantation.
- Postimplantation visits should include interval history and neurologic exam. Other signs to assess for:
  - Diminishing analgesic effect
  - Unusual increases in patient's underlying pain
  - Need for steep dose escalations
  - Changes in bowel/bladder function
- Changes in neurologic status should warrant immediate imaging to rule out malfunction in the pump or catheter system or formation of a catheter-tip mass.
- If all of the above have been ruled out, and the patient is still experiencing the need for drug escalation, then consider drug tolerance. Either increase dose or consider a drug holiday.

Superficial wound infections are generally abated with oral antibiotics; however, more serious infections involving the catheter, pocket, or intraspinal space require removal of implanted hardware and administration of IV antibiotics. Failure to do so could lead to epidural abscess formation, meningitis, or other neurologic complications, such as transverse myelitis.[31] It is also important to exercise sterile technique during pump refills, because delivery of contaminated drug solution can increase the risk of meningitis.

Cerebrospinal fluid (CSF) leakage, with the development of seromas, hygromas, and spinal headaches, may occur in as many as 20% of patients who have an IDDD.[9] The use of a large-bore Tuohy needle to access the epidural space and subsequent puncture of the intrathecal space can cause a post-dural-puncture headache. Headaches are self-limiting and can be managed conservatively; however, some patients develop severe symptoms that impair activities of daily living, necessitating a fluoroscopically guided epidural blood patch. A hygroma (an accumulation of CSF that develops near the incision site or in the pump pocket) may develop with severe CSF leaks and is often self-limiting.

Mechanical

Failure of the IDDD is rare. Device malfunction is most often due to catheter kinking, obstruction, disconnection, or shearing, resulting in failure of drug delivery. Dickerman et al.[32] published a study that showed that intra-abdominal positioning of the ITP may lead the pump catheter neck to prematurely fracture, causing leakage. Use of fluoroscopy to confirm proper placement and position of the catheter, visualization of CSF flow to rule out obstructions, and proper suture technique of the catheter to avoid CSF leaks and catheter migration can help decrease catheter failure.

Pharmacologic

The most common pharmacologic complication is an adverse reaction to the selected drug.[33] Others are due to human error, such as overdose, improper pump settings, incorrect dilution of drug from the pharmacy, or contaminated drug. When refilling a pump with a side port intended for bolus drugs or testing catheter patency, caution must be taken not to inadvertently deposit medication outside the reservoir into the pump pocket, leading to systemic toxicity and potential overdose or death.

Inflammatory Mass/Catheter-Tip Granuloma

Granulomas are a noninfectious collection of cells that can expand and have the potential for spinal cord compression. The etiology of granuloma formation is unclear; however, the most widely accepted theory is that granulomas form due to high-dose opioid infusions, specifically morphine.[34–36] Patients receiving ITDD for nonmalignant pain are more likely to experience this complication, most likely due to their longer life expectancy and thus exposure to higher opioid concentrations over a greater period of time. Clinicians should be vigilant for diminishing analgesic effects despite escalation in opioid therapy or any new-onset neurologic symptoms. Pain upon injection into the catheter or radicular pain that corresponds to the level of the catheter tip necessitates a low threshold for imaging. Obtaining either an MRI or CT myelogram is acceptable and will show the catheter tip in a mass-enhancing lesion.[37]

Once cather-tip granuloma is recognized, a neurosurgery consult for possible decompression and catheter removal is indicated in patients with neurologic deficit. The catheter can be replaced or repositioned below the mass, or it may be removed while leaving the pump intact for future use. If no neurologic deficits are appreciated, the pump infusion should be replaced with low-dose hypertonic saline and serial MRIs should be taken to observe for mass regression. Once the granuloma has resolved, a nonoffending opioid should be started. The patient should be carefully monitored for recurrence with serial MRIs every 3 months.[38] It is recommended that the concentrations of the medications be kept as low as possible to decrease the incidence of granuloma formation or that the practitioner consider polyanalgesic therapy with the use of nonopioid intrathecal therapy to decrease opioid exposure.[39]

Medical

Chronic use of oral or intrathecal opioids induces endocrine dysfunction. The most common endocrine dysfunction seen is hypogonadotropic hypogonadism.[40] Fluctuations in follicle-stimulating hormone, luteinizing hormone, testosterone, and growth hormone levels may be seen, inducing fatigue, reduced libido, emotional disturbances, and sexual dysfunction. Hormone levels should be monitored during prolonged intrathecal therapy.

CONCLUSIONS

- In order to determine if a patient is a suitable candidate for ITDD, a complete history and physical must be obtained. One must first evaluate for the etiology of the pain and classify the pain as cancer pain or nonmalignant pain.
- If the pain is nonmalignant, the next step is to screen for a psychologic, behavioral, or medical cause for the pain. The patient's history of medical therapies must be evaluated. Failure of maximal medical treatment as well as at least a 50% improvement in pain and functional status after intrathecal drug trial must be documented before IDDD placement.
- If pain is oncologic in nature, a device should be recommended only after pain is noted to be refractory to opiate rotation or after the efficacy of the treatment regimen is limited by intolerable adverse drug effects.
- While the only FDA-approved drugs for ITDD are morphine, ziconotide, and baclofen, several other agents have been utilized to successfully treat nociceptive pain, spasticity, and neuropathic pain. The Polyanalgesic Consensus Conference provides recommendations about which drug and what concentration should be administered via the device.
- After IDDD placement, vigilance should be maintained to monitor for complications. If new neurologic deficits are noted, immediate imaging and neurosurgery consult are warranted to evaluate for spinal cord compression from hematoma, catheter-tip granuloma, or abscess formation.
- If deep tissue infection is suspected, the device must be removed and a course of IV antibiotic therapy should be initiated to ward off adverse neurologic sequelae. If device malfunction is suspected, fluoroscopy can be utilized to evaluate the catheter for kinking, shearing, or disconnection. Care should be taken to avoid pharmacologic errors, such as improper pump settings, incorrect drug dilution, and overdose.

REFERENCES

1. Nanney A, Muro K, Levy RM. Implanted drug delivery systems for the control of chronic pain. In Benzon HT, Raja SN, Liu SS, et al., eds. *Essentials of Pain Medicine*. 3rd ed. Philadelphia, PA: Elsevier Saunders; 2011:451–461.
2. Bier A. Versuche über Cocainisirung des Rückenmarkes. *Deut Z Chir*. 1899;51:361–369.
3. Yaksh T, Rudy T. Analgesia mediated by a direct spinal action of narcotics. *Science*. 1976;192:1357–1358.
4. Pert CB, Snyder SH. Opiate receptor: demonstration in nervous tissue. *Science*. 1973;179:1011–1014.
5. Basbaum AI, Clanton CH, Fields HL. Opiate and stimulus-produced analgesia: functional anatomy of a medullospinal pathway. *Proc Natl Acad Sci USA*. 1976;73:4685–4688.

6. Wang JK, Nauss LA, Thomas JE. Pain relief by intrathecally applied morphine in man. *Anesthesiology.* 1979;50:149–151.
7. Alper MH. Intrathecal morphine. *Anesthesiology.* 1979;51:378–379.
8. Onofrio BM, Yaksh TL, Arnold PG. Continuous low-dose intrathecal morphine administration in the treatment of chronic pain of malignant origin. *Mayo Clin Proc.* 1981;56:516–520.
9. Knight KH, Brand FM, Mchaourab AS, Veneziano G. Implantable intrathecal pumps for chronic pain: highlights and updates. *Croat Med J.* 2007;48:22–34.
10. Deer TR, Levy R, Prager J, et al. Polyanalgesic Consensus Conference—2012: recommendations to reduce morbidity and mortality in intrathecal drug delivery in the treatment of chronic pain. *Neuromodulation.* 2012;15:467–482.
11. Deer TR, Prager J, Levy R, et al. Polyanalgesic Consensus Conference 2012: recommendations for the management of pain by intrathecal (intraspinal) drug delivery: report of an interdisciplinary expert panel. *Neuromodulation.* 2012;15(5):436–466.
12. Doleys DM. Psychological factors in spinal cord stimulation therapy: brief review and discussion. *Neurosurg Focus.* 2006;15(6):E1.
13. Gomes I, Gupta A, Filipovska J, et al. A role for heterodimerization of mu and delta opiate receptors in enhancing morphine analgesia. *Proc Natl Acad Sci USA.* 2004;101:5135–5139.
14. Reisine T. Opiate receptors. *Neuropharmacology.* 1995;34:463–472.
15. Ocana M, Cendan CM, Cobos EJ, et al. Potassium channels and pain: present realities and future opportunities. *Eur J Pharmacol.* 2004;500:203–219.
16. Donck AV, Vranken JH, Puyalert M, Hayek S, Mekhail N, Zundert JV. Intrathecal drug administration in chronic pain syndromes. *Pain Pract.* 2014;14:461–76.
17. Winkelmuller W, Burchiel K, Van Buyten J. Intrathecal opioid therapy for pain: efficacy and outcomes. *Neuromodulation.* 1999;2:67–76.
18. Kumar K, Kelly M, Pirlot T. Continuous intrathecal morphine treatment for chronic pain of nonmalignant etiology: long-term benefits and efficacy. *Surg Neurol.* 2001;55:79–86.
19. Anderson VC, Cooke B, Burchiel KJ. Intrathecal hydromorphone for chronic nonmalignant pain: a retrospective study. *Pain Med.* 2001;7:249–259.
20. Sjoberg M, Nitescu P, Appelgren L, et al. Long-term intrathecal morphine and bupivacaine in patients with refractory cancer pain. Results from a morphine:bupivacaine dose regimen of 0.5:4.75 mg/mL. *Anesthesiology.* 1994;80:284–297.
21. Sjoberg M, Appelgren L, Einarsson S, et al. Long-term intrathecal morphine and bupivacaine in "refractory" cancer pain. I. Results from the first series of 52 patients. *Acta Anaesthesiol Scand.* 1991;35:30–43.
22. Deer TR, Caraway DL, Kim CK, Dempsey CD, Stewart CD, McNeil KF. Clinical experience with intrathecal bupivacaine in combination with opioid for the treatment of chronic pain related to failed back surgery syndrome and metastatic cancer pain of the spine. *Spine J.* 2002;2:274–278.
23. Eisenach JC, Rauck RL, Buzzaneli, et al. Epidural clonidine analgesia for intractable cancer pain: phase I. *Anesthesiology.* 1989;71:647–652.
24. Olivera BM, Gray WR, Zeikus R, et al. Peptide neurotoxins from fish-hunting cone snails. *Science.* 1985;230:1338–1343.
25. Staats PS, Yearwood T, Charapata SG, et al. Intrathecal ziconotide in the treatment of refractory pain in patients with cancer or AIDS: a randomized controlled trial. *JAMA.* 2004;291:63–70.
26. Rushman S, McLaren I. Management of intrathecal baclofen overdose. *Intensive Care Med.* 1999;25:239.
27. Krames ES. Intrathecal infusional therapies for intractable pain: patient management guidelines. *J Pain Symptom Manage.* 1993;8:36–46.
28. Narouze S, Benzon HT, Provenzano DA, et al. Interventional spine and pain procedures in patients on antiplatelet and anticoagulant medications. *Reg Anesth Pain Med.* 2015;40:182–212.
29. Langsam A. A case of spinal cord compression syndrome by a fibrotic mass presenting in a patient with an intrathecal pain management pump system. *Pain.* 1999;83:97–99.
30. Gyssens IC. Preventing postoperative infections: current treatment recommendations. *Drugs.* 1999;57:175–185.
31. Ubogu EE, Lindenberg JR, Werz MA. Transverse myelitis associated with *Acinetobacter baumanii* intrathecal pump catheter-related infection. *Reg Anesth Pain Med.* 2003;28:470–474.
32. Dickerman RD, Stevens QE, Schneider SJ. The role of surgical placement and pump orientation in intrathecal pump system failure: a technical report. *Pediatr Neurosurg.* 2003;38:107–109.
33. Bhatia G, Lau ME, Gulur P, et al. Intrathecal drug delivery (ITDD) systems for cancer pain. Version 4. *F1000Res.* 2013;2:96.
34. Miele VJ, Price KO, Bloomfield S, Hogg J, Bailes JE. A review of intrathecal morphine therapy related granulomas. *Eur J Pain.* 2006;10:251–261.
35. Yaksh TL. Coffey RJ. Spinal opiate toxicity. Paper presented at: ASRA conference; November 18–21, 2004; Phoenix, AZ.
36. Allen JW, Horais KA, Tozier NA, et al. Time course and role of morphine dose and concentration in intrathecal granuloma formation in dogs: a combined magnetic resonance imaging and histopathology investigation. *Anesthesiology.* 2006;105:581–589.
37. Hassenbusch S, Burchiel K, Coffey RJ, et al. Management of intrathecal catheter-tip inflammatory masses: a consensus statement. *Pain Med.* 2002;3:313–323.
38. Rauck R. Management of intrathecal pump complications. Paper presented at: ASRA conference; November 17–20, 2004; Miami, FL.
39. Coffey RJ, Burchiel K. Inflammatory mass lesions associated with intrathecal drug infusion catheters: report and observations on 41 patients. *Neurosurgery.* 2002;50:78–86.
40. Abs R, Verhelst J, Maeyaert J, et al. Endocrine consequences of long-term intrathecal administration of opioids. *J Clin Endocrinol Metab.* 2000;85:2215–2222.
41. Bottros MM, Christo PJ. Current perspectives on intrathecal drug delivery. *J Pain Res.* 2014;7:615–626.
42. Douglas AF, Weiner HL, Schwartz DR. Prolonged intrathecal baclofen withdrawal syndrome. Case report and discussion of current therapeutic management. *J Neurosurg.* 2005;102:1133–1136.
43. Ben Smail D, Hugeron C, Denys P, Bussel B. Pruritus after intrathecal baclofen withdrawal: a retrospective study. *Arch Phys Med Rehabil.* 2005;86:494–497.

REVIEW QUESTIONS

1. Which of the following patients is an ideal candidate for ITP placement?

   A. A 36-year-old female with fibromyalgia and a history of chronic migraine headaches
   B. A 43-year-old male with hepatic cancer and right upper quadrant abdominal and mid back pain
   C. A 16-year-old female with irritable bowel syndrome at postoperative day 1 after cholecystectomy
   D. A 83-year-old male with chronic lumbar pain, workup negative for disk herniation or spinal stenosis but positive for facet arthropathy, with a history of rheumatoid arthritis

2. The following are types of ITDD systems, except:

   A. Percutaneous catheter with internal pump
   B. Percutaneous catheter with subcutaneous access port
   C. Implanted, internalized, fixed-rate pump
   D. Implanted, internalized programmable pump

3. Which of the following medications is not FDA approved for intrathecal delivery?

   A. Baclofen
   B. Morphine sulfate
   C. Hydromorphone
   D. Ziconotide

ANSWERS

1. B. ITDD systems are thought to be best for patients with localized, not diffuse pain. They have not been shown to be particularly effective for axial back pain (especially pain due to arthritis), fibromyalgia, irritable bowel syndrome, or other pain syndromes. ITDD systems are not appropriate for acute postoperative pain or for opioid-naïve patients.[9,10]

2. A. All of the systems listed, except A, are types of ITDD systems.

3. C. All are FDA-approved drugs for intrathecal delivery except choice C, hydromorphone. Clonidine is often added to decrease the incidence of tolerance. Other medications are commonly used intrathecally, including hydromorphone and bupivacaine, but they are not approved for that indication.[10]

QUESTIONS AND ANSWERS

This chapter has accompanying questions and answers that are available to subscribers as part of the Oxford eLearning platform. To access the questions, follow the link below, or go to ✔ http://oxfordmedicine.com/painmanagementreview

31.

KETAMINE USE AND OPIOID-TOLERANT CANCER PATIENTS

Fardin Yousefshahi, Giuliano Michelagnoli, and Juan Francisco Asenjo

STEM CASE AND KEY QUESTIONS

A 49-year-old female with a history of metastatic breast cancer presents to the multidisciplinary cancer pain clinic complaining of a recent increase in her back pain. She is known to have several metastases in her vertebrae, ribs, and pelvic bones. She recently finished radiotherapy and chemotherapy. She describes her pain as severe, diffuse, and continual; mainly in her back, pelvis, and extremities; without radiation or an electric or neuropathic component. Muscle and bone pain are exacerbated by movement. Her pain scaled from 6/10 (static) to 9/10 (dynamic) in the Verbal Rating Scale (VRS) without clear worsening in her disease condition. Recent MRI and bone scan showed diffuse metastases in the spine, retroperitoneum, and psoas muscle, as well as lung nodes.

She takes oral acetaminophen 650 mg every 6 hours, celecoxib 200 mg twice a day, pregabalin 150 mg twice a day, methadone 20 mg twice a day, and oxycodone 5 to 10 mg as needed for breakthrough pain, and her oxycodone use has increased during the last 2 weeks from 30 mg/day to 60 mg/day. She is being followed by her oncologist, palliativist, and psychologist, as well as a nutritionist.

The patient was a high school teacher, and otherwise a healthy woman, when she was diagnosed with breast cancer 18 month ago. She lives with her supportive husband and her 17- and 21-year-old children.

Her sleep pattern has been disturbed in the last 2 weeks by pain. Her bowel movement routine has been preserved by a change in diet, regular polyethylene glycol, and bisacodyl as needed. She reports loss of concentration, tiredness, lack of energy, and sometimes feeling there is somebody around her. However, she has no symptom or sign of psychosis. She feels irritable and angry sometimes, but her mood is otherwise normal.

She is diagnosed with intractable cancer pain and possible opioid tolerance. After ruling out new treatable causes, the pain specialist suggests adjustment of medication, ketamine therapy, and perhaps neurolysis.

WHAT IS INTRACTABLE CANCER PAIN? IS THIS DIAGNOSIS CORRECT?

The term *refractory cancer pain* is usually considered when, in the context of cancer, the VRS is more than 4 out of 10 and the pain is nonresponsive to the conventional treatments, such as maximized World Health Organization (WHO) ladder at level III with opioid co-analgesics. For this patient, the diagnosis is correct, since the breakthrough oxycodone has increased significantly to the point that the patient has started experiencing cognitive side effects (visual hallucinations of an intruder's presence) without obtaining proper relief.

WHAT ARE OTHER POSSIBLE TREATMENTS FOR THIS PATIENT?

Radiotherapy and chemotherapy were recently maxed out without improvement in her pain and opioids are not effective anymore. Other possible treatments (i.e., ketamine therapy, systemic lidocaine or steroids, radioactive compounds like samarium or strontium, cannabinoids, hypnotherapy, psychotherapy, intrathecal infusions and perhaps some nerve blocks) must be considered at this point.

IS THERE ANY CONTRAINDICATION TO KETAMINE THERAPY?

Ketamine is contraindicated or should be used with caution in the presence of allergy or intolerance, patient refusal, intracranial pathology with increased intracranial pressure and/or seizures, hypertension, aortic or cerebral aneurysms, glaucoma, ongoing acute or uncontrolled psychosis, and porphyria.

IS THERE ANY SPECIAL CONSIDERATION FOR KETAMINE ADMINISTRATION?

Ketamine should be administered by trained personnel. Parenteral, first trial dose, or high dose of ketamine should be administered in a hospital monitored bed; intravenous access should be verified and resuscitation and emergency aids should be easily accessible. Family and the patient should be informed about side effects. However, careful use of oral ketamine can be started on an ambulatory basis provided progressive, small doses are tried.

HOW SHOULD KETAMINE BE ADMINISTERED? WHAT ROUTES OF ADMINISTRATION ARE AVAILABLE?

Dose should be titrated based on the balance of therapeutic and side effects. Oral ketamine is used first when possible; its use is limited by low bioavailability, and the patient will need to be made aware of this. Intravenous, subcutaneous, intramuscular, intranasal, and even rectal routes are also possible. A suggested starting dose between 0.1 and 0.5 mg/kg of lean body weight can be used, and may be administered over 1 hour intravenously (in normal saline) or subcutaneously (undiluted) or orally at 0.2 to 0.8 mg/kg.

ARE THERE ANY SIDE EFFECTS OF KETAMINE THERAPY?

The most common side effects of ketamine are psychologic disturbances, followed by cardiovascular (tachycardia and hypertension) and less commonly gastrointestinal (nausea and increase in liver enzymes) and renal (dysuria and hematuria) side effects. Often, cancer patients already on opioids and mild sedatives do not experience psychotropic disturbances with ketamine due to the buffer effect of the sedatives and opioids.

DISCUSSION

DEFINITIONS

Cancer Pain

In spite of all the advances in the quality of care, pain is the most common symptom in cancer patients and affects more than 50% of them. In one-third of patients, pain is rated as moderate to severe.[1]

The WHO three-step ladder for management of cancer pain is the present gold standard: non-opioid medications (e.g., acetaminophen) are the first step, mild opioids (codeine, tramadol) are the second line of treatment, and the strong opioids (morphine, methadone) are the last step. Adjuvant medications are suggested to control constipation, bone or neuropathic pain, anxiety, and fear, as indicated. This protocol advises that the medications be used on a regular basis rather than on demand. For patients who have not achieved satisfactory pain relief with medications, invasive interventions are suggested.[2]

If the three-step analgesic ladder of WHO is applied, 70% to 90% of patients will have effective pain relief, and the remaining 10% to 30% will suffer from suboptimally controlled pain. In light of this reality, some modifications to the WHO pain ladder are required.[3] Some suggestions have been advanced by Ripamonti et al. on behalf of European Society for Medical Oncology (ESMO) Guidelines Working Group.[4]

Cancer Pain and Opioid Tolerance

Intractable cancer pain and opioid tolerance have been a challenge in medicine for many years.[5,6] Traditionally, after failure of optimal opioid use, radiation, and hormone therapy, the next option was invasive treatment like neurotomy, neurolysis, or neurosurgery.[7–11]

But, recently, Vayne-Bossert et al., in a review of interventional treatments for refractory cancer pain, couldn't find good supportive evidence for the majority of the interventional treatments,[12] which means that advances in interventional treatments for cancer pain couldn't diminish the importance of opioid.

Treatments for Intractable Cancer Pain

A multidisciplinary approach to cancer pain is generally considered the treatment of choice for all cancer patients with intractable pain and opioid tolerance. In 1970, Robbies[13] suggested a combination of medications (opioids, sedatives, antidepressants, hypnotics, and alcohol), psychotherapy and social welfare, hypnotherapy, nerve blocks, and neurolysis for the treatment of intractable cancer pain. Table 31.1 summarizes the pharmacologic management of cancer pain.

KETAMINE USE IN CANCER PATIENTS

Introduction

Ketamine was introduced 1962 as a rapid-onset general anesthetic. In 1970, it was approved by the federal government for use in humans; its popularity as the anesthetic of choice in battlefield situations rose rapidly.[14]

Ketamine is a phencyclidine anesthetic mainly used for the induction of anesthesia. It is especially of interest for its perceived analgesic effects; even in subanesthetic doses, ketamine has the potential to effectively produce pain relief. This useful property has encouraged use of ketamine as an adjuvant and supplemental drug to control acute, severe, intraoperative and postoperative pain or postprocedural pain. Ketamine has also been used extensively as a sedative outside of the operation room; it has also proven its value in trauma patients and for patients in critical care units.

Ketamine can be administered intravenously, intramuscularly, orally, and intrarectally. Furthermore, topical, subcutaneous, nasal, neuraxial, and intra-articular routes have been used in chronic pain patients.[15–17] However, oral administration seems to be the best choice for long-term prescription.[18]

Ketamine has a bioavailability of 16% to 20% orally, 30% sublingually, 45% nasally, and 93% intramuscularly. It is metabolized in the liver to norketamine by the cytochrome P450 system; norketamine is subsequently excreted in urine and bile. The onset of action of ketamine is 1 to 5 min with intravenous administration, 5 min in intramuscular use, 15 to 30 min with the subcutaneous route, and 30 min orally.[19–23]

Table 31.1. PHARMACOLOGIC APPROACH TO THE TREATMENT OF INTRACTABLE CANCER PAIN

DRUG	ADMINISTRATION ROUTE	TIPS	BENEFITS	DRAWBACKS
Short-acting opioids (morphine, fentanyl)	• Oral is favorite • Switch to parenteral if oral or transdermal is not effective • Same effect with subcutaneous and intravenous	• Opioid rotation • Opioid combination	• First-line drugs	• Tolerance • Side effects
Methadone	• Oral • In epidural with local anesthetics, reduces the need for oral rescue morphine	• Useful for neuropathic pain • Less need for escalation	• Second-line therapy in difficult pain—instead of, or in conjunction with, other opioids	• Low therapeutic index and adverse effects
Buprenorphine	• Transdermal route (extended release)	• Useful for neuropathic pain • Option in opioid rotation • Useful for breakthrough pain	• Transdermal buprenorphine achieved better quality of life and pain control than extended-release morphine	• Low evidence of effectiveness due to poor quality of studies
Acetaminophen and NSAIDs	• Oral	• Effective in mild/moderate pain	• Opioid-sparing effect • Improvement in analgesia (multimodal context)	• Escalation restricted due to adverse effects in severe pain
Antidepressants (amitriptyline, duloxetine, venlafaxine)	• Oral	• Effective in neuropathic pain • Duloxetine useful in chemotherapy-induced neuropathic pain	• Recommended for neuropathic pain in cancer patients with mood disorders	
Anticonvulsants (gabapentin, pregabalin)	• Oral	• Pregabalin provided better control of neuropathic cancer pain than placebo, gabapentin, or amitriptyline • Strong evidence supporting the combination with opioids for neuropathic pain	• First-line therapy in neuropathic pain	• Side effects
NMDA-receptor antagonists (ketamine)	• Oral • Intravenous • Subcutaneous • Intrathecal • Intranasal		• Opioid-sparing effect • Prevention and treatment of central sensitization	• Evidence not clear • Potential adverse effects
Cannabinoids	• Oromucosal spray	• Effective in neuropathic pain in multiple sclerosis and refractory cancer pain	• Low to medium doses improve analgesia in opioid-unresponsive refractory cancer pain	• Potential addiction/abuse • Drowsiness, somnolence
Lidocaine	• Parenteral • Oral (analogs)	• Useful in treatment of neuropathic pain		

Hijazi et al. compared the pharmacokinetics of ketamine in intensive care patients with previously reported values in healthy volunteers. Clearance of ketamine is about 36.0 mL/min/kg in intensive care patients and 19.1 mL/min/kg in healthy volunteers. The volume of distribution is 16.0 L/kg and 5.1 L/kg, and its elimination half-life is 4.9 hours and 3 hours, in intensive care patients and healthy volunteers, respectively.[24] Cancer patients are frequently ill and it's logical to expect the pharmacokinetic values to differ between intensive care patients and healthy individuals.

Ketamine has been effective in controlling neuropathic pain in postherpetic neuralgia,[25] diabetic neuralgia,[26,27] glossopharyngeal neuropathy,[25] complex regional pain syndrome (CRPS),[17,28] and phantom limb pain,[29] as well as neoplastic neuropathic pain.[30,31]

Recently, ketamine is used to treat intractable cancer-induced chronic pain as an add-on to opioids and WHO level III.[32] Most studies of ketamine use in pain medicine are about chronic pain syndromes and few articles are focused on ketamine use in cancer pain.

Mechanism of Action

Different mechanisms have been considered to explain the analgesic effect of ketamine.

Ketamine acts by blocking *N*-methyl-D-aspartate (NMDA) receptors. It binds to a specific subunit of NMDA receptors.[20,33] Activation of these receptors is reported in central sensitization, the pathogenesis of chronic pain and neuropathic pain.[32]

Central sensitization and development of allodynia and hyperalgesia in neuropathic or chronic pain patients are mediated by NMDA receptors, and could be reversed by placing ketamine in the receptors' environment, inducing the classic anti-hyperalgesic effects of ketamine.[33–36]

A relationship between anti-inflammatory effects of ketamine and its anti-hyperalgesic properties had been suggested.[36,37]

Ketamine binds to opioid receptors ($\mu > \kappa > \delta$) and has an agonist effect on them; this effect is resistant to naloxone administration.[35] Recent studies reported the effect of ketamine on descending inhibitory pathways, too.[38]

Ketamine Side Effects

Given the smaller doses of ketamine used in pain management, the incidence of side effects is lower than when it is used in anesthesia.[39,40] The most common and worst side effects of ketamine are related to its effect on the central nervous system (CNS), including altered scary perceptions (vivid dreams), illusions, hallucinations, paranoia, panic attacks, nightmares, vertigo, blurred vision, dizziness, and loss of memory.[39] All of these effects are uncommon when the drug is used orally or in small parenteral doses, especially in patients already using opioids and/or benzodiazepines.

Other side effects of ketamine are rarely reported in cancer pain management. These uncommon side effects are gastrointestinal (nausea and an increase in liver enzymes), renal (dysuria and hematuria), and cardiovascular (tachycardia and hypertension).[39] In a retrospective study, Kator et al. found that, by using higher doses of ketamine infusion, the reduction in pain scores could be improved, but, there is an enhanced risk of cardiopulmonary complication, which occurs in more than 20% of cases, including respiratory depression in 6.3% of patients.[41] In another study, by Hardy et al., the rate of adverse effects was higher than in the placebo group, but the majority of side effects were not serious.[42] In both of the studies ketamine was administered to inpatients.

Others did not report a high rate of serious side effects in ketamine-treated pain patients.[43–45]

Carter et al. reported the successful use of ketamine as a sedative medication in palliative care, without compromising hemodynamic or respiratory function.[46]

Indications and Effect

Ketamine is commonly used as an adjuvant medication in intractable cancer and neuropathic pain, which are resistant to high-dose opioids and have predictable breakthrough behavior.[4,47] It is suspected that its analgesic effects in those situations are related to changes in NMDA receptors.[4,47]

In a systematic review of randomized clinical trials, Bell et al. concluded that ketamine administration in cancer pain is effective in enhancing morphine effects and could reduce morphine requirements.[18] Wick mentioned the supporting data for adding low-dose ketamine to patient-controlled morphine analgesia and its beneficial effects on management of intractable cancer pain.[48] Zgaia et al., in a review article, concluded that ketamine can decrease opioid requirement and manage opioid tolerance in patients with uncontrolled cancer pain, but they recommended ketamine as a third-line analgesic option, caution in its use, and careful monitoring of patients.[32] Table 31.2 presents some evidence about ketamine use.

Oral Ketamine

A common and simple way to administer ketamine in pain management is orally. It is safe and noninvasive and it does not require routine nursing care. In a small study, in 1999, Lauretti et al. reported on the efficacy of low-dose oral ketamine as well as transdermal nitroglycerin as analgesic adjuvants with low-dose morphine in 60 chronic cancer pain patients.[50] In a randomized double-blind trial (RDBT) in 30 patients with severe cancer pain, Ishizuka et al. concluded that side effects of oral S(+)-ketamine, when administered with oral morphine, are comparable to placebo effects.[43]

In a literature review published by Blonk et al. in 2009, the authors found limited evidence regarding ketamine use in chronic pain patients. They concluded that oral ketamine could have a limited role in chronic pain patients as an additive treatment, when other therapeutic strategies for pain control had failed.[53] In a cohort study by Chaudhry et al., the authors concluded that ketamine was effective in improving pain control in cancer patients, as an analgesic adjuvant when opioids provided ineffective pain control. They recommended the oral route of administration for ketamine.[54] Marchetti et al., in a retrospective study of 51 patients with chronic cancer or noncancer pain, found beneficial effects of oral ketamine added to opioid medications. Furthermore, the authors found that, with longer duration of opioid treatment, the response to ketamine was better and the incidence of side effects was lower.[55]

Overall, it seems that oral ketamine could be the first option for managing opioid tolerance in cancer patients.

Intravenous Ketamine

In using parenteral routes of administration, all absorption limitations are bypassed, so faster, more reliable, and predictable effects are expected from ketamine administration. Mercadante et al., in a randomized study of 10 cancer patients with intractable neuropathic pain, added ketamine infusion to morphine and found a significant improvement in severity of the pain.[52] In a randomized double-blind (RDB) placebo-controlled study of cancer pain patients, Schwartzman et al. administered intravenous ketamine for 10 days and showed a decrease in pain scores in comparison with the placebo group.[44]

Table 31.2. EVIDENCE-BASED USE OF KETAMINE IN CANCER PAIN

PUBLICATION: DATE AND STUDY DESIGN*	POPULATION	INTERVENTION	CONTROL	OUTCOME 1°	MAIN RESULTS
1996 RCT[49]	Hospitalized patients with intractable cancer pain (n = 20 per group)	• Intrathecal ketamine (n = 20) • Intrathecal ketamine + morphine (n = 20)	Crossover study	Pain intensity	Low dose of intrathecal ketamine reduces the dose of morphine required
1999 RCT[50]	Cancer patients with pain refractory to tramadol and NSAIDs (N = 60)	• Oral ketamine (15 patients) • Dipyrone (15 patients) • Nitroglycerin (15 patients)	Oral morphine (n = 15)	Pain intensity	Ketamine reduces pain intensity and opioid consumption
1999 RCT[51]	Cancer patients with refractory pain (N = 48)	• Epidural ketamine + morphine (n = 12) • Epidural midazolam+ morphine (n = 12) • Epidural neostigmine + morphine (n = 12)	Epidural morphine (n = 12)	Pain intensity	• Ketamine reduces pain intensity and opioid consumption • Neostigmine reduces pain intensity
2000 RCT[52]	Cancer patients with refractory pain on morphine treatment (N = 10)	• Low-dose ketamine • High-dose ketamine • Normal saline	Crossover study	Pain intensity	Ketamine improves opioid analgesia, mostly in neuropathic pain
2012 RCT[42]	Cancer patients with refractory pain (N = 185)	Parenteral ketamine (n = 93 patients)	Placebo (n = 92)	Clinically relevant pain relief	• No difference between the two groups • Significantly more adverse effects
2012 RCT[45]	Cancer patients with pain refractory to opioids (N = 20)	Continuous intravenous ketamine infusion (11 patients)	Placebo (9 patients)	Pain intensity	• No difference between the two groups • Low statistical power • No remarkable adverse effects

*RCT, randomized controlled trial.

In a RDB placebo-controlled trial in palliative care units, Salas et al. could not confirm the efficacy of an intravenous infusion of ketamine and morphine combination to treat intractable cancer pain. However, they found a group of patients who were "good responders" to a morphine and ketamine combination.[45]

Moira et al., in a case series, reported that the infusion of 0.5 to 4 μg/kg/min of ketamine in critical care patients could be helpful to diminish agitation, pain, depression, and anxiety and prevented respiratory depression.[56]

Briefly, it seems that intravenous ketamine administration is effective in managing intractable cancer pain, especially in patients who are not good candidates for oral medications.

Subcutaneous Ketamine

Subcutaneous injection of ketamine is an acceptable alternative to intravenous administration when there is no suitable vascular access or there is an interest in blunting the peak effect and unwanted effects of the medication.

Jackson et al., in a small, multicenter, randomized clinical trial reported the efficacy of subcutaneous ketamine in management of intractable cancer pain patients. According to well-defined therapeutic targets, they divided patients into responders and nonresponders. They reported a 50% response rate, for 2 to 6 weeks, and 9% of patients were pain-free.[57]

Hardy et al. enrolled 185 patients in a multicenter DBRT to evaluate the efficacy of subcutaneous ketamine added to opioids and other co-analgesic medications to treat intractable cancer pain in palliative care. This study showed a significant placebo effect in the placebo group (27%), and the response was not statistically significant different from the ketamine group (31%).[42] Such a high placebo effect is uncommon; therefore, the results of the study are discouraging for subcutaneous ketamine use in management of cancer pain.

Intranasal Ketamine

Ketamine can be easily and rapidly absorbed from mucous membranes, without irritation or a major unpleasant feeling. This makes ketamine acceptable as an intranasal medication, especially in breakthrough pain.

Carr et al., in their placebo-controlled, RDB, crossover clinical trial, showed the rapid efficacy and safety of intranasal ketamine in controlling breakthrough pain in chronic pain patients at 10 to 60 min after administration. However, the low power of the study limited its results' interpretation.[58]

Huge et al. reported the significant efficacy of low doses of intranasal S-isomer ketamine in rapid management of neuropathic pain.[59] It seems that intranasal ketamine use should be investigated further because it could be an amazing, rapid method for overcoming pain episodes.

PROTOCOLS FOR KETAMINE ADMINISTRATION

McGill University Health Centre,[60] the New York State Education Department,[61] North of Tyne Shred Care Group[62] and many other medical centers have guidelines for ketamine use in intractable chronic or cancer pain and some are accessible online.

Considering the current variable evidence about indications, effects, prescription, and administration of ketamine, a consensus is yet to be agreed upon by pain specialists. A universal protocol, if developed, would be invaluable in providing clinicians with data on safety and ethical issues.

Table 31.3 is a summary of our institution's advisory regarding ketamine use in intractable cancer pain.

CONCLUSIONS

- While it is not possible to recommend the routine use of ketamine in all chronic cancer pain patients, the current overall trend favors its benefit for this specific patient population.
- Ketamine should be used in cancer pain patients who are developing tolerance to conventional opioid treatments. In this situation, oral ketamine could be the first option. It can also be recommended when patients are maxed out on the WHO ladder analgesic protocols and when increasing opioid or co-adjuvant therapy does not control their pain.
- There is great variability in the effective dose of ketamine in different pain syndromes; therefore, it should be used with caution.
- Adverse effects of ketamine are primarily reported in hospitalized patients, when ketamine is used in a higher-bolus doses for inducing and/or maintaining general anesthesia.[41,42] Given the low doses of ketamine used in pain management, side effects or adverse reactions are virtually absent.
- There is no comparison between the risk and benefits of ketamine and those of opioid or non-opioid analgesics. However, ketamine should be used with caution and surveillance, and higher parenteral doses should be administered under cardiorespiratory monitoring.
- Some patients are nonresponders to ketamine, and they should be recognized and withdrawn from ketamine treatment, while in responders to ketamine, treatment should be adjusted based on response and therapeutic targets.[48]

Table 31.3. **TIPS FOR USE OF KETAMINE IN REFRACTORY CANCER PAIN**

Indications and patient selection	• Moderate to severe cancer pain unresponsive to well-designed individualized combination of opioids and co-analgesics. • No indication for, or no response to, more effective or definitive treatments or interventions.
Contraindications	• Allergy or intolerance • Patient refusal • Intracranial pathology, increased intracranial pressure, and/or seizure history • Hypertension, ischemic heart disease, uncompensated congestive heart failure, arrhythmia, severe vascular or valvular stenosis, or unstable hemodynamics • Aortic or cerebral aneurysms • Raised intraocular pressure and glaucoma • Ongoing acute or uncontrolled psychosis • Porphyria
Administration	• Ketamine should be administered by trained personnel. • Parenteral use, any first trial dose, or high dose of ketamine should be prescribed in a hospital monitored bed, intravenous access should be verified, and resuscitation and emergency aids should be easily accessible. • Dose should be titrated based on the balance of therapeutic and side effects. • Intravenous dose should be between 0.1 and 0.5 mg/kg of ideal body weight over 1 hour, or equivalent doses for enteral routes (i.e., 0.3–0.6 mg/kg orally). Higher doses will increase side effects.
Post-administration cares	• In day admission, patient should be accompanied and patient should avoid any activity that needs complete alertness up to 24 hours later. • Patient can be monitored by plasma level (very uncommonly done). • Family should be informed about side effects, especially psychologic effects. • General discharge rules should be applied for ketamine infusion, too. • Patient should avoid other sedatives for one night.

- Ketamine use in pain medicine is an off-label indication, and the current approach to using it should be based on clinical judgment and balancing the risks and benefits of the treatment.

REFERENCES

1. van den Beuken-van Everdingen MH, de Rijke JM, Kessels AG, Schouten HC, van Kleef M, Patijn J. Prevalence of pain in patients with cancer: a systematic review of the past 40 years. *Ann Oncol.* 2007;18(9):1437–1449.

2. World Health Organization (WHO). *WHO's cancer pain ladder for adults*. Available at http://www.who.int/cancer/palliative/painladder/en/.
3. Vargas-Schaffer G. Is the WHO analgesic ladder still valid? Twenty-four years of experience. *Can Fam Physician*. 2010;56(6):514–517, e202–515.
4. Ripamonti CI, Santini D, Maranzano E, Berti M, Roila F, Group EGW. Management of cancer pain: ESMO Clinical Practice Guidelines. *Ann Oncol.* 2012;23(suppl 7):139–154.
5. Kenny M. Relief of pain in intractable cancer of the pelvis. *Br Med J.* 1947;2(4534):862.
6. Potter JF. Management of intractable pain in metastatic cancer. *Med Ann Dist Columbia*. 1961;30:60–63.
7. Hyndman OR. Intractable pain due to cancer; treatment by neurosurgical methods. *Am J Surg.* 1948;75(1):187–199.
8. Nocito FJ, Diez ED. [Splanchnicectomy and lumbar gangliectomy in intractable pain in abdominal cancer]. *Prensa Med Argent.* 1952;39(17):859–869.
9. Ferey D. [Partial coagulation of anterior thalamic peduncle; a trial in intractable pain particularly in inoperable cancer and in psychosurgery]. *Mem Acad Chir (Paris).* 1955;81(25-26):749–753.
10. Hay RC, Yonezawa T, Derrick WS. Control of intractable pain in advanced cancer by subarachnoid alcohol block. *J Am Med Assoc.* 1959;169(12):1315–1320.
11. Espey FF. Treatment of intractable pain secondary to cancer by cordotomy. *Am Surg.* 1962;28:377–380.
12. Vayne-Bossert P, Afsharimani B, Good P, Gray P, Hardy J. Interventional options for the management of refractory cancer pain—what is the evidence? *Support Care Cancer.* 2016;24(3):1429–1438.
13. Robbie DS. Management of intractable pain in advanced cancer of the rectum. *Proc R Soc Med.* 1970;63(suppl):115–116.
14. Jansen KL. A review of the nonmedical use of ketamine: use, users and consequences. *J Psychoactive Drugs.* 2000;32(4):419–433.
15. Azevedo VM, Lauretti GR, Pereira NL, Reis MP. Transdermal ketamine as an adjuvant for postoperative analgesia after abdominal gynecological surgery using lidocaine epidural blockade. *Anesth Analg.* 2000;91(6):1479–1482.
16. Kronenberg RH. Ketamine as an analgesic: parenteral, oral, rectal, subcutaneous, transdermal and intranasal administration. *J Pain Palliat Care Pharmacother.* 2002;16(3):27–35.
17. Finch PM, Knudsen L, Drummond PD. Reduction of allodynia in patients with complex regional pain syndrome: a double-blind placebo-controlled trial of topical ketamine. *Pain.* 2009;146(1-2):18–25.
18. Bell RF, Eccleston C, Kalso EA. Ketamine as an adjuvant to opioids for cancer pain. *Cochrane Database Syst Rev.* 2012;11:CD003351.
19. Clements J, Nimmo W. Pharmacokinetics and analgesic effect of ketamine in man. *Br J Anaesth.* 1981;53(1):27–30.
20. Arendt-Nielsen L, Nielsen J, Petersen-Felix S, Schnider T, Zbinden A. Effect of racemic mixture and the (S+)-isomer of ketamine on temporal and spatial summation of pain. *Br J Anaesth.* 1996;77(5):625–631.
21. Hijazi Y, Boulieu R. Contribution of CYP3A4, CYP2B6, and CYP2C9 isoforms to *N*-demethylation of ketamine in human liver microsomes. *Drug Metab Dispos.* 2002;30(7):853–858.
22. Quibell R, Prommer EE, Mihalyo M, Twycross R, Wilcock A. Ketamine*. *J Pain Symptom Manag.* 2011;41(3):640–649.
23. Quibell R, Fallon M, Mihalyo M, Twycross R, Wilcock A. Ketamine. *J Pain Symptom Manag.* 2015;50(2):268–278.
24. Hijazi Y, Bodonian C, Bolon M, Salord F, Boulieu R. Pharmacokinetics and haemodynamics of ketamine in intensive care patients with brain or spinal cord injury. *Br J Anaesth.* 2003;90(2):155–160.
25. Eide PK, Stubhaug A, Øye I, Breivik H. Continuous subcutaneous administration of the *N*-methyl-D-aspartic acid (NMDA) receptor antagonist ketamine in the treatment of post-herpetic neuralgia. *Pain.* 1995;61(2):221–228.
26. Bell RF. Ketamine for chronic non-cancer pain. *Pain.* 2009;141(3):210–214.
27. Noppers I, Niesters M, Aarts L, Smith T, Sarton E, Dahan A. Ketamine for the treatment of chronic non-cancer pain. *Expert Opin Pharmacother.* 2010;11(14):2417–2429.
28. Kiefer RT, Rohr P, Ploppa A, et al. Efficacy of ketamine in anesthetic dosage for the treatment of refractory complex regional pain syndrome: an open-label phase II study. *Pain Med.* 2008;9(8):1173–1201.
29. Eichenberger U, Neff F, Sveticic G, et al. Chronic phantom limb pain: the effects of calcitonin, ketamine, and their combination on pain and sensory thresholds. *Anesth Analg.* 2008;106(4):1265–1273.
30. Kotlinska-Lemieszek A, Luczak J. Subanesthetic ketamine: an essential adjuvant for intractable cancer pain. *J Pain Symptom Manag.* 2004;28(2):100–102.
31. Persson J. Ketamine in pain management. *CNS Neurosci Ther.* 2013;19(6):396–402.
32. Zgaia AO, Irimie A, Sandesc D, et al. The role of ketamine in the treatment of chronic cancer pain. *Clujul Med.* 2015;88(4):457–461.
33. Attal N. Neuropathic pain: mechanisms, therapeutic approach, and interpretation of clinical trials. *Continuum (Minneap Minn).* 2012;18(1):161–175.
34. Mao J, Sung B, Ji RR, Lim G. Chronic morphine induces downregulation of spinal glutamate transporters: implications in morphine tolerance and abnormal pain sensitivity. *J Neurosci.* 2002;22(18):8312–8323.
35. White PF, Way WL, Trevor AJ. Ketamine—its pharmacology and therapeutic uses. *Anesthesiology.* 1982;56(2):119–136.
36. Esin E, Yalcin S. Neuropathic cancer pain: What we are dealing with? How to manage it? *Oncotargets Ther.* 2014;7:599–618.
37. Subramaniam K, Subramaniam B, Steinbrook RA. Ketamine as adjuvant analgesic to opioids: a quantitative and qualitative systematic review. *Anesth Analg.* 2004;99(2):482–495.
38. Niesters M, Aarts L, Sarton E, Dahan A. Influence of ketamine and morphine on descending pain modulation in chronic pain patients: a randomized placebo-controlled cross-over proof-of-concept study. *Br J Anaesth.* 2013;110(6):1010–1016.
39. Cvrcek P. Side effects of ketamine in the long-term treatment of neuropathic pain. *Pain Med.* 2008;9(2):253–257.
40. Niesters M, Martini C, Dahan A. Ketamine for chronic pain: risks and benefits. *Br J Clin Pharmacol.* 2014;77(2):357–367.
41. Kator S, Correll DJ, Ou JY, Levinson R, Noronha GN, Adams CD. Assessment of low-dose i.v. ketamine infusions for adjunctive analgesia. *Am J Health Syst Pharm.* 2016;73(5)(suppl 1):S22–S29.
42. Hardy J, Quinn S, Fazekas B, et al. Randomized, double-blind, placebo-controlled study to assess the efficacy and toxicity of subcutaneous ketamine in the management of cancer pain. *J Clin Oncol.* 2012;30(29):3611–3617.
43. Ishizuka P, Garcia JB, Sakata RK, Issy AM, Mulich SL. Assessment of oral S+ ketamine associated with morphine for the treatment of oncologic pain. *Rev Bras Anestesiol.* 2007;57(1):19–31.
44. Schwartzman RJ, Alexander GM, Grothusen JR, Paylor T, Reichenberger E, Perreault M. Outpatient intravenous ketamine for the treatment of complex regional pain syndrome: a double-blind placebo controlled study. *Pain.* 2009;147(1-3):107–115.
45. Salas S, Frasca M, Planchet-Barraud B, et al. Ketamine analgesic effect by continuous intravenous infusion in refractory cancer pain: considerations about the clinical research in palliative care. *J Palliat Med.* 2012;15(3):287–293.
46. Carter MJ, Gibbins J, Senior-Smith G, Thomas S, Guest P, Forbes K. Ketamine: does it have a role in palliative sedation? *J Pain Symptom Manag.* 2008;36(4):e1–e3.
47. Kurdi MS, Theerth KA, Deva RS. Ketamine: current applications in anesthesia, pain, and critical care. *Anesth Essays Res.* 2014;8(3):283–290.
48. Wick JY. Ketamine: reinventing chronic pain management. *Pharmacy Times.* http://www.pharmacytimes.com/publications/issue/2014/august2014/ketamine-reinventing-chronic-pain-management. Updated August, 2014. Accessed May, 2016.
49. Yang CY, Wong CS, Chang JY, Ho ST. Intrathecal ketamine reduces morphine requirements in patients with terminal cancer pain. *Can J Anaesth.* 1996;43(4):379–383.

50. Lauretti GR, Lima IC, Reis MP, Prado WA, Pereira NL. Oral ketamine and transdermal nitroglycerin as analgesic adjuvants to oral morphine therapy for cancer pain management. *Anesthesiology.* 1999;90(6):1528–1533.
51. Lauretti GR, Gomes JM, Reis MP, Pereira NL. Low doses of epidural ketamine or neostigmine, but not midazolam, improve morphine analgesia in epidural terminal cancer pain therapy. *J Clin Anesth.* 1999;11(8):663–668.
52. Mercadante S, Arcuri E, Tirelli W, Casuccio A. Analgesic effect of intravenous ketamine in cancer patients on morphine therapy: a randomized, controlled, double-blind, crossover, double-dose study. *J Pain Symptom Manag.* 2000;20(4):246–252.
53. Blonk MI, Koder BG, van den Bemt PM, Huygen FJ. Use of oral ketamine in chronic pain management: a review. *Eur J Pain.* 2010;14(5):466–472.
54. Chaudhary K, Gupta P, Gogia AR. A prospective, randomized, double-blind study to compare the efficacy of lidocaine + metoclopramide and lidocaine + ketamine combinations in preventing pain on propofol injection. *J Anesth.* 2013;27(3):402–406.
55. Marchetti F, Coutaux A, Bellanger A, Magneux C, Bourgeois P, Mion G. Efficacy and safety of oral ketamine for the relief of intractable chronic pain: a retrospective 5-year study of 51 patients. *Eur J Pain.* 2015;19(7):984–993.
56. Moitra VK, Patel MK, Darrah D, Moitra A, Wunsch H. Low-dose ketamine in chronic critical illness. *J Intensive Care Med.* 2016;31(3):216–220.
57. Jackson K, Ashby M, Howell D, et al. The effectiveness and adverse effects profile of "burst" ketamine in refractory cancer pain: The VCOG PM 1-00 study. *J Palliat Care.* 2010;26(3):176–183.
58. Carr DB, Goudas LC, Denman WT, et al. Safety and efficacy of intranasal ketamine for the treatment of breakthrough pain in patients with chronic pain: a randomized, double-blind, placebo-controlled, crossover study. *Pain.* 2004;108(1-2):17–27.
59. Huge V, Lauchart M, Magerl W, et al. Effects of low-dose intranasal (S)-ketamine in patients with neuropathic pain. *Eur J Pain.* 2010;14(4):387–394.
60. Perez J LL, Brecht K, Shir Y, Borod M. Low dose ketamine infusion in the pain clinic and in the palliative care unit (PCU). Non-published document, Medication Administration Policy, McGill University Health Centre. 2014:1–13.
61. Zittel B. IV drug administration of ketamine for the treatment of intractable pain. New York State Education Department. http://www.op.nysed.gov/prof/nurse/nurse-iv-ketamine.htm. Published 2011.
62. North of Tyne Area Prescribing Committee. Shared care guidelines for the use of ketamine in palliative care initiated by palliative care specialists. http://www.northoftyneapc.nhs.uk/wp-content/uploads/sites/6/2012/03/Ketamine-in-Palliative-Care-Cancer-pain-2014-Shared-care-V1-Final-May-14.pdf. Published 2014.

REVIEW QUESTIONS

1. What percentage of patients suffering from cancer have moderate to severe pain?

A. 50%
B. 15%
C. 80%
D. None

2. According to the WHO analgesic ladder for cancer pain, when would invasive pain treatment be instituted?

A. Immediately after the diagnosis of cancer is made
B. When second-line therapy with mild opioids is initiated
C. Never; invasive interventions should never be used in cancer patients as many are debilitated and cannot tolerate them
D. For patients who have not have satisfactory relief with medication after following the WHO analgesic ladder

3. Ketamine as a rapid-onset general anesthetic was mentioned for the first time in

A. 1990
B. 1970
C. 1962
D. 1900

ANSWERS

1. B. About 50% of patients with cancer suffer from pain that affects their quality of life; about half of those suffer from moderate to severe pain, requiring interventions by pain management specialists.[1]

2. D. The WHO three-step ladder for management of cancer pain is the present gold standard; non-opioid medications (e.g., acetaminophen) are the first step, mild opioids (codeine, tramadol) are the second line of treatment, and strong opioids (morphine, methadone) are the last step. Adjuvant medications are suggested to control constipation, bone or neuropathic pain, anxiety, and fear, as indicated. The protocol advises use of the medications on a regular basis rather than on demand. For patients who have not had satisfactory pain relief with medications, invasive interventions are suggested.[2] Currently, there is a significant trend toward using interventional invasive treatments early in the course of cancer progression, as the patient's functional status may significantly improve with decreased pain due to interventional modalities. If the three-step analgesic ladder of WHO is applied, 70% to 90% of patients will have effective pain relief, and the remaining 10% to 30% will suffer from suboptimally controlled pain. In light of this reality, some modifications to the WHO pain ladder are required.[3] Some suggestions have been advanced by Ripamonti et al. on behalf of the ESMO Guidelines Working Group.[4]

3. C. The rapid-onset general anesthetic ketamine was mentioned and introduced in clinical practice in 1962; it was used significantly as a battlefield anesthetic starting in 1970 when its utilization received FDA approval for humans.[14] In 1990, the involvement of ketamine with the NMDA receptors and the wind-up phenomenon was discovered.

QUESTIONS AND ANSWERS

This chapter has accompanying questions and answers that are available to subscribers as part of the Oxford eLearning platform. To access the questions, follow the link below, or go to

✔ http://oxfordmedicine.com/painmanagementreview

32.

PATIENTS WITH SUBSTANCE ABUSE AND CHRONIC PAIN

Dmitri Souza, Denis Snegovskikh, and Julia K. Hunter

STEM CASE AND KEY QUESTIONS

A 55-year-old woman presented to the emergency department (ED) with a chief complaint of back pain. The pain had been present for several years, but had worsened over the past 4 weeks despite physical therapy. She described the pain as constant, sharp, and aching. The pain was lumbar, with radiation to the bilateral upper buttocks. Sitting and walking exacerbated the pain and lying down alleviated it.

She smoked one pack of cigarettes per day and had been smoking since age 15. She drank "a few" cocktails daily and denied illicit drug use. She was unemployed. Her home medications included oxycodone 15 mg two times per day. An X-ray in the ED demonstrated chronic degenerative changes. She was diagnosed with lumbar spondylosis and lumbar degenerative disk disease and was admitted to the hospital for pain management.

Pain medicine was consulted for management of "uncontrolled pain in a patient with opioid tolerance." The pain management team noted a preliminary urine drug screen positive for opiates, benzodiazepines, and cocaine. MRI done during this admission showed increased T2 signal at the L4-L5 disk and adjacent bone.

HOW COMMON IS ADDICTION?

Addiction is very common. The lifetime prevalence of substance abuse and substance dependence disorders has been estimated to be about 10.5% in the U.S. population.[1] Addiction affects people of all ages, races, and socioeconomic classes. It is a chronic relapsing and remitting disease like diabetes, hypertension, and asthma, and is similarly considered present even after periods of remission.[2]

Physicians caring for patients with chronic pain and a substance use disorder should be aware of the epidemiology of substance use, drugs' pathophysiologic effects, and pharmacologic treatments available for substance use disorders. Some pain medications and muscle relaxants can be addictive and should therefore be utilized with careful consideration, especially when treating chronic pain.

WHAT ARE THE DEFINITIONS OF ADDICTION AND RELATED TERMS?

It is important to be familiar with the terms used in addiction medicine. *Addiction* is a chronic brain disorder characterized by continued compulsive substance use despite physical, psychologic, and/or social harm to the user.[3] *Physical dependence* is a state of physical adaptation to a substance characterized by the emergence of objective signs of withdrawal during abstinence, which may be relieved totally or in part by re-administration of the substance.[3] A *withdrawal syndrome* is a characteristic constellation of signs and symptoms (for example, rhinorrhea, lacrimation, yawning, sneezing, piloerection, vomiting, and loose stools may be seen in opioid withdrawal) appearing after the abrupt discontinuation of, or rapid decrease in, substance use.[3] *Psychologic dependence* is the use of a psychoactive substance for its positive effects or for the avoidance of the negative and unpleasant emotions associated with its withdrawal. *Abstinence* is the cessation of all drug use, and it particularly applies to a patient's drug of abuse or dependence.[3]

WHAT ARE THE DIFFERENCES BETWEEN OPIOID TOLERANCE, OPIOID-INDUCED HYPERALGESIA, AND DRUG-SEEKING BEHAVIOR?

The patient has invariably complained of inadequate pain relief during this admission, despite escalating doses of intravenous hydromorphone. Did her behavior suggest opioid tolerance, opioid-induced hyperalgesia, or drug-seeking behavior?

Opioid tolerance is a physiologic adaptation (or desensitization) to opioids' effects, so decreased effects are seen at constant opioid doses and constant effects are maintained only with increasing doses.[3] *Opioid-induced hyperalgesia* is a state of nociceptive sensitization caused by exposure to opioids and that decreases overall pain tolerance.[4] In both of these conditions, the patient experiences inadequate pain control.

Providers often consider *drug-seeking behavior* when patients with seemingly adequate pain control ask for more pain medication.[5] In *pseudo-addiction,* patients ask for more pain medication due to inadequate pain control, not for secondary gain.[6]

HOW TO IDENTIFY A CHRONIC PAIN PATIENT WITH A HISTORY OF SUBSTANCE ABUSE

The patient has had a documented history of back pain, but no history of substance abuse prior to her admission. On the detailed interview, however, the patient admitted that she she ran out of her oxycodone supply quite often because "it was not enough to help me with my pain." This statement prompted here physician to order a drug screen panel, which identified substance abuse disorder in the patient.

This case demonstrates that a skillful discussion can reveal a history of substance abuse, prior diagnoses of, or treatments for, substance use disorders, and compliance with previous pain management and/or addiction treatment plans.[7,8] The discussion should be supplemented by a physical exam (often there are no physical clues of substance abuse, but advanced disease can present with obvious manifestations of use, such as needle marks or "tracks").[9] Chart review of notes and urine drug screens as well as validated screens (such as the AUDIT, DAST, and CAGE) can help diagnose substance use disorders.[8] And, of course, urine drug screens help with monitoring for substance abuse and compliance with use of controlled substances.[7,10]

Some patients with past or present substance abuse may not mention it, or may even deny it, either because they do not understand its relevance or they would like to keep it out of the medical record. These patients can be assured that extra confidentiality protection is provided in federally funded addiction specialty treatment programs above that in place for the Health Insurance Portability and Accountability Act (HIPAA). These programs cannot disclose any information about the patient without the patient's written consent, with only a limited number of exceptions.[11] Substance abuse may negatively affect acute care in the hospital, and, therefore, patients and their families should be encouraged to share relevant information to help to provide adequate and safe care for the patient.

Among patients with chronic pain, abuse is often suspected when a patient increases his or her opioid dose without physician consultation, notes intense pain but appears physically comfortable, obtains opioid prescriptions from multiple providers, claims prescription or drug loss, or is unwilling to rotate opioids or to use non-opioid alternatives.[10]

WHAT CLASSES OF SUBSTANCES ARE COMMONLY ASSOCIATED WITH ABUSE?

The classes of substances commonly associated with abuse include depressants, stimulants, hallucinogens, and inhalants. Depressants include alcohol, sedatives, hypnotics, opioids, and anxiolytics, which are discussed in detail elsewhere in this chapter. Commonly abused stimulants are cocaine, amphetamines, and nicotine. Psychedelic hallucinogens (psychotomimetics) include lysergic acid diethylamide (LSD), psilocybin, mescaline, and 3,4-methylenedioxymethamphetamine (MDMA). Dissociative hallucinogens include dextromethorphan (DXM), phencyclidine (PCP), and ketamine. Deliriants include *Atropa belladonna, Datura stramonium,* and *Myristica fragran* as well as antihistamines, such as diphenhydramine and dimenhydrinate. Inhaled anesthetics and solvents are also substances of abuse. The management of pain in a patient with substance abuse depends on the class of the substance being abused. Special attention should be exercised when a combination of substances is suspected, because it may distort the clinical picture. Mixed use of benzodiazepines and opioids is quite commonly observed. Mixing of these two classes of medications is one of the most dangerous combinations.

WHAT ARE THE DIFFERENCES BETWEEN MANAGEMENT OF PAIN IN PATIENTS WITH CURRENT SUBSTANCE ABUSE, PATIENTS ON REPLACEMENT/MAINTENANCE THERAPY, AND PATIENTS IN RECOVERY?

Common clinical presentations involving substance abuse include abstention from all substances of abuse, medication-assisted treatment (including buprenorphine and methadone for opioid use disorder), and current substance abuse. In general, buprenorphine and methadone are continued during a medical admission if there are no contraindications (such as septic shock). With elective surgical procedures, the total methadone dose is often kept unchanged but is given on a divided schedule (twice or three times a day) instead of a daily schedule. Buprenorphine, because of its ceiling effect, is typically stopped 1 to 5 days before elective surgery, with conversion to other opioids in the perioperative period. Reintroduction of buprenorphine commonly occurs after the acute pain is expected to be over, typically within 7 days.[12] In the case of unanticipated surgery, fentanyl is often used to displace buprenorphine from μ-receptors.

Patients with a history of substance abuse may be at risk of relapse with opioid exposure. Therefore, opioids should be used only after a thorough discussion with the patient about the risks and benefits. The use of non-opioid analgesics and nonpharmacologic pain control (including interventional modalities, physical rehabilitation, chiropractic manipulations, pain psychology, and regional analgesia for acute pain) is very important to avoid provocation of a substance use disorder.

If the patient has a history of substance abuse but is currently abstinent, it is helpful to learn about how they are maintaining their sobriety. Patients actively working a recovery program in conjunction with therapists, counselors, addiction specialists, and/or 12-step support groups are less likely to relapse when prescribed addictive substances, particularly when the addiction treatment modalities are included in their pain management plan.[1,8]

Agains, the management of pain in a patient with substance abuse depends on the class of the substance being abused.

DISCUSSION

CHRONIC PAIN MANAGEMENT FOR PATIENTS WITH A HISTORY OF SUBSTANCE ABUSE

Substance use disorder is a chronic disease that can relapse even after a prolonged remission. Patients with chronic nonmalignant pain and a history of substance abuse, even remote, should be advised against long-term opioid treatment because of the increased risk of relapse. In general, these patients should be offered a comprehensive, non-opioid, outpatient chronic pain rehabilitation program that includes physical rehabilitation, chiropractic manipulations if available, pain psychology, and interventional therapy, among other modalities. A variety of non-opioid medications are available for treatment of chronic nonmalignant pain, including nonsteroidal anti-inflammatory drugs (NSAIDs), membrane stabilizers, and antidepressants. It is generally recommended that individualized treatment planning should start with a behavioral assessment by a psychologist, the establishment of realistic treatment goals, and a detailed history of substance abuse. In our practice, a patient with history of substance abuse is denied entry into the chronic pain program if they decline a non-opioid management plan. The exception is the group of patients with tobacco use disorder. They can be prescribed opioids if indicated, but would have to comply with a smoking cessation program offered at the first visit. They may be denied opioid therapy if they continue to use nicotine.

ACUTE PAIN MANAGEMENT FOR PATIENTS WITH A HISTORY OF SUBSTANCE ABUSE

Management of Acute Pain in Patients with Opioid Abuse Disorder on Replacement Therapy

A contract for addiction treatment, established between the patient and the addiction medicine provider, should not affect acute pain management. However, it should preclude prescription of opioids for chronic nonmalignant pain.

The type of replacement/maintenance therapy determines the approach to acute pain management in patients with substance abuse. Replacement therapy includes buprenorphine, buprenorphine-naloxone, methadone, and naltrexone.

Replacement Therapy with Buprenorphine

Buprenorphine is a partial μ-receptor agonist with a strong affinity for this receptor. Suboxone, a sublingual medication, is a combination of buprenorphine and the μ-receptor antagonist naloxone. Naloxone has no effect on buprenorphine when administered sublingually, but it is intended to prevent misuse in case of crushing and injection, as such routes of naloxone administration can precipitate withdrawal in the chronic opioid user.[13] It is suggested that the patient be weaned off buprenorphine before elective surgery.[12] The dose should be gradually decreased over a 1- to 2-week period; if the dose of buprenorphine is low, 2 to 4 mg a day, the weaning can take place over a shorter period, 3 to 7 days.[14] If the dose of buprenorphine is high, cautious replacement with another opioid may be utilized in anticipation of acute postoperative pain.[15] In practice, many facilities discontinue buprenorphine the day before elective surgery and then have to use significantly higher doses of opioids than anticipated in the surgical and immediate postoperative period. To avoid escalation of the opioid dose in case of unanticipated surgery, or other severe acute pain, fentanyl can be utilized because it has a stronger affinity for μ-receptors than buprenorphine. If it is administered intravenously, it is advisable to place the patient in the intensive care or telemetry unit in order to safely titrate the medication.[15] A fentanyl transdermal iontophoretic system can be utilized on a regular hospital floor.

Replacement Therapy with Methadone

Patients taking methadone for opioid dependency should continue replacement therapy with methadone, with additional opioids used during surgery and/or for breakthrough pain in the postoperative period or during an acute pain episode. There are clinical scenarios where the same dose of methadone the patient was taking prior to the admission may be not permissible. For example, if a patient has sepsis, methadone may suppress the sympathetic drive, and, therefore, worsen the hypotension associated with sepsis. In this situation, the dose of methadone can be reduced, and the daily maintenance dose can be given in increments, every 4 to 8 hours, depending on the patient's condition. The dose of opioids needed to control the pain in an opioid-tolerant and opioid-dependent patient will be two to four times more than their baseline dose.[16] Clinicians should be vigilant, and be able to move the patient to monitored settings if side effects from the escalated opioid dose are observed or anticipated (higher-risk populations include morbidly obese patients, patients with obstructive sleep apnea, and opioid-tolerant patients with coexisting benzodiazepine dependence).[12]

MANAGEMENT OF ACUTE PAIN IN PATIENTS WITH CURRENT OPIOID ABUSE

Multimodal and multidisciplinary acute pain management is the key to providing effective pain relief for patients with acute pain and active opioid abuse. It is important to customize acute pain treatment for these patients by titrating the dose of opioids to balance the analgesia and side effects, including life-threatening respiratory depression. Pain scores reported by patients may not always reflect the level of pain control, but sometimes represent the anxiety these patients frequency experience. Patient appearance, speech, vital signs, and nonverbal signs (face expression, posture, and other) may tell providers more about the adequacy of pain control than the patient-reported pain score. At the same time, it is important to monitor these patients closely during their hospitalization because they may experience severe postoperative or other acute pain.

MANAGEMENT OF ACUTE PAIN IN PATIENTS WITH FORMER OPIOID ABUSE

Patients with history of substance abuse are always at risk for relapse.[15] Therefore, the treatment approach for patients with current opioid abuse applies to patients with former opioid abuse or dependence. The use of multimodal and multidisciplinary treatment is recommended. Opioid therapy should be considered for postoperative or acute pain only if the benefits outweigh the risks.[12–16]

MANAGEMENT OF ACUTE PAIN IN PATIENTS WITH BARBITURATES ABUSE

Barbiturates were widely used in the past for treating a variety of conditions (anxiety, insomnia, headaches, and others) and to antagonize the effects of other drugs. Barbiturates are abused by patients to, among other things, self-treat their anxiety and insomnia and to produce euphoric effects. As the use of barbiturates has declined in general practice, so has the number of cases of abuse,[17] but barbiturate abuse is still relatively high in individuals with easy access to these drugs, including healthcare workers.[17] In addition, barbiturates are still commonly prescribed for headache disorders, and are reportedly available for purchase online.

It is important for the pain practitioner to be familiar with the clinical picture of barbiturate abuse, as well as available treatments and relevant drug interactions (Table 32.1).

MANAGEMENT OF ACUTE PAIN IN PATIENTS WITH BENZODIAZEPINES ABUSE

Since benzodiazepine use and abuse is common (25% to 65%) in patients taking opioids, it is important for the physician to be cognizant of the clinical presentation of benzodiazepine abuse and pertinent drug interactions.[18] Benzodiazepines are infrequently the sole drug abused. On average, more than four out of five benzodiazepine addicts present with polysubstance use disorder, which may increase the complexity of the diagnosis and management.[18] For example, benzodiazepine abuse is particularly prevalent in patients who are on methadone, up to 70% of patients. Since many benzodiazepines have a long half-life, comparable to that of methadone, the presentation of benzodiazepine withdrawal may be delayed and may be complicated by the withdrawal from methadone[18] (Table 32.2).

MANAGEMENT OF ACUTE PAIN IN PATIENTS WITH ALCOHOL ABUSE DISORDER ON MAINTENANCE THERAPY

Patients with a history of alcohol abuse who are currently not drinking, or who are taking maintenance therapy with naltrexone, may be prompted to resume drinking alcohol again if exposed to other addictive substances. Therefore, treatment options for acute pain should be weighed against the risks. In addition, physicians should be familiar with the patient's maintenance therapy and possible drug interactions.

Naltrexone is a cyclopropyl derivative of oxymorphone similar in structure to naloxone. It is a pure competitive antagonist at opioid receptor sites, with a higher affinity for μ-receptors than opioid agonists. Naltrexone is commonly used to treat alcohol dependence and abuse because it can curtail the reinforcing effects of drinking alcohol, which are endorphin-mediated.[19] It is administered orally or via intramuscular depot with an extended-release preparation. Naltrexone is used to improve rates of alcohol abstinence.[19] The half-life of immediate-release naltrexone is about 5 hours, and the half-life for depot naltrexone is about 5 days.[20] Therefore, if a procedure is elective, immediate-release naltrexone ought to be discontinued 3 days before surgery, and depot naltrexone should not be injected for 4 to 6 weeks before the elective sutrgery.[21] If discontinuation is not possible, as in emergent surgery, higher than normal doses of opioids will likely be required to provide analgesia. In this case, patients are typically monitored closely. The μ-receptors in a patient taking naltrexone are upregulated; therefore, the patient may become more sensitive to opioids after discontinuation of naltrexone, resulting in a higher chance of respiratory depression and other opioid side effects.[21]

Table 32.1. **BARBITURATE ABUSE**

CLINICAL PICTURE AND INTOXICATION	WITHDRAWAL	TREATMENT OF WITHDRAWAL	DRUG INTERACTIONS
• Euphoria, drowsiness • Overdose results in CNS depression, including respiratory depression	• Anxiety, skeletal muscle tremors, hyperreflexia • Tachycardia, and orthostatic hypotension, diaphoresis • Cardiovascular collapse, hyperthermia, and grand mal seizures	• Phenobarbital, with a dose reduction of 10% per day • Benzodiazepines can be used for acute withdrawal	• Additive CNS depressant effects, especially in alcoholics, who use barbiturates to relieve their nervousness and tremors • Chronic use results in cross-tolerance to other CNS depressants

Adapted with permission from Souzdalnitski, Nada, and Labor.[34]

Table 32.2. **BENZODIAZEPINE ABUSE**

CLINICAL PICTURE AND INTOXICATION	WITHDRAWAL	TREATMENT OF WITHDRAWAL	DRUG INTERACTIONS
• Used to enhance the euphoria effects of opioids • To alleviate withdrawal syndromes • To temper cocaine highs, to augment alcohol **Intoxication:** • Depressant effect on the CNS, with slow breathing to apnea	• Anxiety, jitteriness, insomnia, seizures • The symptoms may not appear until the third day after cessation of the drug and may not reach their peak of severity until the fifth day.	• Gradually taper benzodiazepines over a period of 1 to 2 weeks	• Interact synergistically with other CNS depressants

Adapted with permission from Souzdalnitski, Nada, and Labor.[34]

Nalmefene is another opioid receptor antagonist, but it is not available in the United States. Similar to naltrexone, nalmefene should be discontinued 7 days before elective surgery.[21]

There are other types of medications used to treat alcohol dependence and abuse. Acamprosate reduces neuronal hyperexcitability by opposing the glutamate *N*-methyl-D-aspartate (NMDA) receptors.[19] Disulfiram disrupts the metabolism of alcohol by inhibiting aldehyde dehydrogenase, leading to a buildup of acetaldehyde in the blood, which, in turn, can cause tachycardia, nausea, emesis, pain, vertigo, hypotension, and other undesirable effects.[19] Disulfiram should be stopped 10 days before any anticipated surgery. Patients should be thoroughly evaluated for disulfiram-induced polyneuropathy if regional anesthesia is planned, and the findings should be documented before the administration of regional anesthesia.[22] The patient's coagulation profile should be assessed if axial anesthesia is planned because, in some cases, disulfiram may contribute to platelet dysfunction and increase the chance of bleeding [22] Axial blocks may be accompanied by sudden, unexpected, and otherwise unexplained hypotension that could result from inadequate stores of norepinephrine due to disulfiram-induced inhibition of dopamine β-hydroxylase. This hypotension is treated with direct-acting sympathomimetics, such as phenylephrine[23] Topiramate, gabapentin, and baclofen are considered second-line treatments for alcohol abuse disorders.[19]

MANAGEMENT OF ACUTE PAIN IN PATIENTS WITH CURRENT ALCOHOL ABUSE

When treating patients with an alcohol use disorder, it is important to be aware of the interactions between alcohol and pain medications. It is also important to treat withdrawal symptoms if they occur, as alcohol withdrawal can be life-threatening.[23] As is true with other drugs of abuse, pain practitioners need to be familiar with the presentation of, treatments for, and potential drug interactions in patients with an alcohol use disorder (Table 32.3).

MANAGEMENT OF ACUTE PAIN IN PATIENTS WITH ABUSE OF OTHER SUBSTANCES

Stimulants: Cocaine and Amphetamines

Cocaine induces a sympathetic response by hindering the presynaptic uptake of norepinephrine and dopamine. As a result, the postsynaptic concentration of these mediators increases.[24] It is not uncommon for cocaine abusers to use cocaine to alleviate pain. Polysubstance abuse is common as well. It is observed in more than 40% of drug users, and should be considered when evaluating and treating stimulant-absing patients' acute pain[18] (Table 32.4).

Hallucinogens

Hallucinogens can produce detachment from one's surroundings or a change in one's perception of reality. Psychedelics, dissociatives, and deliriants are accepted categories of hallucinogens.[25]

Psychedelics are also classified as psychotomimetics. They predominantly incite 5-HT2A receptors, while some of them additionally stimulate dopaminergic, as well as adrenergic, receptors. LSD, psilocybin, mescaline, MDMA are typical representatives of this group.[25] These drugs tend to cause delusions, delirium, and other psychotic symptoms.[26]

Dissociative hallucinogens, including DXM, PCP, and ketamine, are NMDA receptor antagonists. Some of these medications (ketamine, magnesium salts, nitrous oxide, and others) have been shown to be effective adjuncts for acute postoperative pain control, as well as severe pain control, in opioid-dependent patients.[12]

Deliriants include antihistamines (diphenhydramine, dimenhydrinate, cyclizine) and tropanes (naturally occurring jimson weed or medicines, including atropine, scopolamine, and hyoscyamine).[25] These medications are commonly used in chronic pain patients for treatment of opioid side effects. The combination of opioids and these drugs may amplify the opioids' sedating effects, and should therefore be used with caution, despite requests of some patients for intravenous push of some of these drugs (for example, diphenhydramine

Table 32.3. ALCOHOL ABUSE

CLINICAL PICTURE AND INTOXICATION	WITHDRAWAL SYNDROME	TREATMENT OF WITHDRAWAL	DRUG INTERACTIONS

• History of heavy drinking
• Smell of alcohol on breath
• Laboratory analysis of breath, blood, or urine positive for presence of alcohol
• Behavioral disinhibition: Initially euphoria or agitation and combativeness
• Flushed, warm skin
• Hypoglycemia may occur
• Vasodilation, hypotension, and reflex tachycardia
• Severe intoxication results in CNS depression and may cause respiratory depression and coma.
	• Early manifestations: Generalized tremors, nausea, vomiting, insomnia, and confusion with agitation
	• Delirium tremens (DT): Hallucinations, disorientation, tachycardia, hypertension, fever, agitation
		• Substitute alcohol or use benzodiazepines with slower onset, as they have less abuse potential
		• Phenothiazines and haloperidol are used as adjuvants to benzodiazepines.
		• Beta-adrenergic blockers and clonidine reduce autonomic manifestations of withdrawal symptoms and convulsive activity.
		• Carbamazepine helps in reducing emotional distress.
			• Alcohol and sedatives: severe depression of the CNS
			• Naltrexone and nalmefene: resistance to opioids
			• Disulfiram
			  • Induces sedation and hepatotoxicity
			  • Reduces the clearance of other drugs
			  • An altered response to sympathomimetic drugs
			• Acetaminophen is safe in patients who chronically abuse, watch for abuse in a patient with active liver disease and chronic acetaminophen use

Adapted with permission from Souzdalnitski, Nada, and Labor.[34]

together with opioids to "better control" their acute pain). The clinical picture of intoxication, withdrawal symptoms, treatment, and relevant drug interactions are presented in Table 32.5.

Cannabis

Cannabis is abused because of its euphoriogenic and anxiolytic effects. It is estimated that about 13% to 19% of chronic pain patients use marijuana intermittently or routinely.[27] Cannabis inhibits glutamatergic transmission, antagonizes the NMDA receptors, and may increase endorphin levels. It also may have an anti-inflammatory effect.[28] Cannabis is thought to be moderately efficacious for treatment of some chronic pain states, including neuropathic pain, but beneficial effects must be carefully weighed against the risks.[29] It is suggested that marijuana should be avoided at least 7 days before elective surgery

Table 32.4. STIMULANT ABUSE

CLINICAL PICTURE AND INTOXICATION	WITHDRAWAL	TREATMENT OF WITHDRAWAL	DRUG INTERACTIONS
Cocaine			
• Intense high followed by dysphoria, sleeplessness, restlessness, anxiety, nasal damage, loss of appetite, chest pain, hypertension, myocardial infarction, life-threatening arrhythmias, seizures, stroke, or sudden death • Concurrent use of cocaine and amphetamines may lead to significant hypertension and tachycardia • Treatment of overdose: Dexmeditomidine, benzodiazepines	• Depression, fatigue • Refractory hypotension or bradycardia	• Symptomatic treatment • Behavioral and social therapy	• Avoid using ketamine • Persons with decreased plasma cholinesterase activity may be at risk of sudden death • Caution with neuraxial anesthesia: cocaine-induced thrombocytopenia can occur
Amphetamines			
• Increased cortical alertness, appetite suppression • With long-term amphetamine abuse: hypertension, arrhythmias, anxiety, violent behavior, psychosis, necrotizing arteritis, leading to cerebral hemorrhage and renal failure, death from overdose	• Extreme lethargy, depression that may be suicidal, increased appetite, and weight gain	Symptomatic treatment	• Avoid using ketamine. • Reduce the morphine doses needed • Refractory hypotension • Amitriptyline: hypertension, CNS stimulation

Adapted with permission from Souzdalnitski, Nada, and Labor.[34]

Table 32.5. HALLUCINOGEN ABUSE

CLINICAL PICTURE AND INTOXICATION	WITHDRAWAL	TREATMENT OF WITHDRAWAL	DRUG INTERACTIONS
• Hallucinations • Anticholinergic effect (tachycardia, hypertension, dilated pupils)	• Psychologic withdrawal • Physical symptoms are rare and occur after chronic abuse in the form of recurring experiences (flashbacks) of going through a "trip." • Some chronic abusers develop diarrhea and chills	• Acute treatment: Benzodiazepines for control of agitation and anxiety reactions • Chronic abuse: Hallucinogen rehabilitation program	• Amplified responses to sympathomimetic drugs are likely.

Adapted with permission from Souzdalnitski, Nada, and Labor.[34]

because intoxication or withdrawal symptoms may distort the clinical picture.[30] Pain practitioners should be familiar with the clinical picture of cannabis use, intoxication, withdrawal symptoms, and relevant drug interactions (Table 32.6).

Tobacco

Nicotine is a widely abused drug with analgesic properties when used in nicotine-naïve patients. It is obtained from the tobacco plant (*Nicotiana tabacum*). Nicotine is a colorless or pale liquid that turns brown upon exposure to air or light.[31] It has a distinctive pungent odor. It is a tertiary amine comprised of a pyridine and a pyrrolidine rings.[31] The chemical name of nicotine is (*S*)-3-[1-methylpyrrolidin-2-yl]pyridine. It works as an agonist at a subtype of acetylcholine (ACh) receptors called nicotinic receptors. Nicotinic acetylcholine receptors (nAChRs) are variable in their structure. The variability of nAChR subunit combinations is responsible for nicotine's diverse and sometimes paradoxical pharmacologic and physiologic effects.[31]

Nicotine is a CNS stimulant that predominantly works on the prejunctional autonomic ganglia. It works by stimulating release of neurotransmitters, including catecholamines and others, into the synapses.[31] Nicotine's rewarding properties are related to its ability to increase release of dopamine and β-endorphin and enkephalins in the mesolimbic system, similar to other drugs of abuse. It is important to note that opiates elicit analgesia, in part, by releasing ACh and stimulating the same nAChR as nicotine. At the same time, nicotine stimulates α_2-noradrenergic receptors in a manner similar to clonidine, which is used as an adjunct during neuraxial analgesia.[31] Nicotine stimulates epinephrine release from the adrenal medulla, as well as the discharge of catecholamines in the sympathetic synapses, activating brain and spinal cord antinociceptive pathways. Nicotine produces an anti-inflammatory effect. It is a powerful stimulator of some types of mechanoreceptors in the skin, lungs, and gastrointestinal tract and stomach, which may add to its analgesic properties.[31] While acute nicotine-induced analgesia has been used to supplement opioids for acute postoperative pain, chronic nicotine users are more likely to experience chronic pain, probably because nicotine causes decreasing pain tolerance in smokers. Chronic nicotine users require more opioid analgesics to control acute or severe pain.[32] Therefore, it is generally advisable to replace nicotine during hospitalization. The replacement can be achieved by using nicotine patches supplemented by gum. Special consideration should be given to smokers deprived of nicotine in the perioperative period. According to one study, they reported more pain and required a greater amount of opiates than nonsmokers.[33] Therefore, it is important to provide nicotine replacement in the perioperative period to avert withdrawal and, possibly, to improve the patient's perception of pain and recovery after surgery (Table 32.7).

Table 32.6. MARIJUANA ABUSE

CLINICAL PICTURE AND INTOXICATION	WITHDRAWAL	TREATMENT OF WITHDRAWAL	DRUG INTERACTIONS
• Increased sympathetic activity initially, followed (in case of intoxication) by drowsiness, red eyes, cannabis odor, yellowing of fingertips, chronic cough, loss of interest and motivation, and weight loss	• Irritability, insomnia, diaphoresis • Nausea, vomiting, and diarrhea • Increased latency to fall asleep • Deleterious mood and behavioral symptoms	• Tetrahydrocannabinol (THC) replacement • Behavioral therapy • Treatment of concurrent nicotine addiction assists in stopping marijuana abuse. • Trazodone helps with insomnia.	• Cross-tolerance with all CNS depressants (produces sedation) • Disulfiram: hypomania • Tricyclic antidepressants: tachycardia, delirium • Anticholinergic agents: sedation

Adapted with permission from Souzdalnitski, Nada, and Labor.[34]

Table 32.7. **TOBACCO USE DISORDER**

CLINICAL PICTURE AND INTOXICATION	WITHDRAWAL	TREATMENT OF WITHDRAWAL	DRUG INTERACTIONS
• History of smoking • Odor of tobacco smoke • Smoker's cough and voice • Face wrinkles • Yellow and brown teeth • Gingivitis and periodontitis • Complications like leukoplakia, certain cancers • Chronic obstructive pulmonary disease • Intoxication produces excessive CNS stimulation, with tremor, insomnia, and nervousness, and cardiac stimulation and arrhythmias. Respiratory paralysis has been described as well.	• Irritability, frustration, or anger, anxiety, difficulty concentrating, increased appetite, restlessness, depressed mood, insomnia	• Nicotine replacement	Nicotine decreases the efficacy of hydrocodone and, probably, other opioids

Adapted with permission from Souzdalnitski, Nada, and Labor.[34]

CONCLUSIONS

- A number of pain medications have abuse potential.
- Patients may abuse substances to treat their pain.
- It is important to ask patients about substance abuse, substance abuse treatment, and their family history of substance abuse.
- Addiction is a chronic relapsing and remitting disease.
- Patients with pain and addiction may be currently abusing substances, abstinent from drugs of abuse, and/or on medication-assisted treatment.
- Treating a patient with a history of substance abuse with any drug of abuse may trigger relapse.
- If the patient has a history of substance abuse but is currently abstinent, it is helpful to learn about how they are maintaining their sobriety. Patients actively working a recovery program in conjunction with therapists, counselors, addiction specialists, and/or 12-step support groups are less likely to relapse when prescribed addictive substances, particularly when the addiction treatment modalities are included in their pain management plan.
- Due to their increased opioid tolerance, it may be challenging to achieve adequate pain control in patients abusing opioids.
- For patients with a history of addiction, it is important to use non-opioid and nonpharmacologic analgesia (including interventional modalities, physical rehabilitation, chiropractic manipulations, pain psychology, and regional analgesia, if applicable) for pain control.
- Care coordination with a patient's addiction medicine provider contributes to the successful treatment of the patient's chronic pain.

REFERENCES

1. Substance Abuse and Mental Health Services Administration. Results from the 2012 National Survey on Drug Use and Health: Mental Health Findings, 2013 edition. Rockville, MD. http://archive.samhsa.gov/data/NSDUH/2k12MH_FindingsandDetTables/2K12MHF/NSDUHmhfr2012.htm.
2. Miller NS, Giannini AJ, Gold MS, Philomena JA. Drug testing: medical, legal, and ethical issues. *J Subst Abuse Treat.* 1990;7:239–244.
3. Rinaldi RC, Steindler EM, Wilford BB, Goodwin D. Clarification and standardization of substance abuse terminology. *JAMA.* 1988;259:555–557.
4. Angst MS, Clark JD. Opioid-induced hyperalgesia: a qualitative systematic review. *Anesthesiology.* 2006;104:570–587.
5. Vukmir RB. Drug seeking behavior. *Am J Drug Alcohol Abuse.* 2004;30:551–575.
6. Weissman DE, Haddox JD. Opioid pseudoaddiction—an iatrogenic syndrome. *Pain.* 1989;36:363–366.
7. Voon P, Karamouzian M, Kerr T. Chronic pain and opioid misuse: a review of reviews. *Subst Abuse Treat Prev Policy.* 2017;12(1):36.
8. Donroe JH, Holt SR, Tetrault JM. Caring for patients with opioid use disorder in the hospital. *CMAJ.* 2016;188(17-18):1232–1239.
9. Darke S, Ross J, Kaye S. Physical injecting sites among injecting drug users in Sydney, Australia. *Drug Alcohol Depend.* 2001;62:77–82.
10. Portenoy RK, Foley KM. Chronic use of opioid analgesics in non-malignant pain: report of 38 cases. *Pain.* 1986;25:171–186.
11. Hu LL, Sparenborg S, Tai B. Privacy protection for patients with substance use problems. *Subst Abuse Rehabil.* 2011;2:227–233.
12. Souzdalnitski D, Halaszynski TM, Faclier G. Regional anesthesia and co-existing chronic pain. *Curr Opin Anesthesiol.* 2010;23(5):662–670.
13. Orman JS, Keating GM. Buprenorphine/naloxone: a review of its use in the treatment of opioid dependence. *Drugs.* 2009;69:577–607.
14. Alford DP, Compton P, Samet JH. Acute pain management for patients receiving maintenance methadone or buprenorphine therapy. *Ann Intern Med.* 2006;144:127–134.

15. Savage SR, Kirsh KL, Passik SD. Challenges in using opioids to treat pain in persons with substance use disorders. *Addict Sci Clin Pract.* 2008;4:4–25.
16. Mitra S, Sinatra RS. Perioperative management of acute pain in the opioid-dependent patient. *Anesthesiology.* 2004;101:212–227.
17. Morgan WW. Abuse liability of barbiturates and other sedative-hypnotics. *Adv Alcohol Subst Abuse.* 1990;9:67–82.
18. Longo LP, Johnson B. Addiction: Part I. Benzodiazepines—side effects, abuse risk and alternatives. *Am Fam Physician.* 2000;61:2121–2128.
19. Johnson BA. Pharmacotherapy of alcohol abuse disorder. *UpToDate.* 2016. http://www.uptodate.com/contents/pharmacotherapy-for-alcohol-use-disorder.
20. Naltrexone drug information. *UpToDate.* 2016. https://www.uptodate.com/contents/naltrexone-drug-information?source=search_result&search=naltrexone&selectedTitle=1~64.
21. Gonzalez JP, Brogden RN. Naltrexone. A review of its pharmacodynamic and pharmacokinetic properties and therapeutic efficacy in the management of opioid dependence. *Drugs.* 1988;35:192–213.
22. Frisoni GB, Di Monda V. Disulfiram neuropathy: a review (1971–1988) and report of a case. *Alcohol Alcohol.* 1989;24:429–437.
23. Diaz JH, Hill GE. Hypotension with anesthesia in disulfiram-treated patients. *Anesthesiology.* 1979;51:366–368.
24. Howell LL, Kimmel HL. Monoamine transporters and psychostimulant addiction. *Biochem Pharmacol.* 2008;75:196–217.
25. Nichols DE. Hallucinogens. *Pharmacol Ther.* 2004;101:131–181.
26. Griffiths R, Richards W, Johnson M, McCann U, Jesse R. Mystical-type experiences occasioned by psilocybin mediate the attribution of personal meaning and spiritual significance 14 months later. *J Psychopharmacol.* 2008;22:621–632.
27. Pesce A, West C, Rosenthal M, et al. Marijuana correlates with use of other illicit drugs in a pain patient population. *Pain Physician.* 2010;13:283–287.
28. Burns TL, Ineck JR. Cannabinoid analgesia as a potential new therapeutic option in the treatment of chronic pain. *Ann Pharmacother.* 2006;40:251–260.
29. Deshpande A, Mailis-Gagnon A, Zoheiry N, Lakha SF. Efficacy and adverse effects of medical marijuana for chronic noncancer pain: systematic review of randomized controlled trials. *Can Fam Physician.* 2015;61(8):e372–e381.
30. May JA, White HC, Leonard-White A, Warltier DC, Pagel PS. The patient recovering from alcohol or drug addiction: special issues for the anesthesiologist. *Anesth Analg.* 2001;92:1601–1608.
31. Souzdalnitski D, Lerman I., Chung KS. Nicotine transdermal. In: Sinatra R, Jahr J, Watkins-Pitchford, eds. *The Essence of Analgesia and Analgesics.* 1st ed. New York: Cambridge University Press; 2010:512–514.
31. Ditre JW, Heckman BW, Zale EL, Kosiba JD, Maisto SA. Acute analgesic effects of nicotine and tobacco in humans: a meta-analysis. *Pain.* 2016;157(7):1373–1381.
33. Creekmore FM, Lugo RA, Weiland KJ. Postoperative opiate analgesia requirements of smokers and nonsmokers. *Ann Pharmacother.* 2004;38:949–953.
34. Souzdalnitski D, Nada E, Labor N. Management of chronic pain patient with history of substance abuse. In: Rosenquist RW, Souzdalnitski D, Urman R, eds. *Chronic Pain Management for the Hospitalized Patient.* New York: Oxford University Press; 2016:281–316.
35. Souzdalnitski D, Cheng J. Postoperative chronic pain management. In: Farag E, ed. *Anesthesia for Spine Surgery.* New York: Cambridge University Press; 2012:312–347.
36. Göröcs TS, Lambert M, Rinne T, Krekler M, Modell S. Efficacy and tolerability of ready-to-use intravenous paracetamol solution as monotherapy or as an adjunct analgesic therapy for postoperative pain in patients undergoing elective ambulatory surgery: open, prospective study. *Int J Clin Pract.* 2009;63(1):112–120.
37. Härkänen L, Halonen J, Selander T, Kokki H. Beta-adrenergic antagonists during general anesthesia reduced postoperative pain: a systematic review and a meta-analysis of randomized controlled trials. *J Anesth.* 2015;29(6):934–943.
38. De Oliveira GS Jr, Agarwal D, Benzon HT. Perioperative single dose ketorolac to prevent postoperative pain: a meta-analysis of randomized trials. *Anesth Analg.* 2012;114(2):424–433.
39. Chou R, Gordon DB, de Leon-Casasola OA, et al. Management of postoperative pain: a clinical practice guideline from the American Pain Society, the American Society of Regional Anesthesia and Pain Medicine, and the American Society of Anesthesiologists' Committee on Regional Anesthesia, Executive Committee, and Administrative Council. *J Pain.* 2016;17(2):131–157.
40. Younger J, Parkitny L, McLain D. The use of low-dose naltrexone (LDN) as a novel anti-inflammatory treatment for chronic pain. *Clin Rheumatol.* 2014;33(4):451–459.
41. Millar J, Sadasivan S, Weatherup N, Lutton S. Lyrica nights–recreational pregabalin abuse in an urban emergency department. *Emerg Med J.* 2013;30:874.doi:10.1136/emermed-2013-203113.20.
42. Loftus S, Wright A. Potential misuse of pregabalin and gabapentin. *BMJ.* 2014;348: g1290. doi:10.1136/bmj.g1290.

REVIEW QUESTIONS

1. Which of the following statements about the prevalence of substance abuse and substance dependence in the United States is most correct:

A. One million people have substance use or substance dependence disorder.
B. Ten million people have substance use or substance dependence disorder.
C. Thirty million people have substance use or substance dependence disorder.
D. Fifty million people have substance use or substance dependence disorder.

2. What is the most appropriate description of addiction?

A. Addiction is a chronic brain disorder characterized by continued compulsive substance use despite physical, psychologic, and/or social harm to the user.
B. Addiction is a state of adaptation to a psychoactive substance characterized by the emergence of withdrawal during abstinence, which may be relieved in total or part by re-administration of the substance.
C. Addiction is the use of a psychoactive substance for its positive effects or for the avoidance of the negative effects associated with its withdrawal.
D. Addiction is a characteristic constellation of signs and symptoms—including altered activity of the CNS—after the abrupt discontinuation of, or rapid decrease in, substance use.

3. A chronic pain patient complained of inadequate pain relief despite escalating doses of intravenous opioids. What is the most appropriate description of opioid tolerance?

A. Opioid tolerance is a state of nociceptive sensitization caused by exposure to opioids, which decreases overall pain tolerance.

B. Opioid tolerance is a state of nociceptive desensitization caused by exposure to opioids, which increases the overall pain tolerance.
C. Opioid tolerance is a state of nociceptive desensitization caused by exposure to opioids, which decreases the overall pain tolerance.
D. Opioid tolerance is a state where patients ask for more pain medication due to anticipation of poor pain control.

ANSWERS

1. D. Addiction and dependency are common. The lifetime prevalence of substance abuse and substance dependence disorders has been estimated at about 10.5% percent in the U.S. population.[1] All ages, races, and socioeconomic classes are affected. Addiction is a chronic disease, similar to other chronic conditions like diabetes, hypertension, and asthma, and is similarly considered present even after prolonged remission.[2]

2. A. Addiction is a chronic brain disorder characterized by continued compulsive substance use despite physical, psychologic, and/or social harm to the user.[3] Answer B describes physical dependence, answer C describes psychologic dependence, and answer D describes withdrawal.[3]

3. C. Opioid tolerance is a physiologic adaptation (or desensitization) to opioids' effects, so decreased effects are seen at constant opioid doses and constant effects are maintained only with increasing doses.[3] Answer A describes opioid-induced hyperalgesia. Answer C is incorrect. Answer D describes pseudoaddiction, where patients ask for more pain medication not due to inadequate pain control, and not for secondary gain, but because of fear or anticipation of uncontrolled pain.

QUESTIONS AND ANSWERS

This chapter has accompanying questions and answers that are available to subscribers as part of the Oxford eLearning platform. To access the questions, follow the link below, or go to
✔ http://oxfordmedicine.com/painmanagementreview

33.

PSYCHIATRIC COMORBIDITIES IN CHRONIC PAIN SYNDROMES

Nancy J. Beckman and Marie B. Tobin

STEM CASE AND KEY QUESTIONS

A 36-year-old woman was referred from gastroenterology for abdominal pain with nausea and vomiting. The patient's medical history included median arcuate ligament surgery (MALS) 5 years earlier, fibromyalgia, and gastrointestinal reflux disease (GERD). The patient experienced initial pain relief from the surgical procedure, but she reported that her abdominal pain had returned and worsened over the past 2 years, with escalating generalized pain. The patient described her pain as present continuously, but she reported that her stomach pain worsened after eating. Pain typically increased throughout the day, but some days she awakened with stabbing pain and pain interfered with her sleep. Imaging revealed no vascular compression. Pain was unrelieved by oral opiates. The patient had visited the emergency department (ED) for intravenous (IV) pain medications multiple times in the preceding 2 years. The patient described increasing pain-related distress and disability. She had stopped working due to pain and was less able to care for her 10-year-old son.

WHY IS IT IMPORTANT TO ADDRESS THE PATIENT'S REPORT OF DISTRESS? HOW MIGHT YOU FURTHER ASSESS DISTRESS?

Pain, as defined by the International Association of Pain, includes an affective component.[1] Consequently, it is very important to evaluate the extent to which psychologic factors, especially depression and anxiety, contribute to the experience of pain. Studies using structured clinical interviews confirm that 50% of patients with chronic pain meet the criteria for major depression,[2] a prevalence 2.5 times greater than that in the general population.[3] Furthermore, interventions that incorporate depression management into pain treatment result in greater pain relief and enhanced functional ability.[4–6] Anxiety is also frequently comorbid with chronic pain: 45% of patients report some anxiety symptoms.[2] Studies suggest that anxiety disorders occur approximately 1.5 to 3 times more often among people with chronic pain than among nonpain populations.[7,8] The presence of comorbid anxiety and depression worsens the pain experience, impairs coping abilities, and leads to greater morbidity.[9] Consequently, screening for the presence of depression or anxiety is an important part of pain assessment.

To further assess distress, the clinical interview should explore past history and treatments and ask directly about sad mood, anhedonia (inability to enjoy things, loss of interest), and neurovegetative symptoms (e.g., sleep, energy, concentration, appetite, libido). The clinical interview can be augmented with a depression or anxiety screening instrument, such as the Patient Health Questionnaire (PHQ-9, PHQ-2)[10,11] or the Generalized Anxiety Disorder scales (GAD-7, GAD-2).[12,13]

It is also crucial to evaluate suicide risk in patients with chronic pain. Studies report that up to 50% of chronic pain patients had suicidal thoughts due to pain, often related to intensity of pain and depression.[14] Risk factors for suicide among pain patients include male sex, increasing age, family history of suicide, prior attempts, history of childhood abuse, comorbid depression, substance abuse, or impulsive and aggressive behaviors.[14] Assessment should ask about plans or intent. Administration of the six-item, Columbia-Suicide Severity Rating Scale (C-SSRS) can improve identification of at-risk patients.[15]

HOW ARE PAIN AND SLEEP DISTURBANCE RELATED? HOW MIGHT YOU FURTHER ASSESS THE PATIENT'S REPORT OF SLEEP DISTURBANCE?

A significant percentage of patients with chronic pain report sleep disturbance.[2] This may include initial insomnia, frequent waking, or terminal insomnia. The etiology of sleep disturbance in chronic pain is multifactorial and may be related to abnormal sleep behaviors, comorbid depression or anxiety, or pain medications. Problems with sleep can contribute to both increased pain and dysregulated mood.[2] The clinical interview should cover duration of sleep, latency, number of awakenings, duration of and activity during periods of wakefulness, and terminal insomnia. It is also important to obtain a general sense of the patient's sleep hygiene (i.e., behaviors around sleep, sleeping with the television on, drinking caffeine at night). A validated scale, such as the self-report Insomnia Severity Index (ISI),[16] can enhance the clinical interview.

WHAT MEDICATION MIGHT YOU CONSIDER TO ADDRESS THIS PATIENT'S PROBLEMS WITH MOOD AND SLEEP? WHAT FACTORS INFLUENCE THE CHOICE OF ANTIDEPRESSANT MEDICATION FOR THIS PATIENT?

If the patient meets criteria for depression or anxiety, then adding the antidepressant duloxetine may be the next best step. Duloxetine augments both the serotonergic and the norepinephrine neurotransmitter systems. It has a proven analgesic effect that is independent of its antidepressant effect.[17] Recommended starting dose is 30 mg (usually in the morning, but it can be in the evening) with titration by 30-mg increments, as tolerated, to a maximum dose of 120 mg daily.

If insomnia is a significant comorbid factor, the tricyclic antidepressant (TCA) amitriptyline is a useful addition, at a dose of 25 mg taken at night. This dose combines analgesic and hypnotic effects. Amitriptyline should be avoided in patients with known cardiac arrhythmias because of the potential effect on cardiac conduction. To rule out other causes of sleep disturbance (e.g., sleep apnea), referral to a sleep medicine specialist or for cognitive-behavioral therapy for insomnia (CBT-I) should be considered.

The patient missed her scheduled follow-up appointments in the pain clinic. She is hospitalized for IV pain medications. Records show that in the previous year, she had five hospitalizations and presented to the ED eight times with worsened pain. There was some evidence of medication nonadherence but no documented history of psychiatric morbidity.

IN WHAT WAY WOULD A PSYCHIATRIC CONSULT BE USEFUL IN THE MANAGEMENT OF THIS CASE?

A full psychiatric evaluation, including detailed review of past history and collateral information, would help to identify comorbid psychiatric syndromes and symptoms. In addition, psychiatric assessment would characterize relevant underlying personality characteristics, associated psychologic defense mechanisms, and coping strategies employed by this patient to deal with her chronic pain. Evaluation could identify patients who self-medicate with opioids, benzodiazepines (BDZs), and alcohol, leading to substance use disorders.[18–20]

Childhood trauma and adversity are strong risk factors for both the propensity to express distress (physical and emotional) in somatic ways and the use of maladaptive coping strategies. In addition, pain and insomnia are both highly correlated with attempted and completed suicide.[3] Therefore, psychiatric consultation is useful to improve understanding of a patient's presentation and treatment response, and to build a comprehensive pain management plan that simultaneously addresses the psychiatric issues. Psychotropic medications can also be initiated to treat psychiatric comorbidity and for additional analgesia.

The patient is started on IV opioids, with some relief of her pain. A full medical workup to identify reversible causes of her chronic abdominal pain is ordered. No abnormalities are identified. A psychiatric consult is also performed and the patient is found to meet criteria for major depressive disorder, somatic symptom disorder with predominant pain, and post-traumatic stress disorder (PTSD) with panic attacks. The patient's pain often serves as a trigger that reminds her of past trauma (childhood sexual abuse) and is associated with much anxiety and sadness. Review of her history and collateral information indicates dependent personality traits (e.g., helplessness, looks to others for solutions), anxiety sensitivity (fear of bodily sensations), and difficulty expressing distress in any way other than somatically. Opioid dependence is also suspected.

WHAT IS SOMATIC SYMPTOM DISORDER?

According to the *Diagnostic and Statistical Manual of Mental Disorders*, Fifth Edition (DSM-V), somatic symptom disorder is characterized by excessive thoughts, feelings, and behaviors related to a somatic symptom, such as pain.[21] The level of thought, time, and energy dedicated to the symptom is excessive, is not better explained by another mental disorder, and results in impairment in social, occupational, and other functioning.[21] Cognitive-behavioral therapy (CBT) and acceptance and commitment therapies are ideally suited for teaching patients how hypervigilance, rumination, and self-imposed behavioral limitations can maintain and exacerbate the experience of the somatic symptoms, as well as help patients develop new pain coping strategies.

WHAT SIGNS SUGGEST SUBSTANCE DEPENDENCE? HOW CAN THE PROVIDER SUPPORT THIS DIAGNOSIS? WHAT ADDITIONAL STRATEGIES CAN BE USED TO ADDRESS OPIATE OVERUSE?

Patients with chronic pain who are treated with long-term opioids are at increased risk of developing aberrant drug-related behaviors. Behaviors can escalate over time, leading to opioid misuse, abuse, addiction, diversion, and overdose, as well as suicide.[19] Providers must assess for risk on a continuing basis, stratify patients accordingly, and connect patients with appropriate services.

Risk factors for abuse and overdose can be related to pharmacologic aspects of the medication (potency, availability), patient variables, both individual and environmental (psychiatric disorders, family history), and prescriber behavior (careless patient selection, dosing, or titration). At-risk patients can be identified using targeted clinical questions (e.g., the CAGE-AID, adapted to include drugs[22]) augmented by a validated screening tool, such as the Screener and Opioid Assessment for Patients with Pain (SOAPP).[23,24] Biologic risk factors include age under 45, female sex, family history of prescription drug or alcohol abuse, pain severity or duration, and sleep disorders. Psychiatric comorbidities include preadolescent sexual abuse and depression, as well as personality, anxiety, or substance use disorders. Social vulnerabilities include social isolation, poor family support, and a history of motor vehicle accidents or legal problems.

Practitioners also have other methods to assess for the emergence of aberrant behaviors, including urine drug testing and prescription-monitoring programs. Furthermore, examination of patterns of use, coupled with collateral information from family, friends, and pharmacists, aids assessment. Some clinics make contracts a standard part of clinical care. The contracts include agreement by the patient not to obtain pain medications elsewhere, an outline of steps to take if dissatisfied with pain relief, and provider agreement to discuss the patient's desire for increased medication. It is important, however, not to mischaracterize pain-relief-seeking behavior that is caused by disease progression, poor opioid responsiveness to pain, opioid-induced hyperalgesia, or opioid tolerance. Early identification of risk through screening allows providers to implement brief interventions that can affect outcome (e.g., offering advice and education about substance use, eliciting the patient's own reasons for change, focusing on small steps the patient is willing to take, referring for specialty treatment).[25]

The patient evidences risk in all three realms, including age less than 45, a history of childhood sexual abuse, and comorbid depression, PTSD, and maladaptive personality traits. Repeated presentations to the ED and the need for increasing IV opioid doses indicate progression toward abuse and addiction. Furthermore, the patient is openly distressed and reports that she needs pain medications to "cope with my life." The patient is transitioned successfully to oral opioids and is started on duloxetine 30 mg, to be titrated as tolerated, and amitriptyline 25 mg at night. Bedside psychotherapy is initiated and the patient is referred upon discharge to follow up with a pain psychologist and the pain clinic.

WHAT ARE THE POTENTIAL RISKS OF PERFORMING SURGERY IN THIS PATIENT RELATED TO HER PSYCHOPATHOLOGY AND WHAT PRECAUTIONS CAN BE TAKEN TO MANAGE THE RISKS?

For spinal surgery, research has identified various psychologic factors that can negatively influence surgery outcomes, leading to failed back surgery, more complications, or increased medication use. Preoperative psychologic evaluations aim to quantify risk and to predict a patient's surgical prognosis based on the risk factors.[26] Psychosocial risk factors that impact surgical outcome include history of depression, anxiety, anger, a tendency toward pain sensitivity or pain catastrophization, lack of psychosocial support, substance use, and issues of abuse and abandonment, as well as litigation and job dissatisfaction.[27] Medical risk factors include duration of pain, history of previous spinal surgeries, smoking, obesity, and other medical problems. Finally, inconsistent presentations, the presence of personality disorders, patients who try to split staff or are threatening, and problems with compliance also serve as poor prognostic indicators.[27] It is also important to ensure that the patient has an accurate understanding of the procedure, risks and benefits, reasonable expectations for treatment, a solid plan for support after surgery, and commitment to engaging in the behaviors that will facilitate recovery. Following evaluation, specific recommendations are made to manage the risk factors (e.g., reduce substance abuse, treat depression, address overly limiting pain beliefs).[27]

DISCUSSION

ETIOLOGY

Biologic Mechanisms

The frequent co-occurrence of psychiatric disorders and pain disorders raises questions about the nature of the relationship between them (i.e., "the chicken or the egg" question). The stress-diathesis model suggests that the stress of the chronic pain experience activates a pre-existing psychologic diathesis that may or may not have been previously expressed.[28,29] The strongest support for the stress-diathesis model is in explaining the relationship between depression and pain,[30] but there can also be a predisposition toward anxiety, somatization, and maladaptive personality traits or coping skills.[31]

Further, shared biologic mechanisms, such as the overlap in neurotransmitters (e.g., serotonin, norepinephrine, and dopamine), are implicated in the etiology of both pain and psychiatric conditions.[31] Antidepressants commonly target deficits in serotonin and norepinephrine (serotonin reuptake inhibitors [SSRIs], serotonin–norepinephrine reuptake inhibitors [SNRIs]) and the same neurotransmitters are involved in the modification of sensory information.[31] Therefore, dysfunction in either of these systems would cause increased vulnerability to both mood disorders and pain.[28,32]

Another possible shared mechanism relates to the release of cortisol with stress as part of the hypothalamic–pituitary–adrenal (HPA) axis. Cortisol not only contributes to "wear and tear" on the body, but also helps to regulate the uptake of serotonin, norepinephrine, and dopamine. Psychiatric disorders, including depression, anxiety, and substance use, are linked to dysfunction of HPA axis. Chronic pain conditions, such as fibromyalgia and temporomandibular joint disorder, are also associated with cortisol dysfunction.[28,31] Vulnerability could also stem from differences in cognitive processing and attention (e.g., hypervigilance, difficulty disengaging, greater emotional processing of sensory pain information),[33,34] related to the overlap in areas of the brain involved in processing information about mood and pain, such as the dorsal anterior cingulate cortex, anterior insula, and amygdala.[35] Figure 33.1 shows places along the pain modulatory pathway where psychotherapies and psychotropics have their effects.

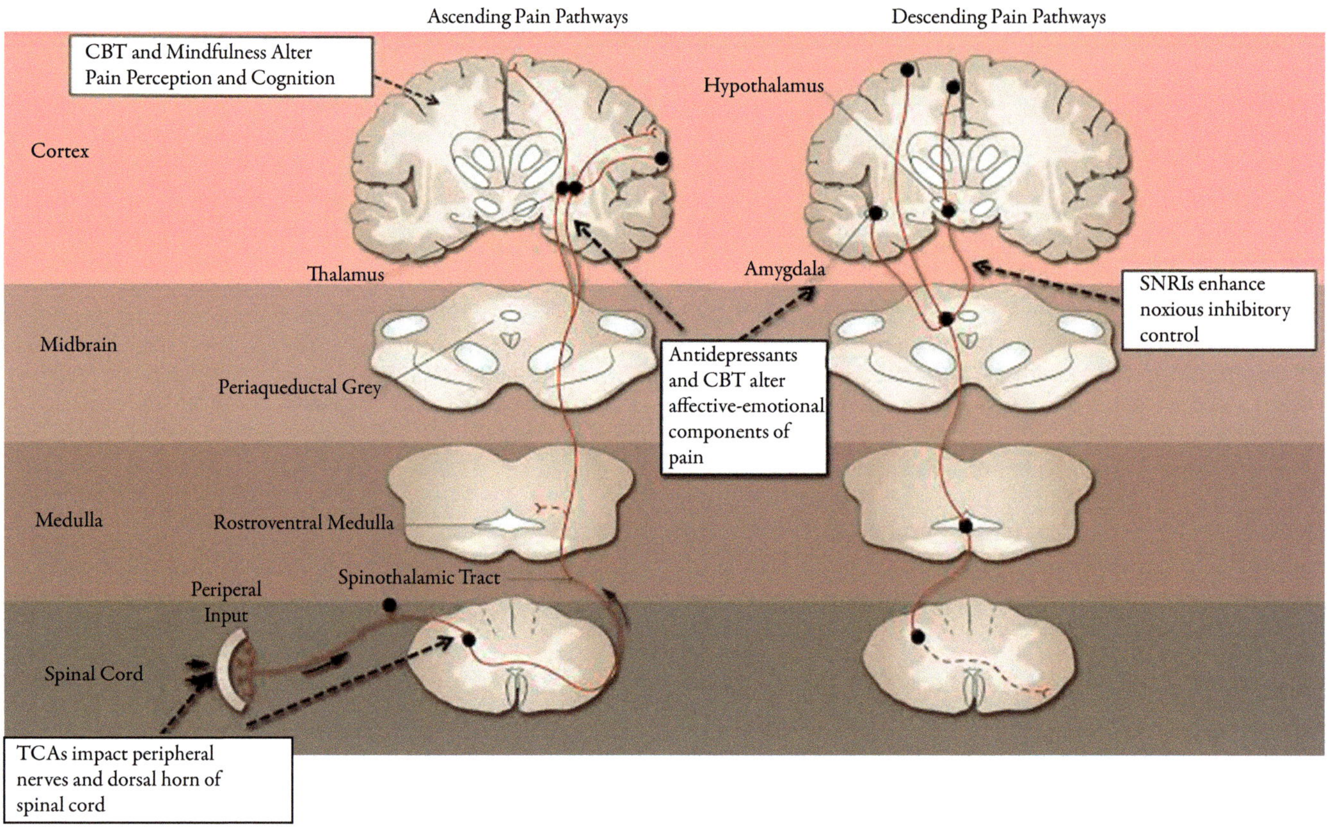

Figure 33.1. Emotion and pain: The role of psychotherapies and psychotropics in pain modulation.

Biopsychosocial Models: Learning and Cognition

Biopsychosocial models incorporate biologic, psychologic, and social/environmental factors to provide a comprehensive framework for understanding the development of comorbid chronic pain and psychiatric disorders. In this model, principles of learning are also relevant in the etiology of both conditions. For example, learned helplessness, a state in which a person stops trying to control an unpleasant stimulus, is implicated in the development of both chronic pain and depression.[28,36]

Another widely cited model explains how the interplay of cognitive variables and learned responses can influence the transition from acute to chronic pain. According to the fear-avoidance model, catastrophic beliefs about pain increase the fear of pain, lead to heightened hypervigilance toward painful stimuli, and drive defensive safety behaviors, such as avoidance of activities that could cause pain.[37,38] Avoidance behavior is negatively reinforcing because, admittedly, it can lessen the pain associated with movement and reduce the anxiety associated with the fear of pain. However, the negative long-term consequences of avoidance and hypervigilance include a lowered threshold for future pain, greater disuse of the affected body part, and increased disability and distress.[38] Avoidance also allows catastrophic beliefs about the meaning of pain to go unchallenged, allowing the beliefs to become more entrenched and limiting over time.

Similarly, anxiety disorders are maintained and exacerbated by hypervigilance about feared stimuli and by anxiogenic thinking patterns, such as overgeneralization and catastrophization (i.e., a cognitive set involving magnification, rumination, and helplessness in response to pain[39]), as well as cognitive and behavioral avoidance of feared stimuli. Another important link is that anxiety triggers the sympathetic nervous system, which can intensify processes involved in the pain condition (e.g., gastrointestinal distress, muscle tension, cortisol release, and inflammation). Conversely, pain can generate anxiety and thereby activate the sympathetic nervous system. Pain can serve as a reminder of a trauma (PTSD), pain can elicit a cascade of worries about the future (GAD), and pain signals can be misinterpreted and trigger a panic attack (panic disorder), especially in individuals with heightened somatic focus and anxiety sensitivity. Anxiety and pain can therefore feed off one another, a situation underscoring the importance of treating both.

Personality Traits and Disorders

Knowledge of personality traits and disorders is also relevant in understanding the etiology of chronic pain, and can be especially helpful for patient management, treatment decisions, and provider communication.[40] A common clinical observation is that chronic pain populations seem to have a large proportion of "difficult" patients with challenging personality characteristics. When confronted with personality pathology, a clinician's own emotional response can be informative, as strong feelings of guilt, frustration, helplessness, anxiety, and aversion are elicited.[41] However, when making judgments about personality, it is also important to remember that unmanaged pain can intensify a patient's responses.[40]

The personality traits of neuroticism (negative affect), anxiety sensitivity (fear of bodily sensations), and harm avoidance (tendency to avoid novelty or frustration) are associated with chronic pain.[42] When personality traits are inflexible and maladaptive, personality disorders are suspected. Personality disorders are defined as patterns of inner experience and behavior (e.g., cognition, affectivity, interpersonal functioning, and impulse control) that deviate from the individual's cultural norms, have onset in adolescence or early adulthood, are stable over time, are pervasive across situations, and lead to distress or impairment.[21]

Personality disorders are generally classified into three broad types: Cluster A, the odd or eccentric, includes paranoid, schizoid, and schizotypal personality disorders; Cluster B, the dramatic or erratic, includes antisocial, borderline, histrionic, and narcissistic personality disorders; and Cluster C, the anxious or fearful, includes avoidant, dependent, and obsessive-compulsive personality disorders.[21] Studies have reported rates of personality disorders among chronic pain patients between 13% and 30%, compared to 10% in the general population.[43] Those with comorbid pain and personality disorders tend to report higher pain scores and distress.[44] See Table 33.1 for core features of selected personality disorders.

Pain Coping Strategies

Pain coping strategies are another important factor that contributes to differences in outcomes. Coping strategies are the efforts employed by a person to alleviate a stressor.[45] Psychoanalytic theory describes four broad categories of psychologic defense mechanisms that serve as the basis of an individual's coping strategies: primitive (e.g., psychotic, conversion), immature (e.g., acting out, somatization), neurotic (e.g., worry, repression), or mature (e.g., acceptance, patience). Other approaches have classified coping strategies as either problem- or emotion-focused or active or passive.[46] While some strategies are more adaptive than others, the coping literature resists classifying strategies as inherently good or bad. Rather, problems tend to arise when coping strategies are applied excessively or inflexibly despite changing needs and context.[47] The most commonly reported coping strategies for dealing with pain include use of medication (73%), exercise (33%), cognitive coping strategies, such as distraction (31%), religious activities (18%), pacing (alternating periods of activity with rest, 15%), and use of heat and cold therapies (13%).[48,49]

ASSESSMENT

It is important to identify patients at risk for comorbid psychiatric disorders and pain, because comorbid presentation is associated with poor treatment response, greater complications, longer duration of illness, higher medical costs, dissatisfaction with treatment, lower quality of life, and more disability.[50] In addition, practitioners at all levels experience greater frustration and devote more time in treating patients with psychiatric comorbidity.[51] Treatment of relevant psychiatric symptoms as part of a comprehensive pain treatment plan not only can help reduce provider frustration, but also can destigmatize the referral to a mental health provider. When patients are referred to a mental health provider only after years of failed medical treatments, they often perceive that their doctors are giving up on them or that the doctors have come to believe that their problem is "in their head."[40,50]

Screening can help pain providers quickly identify patients at risk of having a comorbid psychiatric disorder. Systematically integrating standardized screening into clinic processes (e.g., at check-in) can be an effective method for identifying patients at risk. Additionally, there are validated, ultra-brief screens that require providers to ask only one or two questions during their encounter in order to screen patients. Table 33.1 contains a list of brief screens and assessment tools that can be used for common psychiatric diagnoses.

If indicated, screens can be followed by more in-depth assessment and referral to a mental health professional. The goal of a psychologic assessment of pain is to gain a thorough understanding of the biopsychosocial factors involved in the patient's presenting problem. This information allows the mental health professional to construct a tailored treatment plan that targets problematic areas and improves functioning in alignment with the patient's specific behavioral goals. Provision of feedback can also help providers understand the psychiatric risks and alternative methods for managing their patient's needs.

TREATMENT

Psychotropic Prescribing in Patients with Pain

Patients with pain often receive psychotropic medications to address psychiatric comorbidity, but psychotropics are also widely used as analgesic adjuvants (Table 33.2). In a national study of veterans, Barry and colleagues found that 77% of patients receiving chronic opioids also received psychotropic medications (74% antidepressants, 55% anxiolytics/sedative-hypnotics).[52] The psychotropic drugs were frequently prescribed in mental health clinics, which necessitated coordination of services around the risks of co-prescribing.[52]

Antidepressants

Antidepressants are a major therapeutic tool in the management of chronic pain. Therapeutic effects are achieved by addressing comorbid depression and anxiety and thereby reducing the focus on, and perception of, pain. However, analgesic effects are also achieved independent of the mood-altering effects, specifically with SNRIs, especially duloxetine, and with the TCAs, especially amitriptyline.[17,53] In addition, TCAs have therapeutic effects when applied topically, an effect produced by peripheral mechanisms rather than central effects.[17,53]

Table 33.1. PSYCHIATRIC DIAGNOSES, CORE FEATURES, AND SCREENING TOOLS

PSYCHIATRIC DISORDER	CORE FEATURES	SCREENING TOOLS
Mood Disorders		
Major depressive disorder	Low mood, anhedonia, neurovegetative symptoms lasting 2+ weeks	PHQ-9, PHQ-2[10,11] SIGECAPS: Sad mood, loss of Interest, Guilt, low Energy, Concentration, change in Appetite, Psychomotor behavior, change in Sleep Over the past 2 weeks, have you felt down, depressed, or hopeless? Over the past 2 weeks, have you felt little interest or pleasure in doing things?
Dysthymic disorder	Low-level depressive symptoms, lasting 2+ years	Depressed mood more days than not for at least 2 years and two or more symptoms: change in appetite, change in sleep, low energy, low self-esteem, poor concentration or difficulty making decisions, feelings of hopelessness. Can use screens for major depressive disorder for guidance.
Bipolar I or II disorder	At least one episode of mania (bipolar I) or hypomania and at least one depressive episode (bipolar II)	The Altman Self-Rating Mania Scale (ASRM)[64] Have you ever had so much energy that you felt like you didn't need to sleep much at all?
Suicide	Desire to intentionally cause one's own death, with ideation and intent	PHQ-9 item #9 C-SSRS[15] <u>Ideation</u>: Have you had thoughts about killing yourself? <u>Plan</u>: Do you have a plan or have you started to make preparations? <u>Intent</u>: How intent are you on following through with suicide? 0 is no intent and 10 is total intent.
Insomnia	Dissatisfaction with sleep quality or quantity. Difficulty initiating or maintaining sleep, or early morning awakening, at least three nights per week, lasting at least 3 months.	ISI[16] Pittsburgh Sleep Quality Index (PSQI)[65]
Anxiety Disorders		
Generalized anxiety disorder (GAD)	Psychologic: anxiety, excessive worry, irritability, difficulty concentrating Physical: restlessness, muscle tension, easy startle, sleep disturbance	GAD-7, GAD-2[12,13] Penn State Worry Questionnaire (PSWQ)[66] Are you a worrier? Have you been bothered by feeling nervous, anxious, or on edge? Not being able to stop or control worrying?
Obsessive compulsive disorder (OCD)	Presence of obsessions, compulsions, or both Obsessions: recurrent, persistent thoughts, images, or urges that cause distress and that resist attempts made to ignore, suppress, or neutralize them Compulsions: repetitive behaviors or mental acts (e.g., washing, checking, counting) that a person feels compelled to perform in response to an obsession and that are time-consuming	Yale-Brown Obsessive Compulsive Scale (Y-BOCS)[67] Do you have thoughts or images that keep coming back to you and are difficult to put out of your head? Do you ever feel the need to perform certain actions that don't make sense or that you don't want to do, such as washing, cleaning, counting, or checking things over and over?
Panic disorder	Recurrent and unexpected panic attacks (i.e., abrupt surge of fear/discomfort with physical and cognitive symptoms of anxiety that peak within minutes), fear of having another attack, related avoidance behavior	Anxiety Sensitivity Index (ASI)[68] Brief Panic Disorder Screen (BPDS)[69] Have you ever had a panic attack? Does it scare you when you feel shaky, faint, your heart beats rapidly, or you become short of breath?
Trauma and Stressor-Related Disorders		
PTSD	Experience of a traumatic event, followed by recurrent intrusive thoughts/dreams, avoidance of reminders, changes in mood and cognitions related to the event, and changes in reactivity (e.g., hypervigilance, easy startle, irritability), lasting more than 1 month	Post-Traumatic Checklist (PCL)[70] Primary Care-PTSD Screen (PC-PTSD)[71] In your life, have you ever had any experience that was so frightening, horrible, or upsetting that, in the past month, you had intrusive thoughts or nightmares, tried to avoid reminders of it, felt on guard, easily startled, or numb and detached?

Table 33.1. CONTINUED

PSYCHIATRIC DISORDER	CORE FEATURES	SCREENING TOOLS
Acute stress disorder	As above, but duration is shorter, lasting 3 days to 1 month after trauma	As above
Somatoform Disorders		
Somatic symptom disorder	1+ somatic symptoms that are distressing, with excessive thoughts, feelings, and behaviors related to these somatic concerns	PHQ-15[72] PHQ-SADS (Somatoform, Anxiety, Depression Scales)[72]
Illness anxiety disorder	Preoccupation with having or acquiring a serious illness when somatic symptoms are absent or mild, high level of health anxiety, excessive health-related behaviors (i.e., avoidance or checking/reassurance seeking)	Health Anxiety Inventory (HAI)[73]
Conversion disorder	1+ symptoms of altered motor or sensory function with incompatible findings	
Factitious disorder	Falsification of physical signs or symptoms associated with deception; individual presents self as ill or injured, with no obvious external reward	
Psychologic factors affecting medical conditions	Psychologic or behavioral factors increase medical risk (e.g., poor adherence) or aggravate underlying disease (e.g., anxiety affecting asthma)	
Substance Use Disorders		
Alcohol use disorder	• Problematic pattern of alcohol use leading to impairment or distress • Larger amounts taken than intended • Unsuccessful attempts to cut down • Great deal of time spent obtaining or recovering • Social or occupational problems • Recurrent use in dangerous situations or despite health risks • Cravings • Tolerance, withdrawal	Alcohol Use Disorders Identification Test (AUDIT, AUDIT-C)[74,75] CAGE (Cut down, Annoyed by criticism of your drinking, Guilty about your drinking, Eye-opener)[22] In the last year, have you ever drunk or used drugs more than you meant to? And Have you felt you wanted or needed to cut down on your drinking or drug use in the last year?
Substance use disorder (illicit or prescription)	• Problematic pattern of substance use leading to impairment or distress • Larger amounts taken than intended • Unsuccessful attempts to cut down • Great deal of time spent obtaining or recovering • Social or occupational problems • Recurrent use in dangerous situations or despite health risks • Cravings • Tolerance and withdrawal criteria do not apply to those using substances appropriately with medical supervision	CAGE-AID[76] How many times in the past year have you used an illegal drug or used a prescription medication for nonmedical reasons?
Schizophrenia Spectrum and Psychotic Disorders		
Schizophrenia	Delusions, hallucinations, disorganized thinking or behavior, catatonia, diminished emotional expression	Have people been harassing you or trying to harm you? Have you ever heard sounds or voices that others could not hear?
Schizoaffective disorder	Delusions, hallucinations, disorganized thinking, and a mood episode (depressive or manic)	As above

(*continued*)

Table 33.1. CONTINUED

PSYCHIATRIC DISORDER	CORE FEATURES	SCREENING TOOLS
Delusional disorder	Persistent delusions, otherwise functioning is not impaired or obviously bizarre	
Personality Disorders		
Diagnosed ≥ 18 years of age		
Borderline	Affective lability, unstable relationships and self-image, impulsivity, temper, emptiness, difficulty with perceived/real abandonment, suicidal behavior	Careful history and corroborating information are crucial for accurate diagnosis, possibly including a structured assessment, such as the Minnesota Multiphasic Personality Inventory, Second Edition (MMPI-2)[77] Standardized Assessment of Personality: Abbreviated Scale (SAPAS)[78]
Narcissistic	Grandiosity, need for admiration, lack of empathy, exploitative, sense of entitlement	
Histrionic	Excessive emotionality, rapidly shifting and shallow, attention-seeking, dramatic	
Antisocial	Pattern of disregard and violation of the rights of others, unlawful behaviors, deceitful, impulsive, irritable/aggressive, irresponsible, lack of remorse	
Dependent	Strong need to be cared for; submissive, clinging behavior; difficulty making independent decisions, initiating projects, or expressing disagreement	
Avoidant	Social inhibition, inadequacy, and hypersensitivity to criticism	
Obsessive compulsive	Preoccupied with orderliness, perfectionism, and mental/interpersonal control; rigid/inflexible	
Schizotypal	Social deficits, reduced capacity for close relationships, cognitive or perceptual distortions, and eccentric behavior, including ideas of reference, magical thinking, unusual perceptual experiences, odd thinking and speech, suspicion	

BDZs

Despite the widespread use of BDZs in chronic pain, there is little evidence for their effectiveness. Furthermore, chronic use in conjunction with high-dose opioids greatly heightens the risks of overuse, dependence, and mortality. BDZs may result in impaired cognitive and physical performance, respiratory suppression, sedation, and overdose. There is also mounting evidence for increased risk of death by overdose in patients treated with opioids and chronic BDZs.[20] Consequently, BDZ use should be limited in the treatment of chronic pain, and a careful, coordinated review of chronic BDZ use is warranted.

Anticonvulsants

Carbamazepine is FDA approved for the treatment of trigeminal neuralgia. The analgesic effect is achieved through the inhibition of voltage-gated sodium channels, resulting in reduced neuronal activity of A-delta and C-fibers. Careful observation for the emergence of serious adverse effects, such as Stevens-Johnson syndrome, toxic epidermal necrolysis, or blood dyscrasia (7.2 per 10,000 patients treated), is warranted.[54]

Both gabapentin and pregabalin have proven efficacy in a wide variety of neuropathies. Their effects are achieved through reduced excitatory neurotransmitter release and decreased pain signaling. Both have high safety profiles and are recommend as first-line agents in the treatment of chronic pain.[54] Absorption of pregabalin is linear, with increasing bioavailability with increased dose, as compared to gabapentin, which has a saturable absorption process, with a decrease in absolute bioavailability from 60% to 33% as the dose increases from 900 to 3600 mg/day.[54]

Table 33.2. PSYCHOTROPIC ANALGESIC ADJUVANT MEDICATIONS

MEDICATION	PAIN TYPE	EFFECTS
Antidepressants *TCAs* Amitriptyline Imipramine Nortriptyline Desipramine	Neuropathic pain Postherpetic neuralgia Painful polyneuropathy Postmastectomy pain Central poststroke pain	• Descending inhibitory effect • Treat comorbid psychiatric disorder (anxiety) • Reduce psychologic distress which can amplify pain • Improve health behaviors (adherence)
SNRIs Duloxetine Venlafaxine	Painful diabetic peripheral neuropathy Neuropathic pain Fibromyalgia	Inactivation of $alpha_2$-delta voltage-gated calcium channels in CNS, decreasing excitatory transmitter release
SSRIs Citalopram Escitalopram Fluoxetine Sertraline	Painful diabetic peripheral neuropathy Neuropathic pain Fibromyalgia	Treatment of comorbid anxiety and depression
Anticonvulsants Carbamazepine Oxcarbazepine	Trigeminal neuralgia	• Inhibition of neuronal sodium channels, reducing repetitive firing of action potentials • Decreased neuronal activity of the A-delta and C-fibers
Gabapentin Pregabalin	Diabetic neuropathic pain Postherpetic neuralgia Painful polyneuropathy Noncancer pain Central poststroke pain Spinal cord injury pain	Inactivation of $alpha_2$-delta voltage-gated calcium channels in CNS, decreasing excitatory transmitter release
Antipsychotics	Headaches Neuralgic pain	• Antidopaminergic effects mediate analgesic effects • Serotonin antagonism mediates analgesic effects • Antagonism at $alpha_2$-adrenoreceptors

PSYCHOLOGIC TREATMENTS FOR PATIENTS WITH CHRONIC PAIN

Psychoeducation and Motivational Enhancement

Psychologic management is not solely the task of psychologists; pain specialists can begin by using brief techniques, such as reflective listening, psychoeducation, and motivational enhancement, to gain patient commitment to engage in the treatment plan. Providing psychoeducation about the differences between acute and chronic pain can validate a patient's experience of having struggled with pain for a long time and help the patient better understand treatment options (e.g., recommendation for rest or medication might differ with acute versus chronic pain). Other helpful education includes explanation of the anatomy of pain (brain, spinal cord, nerves) and of Melzack and Wall's gate-control theory of pain: when pain signals travel up the spinal cord to the brain and back down, they pass through "gates" (physical, affective, cognitive, social) that can inhibit or enhance the pain experience.[32] Finally, psychoeducation about the impact of activity, sleep, depression, etc., on pain can help patients understand the biologic reasons why these issues must be treated to improve pain, and offer a cogent rationale for self-management and referral to outpatient psychotherapy.

CBT

There is a strong evidence base for the use of cognitive and behavioral interventions to improve pain from a variety of medical conditions. Drawn from treatments for depression and anxiety, CBT emphasizes the relationship between thoughts, feelings, and behavior. It attempts to improve mood and pain by teaching patients to identify, challenge, and reinterpret thoughts and pain sensations in a more adaptive or less extreme way. Common goals in CBT are to increase activities that provide pleasure or contribute to self-esteem, to engage in graded or paced activities to maximize physical functioning while increasing pain tolerance, to improve other health behaviors (e.g., sleep, exercise, healthy diet, decreased use of alcohol, drugs, and tobacco), and to employ more pain self-management strategies, such as relaxation, problem solving, and assertive communication. Ultimately, the goal of CBT is to accumulate evidence from an expanding behavioral repertoire to alter a patient's limiting pain beliefs (e.g., "The only way to deal with my pain is to stay in bed or take medication." "I am helpless with regard to my pain." "Pain is always unbearable." "Pain should always be avoided.").[55]

Meta-analyses of CBT for pain show that it is an efficacious treatment[4] in decreasing depression, anxiety, disability, pain behaviors, catastrophic thinking, and sometimes, pain.

Improvement in broad domains, but not necessarily pain severity, is consistent with the goals of treatment: to help patients live more satisfying, healthier lives despite their pain.[55] However, more research needs to be done to characterize treatment responders and nonresponders so that better treatments can be developed to reach nonresponders.

Acceptance and Commitment Therapy

There is also growing evidence to support acceptance and commitment therapy as a treatment for chronic pain.[56,57] This is a treatment that focuses on acceptance of pain with the understanding that attempts to control/avoid pain increasingly limit activities and quality of life over time. Using strategies such as mindfulness, thought defusion, values clarification, and committed action, patients are encouraged to relate differently to their pain and to choose to engage in activities that give their life meaning, knowing that pain and difficulties are to be expected in the service of these goals.[57]

Mindfulness

Mindfulness (mindfulness-based stress reduction [MBSR]) has gained increasing popularity as an important psychologic tool to enhance well-being, especially in the face of medical illness. Mindfulness is a set of techniques that encourage purposeful, nonjudgmental, present-moment awareness.[58] The techniques have been shown to be effective in reducing stress, depression, fatigue, pain perception, and disability. People who practice mindfulness show quicker recovery from stressors, reduced cortisol levels, and decreased markers of inflammation. They have also shown improved attention, working memory, and executive functioning. These outcomes have implications for targeting many of the mechanisms believed to underlie the development of chronic pain.[59,60]

Biofeedback

Biofeedback-assisted relaxation training uses noninvasive equipment that monitors information about the body (e.g., respiration rate and quality, heart rate and heart rate variability, EMG muscle tension, brain waves, skin conductance, skin temperature).[61] "Feeding this information back" to the patient, along with guidance on ways to alter thoughts and behaviors, allows patients to learn how to change their physiologic responses that may be contributing to their pain, such as patients with temporomandibular disorders (TMD) learning to reduce muscle tension in the jaw.[62] Biofeedback has proven to be efficacious with anxiety, adult headache, and TMD, and has been classified as probably or possibly efficacious for other pain-related conditions, including fibromyalgia, arthritis, pediatric headache, and depression.[63]

Multidisciplinary Pain Treatment

Optimal treatment of pain utilizes a multidisciplinary team to address the multiple biopsychosocial components of pain (see Figure 33.2). Operating within this model, each member reinforces the goals of the other members and coordinates care among them.

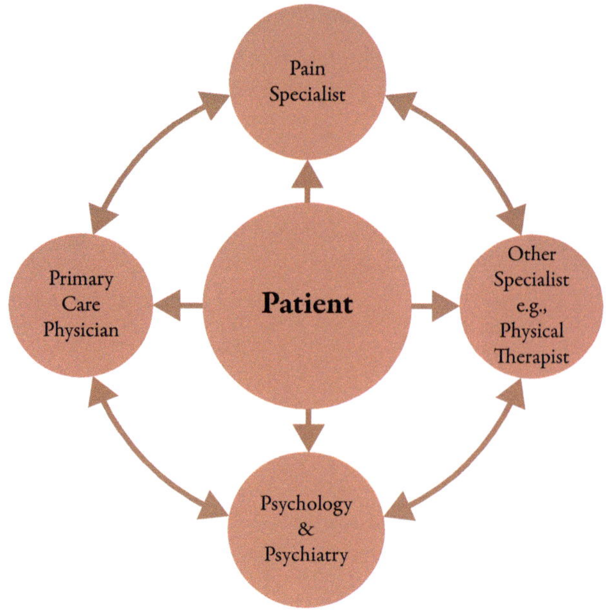

Figure 33.2. The multidisciplinary team approach.

The most intense level of psychologic treatment for pain is the multidisciplinary pain management program. Often considered the gold standard, multidisciplinary programs take a comprehensive approach, with medicine, psychology, and physical, occupational, and vocational therapy working together in one location. Goals are to help the patient take an active role in pain management, to reduce emphasis on narcotic and other pain medications, to improve sleep, to provide intensive physical rehabilitation, and to help patients develop more balanced, evidence-based thoughts and expectancies about pain and activity.[55] Meta-analyses of multidisciplinary treatment for chronic pain show that although pain reduction occurs at a level similar to that achieved with other treatments, these programs successfully reduce medication and healthcare utilization, and increase activity level, return to work, and functioning more than component treatments.[55]

CONCLUSIONS

- Pain is an unpleasant sensory and emotional experience that is highly comorbid with psychiatric disorders.
- Comorbid depression occurs in up to 50% of pain patients and includes sad mood, anhedonia, and neurovegetative symptoms; comorbid anxiety occurs in up to 45% of pain patients.
- Sleep disturbance, such as insomnia, worsens both pain and mood and can be treated with the TCA amitriptyline.
- Somatic symptom disorder with predominant pain is diagnosed when a patient has excessive thoughts, feelings, and behaviors related to pain, resulting in significant distress and disruption to daily life.

- The high rates of pain and psychiatric comorbidity can be explained in part through overlapping mechanisms, such as similar neurotransmitter systems, neural areas that process pain and emotion, and dysfunction of the HPA axis.
- The fear-avoidance model explains how pain becomes chronic in some individuals based on cognitive variables and learning mechanisms.
- Patients with chronic pain treated with long-term opioids are at increased risk of developing aberrant drug-related behaviors that can escalate over time, leading to opioid misuse, abuse, addiction, diversion, overdose, and suicide.
- Ultra-brief oral or written screens are available to identify psychiatric comorbidities, and when combined with brief interventions or referral to treatment, can significantly help mitigate untreated risk factors (e.g., substance use, suicidality).
- Referral to a mental health professional is useful to gain a better understanding of the biopsychosocial factors that contribute to a patient's presentation, to build a comprehensive pain management plan that addresses possible psychiatric issues, and to inform optimal use of psychotropic medication.
- Antidepressants are a major therapeutic tool in the management of chronic pain, with analgesic effects independent of their mood-altering effects.
- Gabapentin and pregabalin have proven efficacy in a wide variety of neuropathies.
- There is evidence for increased risk of death by overdose in patients treated with chronic opioids and BDZs.
- Longer-term psychologic treatments that are empirically supported include CBT, acceptance and commitment therapy, MBSR, and biofeedback-assisted relaxation training.

REFERENCES

1. Derbyshire SWG. The IASP definition captures the essence of pain experience. *Pain Forum.* 1999;8(2):106–109.
2. Annagür BB, Uguz F, Apiliogullari S, Kara İ, Gunduz S. Psychiatric disorders and association with quality of sleep and quality of life in patients with chronic pain: a SCID-based study. *Pain Med.* 2014;15(5):772–781. doi:10.1111/pme.12390.
3. Von Korff M, Crane P, Lane M, et al. Chronic spinal pain and physical–mental comorbidity in the United States: results from the national comorbidity survey replication. *Pain.* 2005;113(3):331–339. doi:10.1016/j.pain.2004.11.010.
4. Williams AC de C, Eccleston C, Morley S. Psychological therapies for the management of chronic pain (excluding headache) in adults. *Cochrane Database Syst Rev.* 2012;11:CD007407. doi:10.1002/14651858.CD007407.pub3.
5. Roditi D, Robinson ME. The role of psychological interventions in the management of patients with chronic pain. *Psychol Res Behav Manag.* 2011;4:41–49. doi:10.2147/PRBM.S15375.
6. Scott EL, Kroenke K, Wu J, Yu Z. Beneficial effects of improvement in depression, pain catastrophizing, and anxiety on pain outcomes: a 12-month longitudinal analysis. *J Pain.* 2016;17(2):215–222. doi:10.1016/j.jpain.2015.10.011.
7. Asmundson GJG, Katz J. Understanding the co-occurrence of anxiety disorders and chronic pain: state-of-the-art. *Depress Anxiety.* 2009;26(10):888–901. doi:10.1002/da.20600.
8. Demyttenaere K, Bruffaerts R, Lee S, et al. Mental disorders among persons with chronic back or neck pain: results from the World Mental Health Surveys. *Pain.* 2007;129(3):332–342. doi:10.1016/j.pain.2007.01.022.
9. Romão APMS, Gorayeb R, Romão GS, et al. High levels of anxiety and depression have a negative effect on quality of life of women with chronic pelvic pain. *Int J Clin Pract.* 2009;63(5):707–711. doi:10.1111/j.1742-1241.2009.02034.x.
10. Kroenke K, Spitzer RL, Williams JBW. The PHQ-9: validity of a brief depression severity measure. *J Gen Intern Med.* 2001;16(9):606–613. doi:10.1046/j.1525-1497.2001.016009606.x.
11. Kroenke K, Spitzer RL, Williams JBW. The Patient Health Questionnaire-2: validity of a two-item depression screener. *Med Care.* 2003;41(11):1284–1292. doi:10.1097/01.MLR.0000093487.78664.3C.
12. Spitzer RL, Kroenke K, Williams JBW, Löwe B. A brief measure for assessing generalized anxiety disorder: the GAD-7. *Arch Intern Med.* 2006;166(10):1092. doi:10.1001/archinte.166.10.1092.
13. Kroenke K, Spitzer RL, Williams JB, et al. Anxiety disorders in primary care: prevalence, impairment, comorbidity, and detection. *Ann Intern Med.* 2007;146(5):317–325.
14. Stenager E, Christiansen E, Handberg G, Jensen B. Suicide attempts in chronic pain patients. A register-based study. *Scand J Pain.* 2014;5(1):4–7. doi:10.1016/j.sjpain.2013.09.001.
15. Posner K, Brown GK, Stanley B, et al. The Columbia-Suicide Severity Rating Scale: initial validity and internal consistency findings from three multisite studies with adolescents and adults. *Am J Psychiatry.* 2011;168(12):1266–1277. doi:10.1176/appi.ajp.2011.10111704.
16. Bastien CH, Vallières A, Morin CM. Validation of the Insomnia Severity Index as an outcome measure for insomnia research. *Sleep Med.* 2001;2(4):297–307. doi:10.1016/S1389-9457(00)00065-4.
17. Perahia DGS, Pritchett YL, Desaiah D, Raskin J. Efficacy of duloxetine in painful symptoms: an analgesic or antidepressant effect? *Int Clin Psychopharmacol.* 2006;21(6):311–317. doi:10.1097/01.yic.0000224782.83287.3c.
18. Wang KH, Becker WC, Fiellin DA. Prevalence and correlates for nonmedical use of prescription opioids among urban and rural residents. *Drug Alcohol Depend.* 2013;127(1-3):156–162. doi:10.1016/j.drugalcdep.2012.06.027.
19. Webster LR, Webster RM. Predicting aberrant behaviors in opioid-treated patients: preliminary validation of the Opioid Risk Tool. *Pain Med.* 2005;6(6):432–442. doi:10.1111/j.1526-4637.2005.00072.x.
20. Jones CM, McAninch JK. Emergency department visits and overdose deaths from combined use of opioids and benzodiazepines. *Am J Prev Med.* 2015;49(4):493–501. doi:10.1016/j.amepre.2015.03.040.
21. *Diagnostic and Statistical Manual of Mental Disorders.* 5th ed. Arlington, VA: American Psychiatric Publishing; 2013.
22. Mayfield D, McLeod G, Hall P. The CAGE questionnaire: validation of a new alcoholism screening instrument. *Am J Psychiatry.* 1974;131(10):1121–1123. doi:10.1176/ajp.131.10.1121.
23. Akbik H, Butler SF, Budman SH, Fernandez K, Katz NP, Jamison RN. Validation and clinical application of the Screener and Opioid Assessment for Patients with Pain (SOAPP). *J Pain Symptom Manag.* 2006;32(3):287–293. doi:10.1016/j.jpainsymman.2006.03.010.
24. Butler SF, Fernandez K, Benoit C, Budman SH, Jamison RN. Validation of the Revised Screener and Opioid Assessment for Patients with Pain (SOAPP-R). *J Pain.* 2008;9(4):360–372. doi:10.1016/j.jpain.2007.11.014.
25. SBIRT/SAMHSA-HRSA. http://www.integration.samhsa.gov/clinical-practice/SBIRT.
26. Block AR, Ohnmeiss DD, Guyer RD, Rashbaum RF, Hochschuler SH. The use of presurgical psychological screening to predict the

outcome of spine surgery. *Spine J.* 2001;1(4):274–282. doi:10.1016/S1529-9430(01)00054-7.
27. Block A, ed. *The Psychology of Spine Surgery.* Washington, DC: American Psychological Association; 2003.
28. Dersh J, Polatin PB, Gatchel RJ. Chronic pain and psychopathology: research findings and theoretical considerations. *Psychosom Med.* 2002;64(5):773–786.
29. Gatchel RJ, Peng YB, Peters ML, Fuchs PN, Turk DC. The biopsychosocial approach to chronic pain: scientific advances and future directions. *Psychol Bull.* 2007;133(4):581–624. doi:10.1037/0033-2909.133.4.581.
30. Fishbain DA, Cutler R, Rosomoff HL, Rosomoff RS. Chronic pain-associated depression: antecedent or consequence of chronic pain? A review. *Clin J Pain.* 1997;13(2):116–137.
31. Gatchel R, Howard K, Kishino N. Etiology of chronic pain and mental illness: the biopsychosocial component. *Pract Pain Manag.* 2008;8(4). http://www.practicalpainmanagement.com/treatments/psychological/etiology-chronic-pain-mental-illness-biopsychosocial-component. Accessed April 24, 2016.
32. Gatchel-Biopsychosocial Approach to Chronic Pain.pdf. http://enniscentre.com/Presentations/Gatchel-Biopsychosocial%20Approach%20to%20Chronic%20Pain.pdf. Accessed April 26, 2016.
33. Pincus T, Morley S. Cognitive-processing bias in chronic pain: a review and integration. *Psychol Bull.* 2001;127(5):599–617.
34. Van Damme S, Crombez G, Eccleston C. Disengagement from pain: the role of catastrophic thinking about pain. *Pain.* 2004;107(1-2):70–76.
35. Borkum JM. Chronic headaches and the neurobiology of somatization. *Curr Pain Headache Rep.* 2010;14(1):55–61. doi:10.1007/s11916-009-0084-z.
36. Banks SM, Kerns RD. Explaining high rates of depression in chronic pain: a diathesis-stress framework. *Psychol Bull.* 1996;119(1):95–110. doi:10.1037/0033-2909.119.1.95.
37. Vlaeyen JW, Linton SJ. Fear-avoidance and its consequences in chronic musculoskeletal pain: a state of the art. *Pain.* 2000;85(3):317–332.
38. Lethem J, Slade PD, Troup JD, Bentley G. Outline of a fear-avoidance model of exaggerated pain perception—I. *Behav Res Ther.* 1983;21(4):401–408.
39. Sullivan MJL, Bishop S, Pivik J. The Pain Catastrophizing Scale: development and validation. *Psychol Assess.* 1995;7(4):524–532. doi:10.1037/1040-3590.7.4.524.
40. Weisberg JN, Keefe FJ. Personality disorders in the chronic pain population. *J Pain.* 1997;6(1):1–9. doi:10.1016/S1082-3174(97)70001-1.
41. Meyer F, Block S. Personality disorders in the oncology setting. *J Support Oncol.* 2011;9(2):44–51.
42. Conrad R, Wegener I, Geiser F, Kleiman A. Temperament, character, and personality disorders in chronic pain. *Curr Pain Headache Rep.* 2013;17(3):318. doi:10.1007/s11916-012-0318-3.
43. Dixon-Gordon KL, Whalen DJ, Layden BK, Chapman AL. A systematic review of personality disorders and health outcomes. *Can Psychol Can.* 2015;56(2):168–190. doi:10.1037/cap0000024.
44. Sansone RA, Sansone LA. Chronic pain syndromes and borderline personality. *Innov Clin Neurosci.* 2012;9(1):10–14.
45. Folkman S, Lazarus RS. If it changes it must be a process: study of emotion and coping during three stages of a college examination. *J Pers Soc Psychol.* 1985;48(1):150–170.
46. Carver CS, Scheier MF, Weintraub JK. Assessing coping strategies: a theoretically based approach. *J Pers Soc Psychol.* 1989;56(2):267–283. doi:10.1037/0022-3514.56.2.267.
47. Carver CS, Scheier MF. Situational coping and coping dispositions in a stressful transaction. *J Pers Soc Psychol.* 1994;66(1):184–195.
48. Barry LC, Kerns RD, Guo Z, Duong BD, Iannone LP, Carrington Reid M. Identification of strategies used to cope with chronic pain in older persons receiving primary care from a Veterans Affairs medical center: pain-related coping strategies in older adults. *J Am Geriatr Soc.* 2004;52(6):950–956. doi:10.1111/j.1532-5415.2004.52263.x.
49. Peres MFP, Lucchetti G. Coping strategies in chronic pain. *Curr Pain Headache Rep.* 2010;14(5):331–338. doi:10.1007/s11916-010-0137-3.
50. Maizels M, Smitherman TA, Penzien DB. A review of screening tools for psychiatric comorbidity in headache patients. *Headache.* 2006;46(suppl 3):S98-S109. doi:10.1111/j.1526-4610.2006.00561.x.
51. Jackson JL, Kroenke K. Difficult patient encounters in the ambulatory clinic: clinical predictors and outcomes. *Arch Intern Med.* 1999;159(10):1069–1075.
52. Barry DT, Sofuoglu M, Kerns RD, Wiechers IR, Rosenheck RA. Prevalence and correlates of co-prescribing psychotropic medications with long-term opioid use nationally in the Veterans Health Administration. *Psychiatry Res.* 2015;227(2-3):324–332. doi:10.1016/j.psychres.2015.03.006.
53. Nelson J. Tricyclic and tetracyclic drugs. In: Schatzberg A, Nemeroff C, eds. *Essentials of Clinical Psychopharmacology.* 3rd ed. Washington, DC: American Psychiatric Publishing; 2013:5–28.
54. Smith HS, Argoff CE, Kaur M, Nagaraja, H. Gabapentinoids and other anticonvulsants. In: Toth C, Moulin DE, eds. *Neuropathic Pain: Causes, Management and Understanding.* Cambridge, United Kingdom: Cambridge University Press; 2013:225–239.
55. Levin J, Janata J. Psychological interventions. In: Waldman SD, ed. *Pain Management.* Vol 2. Philadelphia, PA: Saunders/Elsevier; 2007:1003–1009.
56. Ost L-G. The efficacy of acceptance and commitment therapy: an updated systematic review and meta-analysis. *Behav Res Ther.* 2014;61:105–121. doi:10.1016/j.brat.2014.07.018.
57. Dahl J, Lundgren T. *Living beyond Your Pain: Using Acceptance and Commitment Therapy to Ease Chronic Pain.* Oakland, CA: New Harbinger Publications; 2006.
58. Kabat-Zinn J. *Wherever You Go, There You Are: Mindfulness Meditation in Everyday Life.* New York, NY: Hyperion; 2005.
59. Carlson LE. Mindfulness-based interventions for physical conditions: a narrative review evaluating levels of evidence. *ISRN Psychiatry.* 2012;1–21. doi:10.5402/2012/651583.
60. Rosenkranz MA, Davidson RJ, Maccoon DG, Sheridan JF, Kalin NH, Lutz A. A comparison of mindfulness-based stress reduction and an active control in modulation of neurogenic inflammation. *Brain Behav Immun.* 2013;27(1):174–184. doi:10.1016/j.bbi.2012.10.013.
61. Giggins OM, Persson UM, Caulfield B. Biofeedback in rehabilitation. *J NeuroEng Rehabil.* 2013;10:60. doi:10.1186/1743-0003-10-60.
62. Crider A, Glaros AG, Gevirtz RN. Efficacy of biofeedback-based treatments for temporomandibular disorders. *Appl Psychophysiol Biofeedback.* 2005;30(4):333–345. doi:10.1007/s10484-005-8420-5.
63. La Vaque TJ, Hammond DC, Trudeau D, et al. Template for developing guidelines for the evaluation of the clinical efficacy of psychophysiological interventions. *Appl Psychophysiol Biofeedback.* 2002;27(4):273–281. doi:10.1023/A:1021061318355.
64. Altman EG, Hedeker D, Peterson JL, Davis JM. The Altman Self-Rating Mania Scale. *Biol Psychiatry.* 1997;42(10):948–955. doi:10.1016/S0006-3223(96)00548-3.
65. Buysse DJ, Reynolds CF III, Monk TH, Berman SR, Kupfer DJ. The Pittsburgh Sleep Quality Index: a new instrument for psychiatric practice and research. *Psychiatry Res.* 1989;28(2):193–213. doi:10.1016/0165-1781(89)90047-4.
66. Meyer TJ, Miller ML, Metzger RL, Borkovec TD. Development and validation of the Penn State Worry Questionnaire. *Behav Res Ther.* 1990;28(6):487–495. doi:10.1016/0005-7967(90)90135-6.
67. Goodman WK, Price LH, Rasmussen SA, et al. The Yale-Brown Obsessive Compulsive Scale: I. development, use, and reliability. *Arch Gen Psychiatry.* 1989;46(11):1006–1011. doi:10.1001/archpsyc.1989.01810110048007.
68. Reiss S, Peterson RA, Gursky DM, McNally RJ. Anxiety sensitivity, anxiety frequency and the prediction of fearfulness. *Behav Res Ther.* 1986;24(1):1–8. doi:10.1016/0005-7967(86)90143-9.
69. Apfeldorf WJ, Shear MK, Leon AC, Portera L. A brief screen for panic disorder. *J Anxiety Disord.* 1994;8(1):71–78. doi:10.1016/0887-6185(94)90024-8.
70. Blanchard EB, Jones-Alexander J, Buckley TC, Forneris CA. Psychometric properties of the PTSD checklist (PCL). *Behav Res Ther.* 1996;34(8):669–673. doi:10.1016/0005-7967(96)00033-2.

71. Ouimette P, Wade M, Prins A, Schohn M. Identifying PTSD in primary care: comparison of the Primary Care-PTSD screen (PC-PTSD) and the General Health Questionnaire-12 (GHQ). *J Anxiety Disord.* 2008;22(2):337–343. doi:10.1016/j.janxdis.2007.02.010.
72. Kroenke K, Spitzer RL, Williams JBW, Löwe B. The Patient Health Questionnaire Somatic, Anxiety, and Depressive Symptom Scales: a systematic review. *Gen Hosp Psychiatry.* 2010;32(4):345–359. doi:10.1016/j.genhosppsych.2010.03.006.
73. Salkovskis PM, Rimes KA, Warwick HMC, Clark DM. The Health Anxiety Inventory: development and validation of scales for the measurement of health anxiety and hypochondriasis. *Psychol Med.* 2002;32(05). doi:10.1017/S0033291702005822.
74. Bohn MJ, Babor TF, Kranzler HR. The Alcohol Use Disorders Identification Test (AUDIT): validation of a screening instrument for use in medical settings. *J Stud Alcohol.* 1995;56(4):423–432.
75. Smith PC, Schmidt SM, Allensworth-Davies D, Saitz R. primary care validation of a single-question alcohol screening test. *J Gen Intern Med.* 2009;24(7):783–788. doi:10.1007/s11606-009-0928-6.
76. Brown RL, Rounds LA. Conjoint screening questionnaires for alcohol and other drug abuse: criterion validity in a primary care practice. *Wis Med J.* 1995;94(3):135–140.
77. Butcher J, Dahlstrom W, Graham J, Tellegen A, Kaemmer B. *Manual for Administration and Scoring: MMPI-2.* Minneapolis: University of Minnesota Press; 1989.
78. Moran P, Leese M, Lee T, Walters P, Thornicroft G, Mann A. Standardised Assessment of Personality—Abbreviated Scale (SAPAS): preliminary validation of a brief screen for personality disorder. *Br J Psychiatry.* 2003;183(3):228–232. doi:10.1192/bjp.183.3.228.
79. Moulton EA, Schmahmann JD, Becerra L, Borsook D. The cerebellum and pain: passive integrator or active participator? *Brain Res Rev.* 2010;65(1):14–27. doi:10.1016/j.brainresrev.2010.05.005.
80. Moulton EA, Elman I, Pendse G, Schmahmann J, Becerra L, Borsook D. Aversion-related circuitry in the cerebellum: responses to noxious heat and unpleasant images. *J Neurosci.* 2011;31(10):3795–3804. doi:10.1523/JNEUROSCI.6709-10.2011.
81. Quartana PJ, Campbell CM, Edwards RR. Pain catastrophizing: a critical review. *Expert Rev Neurother.* 2009;9(5):745–758. doi:10.1586/ERN.09.34.
82. Barlow DH, Sauer-Zavala S, Carl JR, Bullis JR, Ellard KK. The nature, diagnosis, and treatment of neuroticism: back to the future. *Clin Psychol Sci.* 2014;2(3):344–365. doi:10.1177/2167702613505532.
83. Terr, LC. Childhood traumas: an outline and overview. *Am J Psychiatry.* 1991;148(1):10–20.
84. Turk DC. Clinical effectiveness and cost-effectiveness of treatments for patients with chronic pain. *Clin J Pain.* 2002;18(6):355–365.

REVIEW QUESTIONS

1. The analgesic effects of SNRIs, such as duloxetine,

   A. Are the result of treating depression.
   B. Occur independently of antidepressant effects.
   C. Are equal to those of SSRIs.
   D. Are related primarily to relief of anxiety.

2. The TCA amitriptyline should be avoided in

   A. Patients with known cardiac risk.
   B. Patients with skin disorders.
   C. Patients with obsessive-compulsive disorders.
   D. Patients with enuresis.

3. Which of the choices below presents the greatest risk factor for suicide in patients with chronic pain?

   A. Younger age
   B. Female sex
   C. Concrete suicide plan
   D. Negative family history for suicide

ANSWERS

1. B. SNRIs achieve their analgesic effect independent of antidepressant effects.[17] Answer A is not correct because, while relief of depression likely also contributes to pain reduction, it does not account for the full analgesic effect. Answer D is not correct because relief of anxiety symptoms does not account for full analgesia. Answer C is incorrect because SNRIs block reuptake of both serotonin and norepinephrine in a balanced manner and this is thought to account for their superior analgesic effect when compared with pure serotonergic agents.

2. A. Amitriptyline belongs to the TCAs, which are known to affect cardiac conduction and increase the risk of arrhythmias. Consequently, they should be avoided in patients with known cardiac risk, especially elderly patients.[53] Answers B and C are incorrect because in certain skin conditions (e.g., skin picking) and obsessive compulsive disorder, TCAs with serotonin activity (e.g., clomipramine) are indicated. Finally, D is incorrect because the TCA imipramine is the treatment indicated for enuresis.

3. C. The correct selection from the risk factors listed is a concrete plan for suicide.[14] Answers A and B are incorrect because increasing age, not younger age, and male sex, not female sex, have been shown to be associated with increased suicide risk. Similarly, a negative family history for completed suicide is associated with less risk.

QUESTIONS AND ANSWERS

This chapter has accompanying questions and answers that are available to subscribers as part of the Oxford eLearning platform. To access the questions, follow the link below, or go to
✔ http://oxfordmedicine.com/painmanagementreview

34.

THE TREATMENT OF PAIN IN PREGNANCY AND LACTATION

Ali Ebrahimi and Geeta Nagpal

STEM CASE AND KEY QUESTIONS

A 35-year-old female with a history of chronic low back pain and anxiety would like to get pregnant. She is concerned about the effects of her medications on her fetus. She has been referred to your clinic by her primary care physician to evaluate the safety profile of her current medications during pregnancy.

WHAT ARE THE FACTORS THAT INFLUENCE FETAL EXPOSURE TO MEDICATIONS?

The patient has taken an array of medications in the past to control her pain symptoms, including opioids and opioid analogs, acetaminophen, NSAIDs (nonsteroidal anti-inflammatory drugs), neuroleptic agents, and benzodiazepines. She is currently taking diclofenac and hydrocodone/acetaminophen for her pain and duloxetine for anxiety. She is willing to make changes to her treatment plan if some medications are considered safer than others during pregnancy.

WHAT ARE THE RISKS, IF ANY, OF TAKING NSAIDS, ASPIRIN, ACETAMINOPHEN, OPIOIDS AND THEIR ANALOGS, NEUROLEPTIC MEDICATIONS, OR BENZODIAZEPINES FOR PAIN CONTROL DURING PREGNANCY?

The patient has now missed her menstrual cycle and thinks she may be pregnant. She has continued her initial regimen and is concerned that if she is pregnant, the child will be at risk of harm after exposure to the medications.

AT WHAT POINT IN PREGNANCY IS THE FETUS MOST AT RISK OF DEVELOPING PROBLEMS WITH DRUG EXPOSURE?

After a urine HCG is done, the patient is told she is pregnant. She no longer wants to take hydrocodone for pain control and asks about alternative opioid medications that may be safer. Her friend had taken methadone during pregnancy, but she has heard that there may be newer medications that are supposed to be safer.

WHAT ARE THE SAFETY PROFILES OF METHADONE AND BUPRENORPHINE DURING PREGNANCY?

Your patient also considers stopping her SNRI (serotonin-norepinephrine reuptake inhibitor), which she takes for anxiety and pain. Both symptoms have been well controlled for 2 years with the medication, but she is concerned about the effects on her developing fetus. She asks you if she should continue the medication or not. She also wonders if she can start taking "Xanax" for her anxiety if she stops the duloxetine.

ARE ANTIDEPRESSANTS AND BENZODIAZEPINES SAFE DURING PREGNANCY? ARE THEY SAFE TO BE DISCONTINUED DURING PREGNANCY?

Your patient is now in her second trimester at 14 weeks of pregnancy and her pain control has been adequate to this point. She reports sudden-onset radicular pain in her low back, right buttock, and down the side of her right leg to the dorsum of the right foot. She says that the pain started when she bent over to pick up an object off the ground. The pain has been present for 2 weeks and is not remitting.

WHAT TREATMENT OPTIONS ARE AVAILABLE? ARE THERE DIAGNOSTIC TESTS THAT YOU MAY CONSIDER? WHAT IMAGING MODALITIES ARE SAFE FOR PREGNANT WOMEN?

The patient recalls having similar symptoms approximately 2 years ago and she remembers receiving an epidural steroid injection, which gave her significant pain relief. She is interested in having another injection, but is concerned about the effects of steroid on the developing baby.

CAN A PREGNANT WOMAN HAVE AN EPIDURAL STEROID INJECTION? ARE STEROIDS CONTRAINDICATED?

Your patient is now 19 weeks pregnant. Her interim health has been good and her pregnancy has been progressing very well. She last saw her obstetrician 2 weeks ago. She comes in today complaining of 3 days of moderate to severe abdominal pain that is radiating along her groin and to the pubic tubercle. She is worried that something is wrong with the fetus.

WHAT IS THE DIFFERENTIAL DIAGNOSIS FOR ABDOMINAL PAIN IN A PREGNANT WOMAN AND WHAT SHOULD BE THE NEXT STEP IN HER MANAGEMENT? SHOULD YOU SEND HER TO THE EMERGENCY DEPARTMENT? SHOULD SHE SEE HER OBSTETRICIAN?

The patient is now in the third trimester of her pregnancy and is very excited about the progress of her pregnancy. However, she has gradually developed dull and achy low back pain across her beltline bilaterally. She states that standing for prolonged periods of time exacerbates the pain and sitting relieves the pain. She states that the aching is different from the radiating pain she had earlier in her pregnancy.

WHAT IS THE DIFFERENTIAL DIAGNOSIS FOR LOW BACK PAIN AT THIS STAGE OF HER PREGNANCY?

As you are about to end the visit, she also mentions recent severe unilateral headaches that are accompanied by nausea and photophobia. She says they are similar to the migraines she had on occasion prior to pregnancy. She typically rests in a dark room in her bed until the headaches subside. She denies any neurologic changes, including blurry vision, tinnitus, weakness, or dizziness. The episodes usually last about 6 hours. Prior to her pregnancy, she would take ergotamine for her migraine headaches.

WHAT ARE TREATMENT OPTIONS FOR MIGRAINES DURING PREGNANCY? IS IMAGING NECESSARY FOR A NEW AND SEVERE HEADACHE?

Your patient successfully delivers her baby safely and comfortably. She is thrilled that the pregnancy went without any issues. She would like to breastfeed her child but is concerned about the effects of her medications on breast milk. She has heard the term "pump and dump," but is unsure of what this means. She does not want her baby receiving any unnecessary chemicals.

DISCUSSION

WHAT ARE THE EFFECTS OF HER MEDICATIONS ON LACTATION AND BREASTFEEDING?

Pain during pregnancy is common and can have a number of causes, ranging from serious problems of pregnancy and musculoskeletal pain to exacerbation of a previous painful syndrome. For nonpregnant patients with pain, an array of treatments can be offered, including medications and interventions. However, the effects of these options upon the developing fetus are not well known.[1]

Approximately half of pregnant women will experience low back pain during pregnancy. In approximately one-third of all pregnancies, the pain is so severe that daily activities are affected.[2] In fact, back pain is so common in pregnancy that many obstetricians consider it a normal finding of pregnancy.[3] An obstetrician should be involved in evaluating the patient in order to exclude the dangerous diagnoses, such as preterm labor, miscarriage, placental abruption, and chorioamnionitis. Urologic disorders, such as renal calculi, hydronephrosis, and pyelonephrosis, are also common and must be ruled out.[4]

Lumbar lordosis is exaggerated during pregnancy as the weight of the uterus shifts the center of gravity forward. Low back pain in pregnant women can be categorized as pelvic girdle pain (PGP) or lumbar pain (LP). PGP is four times as likely in pregnant women as LP.[5] It is described as deep, stabbing, recurrent or continuous pain, and presents between the posterior iliac crest and the gluteal fold. It can occasionally radiate to the posterolateral thigh to the knee and calf.[6] LP tends to present over the lumbar spine, above the sacrum. Tenderness over the paravertebral muscles may also be present and the pain may also radiate into the lower extremities. Despite the radiating symptoms, acute herniated nucleus pulposus is very rare during pregnancy.[7] It is thought that fetal compression of lumbosacral nerves is the cause of the radiculitis. A thorough neurologic examination must be a part of the physical examination. Unilateral change in reflex, motor, or sensory exam is indicative of nerve root involvement. One must also consider sacroiliac pain in the pregnant population. Unilateral low back pain well localized over the sacroiliac joint suggests sacroiliitis, likely secondary to ligamentous laxity of the superior portion of the joint.

Back pain usually starts halfway into pregnancy and is worst in the last trimester.[5] Unfortunately, one in six women has persistent pain even 6 years after pregnancy.[8] It is possible that the polypeptide relaxin contributes to this ongoing back pain. The peptide is produced to soften the ligaments of the pelvic joints and cervix; however, its effect translates onto musculoskeletal joints and may cause hypermobility of the low back.[8]

Abdominal pain during pregnancy is of great concern and should be evaluated immediately. The most urgent concerns are miscarriage, ovarian torsion, or ectopic pregnancy, all of which require evaluation by an obstetrician. Once these potential sources of pain are ruled out, other myofascial causes of pain should be considered. For one, the growing uterus can stretch the round ligaments. Should this occur too quickly, a hematoma can form, often presenting as pain radiating into the pubic tubercle.[9] Safe oral analgesics and bed rest are the treatments of choice. Another painful syndrome of the growing uterus is tearing of the rectus abdominis muscle, or overstretching of the abdominal wall causing hematoma formation. Ultrasonography can be helpful in diagnosing hematoma formation. Again, heat and bed rest are the treatments of choice. The typical time period for pain caused by abrupt stretching of the uterus is typically within 16 to 20 weeks of gestation.[9]

DIAGNOSTICS

Diagnosis is usually through history and physical examination in the pregnant patient, and radiation exposure is to be avoided unless necessary. The main concerns are an increased risk of congenital malformations and increased risk of cancer later in life for the fetus.[10] However, certain situations allow for radiation exposure if the mother's safety is in question, such as presentation of cauda equina syndrome. Other reasons to use imaging modalities are to diagnose possible broken bones or destructive lesions of bones. The mother and fetus should be exposed to radiation only when the benefits outweigh the risks. The threshold at which a fetus will develop a malformation is thought to be around 100 mGy; however, the risk of developing cancer later in life can occur with any dose of radiation.[10]

CT and X-rays are not ideal during pregnancy. With the advent of MRI, it has become possible to image without exposing patients to radiation. Although it is theoretically safe, there are no long-term studies evaluating the risk of adverse effects of MRI on pregnancy.[11] EMG (electromyography) is an alternative diagnostic tool that does not require radiation when a patient has new-onset low back pain with sensory or motor symptoms.

TREATMENT

The treatment of low back pain in all pregnant patients first starts with conservative measures. Activity adjustments and education about ergonomics are ideal to start with, typically with evaluation by a physical therapist. In some cases, braces may be helpful to help with posture. There is some evidence that acupuncture may be useful for treating pain in pregnant women[12] and can be used as an adjunct with physical therapy.

If conservative measures fail, it may be necessary to prescribe medications. During pregnancy, attempts should be made to minimize the number of medications taken by the expectant mother. However, in some cases, medical therapy may be necessary. When administering or prescribing a medication to a pregnant patient, the degree of medication exposure to the fetus must be considered. Factors such as protein binding, lipid solubility, rate of metabolism by the mother, molecular weight, and polarity of the medication all affect the amount transferred across the placenta. Typically, large, ionized, water-soluble drugs with high protein binding have a lower rate of crossing the placenta. Almost all medications will pass through the placenta to some degree.[13]

Although complications secondary to medication intake can arise at any point during pregnancy, the most critical period is early in pregnancy, when organogenesis is occurring. The period after conception, known as the "all-or-none" period (the first 2 to 4 weeks after conception), is when the fetus either develops without abnormality or is spontaneously aborted.[13] The remainder of the first trimester is critical for anatomic and organ development, and medications can potentially have a teratogenic effects.[13] After the first trimester, once organogenesis is complete, drug exposure is more likely to cause single-organ problems, developmental issues, or intrauterine growth restriction (IUGR).[14]

NSAIDS AND ACETAMINOPHEN

NSAIDs are one of the most commonly used medications in the treatment of pain. They decrease pain by acting as nonselective cyclooxygenase inhibitors, disrupting the function of prostaglandin synthetase, thereby decreasing the production of prostaglandins.[15] However, prostaglandins play a significant role in the physiology of pregnancy at multiple stages. For example, prostaglandins are known to stimulate uterine activity, maintain patency of the fetal ductus arteriosus, and promote fetal urine production.[15] The ductus arteriosus is a vessel connecting the main pulmonary trunk with the descending aorta, and it is essential during fetal life to shunt blood away from the high-resistance pulmonary circulation. Ductal closure in utero may lead to fetal demise and/or pulmonary hypertension. After birth, the ductus normally constricts within 96 hours due to a drop in circulating prostaglandin E2 levels.[16] Previous studies have demonstrated that using indomethacin for more than 48 hours in the third trimester of pregnancy may be associated with narrowing of the ductus arteriosus[17] and oligohydramnios.[18] Currently, the general recommendation is that women avoid NSAIDs during the first trimester of pregnancy, and if they are taken, they should be stopped by 30 to 32 weeks of gestation. Furthermore, if NSAID use is necessary, it is recommended that its use be for a short duration, less than 48 to 72 hours, and ideally delivery should not occur within 48 hours of NSAID intake.[18] Nonpharmacologic management or acetaminophen is recommended as first-line therapy for pain during pregnancy before the consideration of NSAIDs. If pain control is inadequate, the use of mild opioids may be considered next. If the symptoms are not controlled with this, an NSAID or aspirin may be considered; however, close fetal monitoring during the second trimester must be instituted if high doses are required.[1] Fetal echocardiography should be utilized to monitor amniotic fluid volume and patency of the ductus arteriosus.

Aspirin is another nonspecific cyclooxygenase inhibitor occasionally used for pain control, and it is known to inhibit platelet function. Therefore, aspirin intake around the time of labor may increase the risk of peripartum hemorrhage and may inhibit neonatal platelet function for several days after birth.[19] Furthermore, higher doses (> 81 mg/day) of aspirin have been shown to increase the risk of intracranial hemorrhage in neonates who are born prior to 35 weeks' gestation,[20] while lower doses have no had such an association.[20] In certain cases, such as pre-eclampsia and antiphospholipid syndrome, low-dose aspirin (60–150 mg/day) has been shown to improve outcomes.[21] Furthermore, it can modestly reduce the risks of preterm birth, IUGR, and possibly perinatal mortality.[21] Conversely, retrospective meta-analyses have demonstrated a link between aspirin exposure and gastroschisis, but this remains an uncertain finding.[22] Overall, low- dose aspirin has not been shown to increase the risk of poor outcomes during pregnancy, and it may have a significant protective effect.[21] Whether aspirin can or should be used for pain control during pregnancy has yet to be determined.

Acetaminophen has similar analgesic potency to aspirin, but it is not a salicylate[23] or an NSAID. It appears to be a safe medication during all stages of pregnancy in standard doses, and it appears to be efficacious in treating pain. In a study of thousands of women who used acetaminophen, no increase in risk of congenital abnormalities or adverse pregnancy outcomes was seen.[24]

OPIOIDS

When acetaminophen and conservative measures have failed to control pain in a pregnant woman, it may be reasonable to consider an opioid. Medications in this category include morphine, hydromorphone, hydrocodone, codeine, oxycodone, meperidine, and synthetic analogues, such as tramadol. Epidemiologic data from chronic opioid and illicit drug users who became pregnant suggest an association with low birth weight and decreased head circumference in the neonate.[25] However, the Collaborative Perinatal Project identified 448 morphine exposures at various stages of pregnancy and no increased risk of teratogenesis was found.[26] Prior to the 2015 FDA (U.S. Food and Drug Administration) labeling change, all opioids were teratogenic risk category C when used acutely, and risk category D when used chronically; the increased risk is due to the possibility of neonatal opioid dependence with prolonged use[1] (Table 34.1).

The FDA has now instituted a gradual change in labeling requirements, and in place of letter categories, there will be descriptive subsections defining the pregnancy and lactation exposure and risk. The fetus of an opioid-dependent mother is at risk of withdrawal if the opioid is abruptly stopped, and abrupt cessation can even result in fetal death.[27] Therefore, patients on opioids should not stop the medication without supervision. If the patient is addicted or abusing opioids, it is suggested that she be monitored on methadone or buprenorphine in a treatment program.[28] After delivery and for a few days thereafter, a neonate may be opioid dependent and exhibit signs of withdrawal. These symptoms may range from irritability to seizures. The term for this condition is *neonatal abstinence syndrome* (NAS), and NAS usually manifests within 48 hours of birth.[29]

A commonly prescribed opioid for chronic pain is the fentanyl patch; however, there is very little information about its use in pregnancy. One case report documented 125 μg/hr throughout pregnancy, and the newborn had mild withdrawal symptoms 24 to 72 hours after birth.[30] The safety of fentanyl patches in pregnancy is still not known.

Buprenorphine is an interesting opioid because its unique pharmacology as a competitive partial μ-opioid receptor agonist and a partial κ-opioid receptor antagonist.[31] As a result, buprenorphine has a ceiling effect, diminishes dysphoria, and inhibits other opioids from binding to the μ-opioid receptor. In 2000, it became the only opioid that physicians could legally prescribe for opioid addiction, but despite its unique pharmacology, buprenorphine has largely failed to overtake methadone in managing addiction.[32] In pregnancy, however, the data may indicate some advantages to the use of buprenorphine. A randomized double-blind comparison between the two medications in neonates of mothers using one of the two medications showed that neonates exposed to methadone had a higher morphine requirement and had a longer period of NAS.[33] The number of neonates requiring NAS treatment and their peak NAS scores were not significantly different in the two groups. Another advantage is that buprenorphine does not readily cross into breast milk and is poorly available orally. Therefore, it is safer for the neonates of breastfeeding mothers. Despite this, the drug manufacturer does not recommend buprenorphine during breastfeeding.[34]

Tramadol is a synthetic analog of codeine that is commonly used to treat mild to moderate somatic pain, visceral pain, and neuropathic pain. Given its pharmacology, its abuse potential is low.[35] During its phase 1 to 3 clinical trials, pregnant and breastfeeding women were excluded from studies. Therefore, little is known about its effect on pregnant or lactating women. At this time, it is recommended that women be advised against using tramadol during the first trimester of pregnancy.[35] Currently, there is insufficient evidence regarding the medication's safety or risk during pregnancy. If the medication has been used during pregnancy, one must be cognizant of neonatal withdrawal syndrome.

BENZODIAZEPINES

The data on the effects of benzodiazepines on pregnancy are mixed. Initially, diazepam in the first trimester was associated with cleft palate and cleft lip. Later, large epidemiologic studies looking at population data from before and after the introduction of diazepam to the public showed no change in the rates of these malformations.[36] The same epidemiologic studies confirmed the association between diazepam and congenital inguinal hernias. The cause of the mixed data is unknown, but it may be due to a higher prevalence of alcohol and illicit drug use in those taking benzodiazepines. Neonatal withdrawal after birth is well documented in those exposed to benzodiazepines in utero.[37] Furthermore, diazepam and its active metabolites are known to linger in a neonate's circulation up to 10 days after a single maternal dose, due to the drug's limited metabolism in infants.[38] In general, it is best to avoid all benzodiazepines during pregnancy and lactation.

Table 34.1. **FOOD AND DRUG ADMINISTRATION DRUG CATEGORIES FOR PREGNANCY RISK**

FDA CLASSIFICATION[a]	DEFINITION	EXAMPLES
Category A	Controlled human studies indicate no apparent risk to fetus. The possibility of harm to the fetus seems remote.	Multivitamins
Category B	Animal studies do not indicate a fetal risk or animal studies do indicate a teratogenic risk but well-controlled human studies have failed to demonstrate a risk.	Acetaminophen Caffeine Metoprolol Prednisolone, prednisone
Category C	Studies indicate teratogenic or embryocidal risk in animals, but no controlled studies have been done in women or there are no controlled studies in animals or humans.	Aspirin, ketorolac, ibuprofen, naproxen, indomethacin[b] Butorphanol, nalbuphine[c] Codeine, propoxyphene, fentanyl, hydrocodone, methadone, meperidine, morphine, oxycodone, oxymorphone[c] Gabapentin, pregabalin Fluoxetine, duloxetine Lidocaine, mexiletene Nifedipine Propranolol Sumatriptan
Category D	Positive evidence of human fetal risk, but in certain circumstances, the benefits of the drug may outweigh the risks involved.	Amitriptyline, imipramine Diazepam Paroxetine Phenobarbital Phenytoin Valproic acid
Category X	Positive evidence of significant fetal risk, and risk clearly outweighs any possible benefit.	Ergotamine

[a] Adapted from the Food and Drug Administration website: www.fda.gov/Drugs/DrugSafety (prior to FDA classification change).

[b] All NSAIDs are Risk Category D after 30 weeks of gestation.

[c] All opioid analgesics are Risk Category D if used for prolonged periods or in large doses near term.

ANTIEPILEPTICS

Gabapentin and pregabalin are now commonly used antiepileptic medications for the treatment of neuropathic pain. Although other anticonvulsants, such as valproate, are known teratogens, the effects of the newer drugs are currently under investigation. Gabapentin and pregabalin are designed to treat partial seizures and are gamma-aminobutyric acid analogs.[39] The European Gabapentin Registry looked at prospective and retrospective data from pregnant women with epilepsy and other disorders where gabapentin was the treatment of choice. Data from a total of 51 outcomes and 44 live births were obtained, and two major malformations were detected in infants exposed to gabapentin in the first trimester.[40] More recently, the North American Antiepileptic Drug (AED) Pregnancy Registry documented one major malformation in 145 fetuses in the registry.[41] Similarly, the effects of pregabalin are currently unknown, and it is categorized as FDA pregnancy risk C.

Another commonly used medication is topiramate. Epidemiologic information from 1997 to 2009 from the National Birth Defects Prevention Study (NBDPS) compared first-trimester topiramate monotherapy to no antiepileptic drug use. The study found that the risk of developing cleft lip or palate was five times higher in the population that used topiramate than in the group that did not.[42]

Finally, carbamazepine has a role in chronic pain conditions, most famously trigeminal neuralgia, but other uses include treatments for bipolar disorder and seizures. There are mixed data on the use of this medication during pregnancy. A review in 2008 concluded that, when used alone, carbamazepine has one of the lower risks of teratogenicity among antiepileptic drugs.[43] The review summarized nine studies, and only one of the nine showed a significant increase in the relative risk of congenital malformations in the newborns of mothers taking the medication.

ANTIDEPRESSANTS

The use of antidepressants has risen dramatically and they are very widely used for the treatment of depression, anxiety, and chronic pain states, such as migraines. Initially, selective serotonin reuptake inhibitors (SSRIs) were thought to be safe and were considered class B during pregnancy; however, more recent epidemiologic reports indicate that there may be a risk of congenital abnormalities and NAS associated with paroxetine intake during pregnancy.[44] Among 3,581 patients exposed to paroxetine or other antidepressants during the first trimester of pregnancy, there was an increased risk for overall major congenital malformations, including major cardiovascular malformations, in infants of mothers taking paroxetine. Furthermore, seizures and jitteriness have been documented in newborns of mothers who took paroxetine late in pregnancy.[45] It is important to note that, although the relative risk increase with paroxetine was found to be significant, the overall rates of the congenital abnormalities were low; as such, the absolute risk increase may be small. Another review in 2013 of over 1.6 million births in Nordic countries from 1996 to 2007 found that there was no significant increase in the rate of stillbirth, neonatal mortality, or postneonatal mortality in cases where mothers took SSRIs during pregnancy.[46] Given the conflicting information, it is getting progressively more challenging for providers to decide on how to prescribe antidepressants.

Older antidepressants, such as tricyclic antidepressants (TCAs), play an important role in chronic pain management. Examples include nortriptyline and amitriptyline, which are categorized as pregnancy risk group D. Most of the data surrounding this assignment have been derived from studies mammals, but convincing data are not available for humans.[20]

In terms of lactating women, again there is insufficient data to assess the risk of taking these medications while breastfeeding. TCAs do not accumulate to a great degree in breast milk; however, it is important to note that neonatal metabolism of the medications may be different from that of adults, and accumulation may still occur.[47] Overall, the risk is unknown and no recommendation can be made. The physician should weigh the risks and benefits in a case-by-case manner.

Special consideration should be given to duloxetine, a serotonin–norepinephrine reuptake inhibitor that is effective in the treatment of neuropathic pain. It is currently categorized as group C for pregnancy risk. In 2013, Hoog et al. reported on 400 cases of duloxetine exposure during pregnancy for which outcomes were available. The cases were obtained through the Eli Lilly Safety System database. Most women received duloxetine for depression. Within the study, the women who had abnormal outcomes (spontaneous abortions, premature births, congenital malformations) were also more likely to be taking unsafe medications, such as benzodiazepines, NSAIDs, and anticonvulsants, and were also more likely to have past or current history of medical issues, such as miscarriage, smoking, and substance abuse.[48] The pharmaceutical company advises against duloxetine use during breastfeeding, although there are minimal data for or against its use during this period.

MIGRAINES

The clinician is often confronted with headache in a pregnant patient, as recurring headaches happen most commonly during the childbearing years. Migraine can be a disabling disorder that is more prevalent among women than men, which is thought to be due in part to the influence of female sex hormones. Migraine headaches vary with female reproductive events, including menarche, menstruation, oral contraceptive use, pregnancy, and menopause.[49] Eighty percent of female migraineurs report the onset of migraine during the ages of 10 to 39 years, suggesting that the sex hormones do play a significant role in the pathogenesis.[50] Migraines typically improve in the first trimester of pregnancy, when there is a sudden and sustained increase in estradiol levels. In fact, 50% to 80% of patients who suffer from migraines experience a significant reduction in frequency or total cessation of migraine attacks during pregnancy. However, women with headaches persisting into the second trimester are less likely to improve thereafter.

For pregnant women with a history of migraines prior to pregnancy and a normal neurologic examination, the therapeutic challenge is to achieve control of the headaches while minimizing risk to the fetus. Nonpharmacologic techniques, including relaxation, biofeedback, and elimination of certain foods, often suffice for treatment. If pharmacologic therapy appears warranted, acetaminophen with or without caffeine (both category B rated) is safe and effective.[51] A drawback to acetaminophen is the potential for medication overuse and rebound headache, which could develop into daily chronic headaches. Ibuprofen and naproxen are the most commonly used NSAIDs for abortive management of migraines; however, they carry a category C risk rating prior to 30 weeks and a category D rating in the third trimester. Like acetaminophen, NSAIDS are safe in the postpartum period with breastfeeding. The short-term use of mild opioid analgesics like hydrocodone, alone or in combination with acetaminophen, also appears to carry little risk.

Most patients with refractory migraines are treated with ergotamine and triptans. Ergot preparations should be avoided during pregnancy and lactation. Ergotamines are known to cause uterine contractions, spontaneous abortions, and teratogenesis[52] and their use during lactation is known to cause neonatal convulsions.[20] The alternative group of medications, the triptans, do not appear to increase the risk of birth defects compared to the risk in the general population.[53] To date, multiple comparative studies and systematic reviews have shown no difference in the reporting of major malformations between women who took or did not take triptans during pregnancy.[54–58] Thus far, triptans have been deemed safe and are categorized as class C. The effects of sumatriptan on lactation and breastfeeding are currently unknown. However, the medication does not freely cross into breast milk, and gastrointestinal absorption in neonates is low.[53]

LACTATION AND BREASTFEEDING

Much like placental drug transfer, drug accumulation in breast milk is affected by the physical properties of the drugs. Large, ionized molecules with high protein binding and low lipid solubility are much less likely to accumulate in breast milk. However, it is critical to keep in mind that neonates may have much slower metabolism of certain medications, and medications may accumulate in their systems, even at low doses. For example, salicylates cross into breast milk in very small amounts due to high ionization and high protein binding. However, neonates have very slow elimination of salicylates.[59] Therefore, salicylate intake by mothers can lead to rashes, platelet abnormalities, and bleeding in nursing infants. The majority of breast milk is produced and stored immediately after feeding. Avoiding medications immediately after breastfeeding and avoiding long-acting medications in general are the best way to reduce drug transfer into breast milk.[60]

EPIDURAL STEROID INJECTIONS

There are currently no recommendations for or against epidural steroid injections in a pregnant patient. What is known is that women with acute disk pathology and radiculopathy respond the best to epidural steroid injections.[61] The dose of steroid in a single epidural injection is unlikely to affect the fetus.[1] Therefore, it is generally agreed that pregnant patients with acute radiculopathy can receive an epidural steroid injection for treatment.[62] However, one should avoid using radiation in performing the procedure; alternative modalities are ultrasound guidance or use of anatomic landmarks.

CONCLUSIONS

Overall, the prognosis for a pregnant woman is that her pain symptoms will improve.[63] It is thought that approximately 20% of women will continue to have pain after pregnancy.[64] Being able to evaluate and assess a pregnant patient with pain, and having thorough knowledge about treatment options, will help the clinician provide the best care possible for these patients.

- Almost all women will experience pain during pregnancy and lactation. Low back pain can be categorized as LP or PGP.
- Low back pain typically starts halfway through the pregnancy and is worst in the last trimester. One in six women will have persistent pain after pregnancy.
- If diagnostic studies are required for the evaluation of pain, radiation exposure should be avoided, weighing the risks and benefits.
- Treatment should always begin with conservative therapy and then the use of acetaminophen. Opioids can be used for short time periods, but with prolonged use, the fetus can become physiologically dependent and suffer from NAS.
- NSAIDs disrupt prostaglandin synthesis and can interfere with uterine activity, the fetal ductus arteriosus, and fetal urine production. They should be avoided in the first trimester as well as from 30 to 32 weeks until birth. NSAIDs are considered safe in breastfeeding and lactation.
- Ergot preparations should be avoided in lactation and pregnancy because they are known to cause uterine contractions, spontaneous abortions, teratogenesis, and neonatal convulsions.

REFERENCES

1. Nagpal G, Rathmell JP. Managing pain during pregnancy and lactation. In: Benton HT, Rathmell JR, Wu CL, Turk DC, Argoff CE, Hurley RW, eds. *Practical Management of Pain.* 5th ed. Philadelphia, PA: Elsevier Mosby; 2014:474–490.
2. Mogren I, Pohjanen A. Low back pain and pelvic pain during pregnancy: prevalence and risk factors. *Spine.* 2005;30:983–991.
3. Mack KA, Jones CM, Paulozzi LJ. Vital signs: overdoses of prescription opioid pain relievers and other drugs among women—United States, 1999–2010. *MMWR,* 2013;62(26):537–542.
4. Roy C, Sussine C, LeBras Y, et al. Assessment of painful ureterohydronephrosis during pregnancy by MR urography. *Eur Radiol.* 1996;334–338.
5. Katonis P, Kampouroglou A, et al. Pregnancy-related low back pain. *Hippokratia.* 2011;15(3):205–210.
6. Ostgaard HC, Zetherstrom G, Roos-Hansson E, Svanberg B. Reduction of back and posterior pelvic pain in pregnancy. *Spine.* 1994;19:894–900.
7. LaBan MM, Perrin JCS, Latimer FR. Pregnancy and the herniated lumbar disc. *Arch Phys Med Rehabil.* 1983;64:319–321.
8. Gutke A, Ostgaard H, Oberg B. Predicting persistent pregnancy related low back pain. *Spine.* 2008;33:386–393.
9. Chamberlain G. ABC of antenatal care: abdominal pain in pregnancy. *Br Med J.* 1991;302:1390–1394.
10. Akintomide AO, Ikpeme AA. Radiation safety of women of the reproductive age: evaluation of the role of referring physicians. *J Family Med Prim Care.* 2014;3(3):243–246.
11. Kanal E. Pregnancy and the safety of magnetic resonance imaging. *Magn Reson Imaging Clin North Am.* 1994;2:309–317.
12. Pennick V, Liddle SD. Interventions for preventing and treating pelvic and back pain in pregnancy. *Cochrane Database Systematic Rev.* 2013;8:CD001139.
13. Rice SA. Anaesthesia in pregnancy and the fetus: toxicology aspects. In: Reynolds F, ed. *Effects on the Baby of Maternal Analgesia and Anaesthesia.* London: Saunders; 1993:88–89.
14. Niebyl JR. Nonanesthetic drugs during pregnancy and lactation. In: Chestnut DH, ed. *Obstetric Anesthesia: Principles and Practice.* St. Louis, MO: Mosby; 1994:229–240.
15. Antonucci R, Zaffanello M, Puxeddu E, et al. Use of non-steroidal anti-inflammatory drugs in pregnancy: impact on the fetus and newborn. *Curr Drug Metab.* 2012;13(4):474–490.
16. Van Overmeire B, Chemtob S. The pharmacologic closure of the patent ductus arteriosus. *Semin Fetal Neonatal Med.* 2005;10(2):177–184.
17. Moise KJ, Huhta JC, Sharif DS, et al. Indomethacin in the treatment of premature labor: effects on the fetal ductus arteriosus. *N Engl J Med.* 1988;319:327–331.
18. Goffinet F. Indomethacin: come back of a controversial tocolytic? Obstetrical point of view. *Arch Pediatr.* 2010;Suppl 3:S105–S109.
19. Werler MM, Mitchell AA, Moore CA, Honein MA. Is there epidemiologic evidence to support vascular disruption as a pathogenesis of gastroschisis? *Am J Med Genet A.* 2009;149A(7):1399–1406.
20. Briggs GG, Freeman RK, Yaffe SJ. *Drugs in Pregnancy and Lactation.* Baltimore, MD: Williams & Wilkins; 1990.
21. Henderson JT, Whitlock EP, O'Connor E, et al. Low-dose aspirin for the prevention of morbidity and mortality from preeclampsia—a systematic evidence review for the US Preventive Services Task Force. *Ann Intern Med.* 2014;160(10):695–703.
22. Werler M, Sheehan J, Mitchell A. Maternal medication use and risks of gastroschisis and small intestinal atresia. *Am J Epidemiol.* 2002;155:26–31.
23. Babb M, Koren G, Einarson A. Treating pain during pregnancy. *Can Fam Physician.* 2010;56(1):25–27.
24. Rebordosa C, Kogevinas M, Bech BH, Sorensen HT, Olsen J. Use of acetaminophen during pregnancy and risk of adverse pregnancy outcomes. *Int J Epidemiol.* 2009;38(3):706–714.

25. MacGregor SN. Drug addiction and pregnancy. In: Dilts PV, Sciarra JJ, eds. *Gynecology and Obstetrics*. Philadelphia, PA: Lippincott; 1976:1–18.
26. Heinonen OP, Slone D, Shapiro S. *Birth Defects and Drugs in Pregnancy*. Littleton, MA: Publishing Sciences Group; 1977.
27. Rementeria JL, Nunaq NN. Narcotic withdrawal in pregnancy: stillbirth incidence with a case report. *Am J Obstet Gynecol.* 1973;116:1153–1156.
28. Rayburn WF, Bogenschutz MP. Pharmacotherapy for pregnant women with addictions. *Am J Obstet Gynecol.* 2004;191:1885–1897.
29. Zelson M, Lee SJ, Casalino M. Neonatal narcotic addiction. *N Engl J Med.* 1973;289:1216–1220.
30. Regan J, Chambers F, Gorman W, MacSullivan R. Neonatal abstinence syndrome due to prolonged administration of fentanyl in pregnancy. *BJOG.* 2000;107(4):570–572.
31. Lutfy K, Cowan A. Buprenorphine: a unique drug with complex pharmacology. *Curr Neuropharmacol.* 2004;2(4):395–402.
32. Whelan PJ, Remski K. Buprenorphine vs methadone treatment: A review of evidence in both developed and developing worlds. *J Neurosci Rural Pract.* 2012;3(1):45–50.
33. Jones H, Kaltenbach K, Heil S. Neonatal abstinence syndrome after methadone or buprenorphine exposure. *N Engl J Med.* 2010;363:2320–2330.
34. Alto W, O'Connor A. Management of women treated with buprenorphine during pregnancy. *Am J Obstet Gynecol.* 2011;205:302–308.
35. Bloor M, Paech MJ, Kaye R. Tramadol in pregnancy and lactation. *Int J Obstet Anesth.* 2012;21(2):163–167.
36. Rosenberg L, Mitchell AA, Parsells JA, et al. Lack of relation of oral clefts to diazepam use during pregnancy. *N Engl J Med.* 1983;309:1282–1285.
37. Athinarayanan P, Pierog SH, Nigm SK, et al. Chlordiazepoxide withdrawal in the neonate. *Am J Obstet Gynecol.* 1976;124:212–213.
38. Erkolla R, Kanto J. Diazepam and breast-feeding. *Lancet.* 1972;1:1235–1236.
39. Fujii H, Goel A, Bernard N, et al. Pregnancy outcomes following gabapentin use. *Neurology.* 2013;80:1565–1570.
40. Montouris G. Gabapentin exposure in human pregnancy: results from the Gabapentin Pregnancy Registry. *Epilepsy Behav.* 2003;4:310–317.
41. Hernandez-Diaz S, Smith CR, Shen A, et al. Comparative safety of antiepileptic drugs during pregnancy. *Neurology.* 2012;78:1692–1699.
42. Margulis AV, Mitchell AA, Gilboa SM, et al. Use of topiramate in pregnancy and risk of oral clefts. *Am J Obstet Gynecol.* 2012;5:405.e1–405.e7.
43. Eadie MJ. Antiepileptic drugs as human teratogens. *Expert Opin Drug Safety.* 2008;7(2):195–209.
44. Williams M, Wooltorton E. Paroxetine (Paxil) and congenital malformations. *CMAJ.* 2005;173:1320–1321.
45. Moses-Kolko EL, Bogen D, Perel J, et al. Neonatal signs after late in utero exposure to serotonin reuptake inhibitors: literature review and implications for clinical applications. *JAMA.* 2005;293:2372–2385.
46. Stephansson O, Kieler H, Haglund B, et al. Selective serotonin reuptake inhibitors during pregnancy and risk of stillbirth and infant mortality. *JAMA.* 2013;309(1):48–54.
47. Wisner KL, Perel JM, Findling RL. Antidepressant treatment during breast-feeding. *Am J Psychiatry.* 1996;153:1132–1137.
48. Hoog SL, Cheng Y, Elpers J, et al. Duloxetine and pregnancy outcomes: safety surveillance findings. *Int J Med Sci.* 2013;10(4):413–419.
49. Kvisvik EV, Stovner LJ, Helde G, Bovim G, Linde M. Headache and migraine during pregnancy and puerperium: the MIGRA study. *J Headache Pain.* 2011;12(4):433–451.
50. Menon R, Bushnell C. Headache and pregnancy. *Neurologist.* 2008;14:108–119.
51. Silverstein SD. Headaches and women: treatment of the pregnant and lactating migraineur. *Headache.* 1993;33:533–540.
52. Hainline B. Neurologic complications of pregnancy: headache. *Neurol Clin.* 1994;12:443–460.
53. Duong S, Bozzo P, Nordeng H, Einarson A. Safety of triptans for migraine headaches during pregnancy and breastfeeding. *Can Fam Physician.* 2010;56(6):537–539.
54. Kallen B, Lygner PE. Delivery outcome in women who use drugs for migraine during pregnancy with special reference to sumatriptan. *Headache.* 2001;41(4):351–356.
55. O'Quinn S, Ephross SA, Williams V, Davis RL, et al. Pregnancy and perinatal outcomes in migraineurs using sumatriptan: a prospective study. *Arch Gynecol Obstet.* 1999;263(1-2):7–12.
56. Shuhaiber S, Pastuszak A, Schick B, Matsui D, et al. Pregnancy outcome following first trimester exposure to sumatriptan. *Neurology.* 1998;51(2):581–583.
57. Fox AW, Chambers CD, Anderson PO, Diamond ML, Spierings EL. Evidence-based assessment of pregnancy outcome after sumatriptan exposure. *Headache.* 2002;42(1):8–15.
58. Loder E. Safety of sumatriptan in pregnancy: a review of data so far. *CNS Drugs.* 2003;17(1):1–7.
59. Levy G, Garrettson JK. Kinetics of salicylate elimination by newborn infants of mothers who ingested aspirin before delivery. *Pediatrics.* 1974;62:201–220.
60. Vorherr H. Drug excretion in breast milk. *Postgrad Med.* 1974;5:97–104.
61. Benzon HT. Epidural steroid injections for low back pain and lumbosacral radiculopathy. *Pain.* 1986;24(3):277–295.
62. Shah S, Banh ET, Koury K, Bhatia G, Nandi R, Gulur P. Pain management in pregnancy: multimodal approaches. *Pain Res Treat.* 2015;987483.
63. Sabino J, Grauer JN. Pregnancy and low back pain. *Curr Rev Musculoskelet Med.* 2008;1(2):137–141.
64. Noren L, Ostgaard S, Johansson G, Ostgaard C. Lumbar back and posterior pelvic pain during pregnancy: a 3-year follow up. *Eur Spine J.* 2002;11(3):267–271.

REVIEW QUESTIONS

1. A 32-weeks-pregnant patient comes to your office complaining of new-onset low back pain with radiating pain into the right lower extremity. She had a similar episode a few years ago and used meloxicam. She asks for a refill of this medication. Intrauterine exposure to NSAIDs is associated with which of the following problems?

   A. Cleft palate
   B. Spina bifida
   C. Premature labor
   D. Oligohydramnios

2. A 12-weeks-pregnant patient is referred to your clinic from her obstetrician because she has an addiction to oxycodone. The patient states it started with poorly controlled low back pain and she now buys the drug from friends. She agrees with your plan to start sublingual buprenorphine/naloxone. Buprenorphine is an excellent opioid for the treatment of addiction because:

   A. It is a partial μ-opioid receptor agonist.
   B. It is a partial κ-opioid receptor antagonist.
   C. It competes with the binding of other opioids.
   D. All of the above.

3. The same patient in Question 2 now presents for her weekly appointment with her obstetrician at 37 weeks. The fetus is determined to be in the breech position and cesarean delivery section is scheduled at 38 weeks. The patient has continued buprenorphine/naloxone 8 mg/3mg since she was 12 weeks pregnant. What concern does this treatment cause?

A. Inappropriate surgical level with spinal anesthesia
B. Risk of NAS for the newborn
C. Greater sensitivity of the μ-receptors to intrathecal and intravenous opioids
D. Delayed emergence from general anesthesia

ANSWERS

1. D. During pregnancy, prostaglandins modulate many key processes, including stimulation of uterine activity, maintaining patency of the ductus arteriosus, and promoting fetal urine production. NSAIDs decrease pain by acting as nonselective cyclooxygenase inhibitors, disrupting the function of prostaglandin synthetase and thereby decreasing the production of prostaglandins. With reduced renal output from the fetus, oligohydramnios will result.

2. D. Buprenorphine is an interesting opioid because of its unique pharmacology as a competitive partial μ-opioid receptor agonist and a partial κ-opioid receptor antagonist. This results in an opioid that has a ceiling effect, diminishes dysphoria, and inhibits other opioids from binding to the μ-opioid receptor.

3. B. After delivery and for a few days thereafter, a neonate may be opioid dependent and exhibit signs of withdrawal. These symptoms may range from irritability to seizures. The term for this condition is *neonatal abstinence syndrome* (NAS), and NAS usually manifest within 48 hours. This is a risk with all chronic opioid use during pregnancy. The use of buprenorphine will not affect spinal anesthesia. Buprenorphine is a competitive, partial agonist so it will decrease binding of all opioids to the μ-receptor, making pain management more difficult during the perioperative period.

QUESTIONS AND ANSWERS

This chapter has accompanying questions and answers that are available to subscribers as part of the Oxford eLearning platform. To access the questions, follow the link below, or go to http://oxfordmedicine.com/painmanagementreview

35.

BUPIVACAINE AND GLUCOCORTICOID-INDUCED MYONECROSIS

David Gordon, Ahmad Khattab, and Magdalena Anitescu

STEM CASE AND KEY QUESTIONS

A 25-year-old female is admitted to the hospital complaining of a severe headache. Her pain is generalized and throbbing, with a mild positional component, and the episodes are frequent. The pain is localized over the right supraorbital notch. The patient reports that she has eight to ten frontal headache episodes per week. She has a history of migraine headaches and posterior fossa decompression surgery for symptomatic Chiari malformation. She has been treated with occipital nerve blocks for ongoing occipital neuralgia caused by a long-standing ventriculoperitoneal shunt, but the new symptoms are severe and debilitating. Her occipital neuralgia has been well controlled in the past with oral medications, and she has never required hospitalization. She describes the current pain as a sharp, burning, cramping pain over the right supraorbital notch, superimposed on the occipital neuralgia. It is unresponsive to topiramate and sumatriptan.

WHAT DO YOU THINK IS HAPPENING? DOES SHE HAVE A MALFUNCTIONING SHUNT? WHAT MEDICATIONS MIGHT BE EFFECTIVE IN THIS SITUATION?

Because the headache responds to changes in body position, shunt malfunction with excessive drainage of cerebrospinal fluid is of concern. An oral regimen of butalbital-acetaminophen-caffeine is initiated. Relief of the generalized headache is partial, but there is no effect on the supraorbital and occipital pain.

WHAT SHOULD YOUR DIFFERENTIAL DIAGNOSIS INCLUDE? WHY IS THE OCCIPITAL PAIN, BUT NOT THE FRONTAL PAIN, RELIEVED? WHAT TESTS WOULD YOU ORDER?

Subsequent CT and MRI studies confirm severe intracranial hypotension from excessive shunt drainage. After adjustment of shunt settings, the positional headache improves. Right frontal burning and occipital paroxysmal pain continue. Physical examination of the patient reveals conjunctival injection, uncontrolled tearing, and rhinorrhea. Trigeminal autonomic cephalalgia (TAC) is suspected and the patient is given 100% oxygen via mask. Occipital neuralgia and the burning of the supraorbital pain improve. The patient complains of stabbing pain over the supraorbital notch consistent with neuralgia, likely an entrapment neuropathy of the supraorbital nerve.

WHAT ARE THE TREATMENT OPTIONS FOR THIS PATIENT? WOULD YOU CONSIDER PERFORMING A SUPRAORBITAL NERVE BLOCK? WHAT ARE THE RISKS AND BENEFITS OF THIS PROCEDURE? DO YOU DISCUSS THE COMMON RISKS, THE RARE ONES, OR BOTH? WHAT AGENTS WOULD YOU USE FOR THE BLOCK(S)?

The patient is informed of the risks of a supraorbital block: bleeding, infection, nerve injury, nerve damage, seizures, and cardiac arrhythmias. A right supraorbital nerve block is performed under ultrasound guidance. Triamcinolone 20 mg and 5 mL of 0.5% bupivacaine provide immediate relief of the patient's pain. Pain relief is sustained at 10 weeks' follow-up. At week 15 during a follow-up visit, the patient requests a repeat block.

WOULD YOU CONSIDER REPEATING THE BLOCK? WOULD YOU CHANGE THE SOLUTION INJECTED? WHAT OTHER ADVERSE EFFECTS OF GLUCOCORTICOID INJECTION SHOULD YOU INFORM THE PATIENT ABOUT? DOES THE GLUCOCORTICOID CHOSEN AFFECT THE RISK OF ADVERSE EFFECTS? WOULD YOU ADD ANY OTHER MEDICATIONS? IS ADDITIONAL WORKUP NEEDED?

The patient's occipital neuralgia has been under control with baclofen 10 mg three times a day. The generalized, throbbing pain is much improved after the shunt adjustment, but the supraorbital neuralgia is debilitating. She has a difficult time falling asleep and her graduate studies are affected. A repeat supraorbital nerve block with triamcinolone 40 mg and 6 mL of 0.25% bupivacaine relieves pain for only 6 weeks. At the follow-up visit, the patient again requests a supraorbital block. There are small areas of mild depigmentation and a barely visible asymmetry in her forehead. Given the possible risk of systemic uptake of the glucocorticoid with risk of infection, poor healing, and adrenal suppression, the patient agrees to a local anesthetic-only block. Under an ultrasound-guided technique, 8 mL of 0.5% bupivacaine is injected. The relief of pain is immediate and lasts about 4 weeks.

WHAT OTHER TREATMENTS MAY BE AVAILABLE? WOULD YOU CONSIDER DEPOT PREPARATIONS OF LOCAL ANESTHETIC? CONSIDER FREQUENT ADMINISTRATION OF STEROIDS AT LOW DOSES? PERIPHERAL NERVE STIMULATION? RADIOFREQUENCY ABLATION?

At a 6-week follow-up visit, the patient reports suffering from pain again. The patient refuses medications and insists on a fourth block. She mentions that the medications she has taken decreased her ability to function because of sedation, nausea, and dizziness. She experienced relief with the local anesthetic-only block and wants another one. Physical examination reveals a little depigmentation and a small depression on the right of her forehead, but she states that the depression is no worse than on the previous visit. Since the last steroid treatment was administered over 12 weeks ago, a repeat injection is now performed under ultrasound guidance using 40 mg of triamcinolone and 4 mL 0.5% bupivacaine.

GIVEN HER RESPONSE TO LOCAL ANESTHETIC ALONE, WOULD YOU ADVISE NERVE BLOCKS AT SHORTER, REGULAR INTERVALS WITH BUPIVACAINE OR WOULD YOU COUNSEL THE PATIENT DIFFERENTLY? IS THERE CONCERN ABOUT THE USE OF LOCAL ANESTHETIC AT AN INTERVAL OF 4 TO 6 WEEKS?

When the patient returns for follow-up in 4 weeks, her pain is well controlled. Now she is concerned about the large area of depigmentation and a visible indentation over the supraorbital notch and forehead measuring approximately 3 cm in diameter. She observed the lesion 1 week after the most recent block; it has continued to enlarge to its current size. The area of interest measures 4 cm long by 3 cm wide; the depression is 5 mm. The starting point of the lesion is the needle entry point over the supraorbital notch, and the lesion extends with irregular borders over most of the forehead on the right. The region is neither tender nor painful.

DO YOU THINK THE INDENTATION IS ANYTHING TO WORRY ABOUT? IS THE INDENTATION ASSOCIATED WITH YOUR INJECTIONS? DO YOU REPEAT THE BLOCK?

Because the mild depigmentation may be an effect of the glucocorticoid, a referral is made to dermatology. The dermatologist assures the patient that her condition is self-limiting and reversible, and most likely is associated with the local anesthetic rather than the glucocorticoid.

HOW WOULD YOU MANAGE THE PATIENT'S PAIN? DO YOU DISCLOSE THAT HER CONDITION IS ASSOCIATED WITH FREQUENT BUPIVACAINE INFILTRATIONS?

The patient's supraorbital pain returns 4 weeks after the visit, approximately 8 weeks after the last nerve block. In addition to her concern about the severe stabbing pain, the patient is now deeply concerned about her appearance. She reports instances of social rejection because of her appearance. The indentation appears to have stabilized; it is 5 cm in diameter and 8 mm deep. The surface is uneven and noticeable even with her hair overlapping the region. Depressed, the patient requests a plastic surgery consultation. Since the regeneration process takes long, the patient undergoes a fat transfer procedure, with excellent cosmetic results. Her pain, however, persists.

WHAT OPTIONS ARE AVAILABLE FOR SUPRAORBITAL ANALGESIA AT THIS POINT? WOULD YOU CONSIDER NEUROMODULATION AFTER THE RECENT FAT TRANSFER? WOULD YOU MODIFY YOUR DISCUSSION OF THE RISKS OF NEUROMODULATORY TECHNIQUES?

The patient's pain persists and is regularly accompanied by tears, rhinorrhea, and conjunctival injection. An oral analgesic regimen with membrane stabilizers, muscle relaxants, antidepressants, and a ketamine infusion provides 50% pain relief from the supraorbital neuralgia. The TAC symptoms are attenuated by a lidocaine infusion.

DISCUSSION

Multimodal analgesic regimens are the mainstay of treating chronic pain syndromes; oral medications are often combined with various interventional procedures to increase the efficacy of treatment. The most common medications used in pain clinics are local anesthetics and glucocorticoids, effective for a variety of conditions but accompanied by adverse effects. Many pain conditions are multifactorial, and the pain generator may change over time, although the distribution of pain is similar. Identifying new elements through history and physical examination is essential for an accurate differential diagnosis, and, ultimately, a comprehensive treatment plan.

LOCAL ANESTHETIC TOXICITY

Local anesthetics are widely used in clinical practice to relieve pain. Before obtaining consent for various procedures, physicians are required to discuss the risks and benefits of a procedure and to inform patients of the potential adverse effects of the medications injected. There are three types of local anesthetic toxicity: systemic toxicity, direct local anesthetic neurotoxicity, and myotoxicity. The most common and feared adverse event is local anesthetic systemic toxicity (LAST). Signs of central nervous system excitation, such as perioral numbness, tinnitus, and progression through a so-called "sense of impending doom," can progress quickly to seizures. The most feared complication is intravascular injection of a large quantity of bupivacaine. Before intralipid treatment was introduced, sudden and profound cardiac arrest resulted from such an injection. Local anesthetic toxicity in the central nervous and vascular systems alerts the physician to impending systemic toxicity (Table 35.1).[1]

LAST may occur after accidental intravascular injection during a peripheral nerve block. It is also likely during lidocaine infusions to treat refractory pain conditions, such as fibromyalgia, headaches, and other chronic pain syndromes. The factors that influence LAST are shown in Table 35.2.[1]

When LAST is suspected, a solution of 20% lipid emulsion (Intralipid 20%, Fresenius Kabi, Hamburg, Germany) is administered in a bolus of 1.5 mL/kg over 1 min followed by a 500 mL continuous infusion over 30 min at a rate of 0.25 mL/kg/min.[2] The lipid emulsion acts as a "sink" for the local anesthetic; this therapy emerged in the 1990s and is used at the earliest signs of local anesthetic cardiotoxicity or neurotoxicity.

Table 35.1. **SIGNS AND SYMPTOMS OF LOCAL ANESTHETIC-INDUCED TOXICITY**

CNS TOXICITY	CARDIOVASCULAR TOXICITY
Initial phase: a. Tinnitus b. Confusion c. Lightheadedness d. Circumoral tingling	Initial events: Hypertension/ tachycardia during CNS excitation phase
Excitation phase: Tonic-clonic convulsions	Intermediate phase: a. Myocardial depression b. Decreased cardiac output c. Mild to moderate hypertension
Depression phase: a. Unconsciousness b. CNS depression c. Respiratory arrest	Terminal phase*: a. Peripheral vasodilation b. Profound hypertension c. Sinus bradycardia d. Conduction defects e. Ventricular dysrhythmias f. Circulatory collapse

Modified from Byrne and Engelbrecht.[1]

* Sequence of events in the terminal phase will depend on the type of local anesthetic.

Table 35.2. **RISK FACTORS FOR LOCAL ANESTHETIC-INDUCED TOXICITY**

PATIENT GROUP AT INCREASED RISK	PROPOSED MECHANISM
Cardiac failure	• Higher proportion of cardiac output to vital organs and • Reduced volume of distribution and clearance
Liver failure	• Reduced plasma clearance • Prolongation of plasma half-life
Renal failure	• Increased absorption due to high output state • Accumulation of metabolites of local anesthetic breakdown
Neonates	• Reduction in $alpha_1$-acid glycoprotein • Increased in unbound local anesthetic concentrations • Reduction in clearance of local anesthetics compared to adult values
Pregnancy	• Reduction in the plasma protein binding of bupivacaine • Rapid absorption due to high cardiac output state • Increased sensitivity of cardiac and nervous tissue

Modified from Byrne and Engelbrecht.[1]

Neurotoxicity is a possible adverse event after administration of local anesthetic. Direct neurotoxicity is a persistent neurologic injury unrelated to needle trauma. This effect was described after administration of high-concentration lidocaine (5%) via microcatheters during continuous spinal anesthesia. The mechanism is direct exposure of the cauda equina, which lacks connective tissue, to the pooled local anesthetic. Serious injury outside the subarachnoid space is not common because of the lower concentration of local anesthetic used for nerve blocks.[3]

The cellular mechanism of neurotoxicity is not well understood, but it appears to be unrelated to sodium channel blockade. Lidocaine, for example, may act at a mitochondrial level, through direct depletion of ATP and production of free radicals by uncoupling of oxidative phosphorylation; bupivacaine may "uncouple" ADP[4] and inhibit the respiratory chain complex.[5] Ropivacaine increases the activity of phospholipase C.[6]

Neurotoxicity may result from a variety of interventions, such as differential spinal blocks and selective nerve root blocks with high concentrations of anesthetics. In some instances, continued neurologic deficit after block regression suggests elements of neurotoxicity in the absence of coexisting nerve injury.

MYOTOXICITY

The first report of local anesthetic myotoxicity as a clinical entity dates back to 1959.[7] During the following years, the effects were described in rats, rabbits, pigs, and humans in multiple clinical and experimental studies.[7–11] Bupivacaine, in various concentrations, has been used in laboratories as a reliable agent to induce and control myotoxicity. A common description of local anesthetic-induced myotoxicity is documented in ophthalmologic surgery: atrophic effects were noted in the extraocular muscles after retrobulbar or peribulbar block.[12]

Although bupivacaine is the most myotoxic agent, all local anesthetics produce some degree of myotoxicity. Procaine and tetracaine seem to be the least myotoxic; lidocaine and ropivacaine have fewer myotoxic effects than bupivacaine.[13] The effects of local anesthetics on striated muscle fibers were first considered in laboratory animals, whose muscle fibers were bathed in high concentrations of local anesthetic drugs. In humans, despite the low volumes of local anesthetic used in regional anesthesia for ultrasound-guided blocks, muscle weakness continues to be reported after surgical procedures. Muscle weakness, after even a single-shot block, may not be attributed entirely to the surgical intervention. Myotoxicity was not reported in one review of complications of peripheral nerve blocks, although the possibility was recognized.[14] There are published case reports of myotoxicity in humans.[15] The majority of human case reports come from the ophthalmology literature that reports diplopia during cataract and other eye surgeries. Other reports involve peripheral nerve catheters and long exposure to local anesthetics, trigger-point injections, and wound infiltration with local anesthetics.[16]

DIAGNOSIS OF MYOTOXICITY

Pain and tenderness around the site of an injection may be the first sign of myotoxicity.[17] Palpation and active and passive range of motion may elicit pain in the muscle. After a local anesthetic injection, the inflammatory response begins within 24 hours and peaks in 3 to 4 days, when swelling and edema may be seen on an MRI.[17] Electromyographic abnormalities (brief, small, polyphasic motor action potentials of suspected myopathy) may be found after 4 weeks.[17] Definitive diagnosis is made with a muscle biopsy to track histologic changes, but a biopsy is rarely required.

An acute inflammatory reaction may also be seen in infection or hematoma. The likelihood of myotoxicity from local anesthetics depends greatly on the medications administered. Corticosteroids also affect myotoxicity. In a study in rats, no histologic changes of myotoxicity were found after an intramuscular corticosteroid injection.[18] Yet the combination of bupivacaine and triamcinolone resulted in a greater degree of myotoxicity than injections of bupivacaine alone, suggesting a synergistic effect on muscle tissue.[19]

PATHOGENESIS

Histologic changes begin with hypercontractility of the myofibrils, which results in edema and calcified necrosis before regeneration commences. If the basal laminae and connective tissue remain intact, the myoblasts regenerate after approximately 4 weeks.[13]

Disruption of mitochondria in muscle cells is the pathway of myotoxicity. Various mechanisms have been proposed for myonecrosis: inhibition of ATP synthase, reduction of respiratory chain protein content, uncoupling of oxidative phosphorylation, and the presence of reactive oxygen species.[20,21] In addition to their action on sodium channels, local anesthetics act on the sarcoplasmic reticulum at the ryanodine receptors. The receptors are channels for calcium release, which increases intracellular calcium by inhibiting calcium reuptake. High concentrations of local anesthetics increase cytosolic calcium, which is associated with cell death.[21] Calcium in the sarcoplasmic reticulum also may be depleted by reactive oxygen species. Increased intracellular calcium results in hypercontractility in a mechanism similar to that in malignant hyperthermia. Local anesthetics, however, have been used safely in patients with malignant hyperthermia.

Myotoxicity has been studied in laboratory animals exposed to supratherapeutic concentrations of local anesthetics. That the concentration of local anesthetic correlates closely with the degree of myotoxicity was demonstrated in rabbit extraocular muscle.[22] The histologic effects of different concentrations of bupivacaine are shown in Figure 35.1.

Histologic changes with the injection of large concentrations of bupivacaine were evaluated 5 days after injection. Muscle fibers appeared normal with saline control and 0.19% concentration of bupivacaine. Degenerative changes were found with 0.38% bupivacaine; 0.75% bupivacaine produced large areas of inflammation, myonecrosis, and fibrous tissue. When the myotoxic effects of ropivacaine and bupivacaine were studied in pigs, single-shot femoral nerve blocks were administered with 0.75% ropivacaine or 0.5% bupivacaine and followed by a continuous catheter infusion of 0.375% ropivacaine or 0.25% bupivacaine at 8 mL/hr for 6 hours. Muscle biopsies performed at 7 and 28 days showed the spectrum of necrosis and regeneration. The greatest damage was along the spread of local anesthetic on the surface of the muscle fascicles. The degree of damage was significantly greater with bupivacaine than with ropivacaine. The investigators found microscopic calcium deposits, necrotic clusters of myocytes, proliferation of myoblasts with signs of regeneration, and scar formation.[16] A similar study in humans using 1.8 mL of 2% lidocaine with epinephrine injected before radical neck dissection confirmed the histologic changes.[9] The appearance of a patient with myonecrosis after a supraorbital nerve block is shown in Figure 35.2.

The myotoxicity of local anesthetics may be altered and enhanced by several factors: concentration of local anesthetic, duration of exposure, preexisting altered metabolism, and young age.[20] Thus, a continuous local anesthetic infusion via a peripheral nerve catheter or continuous-release or depot preparations, such as extended-release bupivacaine, should increase myonecrosis. Yet there is insufficient evidence in humans to link local anesthetic concentration and duration of administration to myonecrosis.

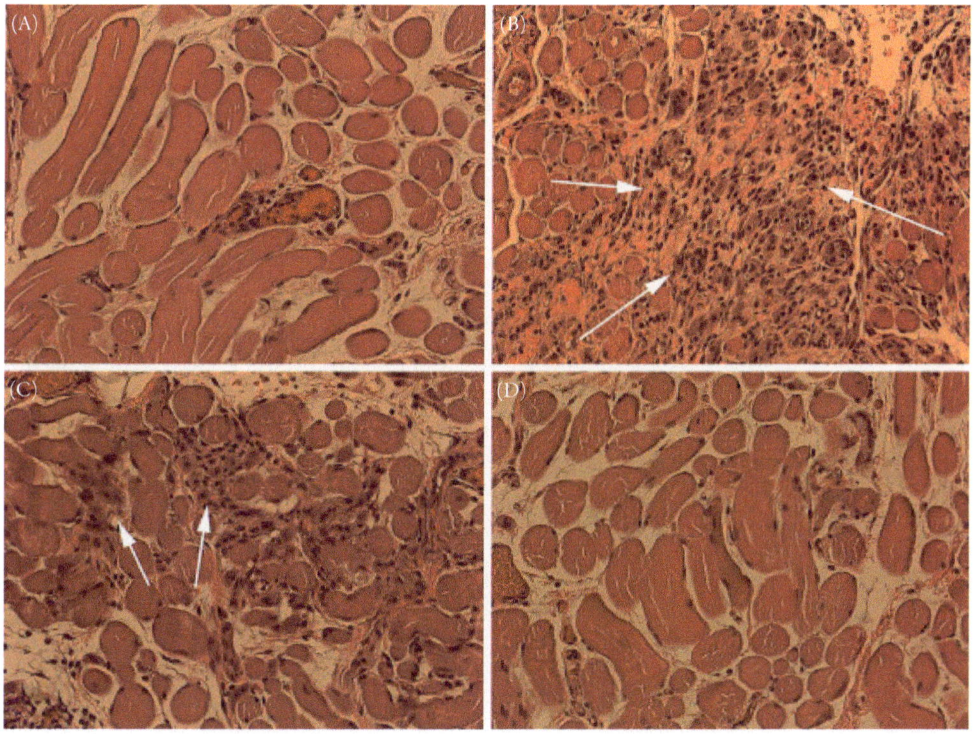

Injection	Effect
A: Saline	Normal appearing muscle fibers
B: Bupivacaine 0.75%	Large area of degenerated muscle tissue Regenerating muscle fibers Inflammatory cell infiltrate Fibrous tissue formation
C: Bupivacaine 0.38%	Scattered degenerated areas Regenerating muscle fibers
D: Bupivacaine 0.19%	Normal appearing muscle fibers

Figure 35.1. Concentration-dependent bupivacaine myotoxicity in rabbit extraocular muscle 5 days after injection of bupivacaine or saline. Reproduced with permission from Elsevier.[23]

PREVENTION

Several measures may prevent myotoxicity. First, the lowest effective concentration of local anesthetic and shortest duration of exposure should be selected for regional techniques. Calcium channel blockers prevented myotoxicity in vitro by targeting the calcium release from the sarcoplasmic reticulum. As an adjunct, dexmedetomidine administered with bupivacaine has the benefit of increasing the duration of a block while preventing myotoxicity. In preclinical trials of recombinant human erythropoietin and antioxidants to reduce reactive oxygen species, an observed protective effect decreased mitochondrial damage.[20]

Since bupivacaine has the greatest potential to produce myotoxicity, alternative local anesthetics like ropivacaine and levobupivacaine have been considered. Ropivacaine and levobupivacaine, similar in onset and duration to bupivacaine, have fewer cardiotoxic effects. There is the potential to decrease the volume of local anesthetic using ultrasound guidance while still achieving an effective nerve block. For patients with mitochondrial disorders or other diseases that predispose to myotoxicity, local anesthetics may not be the best choice. Preventative measures to reduce the risk of myonecrosis are summarized in Table 35.3.

TREATMENT

Myotoxicity is predictable and limited; therefore, treatment is rarely necessary. Additional damage is prevented by discontinuing injections and treating with nonsteroidal anti-inflammatory drugs or systemic steroids.[17] Physical therapy and rehabilitation may be required depending on the muscles affected and the degree of muscle damage.

ADVERSE EFFECTS OF CORTICOSTEROIDS

When glucocorticoids are used with local anesthetics, myonecrosis can be accelerated. A review of the side effects of intra-articular glucocorticoid injections in humans found infection, intra-articular or periarticular calcifications (the most common), cutaneous atrophy, cutaneous depigmentation,

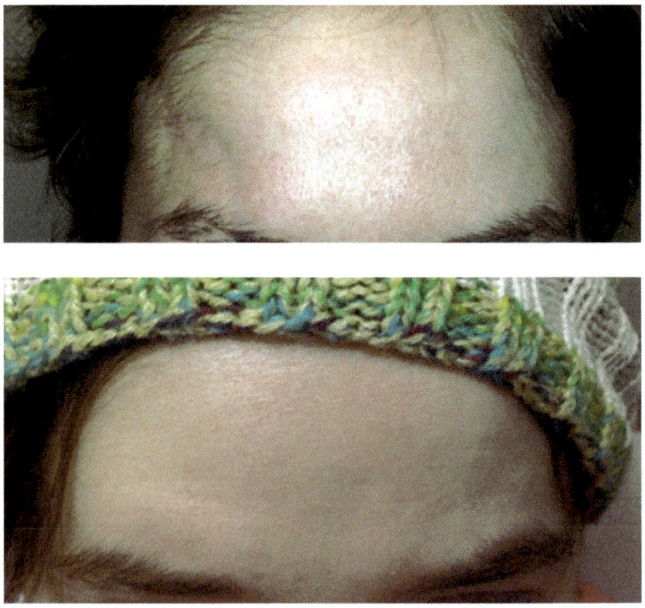

Same patient 2 years after fat transfer to treat myonecrosis

Figure 35.2. Patient with signs of myonecrosis in response to bupivacaine injection.

avascular necrosis, rapid destruction of the femoral head, acute synovitis, Charcot's arthropathy, tendinopathy, and joint dislocation.[23] Common conditions that are part of the differential diagnosis are infection, skin atrophy, and depigmentation.

Infection has been reported after intra-articular injection of glucocorticoids. The clinical signs are swelling and redness, fever, and pain with passive or active motion of the joint. If septic arthritis is suspected, arthrocentesis that reveals a WBC count > 50,000 helps to confirm the suspicion, provided the clinical picture also matches. The reported time frames for developing infection range from 6 days to a few weeks.[23] Infection rates after steroid injections are generally considered to be quite low, ranging anywhere from 1:1,000 to 1:25,000.[24] Antiseptic measures are the standard of care when performing any injection.

With a reported 8% frequency of occurrence, tissue atrophy is one of the more common adverse effects of injecting glucocorticoids.[23] Tissue atrophy usually develops 1 to 4 months after the injection and is common in patients with juvenile idiopathic arthritis. Small joints are prone to this adverse effect because accuracy of injection is not reliable, and the subcutaneous tissue is thinner around small joints than around large joints.[25]

Table 35.3. **FACTORS THAT DECREASE RISK OF MYOTOXICITY**

Tetracaine, procaine < lidocaine, ropivacaine, prilocaine < bupivacaine[13]
Lowest effective concentration
Inject outside the muscle
Avoid serial injections
Avoid injection of epinephrine and steroid
Coadminister dexmedetomidine

Depigmentation, usually hypopigmentation rather than the rarer hyperpigmentation, is another local adverse effect of glucocorticoid injections. The reported frequency is about 5%, and pigmentation change sometimes accompanies tissue atrophy.[20] Depigmentation manifests 2 months after the second injection but can appear as soon as 48 hours after injection.[26] Depigmentation is more common in dark-skinned patients. Most cases resolve within 2 months but some last for many months, or, rarely, become permanent.[23] It is unclear whether depigmentation is caused by the steroid itself or the biologically inactive contents of the vehicle[27] (Figure 35.3).

Soluble and insoluble glucocorticoids are used in clinical practice. Betamethasone sodium phosphate or dexamethasone sodium phosphate, the more soluble agents, are used in soft tissue injections, to the bursae or superficial small joints. Less soluble glucocorticoids, such as triamcinolone acetonide, are favored for intra-articular injections of deeper structures, such as the knee, elbow, or shoulder.[28] Soluble agents are preferred in peripheral nerve blocks for the greater occipital and supraorbital nerve. In a study comparing methylprednisolone

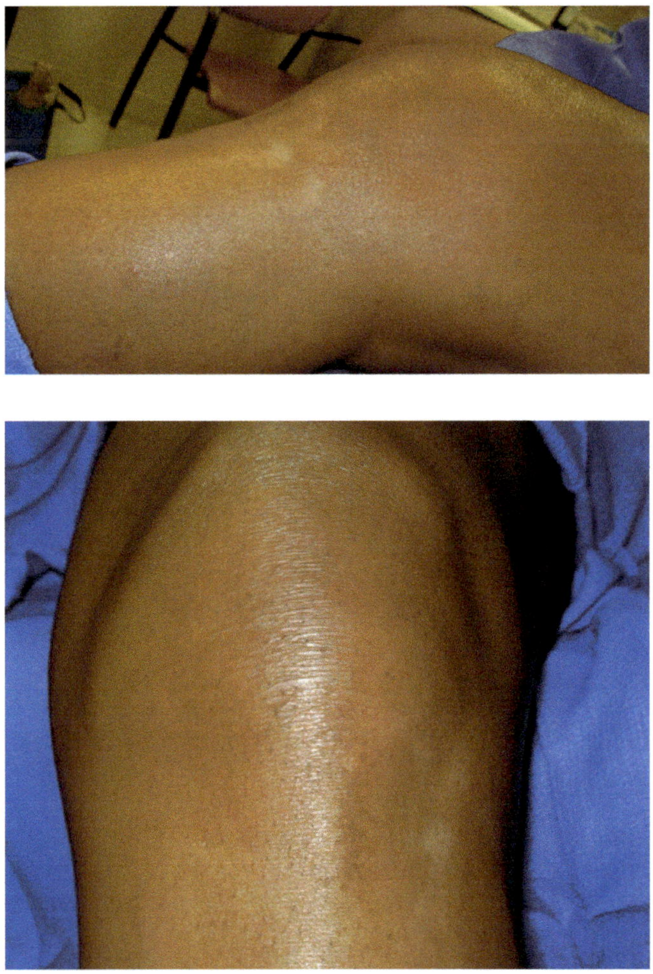

Figure 35.3. Front and lateral view of depigmentation and atrophy in a patient after steroid injections of the knee.

and triamcinolone in lidocaine, only one case of cutaneous complication was observed in more than 800 occipital nerve blocks when methylprednisolone was used. In contrast, four cases of cutaneous atrophy and alopecia were observed when the block was performed with triamcinolone in 100 patients.[29]

SHORT-LASTING UNILATERAL NEURALGIFORM HEADACHE WITH CONJUNCTIVAL INJECTION AND TEARING (SUNCT)

SUNCT is a rare but debilitating condition and a subtype of TAC. SUNCT headaches are characterized by episodes at least once a day of moderate-to-severe, unilateral pain that lasts seconds to minutes and is associated with prominent tearing and redness of the ipsilateral eye.[30] Distinguishing SUNCT from other headache syndromes is essential. Diagnostic criteria for SUNCT are:[30]

A. At least 20 attacks fulfilling criteria B to D

B. Moderate or severe unilateral head pain, with orbital, supraorbital, temporal, or other trigeminal distribution, lasting for 1 to 600 seconds and occurring as single stabs, a series of stabs, or in a sawtooth pattern

C. At least one of the following cranial autonomic symptoms or signs, ipsilateral to the pain:

- Conjunctival injection or lacrimation
- Nasal congestion or rhinorrhea
- Eyelid edema
- Forehead and facial sweating
- Forehead and facial flushing
- Sensation of fullness in the ear
- Miosis or ptosis

D. Attacks occur at a frequency of at least one a day for more than half of the time when the disorder is active

E. The symptoms are not better accounted for by another diagnosis

Differentiating SUNCT from other TACs can be challenging because the symptoms are similar. Many times, patients with SUNCT or other subtypes of TACs are misdiagnosed with cluster headache. The three main TAC subtypes are cluster headache, paroxysmal hemicrania, and SUNCT.

TACs differ from other headaches in duration and frequency. Cluster headaches last 30 to 180 min and attack frequency is one to eight per day. Paroxysmal hemicranias last 2 to 30 min and attack frequency is 20 per day. SUNCT lasts 1 to 5 min and attack frequency is 100 per day.[31] Indomethacin is effective in treating paroxysmal hemicrania. Cluster headaches respond to oxygen therapy, sumatriptan, and verapamil.[32]

One of the classic ways of differentiating between trigeminal neuralgia and SUNCT is to assess for a refractory period between headache attacks. Trigeminal neuralgia attacks will usually have a refractory period, whereas SUNCT will not.

Table 35.4. **PHARMACOLOGIC TREATMENT OPTIONS FOR SUNCT**

TREATMENT	MEDICATION (MAX DOSE REPORTED TO BE EFFECTIVE)
First-line treatment	**Lamotrigine (up to 600 mg/day)**
Second-line treatment	**Oxcarbazepine (up to 2400 mg/day)** **Topiramate (up to 700 mg/day)** **Duloxetine (30–120 mg/day)**
Third-line treatment	**Carbamazepine (up to 1600 mg/day)** **Gabapentin (up to 3600 mg/day)** **Pregabalin (up to 600 mg/day)** **Mexiletine (up to 1200 mg/day)** **Lidocaine patch (5%)**
Transitional treatments	**IV Lidocaine (1.3–3.3 mg/kg/hr for 7–10 days)** **Methylprednisolone (80 mg + 2 mL of 2% lidocaine)** **Oral/IV Corticosteroids**

Modified from Lambru and Matharu.[35]

Yet there have been case reports of exceptions.[33] Predominant distribution of the pain is in the ophthalmic division of cranial nerve V, and attacks triggered by cutaneous stimuli point in the direction of trigeminal neuralgia.[32]

Pharmacologic treatment of SUNCT aims at prevention. The most widely accepted pharmacologic treatment option is lamotrigine. Doses range from 25 to 600 mg/day. Treatment can be effective in 67% of patients.[34] Alternative pharmacologic options include other voltage-gated sodium channel blockers, such as oxcarbazepine, topiramate, and gabapentin.

Pharmacologic treatments can be transitional options (some preventive medications take time to become effective). Lidocaine infusions were effective in making up to 87% of patients pain free, although the effect diminished after the infusion was discontinued.[34] Table 35.4 summarizes the pharmacologic treatment options for SUNCT.[35]

Surgical procedures for SUNCT are ablation of the trigeminal nerve, microvascular decompression of the trigeminal nerve, occipital nerve stimulation, and deep brain stimulation of the posterior hypothalamic region.[35] Occipital nerve stimulation is favored because of fewer side effects than after more invasive techniques.[35]

CONCLUSION

When obtaining informed consent for interventional pain procedures, the possibility for myotoxicity must be discussed. Repeat injections of myotoxic medications increase the risk of myonecrosis, The possible consequences of myotoxic medications must be appreciated to prevent them and to produce favorable outcomes.

- All local anesthetics cause some degree of myotoxicity in clinically relevant concentrations.

- Bupivacaine causes the greatest myotoxicity.
- Myotoxicity results from the disruption of mitochondria in muscle cells.
- The degree of myotoxicity of a local anesthetic correlates with the concentration, time of exposure, young patient age, and preexisting altered metabolism.
- The effect with local anesthetics and glucocorticoids in myotoxicity is synergistic.
- Infection, tissue atrophy, and skin depigmentation may obscure myotoxicity from glucocorticoids.
- Muscles generally regenerate over time after an insult; however, irreversible myonecrosis may result from repeated injections of myotoxic medications.
- SUNCT is a type of TAC. Attacks are treated with methods distinct from those used for other TACs.

REFERENCES

1. Byrne K, Engelbrecht C. Toxicity of local anesthetic agents. *Trends Anaesth Crit Care.* 2013;3:25–30.
2. Neal JM, Bernards CM, Butterworth JF IV, et al. ASRA practice advisory on local anesthetic systemic toxicity. *Reg Anesth Pain Med.* 2010;35(2):152–161.
3. Drasner K. Models for local anesthetic toxicity from continuous spinal anesthesia. *Reg Anesth.* 1993;18(suppl 6):434–438.
4. Sztark F, Ouhabi R, Dabadie P, Mazat JP. Effects of the local anesthetic bupivacaine on mitochondrial energy metabolism: change from uncoupling to decoupling depending on the respiration state. *Biochem Mol Biol Int.* 1997;43:997–1003.
5. Cela O, Piccoli C, Scrima R, et al. Bupivacaine uncouples the mitochondrial oxidative phosphorylation, inhibits respiratory chain complexes I and III and enhances ROS production: results of a study on cell cultures. *Mitochondrion.* 2010;10:487–496.
6. Lin PL, Fan SZ, Tsai FF, Tsai MC, Lin CH, Huang CH. Neurotoxicity of a novel local anesthetic agent, ropivacaine: the possible roles of bursts of potential and cytoplasmic second messenger. *J Formos Med Assoc.* 2007;106:815–825.
7. Brun A. Effect of procaine, carbocaine and xylocaine on cutaneous muscle in rabbits and mice. *Acta Anaesthesiol Scand.* 1959;3:59–73.
8. Zink W, Seif C, Bohl JR, et al. The acute myotoxic effects of bupivacaine and ropivacaine after continuous peripheral nerve blockades. *Anesth Analg.* 2003;97:1173–1179.
9. Yagiela JA, Benoit PW, Buoncristiani R, et al. Comparison of myotoxic effects of lidocaine with epinephrine in rats and humans. *Anesth Analg.* 1981;60:471–480.
10. Carlson BM, Shepard B, Komorowski TE. A histological study of local anesthetic-induced muscle degeneration and regeneration in the monkey. *J Orthop Res.* 1990;8:485–494.
11. Karpie JE, Chu CR. Lidocaine exhibits dose and time dependent cytotoxic effects on bovine articular chondrocytes in vitro. *Am J Sports Med.* 2007;25:1621–1627.
12. Guyton DL. Strabismus complications from local anesthetics. *Semin Ophthalmol.* 2008;23(5):298–301.
13. Zink W, Graf BM. Local anesthetic myotoxicity. *Reg Anesth Pain Med.* 2004;29(4):333–340.
14. Berg AP, Rosenquist RW. Complications of peripheral nerve blocks. *Techn Reg Anesth Pain Manage.* 2007;11(3):133–140.
15. Hogan Q, Dotson R, Erickson S, et al. Local anesthetic myotoxicity: a case and review. *Anesthesiology.* 1994;80:942–947.
16. Zink W, Bohl J, Hacke N, et al. The long term myotoxic effects of bupivacaine and ropivacaine after continuous peripheral nerve blocks. *Anesth Analg.* 2005;101(2):548–554.
17. Neal JM, Rathmell JP. *Complications in Regional Anesthesia and Pain Medicine.* Philadelphia, PA: Lippincott Williams & Wilkins; 2013:170–173.
18. Reurink G, Goudswaard GJ, Maen MH, et al. Myotoxicity of injections for acute muscle injuries: a systematic review. *Sports Med.* 2014;44(7):943–956.
19. Guttu RL, Page DG, Laskin DM. Delayed healing of muscle after injection of bupivacaine and steroid. *Ann Dent.* 1990;49(1):5–8.
20. Nouette-Gauhlain K, Jose C, Capdevila X, et al. From analgesia to myopathy: when local anesthetics impair the mitochondrion. *Int J Biochem Cell Biol.* 2011;43(1):14–19.
21. Nouette-Gauhlain K, Capdevila X, Rossignol R. Local anesthetic "in-situ" toxicity during peripheral nerve blocks: update on mechanisms and prevention. *Curr Opin Anaesthesiol.* 2012;25(5):589–595.
22. Zhang C, Phamanvaechavan P, Rajan R, et al. Concentration-dependent bupivacaine myotoxicity in rabbit extraocular muscle. *J AAPOS.* 2010;14(4):323–327.
23. Habib GS, Saliba W, Nashashibi M. Local effects of intra-articular corticosteroids. *Clin Rheumatol.* 2010;29(4):347–356.
24. Pal B, Morris J. The perceived risks of joint infection following intra-articular corticosteroid injection: a survey of rheumatologists. *Clin Rheumatol.* 1999;18:264–265.
25. Cassidy JT, Bole GG. Cutaneous atrophy secondary to intra-articular corticosteroid administration. *Ann Intern Med.* 1966; 65:1008–1018.
26. Rogojan D, Hetland ML. Depigmentation—a rare side effect of intra-articular glucocorticoid treatment. *Clin Rheumatol.* 2004;23:373–375.
27. Newman RJ. Local skin depigmentation due to corticosteroid injection. *Br Med J (Clin Res Ed).* 1984;288(6432):1725–1726.
28. Papadopoulos PJ, Edison JD. The clinical picture: soft tissue atrophy after corticosteroid injection. *Cleve Clin J Med.* 2009;76(6):373–374.
29. Lambru G, Lagrata S, Matharu S. Cutaneous atrophy and alopecia after greater occipital nerve injection using triamcinolone. *Headache.* 2012;52:1596–1599.
30. Headache Classification Committee of the International Headache Society. The international classification of headache disorders, 3rd ed. (beta version). *Cephalalgia.* 2013;33(9):629–808.
31. Goadsby PJ, Cittadini E, Burns B, Cohen AS. Trigeminal autonomic cephalalgias: diagnostic and therapeutic developments. *Curr Opin Neurol.* 2008;21(3):323–330.
32. Cohen AS. Short-lasting unilateral neuralgiform headache attacks with conjunctival injection and tearing (SUNCT) or cranial autonomic features (SUNA)—a prospective clinical study of SUNCT and SUNA. *Brain.* 2006;129(10):2746–2760.
33. Paliwal VK, Singh P, Kumar A, Rahi SK, Gupta RK. Short-lasting unilateral neuralgiform headache with conjunctival injection and tearing (SUNCT) with preserved refractory period: report of three cases. *J Headache Pain.* 2012;13(2):167–169.
34. Lambru G, Shanahan P, Matharu MS. Medical treatments for short-lasting unilateral neuralgiform headache attacks with conjunctival injection and tearing (SUNCT) and short-lasting unilateral neuralgiform headache attacks with cranial autonomic symptoms (SUNA). *Cephalalgia.* 2011;31(suppl 1):169.
35. Lambru G, Matharu MS. SUNCT and SUNA: medical and surgical treatments. *Neurol Sci.* 2013;34(suppl 1):75–81.

REVIEW QUESTIONS

1. A 20-year-old female with chronic occipital neuralgia has significant relief from regular nerve blocks with local

anesthetic. Which of the following will decrease the risk of local anesthetic myonecrosis?

A. Choosing a long-acting local anesthetic, such as bupivacaine
B. Adding corticosteroid to the local anesthetic
C. Coadministration with dexmedetomidine
D. Performing the block with higher concentration and lower volume

2. Which local anesthetic is associated with the greatest risk of myonecrosis?

A. Lidocaine
B. Bupivacaine
C. Ropivacaine
D. Tetracaine

3. What is the first sign that a patient may have local anesthetic-induced myotoxicity after a peripheral nerve block with 0.5% bupivacaine with epinephrine?

A. Muscle weakness
B. Pain around the injection site
C. Swelling and edema seen on MRI
D. EMG abnormalities

ANSWERS

1. C. Answer A is incorrect because bupivacaine has the highest degree of myotoxicity.[7] The effects of local anesthetics combined with glucocorticoids are known to increase muscle breakdown; therefore, answer B is incorrect. When coadministered, dexmedetomidine has been shown to decrease the degree of bupivacaine-induced neurotoxicity and extend the duration of the block; therefore, answer C is correct. The effect of concentration, even at commonly used levels, correlates with the degree of myotoxicity, and lower volumes using ultrasound-guided techniques have not been associated with decreased rates of muscle weakness. Therefore, answer D is incorrect.

2. B. All local anesthetics produce some degree of myotoxicity, with bupivacaine causing the worst effects and procaine the least.[7] The risk of local anesthetic-induced myonecrosis, in order from least to greatest, is: tetracaine, procaine < lidocaine, ropivacaine, prilocaine < bupivacaine.[13]

3. B. The initial sensation of myotoxicity may be pain and tenderness around the site of the injection.[11] Swelling and edema may be seen on MRI during the period of inflammation, which peaks 3 to 4 days after injection, making it a later sign. After 4 weeks, myopathy may be revealed by EMG abnormalities, including small, brief, polyphasic motor action potentials.[11] Therefore, although all the choices given can be present in the condition described, B, pain around the injection site, is the earliest sign in suspected local anesthetic-induced myotoxicity.

QUESTIONS AND ANSWERS

This chapter has accompanying questions and answers that are available to subscribers as part of the Oxford eLearning platform. To access the questions, follow the link below, or go to http://oxfordmedicine.com/painmanagementreview

36.

EPIDURAL BLOOD PATCH

Kenneth D. Candido, Teresa M. Kusper, Bora Dinc, and Nebojsa Nick Knezevic

STEM CASE AND KEY QUESTIONS

A 28-year-old female at 39 weeks' pregnancy (G2P0) and negative past medical history arrives at the labor and delivery unit for an elective cesarean delivery. Epidural anesthesia was performed for pain control using a sterile technique after an informed consent was obtained and prior to the patient's arrival in the operating room. The subarachnoid space was accidentally entered as the Touhy needle was advanced into the L4-L5 interspace and free flow of clear cerebrospinal fluid (CSF) was observed. The needle was retracted until no additional fluid was identified, and local anesthetic was uneventfully injected. The remainder of the epidural and delivery procedure proceeded uneventfully. The patient was taken to the mother & baby unit and was discharged home 2 days later in stable condition. Seven days later, the patient came back to the emergency department complaining of a severe postural fronto-occipital headache associated with nausea, neck pain, dizziness, and photophobia not responding to oral analgesics. The husband is present at the bedside with the newborn daughter. The patient is in considerable distress because she is unable to care for her newborn.

WHAT IS POST-DURAL-PUNCTURE HEADACHE (PDPH) AND WHAT ARE ITS CHARACTERISTIC FEATURES?

PDPH occurs most frequently after spinal and epidural anesthesia and after diagnostic lumbar puncture techniques. A puncture of the dura mater (unintentional or as a part of an intended spinal technique) results in CSF leak and low CSF pressure, leading to traction on the meninges (membranes enclosing the brain and spinal canal) and intracranial neurovasculature, which combined cause the PDPH. The positional component (pain worsened by the upright position, with resolution in a supine posture) is the distinguishing feature of this common painful entity, which aids the clinician in narrowing down an extensive list of other possible causes of cephalalgia and arriving at the correct diagnosis. The pain can be observed soon after the procedure or it can evolve over several days. It involves the frontal and occipital areas and occasionally radiates to the neck or shoulders, and it can be associated with nausea, emesis, visual and auditory disturbances, tinnitus, vertigo, dizziness, and photophobia. Standing, sitting up, coughing, or straining exacerbates the pain, which can be poorly responsive to conventional analgesics.

WHAT SHOULD BE INCLUDED IN THE DIFFERENTIAL DIAGNOSIS?

Headache pain is one of the most challenging pain complaints. Many clinicians, especially inexperienced ones, continue to be intimidated by even a remote possibility of overlooking a serious pathology disguised as a headache. This is where the art of medicine is integral. Because of the presence of the postural component and the knowledge of a recent spinal or epidural intervention, it is relatively easy to develop tunnel vision, and concentrate all efforts on the management of what appears to be PDPH. Once in a while, one needs to consider "zebras" when hearing "the hoofbeats" in order to avoid missing other dire possibilities requiring emergent interventions. The differential diagnosis is broad and starts with commonly seen primary headaches, such as migraine, cluster, and tension headaches, and culminates with an exhaustive list of secondary headaches due to organic causes (Table 36.1).[1,2]

WHICH METHODS ARE USED FOR DIAGNOSIS? WHAT IS EXPECTED ON DIAGNOSTIC IMAGING?

The complaint of headache ought to be investigated in the context of the clinical picture painted by the patient's story, past medical history, and presentation prior to, and on arrival at, the medical facility. Good history-taking skills and attentiveness to detail allow capture of specific indicators of the etiology of the headache, which helps to guide diagnosis and clinical decision-making. MRI, CT myelography, and radionuclide cisternography (RC) are utilized to support the diagnosis in ambiguous circumstances. These imaging methods can demonstrate characteristic intracranial morphologic changes, such as dural enhancement and contrast involvement, sagging of brain parenchyma, downward displacement of the brain, venous sinus distention, and a specific contrast leakage pattern that might allow localizing and estimating the level of the CSF leak.

Table 36.1. **DIFFERENTIAL DIAGNOSIS OF HEADACHE**

PRIMARY HEADACHES	SECONDARY HEADACHES
Cluster headache	Temporomandibular joint syndrome
Tension or tension-type headache	Neuralgias: trigeminal neuralgia, postherpetic neuralgia, and glossopharyngeal neuralgia
Migraine (with or without aura)	Dehydration and/or electrolyte imbalance
Exercise-induced headache	Caffeine, alcohol, or substance withdrawal
Trigeminal autonomic cephalagias	Carbon monoxide poisoning
	Endocrine or metabolic causes
	Pulmonary causes: sleep apnea or hypercapnea
	Cervicogenic headache
	Infection: meningitis, encephalitis, abscess, sinusitis
	Inflammation: giant cell arteritis, SLE
	Hypertensive urgency/emergency
	Subarachnoid hemorrhage
	Intraparenchymal hemorrhage
	Posttraumatic (epidural/subdural hematoma, skull/facial fracture)
	Arterial dissection (carotid or vertebral)
	Brain aneurysm or arteriovenous malformation
	Pseudotumor cerebri
	Hydrocephalus or Chiari malformation
	Psychiatric illness
	Neoplastic disease

WHAT IS THE ACCEPTED MANAGEMENT OF A PATIENT WITH PDPH? WHAT IS AUTOLOGOUS EPIDURAL BLOOD PATCH (AEBP) AND HOW IS IT APPLIED?

After a detailed interview and thorough neurologic examination, a diagnosis of PDPH was made, and hydration, caffeine, and intravenous analgesics were initiated. These are considered the first line of treatment, and are attempted before resorting to aggressive interventions. A couple of hours later, the patient was re-evaluated, but she reported only a negligible improvement. Subsequently, an AEBP was performed using 12 mL of autologous blood sterilely and aseptically injected (injection was terminated upon onset of transient radicular symptoms) and the patient was discharged home the same evening with satisfactory analgesia and almost complete resolution of the symptoms. An AEBP is an invasive procedure in which the patient's venous blood is injected into the epidural space in the hope of closing the rent in the dura mater of the spinal canal while taking advantage of the anti-inflammatory, clotting, and healing characteristics of the blood. However, because AEBP carries an inherent risk of additional dural puncture, less-invasive measures are undertaken before AEBP is considered.

WHAT ARE THE POSSIBLE COMPLICATIONS OF AEBP?

The most likely complications of AEBP are pain at the injection site, transient fevers, and pain and/or paresthesia or dysethesia in the lower extremities. Other possible complications include repuncturing of the dura mater, stiffness of the neck, stomach cramps, tinnitus, vertigo, dizziness, or asthenia. Rarely, serious neurologic complications can ensue, such as subdural or spinal hematoma, cauda equina syndrome, sinus venous thrombosis (SVT), meningitis, or arachnoiditis. Before her discharge from the hospital, the patient was advised to avoid any strenueous activity, lifting, and bending. Additionally, she was asked to pay close attention if any new symptoms developed and to return promptly to the hospital should she develop any neurologic abnormalities.

DISCUSSION

PDPH

Karl August Bier is credited with describing the first case of PDPH in 1898, after he and his trainee, Hildebrandt, performed spinal anesthesia on each other and both developed significant postural headaches.[3] MacRobert[4] provided the first published definition of spinal headache in 1918. He wrote:

> Lumbar puncture headache differs from all others in that, being present when the patient is sitting up, it completely disappears when he lies down. It is throbbing and severe, and felt mostly in the frontal and occipital regions. No drugs give sufficient relief to allow its victim to walk about and attend to his affairs, or even to sit up.

A few decades later, Gormley[5] and DiGiovanni[6] described the technique of AEBP, which has been perfected over the years and which remains a procedure of choice for treatment of PDPH until the present day.

Different risk factors have been identified that increase the likelihood of developing PDPH. Generally, female sex, young age, pregnancy, multiple dural puncture attempts, low body mass index (BMI), prior history of headaches, and lack of experience of the clinician are all considered risk factors.[7] Although one research study on healthy volunteers found no gender differences in PDPH incidence.[8] In a study of 153 consecutive patients, no differences in PDPH incidence were found between genders or between Caucasian and African-American races, and a negative correlation was found between a smoking history and the incidence of PDPH (13.7% in smokers and 34.1% in nonsmokers).[9] The authors of the study explained that smoking promotes coagulation and clot formation, which might block the CSF leakage after dural puncture and which may subsequently lower the risk of developing the headache.[9] Early ambulation does not increase the risk of developing a low-CSF-pressure headache.[10]

In obstetric patients, employing a lateral decubitus position during the neuraxial technique, using multiple punctures, and dilation of the cervix > 7 cm increase the risk of spinal headache.[11] Factors that lower the CSF pressure, such as the seated position or volumes of extracted CSF > 30 mL are also associated with increased risk of PDPH.[12] Additionally, a drop in intra-abdominal pressure after delivery might contribute to a reduction in the epidural pressure and increased CSF leak, provoking PDPH in these patients.[13] Peralta et al. reported a lower incidence of headache in females with a BMI > 31.5 kg/m^2 compared with a BMI < 31.5 kg/m^2 (39% vs. 56%)[14]; however, this finding has not been corroborated by other reports.[11,15] Additionally, Bardon et al. found no correlation between PDPH and maternal age, mode of delivery, level of the needle insertion, and the timing of the procedure.[11]

Different technical variables that influence the rate of headache onset have also been elucidated, with the most important being the design and size of the needle. A positive relationship has been found between the needle diameter and occurrence of headache.[16] The incidence of PDPH dropped from > 80% to 5% when a 16-G needle was changed to a 26-G needle.[13] In much the same way, use of 17- or 18-G needles increases the incidence of headache.[17] Pencil-point needles result in a smaller dural hole, leading to less potential CSF leakage and lower headache incidence than with cutting (Quincke) needles. This finding was demonstrated by a randomized controlled trial (RCT) that assessed the impact of the needle type on PDPH in 217 patients undergoing lumbar puncture (Figure 36.1); the results showed a higher incidence and longer duration of headache with Quincke needle use than with Sprotte needle use (22.43% vs. 8.51%, and a median headache onset of 4.14 days vs. < 1 day).[18] Five spinal needles were examined in a different RCT (N = 1,002): two cutting needles—26-G Atraucan and 25-G Quincke—and three pencil-point needles—24-G Gertie Marx, 24-G Sprotte, and 25-G Whitacre.[19] The study reported the following incidence of PDPH by needle type, in descending order: Quincke 8.7%, Atraucan 5%, GM 4%, Whitacre 3.1%, and Sprotte 2.8%. No differences in the incidence of PDPH or the rates of blood patch use were found among the pencil-point needles.[19] Based on these results, the pencil-point Sprotte needles exhibited a better safety profile than the other needle designs. Aligning the bevel parallel to the fibers of the dura during insertion, in case of accidental puncture of the dura, decreases the incidence of headache from 75% to 31%,[20] and saline use instead of air during the loss of resistance decreases the incidence from 65% to 10%.[21] In contrast, rotating the Tuohy needle while in the epidural space should be avoided, because it increases the risk of puncturing the dura and precipitating spinal headache.[22,23]

EPIDEMIOLOGY AND PATHOPHYSIOLOGY

The reported incidence of PDPH after neuraxial anesthesia varies among different authors and exceeds 80% in some reports.[14,24–26] The incidence of headache after spinal drain placement is 18.3%,[27] after lumbar puncture it is 21.6%,[12] and after intrathecal pump placement it is 23%.[28] Continuous spinal anesthesia has a 1% incidence of PDPH.[29]

Most commonly, the integrity of the dura is disrupted by a needle, causing CSF leakage, which then results in PDPH, but PDPH can also be triggered by a puncture caused by the migration of an epidural catheter.[30,31] Different theories have emerged to explain the pathogenesis of PDPH. The theme unifying the theories is the loss of CSF and resultant intracranial hypotension after puncture of the dura mater. In humans, CSF is produced at a rate of 0.3 to 0.4 mL/min and the total CSF volume ranges between 90 and 150 mL in adults.[32] Normally, production and absorption of CSF are in a state of equilibrium, which maintains the homeostasis of CSF in the cranium and the spinal canal. CSF is produced in the choroid plexuses of the lateral, third, and fourth ventricles, and is absorbed by the arachnoid granulations (villi) into the sagittal and transverse venous sinuses in the skull (Figure 36.2). A hole formed in the dura results in CSF loss and a reduction in CSF. Rather than "floating" in CSF, the brain sinks

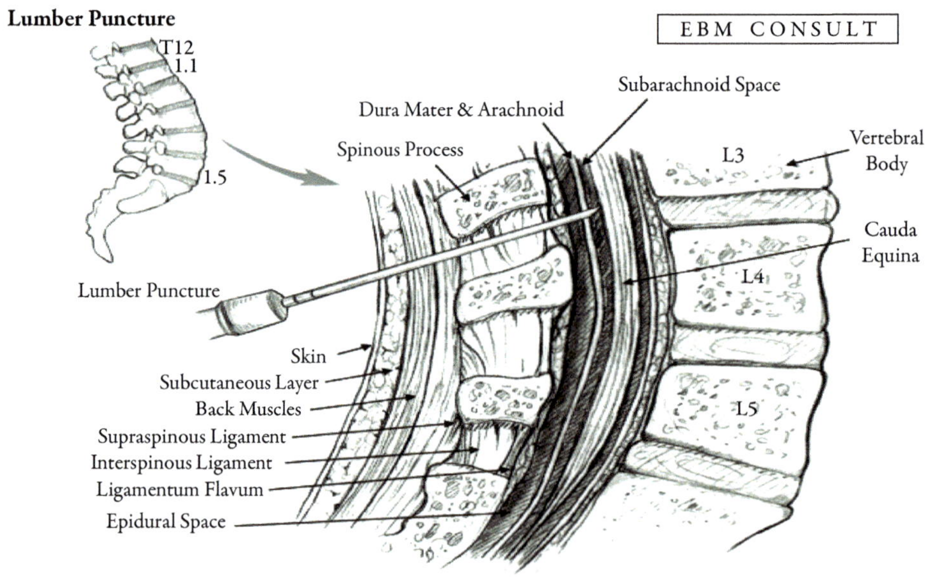

Figure 36.1. Depiction of the lumbar spine anatomy and lumbar puncture.[23] Reproduced with permission from EBM Consult.

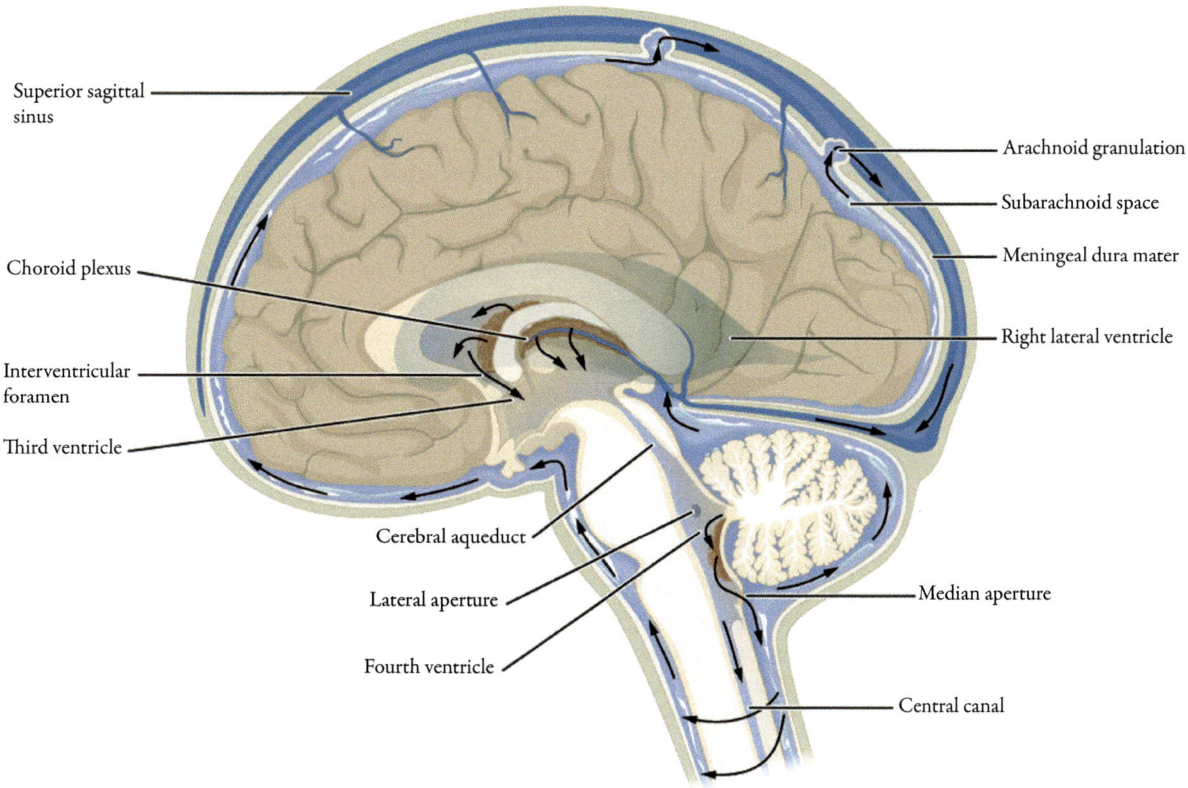

Figure 36.2. The ventricular system involved in production, circulation, and absorption of cerebrospinal fluid. From Anatomy & Physiology, Connexions Web site. http://cnx.org/content/col11496/1.6/.

downward, which stretches the meninges, tentorium, falx cerebri, and the intracranial neurovascular structures, resulting in pain manifesting as PDPH.

CLINICAL PRESENTATION OF PDPH

The characteristic feature of PDPH is a positional component, which is a prerequisite to the diagnosis of PDPH. The pain begins after standing or sitting upright and its magnitude increases as time passes, whereas assuming a supine position and staying in it for nearly 30 minutes reduces the pain.[33,34] Symptom onset is typically within the first 2 days after the procedure, but it may occur as late as 1 week after the procedure. The headache usually resolves spontaneously, although cases of chronic headache lasting for several months (or in rare cases, even for years) have been documented.[13] The pain is typically bilateral, frontal and/or occipital, and may radiate to the neck or the shoulders. It is aggravated by a change in position, coughing, or straining. Associated symptoms include nausea, photophobia, hearing changes, and visual disturbances. Cranial nerve palsies may he evident in severe cases due to the traction on intracranial structures.[35] For example, some patients develop hearing loss or diminished hearing acuity with PDPH, both of which resolve after a successful epidural blood patch (EBP) procedure.[36] Facial paresthesias and numbness may develop due to puncture-induced trigeminal and facial nerve palsies.[37] Traction on the cervical nerve roots might result in development of neck tension.[38]

PREVENTION OF PDPH

Specific measures can be adopted to minimize, but not prevent, PDPH, such as retracting the epidural needle when penetration of the dura is suspected, providing spinal anesthesia via an epidural catheter, or selecting a general anesthetic. Pulling out and attempting the epidural intervention at another interlaminar space, which is routinely done, subjects the patient to the possibility of creating another hole in the dura and further increasing the chance of developing a headache. Cesur et al. showed a decreased incidence of headache after epidural catheter implantation.[39] Prophylactic administration of intrathecal normal saline (5 mL) before administration of bupivacaine is an effective measure to reduce the risk of PDPH in patients undergoing cesarean delivery.[40] In a study of spinal anesthesia (N = 630) comparing the incidence of headache after removal of the needle with and without stylet reinsertion, no protective benefits were demonstrated with reinsertion of the stylet.[41] Ultrasonography and fiberoptics have been used by some to guide the placement of the needle into the epidural space.[42,43] A review of 24 studies with a total of 2,996 participants evaluated the preventive effects of fluid hydration and prolonged bed rest with different body positions after lumbar puncture and revealed no evidence supporting prolonged bed rest, whereas the evidence for supplemental fluids was deemed inconclusive.[44]

Various pharmacologic measures for preventing the development of PHPH have been examined. A double-blind RCT with 210 parturient women looked at the benefits of an antiemetic agent, and found a reduced incidence of PDPH after the administration of ondansetron.[45] Studies on prophylactic administration of dexamethasone 8 mg show discordant results. One trial (N = 160) demonstrated the therapeutic benefits of dexamethasone use in the first 24 hours and during the first week after spinal anesthesia in cesarean delivery.[46] But another study (N = 616) did not support the use of dexamethasone and showed an increased incidence of PDPH in the first 24 hours after dexamethasone administration.[47] On the other hand, prophylactic administration of aminophylline plus dexamethasone reduced PDPH in patients (N = 140) undergoing orthopedic surgery with spinal anesthesia.[48] The alleged benefits of the prophylactic administration of caffeine, magnesium, aminophylline, and postoperative fluid in preventing spinal headaches have not been substantiated.[49]

DIAGNOSTIC MODALITIES FOR PDPH

Diagnosis of PDPH is usually clinical, based entirely on the clinical picture, which includes the positional component and the history of dural puncture. However, the clinical presentation might resemble that with other headaches, and PDPH can easily be confused with migraine, tension headache, cluster headache, blood pressure headache, or cervicogenic headache. Additionally, a multitude of other, potentially life-threatening conditions might present in the same fashion as PDPH, which necessitates vigilance, caution, and careful neurologic examination. In the event that the pain is accompanied by nonresolving or worsening back pain, altered mental status, or progressive neurologic deficits, a low threshold needs to be maintained for excluding other pathologies, such as subdural or spinal hematoma, subarachnoid hemorrhage (SAH), intrathecal hematoma, cauda equina syndrome, sagittal sinus thrombosis, or epidural abscess. A definitive diagnosis must be made with great care, and imaging methods may need to be used. MRI and CT will confirm the diagnosis and rule out other possibilities, with CT being the modality of choice as a starting point.

RC is one of the confirmatory methods for identifying spontaneous intracranial hypotension. However, its utility is limited due to some considerable disadvantages, such as invasiveness, inadequate spatial resolution, risk of contrast extravasation, and low sensitivity.[50,51] Moreover, RC lags behind MRI and CT in revealing anatomic structural abnormalities of the brain.[52] CT myelography is a more reliable method for localizing the CSF leak site and has greater sensitivity than RC; however, traditional CT requires obtaining images of multiple sections of the brain and spine, which is a lengthy, time-consuming, and labor-intensive process.[51] Multidetector CT (MDCT) myelography is a time-saving alternative for confirming spinal headache and for determining the appropriateness of the epidural patch. MDCT myelography can rapidly scan the entire spine, detect CSF leakage, and indicate the level of the leak.[50]

Contrast leakage seen on imaging supports the presence of a dural puncture and the concomitant fluid leak. There are two commonly seen leakage patterns: "pseudo-diverticular sign," a diverticular extension of the contrast beyond the confines of the dural sac, and "gray-rim sign," a less highly attenuated diffuse rim of leaking contrast inside the dural sac (Figure 36.3).[50] MRI is a valuable confirmatory method that demonstrates characteristic morphologic changes and does not subject patients to the radiation exposure that accompanies CT. Intracranial hypotension due to CSF leakage will present on this study as pachymeningeal (dura-arachnoid) enhancement, venous sinus distention, subdural fluid collection or hematoma, downward movement of the brain with displacement of the optic chiasm and cerebellar tonsil, and effacement of the basal cisterns.[51] Although it is rare, it is possible to observe changes in the brain parenchyma resulting in tissue distention and laceration of the meningeal vessels, ultimately causing subdural hematoma.[33,53,54]

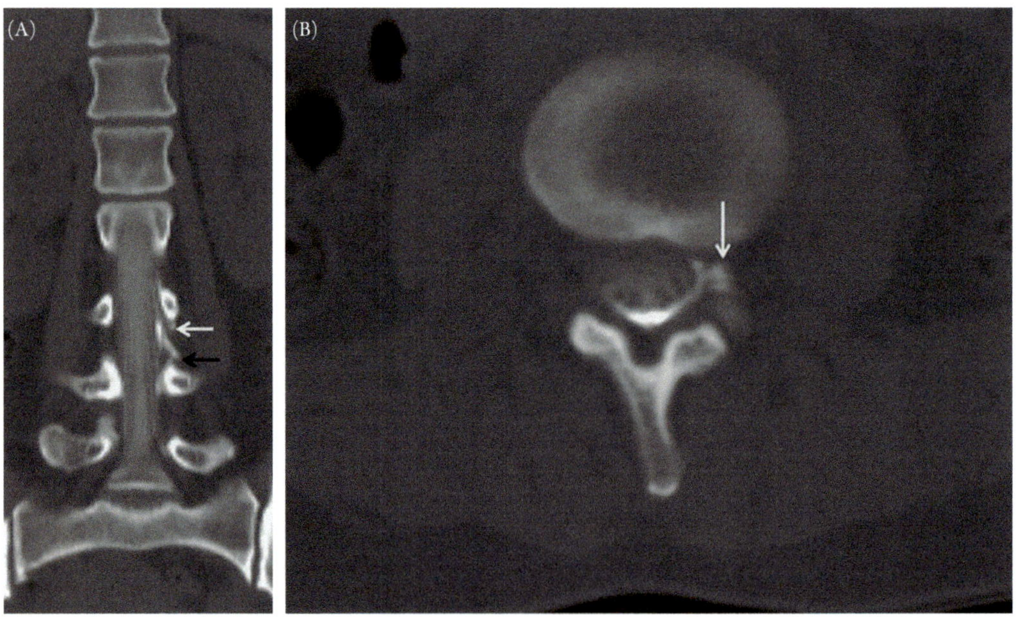

Figure 36.3. Contrast leak identified by multidetector CT (MDCT)-myelography, producing the characteristic pseudo-diverticular sign. From Choi et al.[50] Reproduced with permission from Springer Open.

TREATMENT OF PDPH

The main goal of treatment is to halt the leakage and to bring the CSF pressure back to equilibrium. The majority of PDPHs resolve spontaneously or with conservative treatment within a few days. Initial historical conservative approaches involved bed rest (unproven), intravenous fluids, caffeine, and analgesics. While bed rest is widely recommended to affected patients, a meta-analysis comparing it to immediate mobility failed to demonstrate differences in efficacy.[55]

The efficacy of oral and parenteral caffeine has been examined in a few separate studies. One study assessed oral caffeine 300 mg and although it was superior to placebo in relieving pain at 4 hours from administration, no analgesic difference was found between the two at 24 hours.[56] Parenteral caffeine 500 mg was assessed in a RCT ($N = 41$), and pain reduction was observed in 71% of the patients.[57]

Epidural injections of saline and dextran may be used in cases of refractory PDPH but before the AEBP is considered. Injection of either solution causes a transient pressure increase in the epidural space, which reduces the CSF leak and brings the subarachnoid pressure back up transiently.[35] Dextran injections have a moderate success rate but can precipitate an anaphylactic reaction.[58] The efficacy of saline injections is questionable, due to mixed results, likely caused by lack of sustainability.[59–61]

AEBP

EBP is a therapeutic technique in managing low-CSF-pressure headaches (Figure 36.4). The proposed mechanism is that the blood deposited into the epidural space forms a fibrin clot, which closes the dural defect, stops CSF leakage, and ultimately restores the CSF pressure.[62] Additionally, the blood injected into the epidural space increases the epidural and subarachnoid pressures, which reverse the cerebral venous dilation.[63] The value of the prophylactic EBP in preventing PDPH is debatable, since the available literature shows divergent results.[60,63,64] The reported initial relief obtained with therapeutic EBP ranges from 34% to 91%, and the recorded permanent relief between is about 61% to 73%.[58,65–68] Paech et al. compared different blood volumes used for the patch and found superior pain relief with volumes of 20 mL and 30 mL compared to 15 mL.[69] The authors ultimately concluded that 20 mL of autologous blood is the optimal volume to be used when treating spinal headaches, as the higher volumes are difficult for patients to tolerate and increase the incidence of EBP-related back pain.[69] A review by Schievink et al. showed an 80% success rate for 10 to 15 mL and > 95% for 20 mL volumes of autologous venous blood.[70]

AEBP TECHNIQUE

Candido and Stevens recommended the following approach for AEBP.[35] After other causes of headache are ruled out and contraindications to the procedure are considered, such as infection or anticoagulation, an informed consent is obtained, with risks, benefits, and alternatives to the procedure fully explained. Prophylactic antibiotics are not recommended. Patients are placed in either the sitting or lateral decubitus position, or prone if fluoroscopic guidance is available. A strict adherence to aseptic and sterile technique is mandatory. A skilled anesthesiologist, using mask and sterile gown and gloves, localizes an appropriate interlaminar space, either at the level of the previous injection or the one below it. An epidural needle is introduced into the selected space, while another skilled team member draws at least 20 mL of venous blood from a previously sterilized upper extremity. The timing of the two steps needs to be synchronized to avoid clotting of blood drawn too early. Drawn blood is carefully handed over to the anesthesiologist while taking all precautions not to contaminate the sample. The anesthesiologist slowly injects the autologous blood through the epidural needle until the patient complains of back pain or worsening headache or until a volume of at least 15 mL is successfully injected without the patient's discomfort.[71] The patient is maintained in the supine position (while being monitored) for 30 to 60 mins after the injection to prevent backflow of CSF through the formed hole

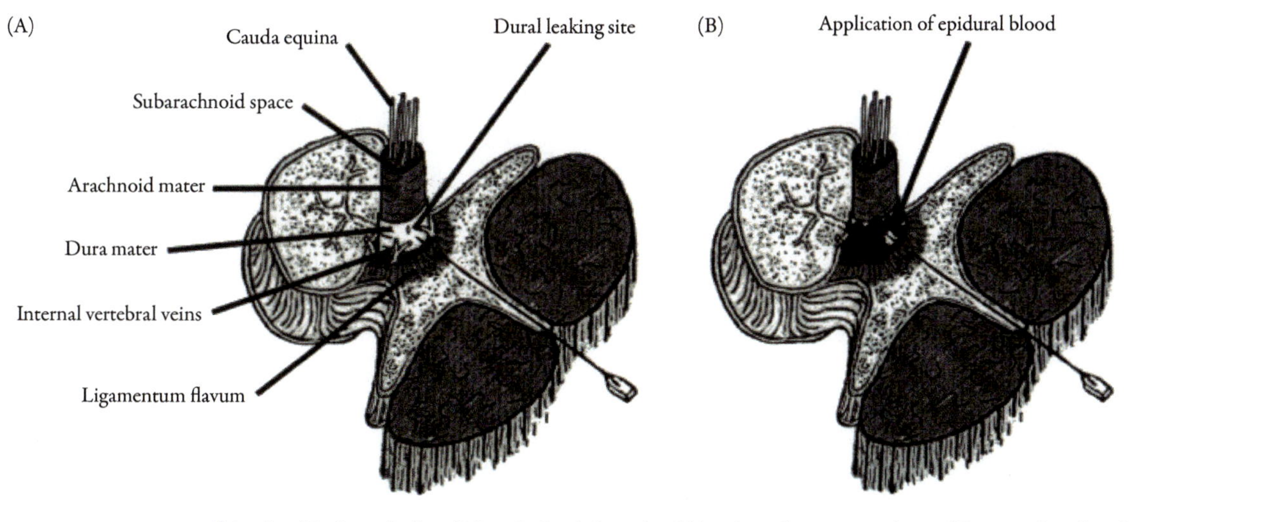

Figure 36.4. Schematic representation of the dural leak site before (A) and after (B) epidural blood patch. From Oedit et al.[71] Reproduced with permission from BioMed Central.

and to allow fibrin clot formation. The patient is advised to avoid bending, lifting, and strenuous activity for the next 2 to 3 days, and is discharged home in a stable, street-fit condition.

COMPLICATIONS OF THE EBP

Common complications of the EBP include back pain, fever, and neck pain lasting for 24 to 48 hours.[35] A records review of 236 EBP patients revealed the following complications as well, in descending order of occurrence: pain at the injection site (37%), lower extremity pain (12%), sensory disturbances (10%) and weakness (8%), sensory changes (6%) and pain in the abdomen (4%), visual and auditory disturbances (4%), and urinary and bowel abnormalities (2%).[72] Additional complications included bleeding, infections, and repeat dural puncture.[35]

Neurologic complications of vital importance, although exceedingly rare, have been reported, such as aseptic meningitis,[73] permanent paraparesis and cauda equina syndrome,[74] SVT,[75] lumbovertebral syndrome,[76] arachnoiditis,[35,77] and seizures.[78] Spinal hematomas have been reported in patients on anticoagulation, in those with thrombocytopenia, and in those with renal or liver failure.[79–83]

CONCLUSIONS

- Predictive factors for development of PDPH include female sex, young age, pregnancy, multiple dural punctures, low BMI, and level of experience of the anesthesiologist.[7]
- It is imperative to investigate other causes of the headache besides PDPH.
- The efficacy of preventive measures is controversial.
- Fluids, caffeine, and analgesics are the first steps in management of PDPH.
- EBP is used for persistent pain and it has a confirmed efficacy.
- An optimal volume of blood for EBP is 20 mL and it is associated with > 90% pain reduction.
- Pain at the injection site, lower extremity pain. and dysesthesias are the most common complications of EBP.

REFERENCES

1. Andreoli TE, Benjamin IJ, Griggs RC, Wing EJ, eds. *Andreoli and Carpenter's Cecil Essentials of Medicine*. 8th ed. Philadelphia, PA: Saunders Elsevier; 2010.
2. Headache Classification Committee of the International Headache Society. The international classification of headache disorders, 3rd ed. (beta version). *Cephalalgia*. 2013;33(9):629–808.
3. Brown DL FB. The history of neural blockade and pain management. *Neural Blockade in Clinical Anaesthesia and Management of Pain*. 3rd ed. Philadelphia, PA: Lippincott-Raven Publishers; 1998:3–27.
4. MacRobert R. The cause of lumbar puncture headache. *JAMA*. 1918;70:1350–1353.
5. Gormley J. Treatment of post spinal headache. *Anesthesiology*. 1960;21:565–566.
6. DiGiovanni AJ, Dunbar BS. Epidural injections of autologous blood for postlumbar-puncture headache. *Anesth Analg*. 1970;49(2):268–271.
7. Jabbari A, Alijanpour E, Mir M, Bani Hashem N, Rabiea SM, Rupani MA. Post spinal puncture headache, an old problem and new concepts: review of articles about predisposing factors. *Caspian J Intern Med*. 2013;4(1):595–602.
8. de Almeida SM, Shumaker SD, LeBlanc SK, et al. Incidence of post-dural puncture headache in research volunteers. *Headache*. 2011;51(10):1503–1510.
9. Dodge HS, Ekhator NN, Jefferson-Wilson L, et al. Cigarette smokers have reduced risk for post-dural puncture headache. *Pain Physician*. 2013;16(1):E25–E30.
10. Tejavanija S, Sithinamsuwan P, Sithinamsuwan N, Nidhinandana S, Suwantamee J. Comparison of prevalence of post-dural puncture headache between six hour- supine recumbence and early ambulation after lumbar puncture in Thai patients: a randomized controlled study. *J Med Assoc Thai*. 2006;89(6):814–820.
11. Bardon J, Le Ray C, Samama CM, Bonnet MP. Risk factors of post-dural puncture headache receiving a blood patch in obstetric patients. *Minerva Anestesiol*. 2016;82(6):641–648.
12. Monserrate AE, Ryman DC, Ma S, et al. Factors associated with the onset and persistence of post-lumbar puncture headache. *JAMA Neurol*. 2015;72(3):325–332.
13. Vandam LD, Dripps RD. Long-term follow-up of patients who received 10,098 spinal anesthetics; syndrome of decreased intracranial pressure (headache and ocular and auditory difficulties). *JAMA*. 1956;161(7):586–591.
14. Peralta F, Higgins N, Lange E, Wong CA, McCarthy RJ. The relationship of body mass index with the incidence of postdural puncture headache in parturients. *Anesth Analg*. 2015;121(2):451–456.
15. Miu M, Paech MJ, Nathan E. The relationship between body mass index and post-dural puncture headache in obstetric patients. *Int J Obstet Anesth*. 2014;23(4):371–375.
16. Ready LB, Cuplin S, Haschke RH, Nessly M. Spinal needle determinants of rate of transdural fluid leak. *Anesth Analg*. 1989;69(4):457–460.
17. Hawkins JL, Koonin LM, Palmer SK, Gibbs CP. Anesthesia-related deaths during obstetric delivery in the United States, 1979–1990. *Anesthesiology*. 1997;86(2):277–284.
18. Castrillo A, Tabernero C, Garcia-Olmos LM, et al. Postdural puncture headache: impact of needle type, a randomized trial. *Spine J*. 2015;15(7):1571–1576.
19. Vallejo MC, Mandell GL, Sabo DP, Ramanathan S. Postdural puncture headache: a randomized comparison of five spinal needles in obstetric patients. *Anesth Analg*. 2000;91(4):916–920.
20. Norris MC, Leighton BL, DeSimone CA. Needle bevel direction and headache after inadvertent dural puncture. *Anesthesiology*. 1989;70(5):729–731.
21. Aida S, Taga K, Yamakura T, Endoh H, Shimoji K. Headache after attempted epidural block: the role of intrathecal air. *Anesthesiology*. 1998;88(1):76–81.
22. Meiklejohn BH. The effect of rotation of an epidural needle. An in vitro study. *Anaesthesia*. 1987;42(11):1180–1182.
23. Busti AJ KD. Procedure: lumbar puncture. 2015. Available from https://www.ebmconsult.com/articles/procedure-lumbar-puncture?action=search&search_box=procedure:%20lumbar%20puncture&search_within=&type_of_search=&onetimeadvanced=auto.
24. Lybecker H, Djernes M, Schmidt JF. Postdural puncture headache (PDPH): onset, duration, severity, and associated symptoms. An analysis of 75 consecutive patients with PDPH. *Acta Anaesthesiol Scand*. 1995;39(5):605–612.
25. Paech M, Banks S, Gurrin L. An audit of accidental dural puncture during epidural insertion of a Tuohy needle in obstetric patients. *Int J Obstet Anesth*. 2001;10(3):162–167.
26. Liu S, Carpenter RL, Neal JM. Epidural anesthesia and analgesia. Their role in postoperative outcome. *Anesthesiology*. 1995;82(6):1474–1506.
27. Riley SP, Donnelly MJ, Khatib D, Warren C, Schroeder KM. Post-dural puncture headaches following spinal drain placement during

thoracoabdominal aortic aneurysm repair: incidence, associated risk factors, and treatment. *J Anesth*. 2015;29(4):544–550.
28. Neuman SA, Eldrige JS, Qu W, Freeman ED, Hoelzer BC. Post dural puncture headache following intrathecal drug delivery system placement. *Pain Physician*. 2013;16(2):101–107.
29. Denny N, Masters R, Pearson D, Read J, Sihota M, Selander D. Postdural puncture headache after continuous spinal anesthesia. *Anesth Analg*. 1987;66(8):791–794.
30. Kalas DB, Hehre FW. Continuous lumbar peridural anesthesia in obstetrics. 8. Further observations on inadvertent lumbar puncture. *Anesth Analg*. 1972;51(2):192–195.
31. Crawford JS. Some maternal complications of epidural analgesia for labour. *Anaesthesia*. 1985;40(12):1219–1225.
32. Brinker T, Stopa E, Morrison J, Klinge P. A new look at cerebrospinal fluid circulation. *Fluids Barriers CNS*. 2014;11:10.
33. Ferrante E, Savino A, Sances G, Nappi G. Spontaneous intracranial hypotension syndrome: report of twelve cases. *Headache*. 2004;44(6):615–622.
34. Park ES, Kim E. Spontaneous intracranial hypotension: clinical presentation, imaging features and treatment. *J Korean Neurosurg Soc*. 2009;45(1):1–4.
35. Candido KD, Stevens RA. Post-dural puncture headache: pathophysiology, prevention and treatment. *Best Pract Res Clin Anaesthesiol*. 2003;17(3):451–469.
36. Wang LP, Fog J, Bove M. Transient hearing loss following spinal anaesthesia. *Anaesthesia*. 1987;42(12):1258–1263.
37. Carrero EJ, Agusti M, Fabregas N, Valldeoriola F, Fernandez C. Unilateral trigeminal and facial nerve palsies associated with epidural analgesia in labour. *Can J Anaesth*. 1998;45(9):893–897.
38. Brownridge P. The management of headache following accidental dural puncture in obstetric patients. *Anaesth Intensive Care*. 1983;11(1):4–15.
39. Cesur M, Alici HA, Erdem AF, Silbir F, Celik M. Decreased incidence of headache after unintentional dural puncture in patients with cesarean delivery administered with postoperative epidural analgesia. *J Anesth*. 2009;23(1):31–35.
40. Faridi Tazeh-Kand N, Eslami B, Ghorbany Marzony S, Abolhassani R, Mohammadian K. Injection of intrathecal normal saline in decreasing postdural puncture headache. *J Anesth*. 2014;28(2):206–209.
41. Sinikoglu NS, Yeter H, Gumus F, Belli E, Alagol A, Turan N. Reinsertion of the stylet does not affect incidence of post dural puncture headaches (PDPH) after spinal anesthesia. Braz J Anesthesiol. 2013;63(2):188–192.
42. Kim SH, Lee KH, Yoon KB, Park WY, Yoon DM. Sonographic estimation of needle depth for cervical epidural blocks. *Anesth Analg*. 2008;106(5):1542–1547.
43. Ting CK, Tsou MY, Chen PT, et al. A new technique to assist epidural needle placement: fiberoptic-guided insertion using two wavelengths. *Anesthesiology*. 2010;112(5):1128–1135.
44. Arevalo-Rodriguez I, Ciapponi A, Roque i Figuls M, Munoz L, Bonfill Cosp X. Posture and fluids for preventing post-dural puncture headache. *Cochrane Database Syst Rev*. 2016;3:CD009199.
45. Fattahi Z, Hadavi SM, Sahmeddini MA. Effect of ondansetron on post-dural puncture headache (PDPH) in parturients undergoing cesarean section: a double-blind randomized placebo-controlled study. *J Anesth*. 2015;29(5):702–707.
46. Hamzei A, Basiri-Moghadam M, Pasban-Noghabi S. Effect of dexamethasone on incidence of headache after spinal anesthesia in cesarean section. A single blind randomized controlled trial. *Saudi Med J*. 2012;33(9):948–953.
47. Yang B, Li DL, Dong P, Zhang XY, Zhang L, Yu JG. Effect of dexamethasone on the incidence of post-dural puncture headache after spinal anesthesia: a randomized, double-blind, placebo-controlled trial and a meta-analysis. *Acta Neurol Belg*. 2015;115(1):59–67.
48. Naghibi K, Hamidi M. Prophylactic administration of aminophylline plus dexamethasone reduces post-dural puncture headache better than using either drug alone in patients undergoing lower extremity surgery. *Adv Biomed Res*. 2014;3:5.
49. Zajac K, Zajac M, Hladki W, Jach R. [Is there any point in pharmacological prophylaxis of PDPH (post-dural puncture headache) after spinal anaesthesia for Caesaren section?]. *Przeglad Lekarski*. 2012;69(1):19–24.
50. Choi SW, Ahn JM, Lee JW, Park KS, Kang HS. The usefulness of MDCT-myelography for patients with spontaneous intracranial hypotension. *Springerplus*. 2016;5:424.
51. Sainani NI, Lawande MA, Pungavkar SA, Desai M, Patkar DP, Mohanty PH. Spontaneous intracranial hypotension: a study of six cases with MR findings and literature review. *Australas Radiol*. 2006;50(5):419–423.
52. Diaz JH. Epidemiology and outcome of postural headache management in spontaneous intracranial hypotension. *Reg Anesth Pain Med*. 2001;26(6):582–587.
53. Kale A, Emmez H, Piskin O, Durdag E. Postdural puncture subdural hematoma or postdural puncture headache? Two cases report. *Korean J Anesthesiol*. 2015;68(5):509–512.
54. Inamasu J, Moriya S, Shibata J, Kumai T, Hirose Y. Spontaneous intracranial hypotension manifesting as a unilateral subdural hematoma with a marked midline shift. *Case Rep Neurol*. 2015;7(1):71–77.
55. Thoennissen J, Herkner H, Lang W, Domanovits H, Laggner AN, Mullner M. Does bed rest after cervical or lumbar puncture prevent headache? A systematic review and meta-analysis. *CMAJ*. 2001;165(10):1311–1316.
56. Camann WR, Murray RS, Mushlin PS, Lambert DH. Effects of oral caffeine on postdural puncture headache. A double-blind, placebo-controlled trial. *Anesth Analg*. 1990;70(2):181–184.
57. Sechzer P. Post-spinal anaesthesia headache treated with caffeine. II. Intracranial vascular distention: a key factor. *Curr Ther Res*. 1979;26:440–448.
58. Stride PC, Cooper GM. Dural taps revisited. A 20-year survey from Birmingham Maternity Hospital. *Anaesthesia*. 1993;48(3):247–255.
59. Rice GG, Dabbs CH. The use of peridural and subarachnoid injections of saline solution in the treatment of severe postspinal headache. *Anesthesiology*. 1950;11(1):17–23.
60. Trivedi NS, Eddi D, Shevde K. Headache prevention following accidental dural puncture in obstetric patients. *J Clin Anesth*. 1993;5(1):42–45.
61. Shah JL. Epidural pressure during infusion of saline in the parturient. *Int J Obstet Anesth*. 1993;2(4):190–192.
62. Rosenberg PH, Heavner JE. In vitro study of the effect of epidural blood patch on leakage through a dural puncture. *Anesth Analg*. 1985;64(5):501–504.
63. Scavone BM, Wong CA, Sullivan JT, Yaghmour E, Sherwani SS, McCarthy RJ. Efficacy of a prophylactic epidural blood patch in preventing post dural puncture headache in parturients after inadvertent dural puncture. *Anesthesiology*. 2004;101(6):1422–1427.
64. Ackerman WE, Juneja MM, Kaczorowski DM. Prophylactic epidural blood patch in parturients. *South Med J*. 1989;82(5):671.
65. Vercauteren MP, Hoffmann VH, Mertens E, Sermeus L, Adriaensen HA. Seven-year review of requests for epidural blood patches for headache after dural puncture: referral patterns and the effectiveness of blood patches. *Eur J Anaesthesiol*. 1999;16(5):298–303.
66. Taivainen T, Pitkanen M, Tuominen M, Rosenberg PH. Efficacy of epidural blood patch for postdural puncture headache. *Acta Anaesthesiol Scand*. 1993;37(7):702–705.
67. Williams EJ, Beaulieu P, Fawcett WJ, Jenkins JG. Efficacy of epidural blood patch in the obstetric population. *Int J Obstet Anesth*. 1999;8(2):105–109.
68. Safa-Tisseront V, Thormann F, Malassine P, et al. Effectiveness of epidural blood patch in the management of post-dural puncture headache. *Anesthesiology*. 2001;95(2):334–339.
69. Paech MJ, Doherty DA, Christmas T, Wong CA, Epidural Blood Patch Trial Group. The volume of blood for epidural blood patch in obstetrics: a randomized, blinded clinical trial. *Anesth Analg*. 2011;113(1):126–133.
70. Schievink WI. Spontaneous spinal cerebrospinal fluid leaks: a review. *Neurosurg Focus*. 2000;9(1):e8.
71. Oedit R, van Kooten F, Bakker SL, Dippel DW. Efficacy of the epidural blood patch for the treatment of post lumbar puncture headache BLOPP: a randomised, observer-blind, controlled clinical trial [ISRCTN 71598245]. *BMC Neurol*. 2005;5(1):12.

72. Tarkkila PJ, Miralles JA, Palomaki EA. The subjective complications and efficiency of the epidural blood patch in the treatment of postdural puncture headache. *Reg Anesth*. 1989;14(5):247–250.
73. Oh J, Camann W. Severe, acute meningeal irritative reaction after epidural blood patch. *Anesth Analg*. 1998;87(5):1139–1140.
74. Diaz JH. Permanent paraparesis and cauda equina syndrome after epidural blood patch for postdural puncture headache. *Anesthesiology*. 2002;96(6):1515–1517.
75. Schievink WI, Maya MM. Cerebral venous thrombosis in spontaneous intracranial hypotension. *Headache*. 2008;48(10):1511–1519.
76. Palmer JH, Wilson DW, Brown CM. Lumbovertebral syndrome after repeat extradural blood patch. *Br J Anaesth*. 1997;78(3):334–336.
77. Aldrete JA, Brown TL. Intrathecal hematoma and arachnoiditis after prophylactic blood patch through a catheter. *Anesth Analg*. 1997;84(1):233–234.
78. Bolton VE, Leicht CH, Scanlon TS. Postpartum seizure after epidural blood patch and intravenous caffeine sodium benzoate. *Anesthesiology*. 1989;70(1):146–149.
79. Owens EL, Kasten GW, Hessel EA II. Spinal subarachnoid hematoma after lumbar puncture and heparinization: a case report, review of the literature, and discussion of anesthetic implications. *Anesth Analg*. 1986;65(11):1201–1207.
80. DeAngelis J. Hazards of subdural and epidural anesthesia during anticoagulant therapy: a case report and review. *Anesth Analg*. 1972;51(5):676–679.
81. Grejda S, Ellis K, Arino P. Paraplegia following spinal anesthesia in a patient with chronic renal failure. *Reg Anesth*. 1989;14(3):155–157.
82. Laglia AG, Eisenberg RL, Weinstein PR, Mani RL. Spinal epidural hematoma after lumbar puncture in liver disease. *Ann Intern Med*. 1978;88(4):515–516.
83. Tekkok IH, Carter DA, Brinker R. Spinal subdural haematoma as a complication of immediate epidural blood patch. *Can J Anaesth*. 1996;43(3):306–309.
84. Errando CL, Peiro CM. Postdural puncture upper back pain as an atypical presentation of postdural puncture symptoms. *Anesthesiology*. 2002;96(4):1019–1020.
85. Patel AR, Alton TB, Bransford RJ, Lee MJ, Bellabarba CB, Chapman JR. Spinal epidural abscesses: risk factors, medical versus surgical management, a retrospective review of 128 cases. *Spine J*. 2014;14(2):326–330.
86. Curry WT Jr, Hoh BL, Amin-Hanjani S, Eskandar EN. Spinal epidural abscess: clinical presentation, management, and outcome. *Surg Neurol*. 2005;63(4):364–371, discussion 371.

REVIEW QUESTIONS

1. A 26-year-old female (G2P1) is admitted to the labor and delivery unit for an elective induction of labor with epidural anesthesia. She is 157 cm tall and weighs 80 kg. She has no prior medical history. Social history includes smoking half a pack a day for 8 years and occasional alcohol use. She denies illicit drugs. How many risk factors are present that increase and decrease the likelihood of PDPH in this patient?

   A. Three increasing, one decreasing
   B. Five increasing, zero decreasing
   C. Four increasing, one decreasing
   D. Three increasing, two decreasing

2. A 37-year-old female with a history of pseudotumor cerebri and who had a spinal tap 8 days earlier presented to the emergency department with a 3-day history of severe, constant, throbbing, bilateral headache, as well as neck pain with stiffness. She denied any neurologic deficits but noted sensitivity to light, blurry vision, nausea, and chills. She had spent previous 2 days lying in bed because moving around intensified her pain. On physical exam, vitals were stable, skin was moist, and PERRLA. She had tenderness to palpation over the scalp and restricted ROM of the cervical spine, and she was unable to extend her knees due to severe pain in her neck. Which of the following is the most likely diagnosis?

   A. Pseudotumor cerebri
   B. Meningitis
   C. PDPH
   D. Cervicogenic headache

3. What is the best next step in management of this patient?

   A. MRI
   B. EBP
   C. Repeat lumbar puncture
   D. Initiate intravenous antibiotics

ANSWERS

1. D. The risk factors for PDPH present in this patient include female sex, young age, and pregnancy, whereas her calculated BMI of 32.6 (> 31.5 kg/m^2) and smoking history decrease the risk of developing PDPH.

2. B. In the context of the recent spinal tap and the current clinical presentation, meningitis is the most likely diagnosis. The patient complained of headache, chills, and neck pain with stiffness, which are strong indicators of both meningitis and PDPH; however, because she was febrile and had a positive Kernig's sign (when the patient is supine with knees and hips flexed, and extension of the knee elicits pain), a diagnosis of meningitis is more probable. Therefore, answer C is incorrect. Pseudotumor cerebri (idiopathic intracranial hypertension) is caused by elevated CSF in the brain, resulting in increased ICP. Symptoms of increased ICP are headache, blurry vision, and neck stiffness, all of which were present in the patient. On monitoring, Cushing reflex (Cushing's triad) would be observed, which is characterized as bradycardia, systolic hypertension, and abnormal respirations. This patient has stable vital signs. Cervicogenic headache can also manifest as headache and neck pain and/or stiffness but fever and meningismus would not be observed.

3. D. This patient needs immediate antibiotic therapy, since meningitis progresses quickly and is associated with high mortality if not addressed promptly.

QUESTIONS AND ANSWERS

This chapter has accompanying questions and answers that are available to subscribers as part of the Oxford eLearning platform. To access the questions, follow the link below, or go to ✔ http://oxfordmedicine.com/painmanagementreview

37.

OPIOID-INDUCED HYPERALGESIA, TOLERANCE, AND CHRONIC POSTSURGICAL PAIN: A DILEMMA COMPLICATING POSTOPERATIVE PAIN MANAGEMENT

Dalia H. Elmofty

STEM CASE AND KEY QUESTIONS

A 38-year-old male with a history of Crohn's disease and substance abuse is scheduled for exploratory laparotomy and total colectomy. He has chronic abdominal pain and a history of multiple lower extremity deep venous thromboses for which he takes warfarin 5 mg at bedtime. He also takes oxycodone 20 mg and gabapentin 600 mg three times a day and amitriptyline 25 mg at bedtime. He has had multiple abdominal surgeries, with several readmissions for poorly controlled pain. He expresses concern about management of his postoperative pain. He states that even very high doses of pain medication do not alleviate his pain.

WHAT WOULD YOU TELL THIS PATIENT IN PREPARATION FOR SURGERY? WHAT ARE YOUR GOALS AND EXPECTATIONS FOR THIS PATIENT?

On the day of surgery, the patient mentions that he forgot to take his morning dose of oxycodone. He is anxious and concerned about pain management. He discontinued warfarin 5 days earlier. Test results show a normal prothrombin time (PT) and international normalized ratio (INR).

WHAT ARE SOME OF THE DIFFERENT PERIOPERATIVE OPTIONS FOR PAIN MANAGEMENT IN THIS PATIENT?

A T10-T11 epidural is placed preoperatively. A 5 mL test dose of lidocaine with epinephrine 1:200,000 is administered. The patient remains hemodynamically stable. A dermatomal distribution is identified from the T7 to the T12 level. General anesthesia with intravenous induction is used. An epidural infusion containing bupivacaine 0.1% and hydromorphone 5 μg/mL is initiated at 8 mL/hr. The patient's surgery lasts approximately 8 hours. He is extubated and brought to the postanesthesia care unit (PACU). He appears comfortable and is transferred to the surgical floor. During acute pain service rounds on postoperative day 2, the patient's warfarin therapy has inadvertently been reinitiated. Results of morning tests showed an INR increase from 1.2 to 1.7. The surgical service requested reinstatement of anticoagulation therapy because of the patient's history of recurrent deep venous thrombosis.

ARE YOU CONCERNED? WILL YOU KEEP OR REMOVE THE EPIDURAL CATHETER? IF YOU DECIDE TO REMOVE IT, WOULD YOU REMOVE IT WHEN HIS INR IS 1.7?

The acute pain service decides to remove the epidural catheter. Repeat labs show a decrease of INR to 1.5. Patient-controlled analgesia (PCA) is initiated with hydromorphone 0.5 mg every 8 min. Approximately 3 hours after epidural catheter removal, the patient is hypertensive and tachycardic. He reports severe pain. Over the next few hours, the patient is given escalating doses of potent opioids. His PCA delivery is increased to 1 mg every 10 min. He continues to complain of excruciating pain, no longer incisional, but a diffuse body ache.

WHY IS THE PATIENT NOT RESPONDING TO THE ADMINISTERED NARCOTICS? IS THIS PATIENT DEMONSTRATING OPIOID-INDUCED HYPERALGESIA (OIH) OR TOLERANCE? ARE SOME PATIENTS MORE PRONE TO OIH, TOLERANCE, OR CHRONIC POSTSURGICAL PAIN? HOW IS OIH DIAGNOSED? HOW WOULD YOU MANAGE OPIOID NONRESPONSIVENESS?

In spite of several adjustments to the patient's pain regimen, he continues to have severe pain. The PCA dosage is reduced and intravenous methadone 2.5 mg is administered every 6 hours for 48 hours. An electrocardiogram shows a normal QTc interval. A ketamine infusion of 3 μg/kg/min is administered for 48 hours. The patient now appears to be more comfortable. He is able to ambulate and to tolerate clear liquids. The surgical service requests recommendations for transitioning to an oral pain regimen.

ARE THERE ANY ADDITIONAL CONSIDERATIONS FOR A PATIENT WITH A HISTORY OF SUBSTANCE ABUSE? WHAT TYPE OF OUTPATIENT MANAGEMENT IS REQUIRED FOR THIS PATIENT?

The patient is reinitiated on his oxycodone 20 mg and gabapentin 600 mg three times a day and amitriptyline 25 mg at bedtime. He is asked to come to the pain clinic in 2 weeks for follow-up.

DISCUSSION

The treatment of acute postoperative pain continues to be a challenge for physicians. In a random sample of 250 adults who underwent a surgical procedure, 80% of the patients reported having acute postoperative pain, and 86% reported moderate to severe pain.[1] Some patients are more vulnerable to severe acute postoperative pain. No treatment or inadequate treatment can have a devastating impact on patients and lead to chronic pain. Pain burdens patients in multiple domains: socioeconomic, psychologic, and qualitative. Anesthesiologists have a crucial role in the perioperative management of pain. Anesthetic technique influences the development of acute postoperative pain, chronic postsurgical pain, OIH, and opioid tolerance. Opioids are conventionally thought of as the first-line treatment for pain. The United States appears to be the main consumer of opioids, accounting for 56% of morphine and 81% of oxycodone global usage.[2] Growing evidence has shown that opioids may have a negative impact on postoperative pain.

PERIOPERATIVE PAIN MANAGEMENT

Perioperative management of pain begins preoperatively. A pain prevention plan focuses on multimodal therapy, education of patients, and assessment. Scoring systems help providers identify patients at risk for severe postoperative pain.[3] Education of the patient is an important component in the management of pain. One of the major sources of presurgical anxiety for patients is the apprehension of experiencing postoperative pain. There should be an emphasis on patient-targeted goals in treatment. Patients must be educated about multimodal analgesia, which decreases opioid-related adverse events, hospital stay, and cost. Options regarding different analgesic agents should be discussed with patients as well as past experience with pain, if applicable. Regional techniques using epidural or peripheral nerve blocks and catheters may be considered. Patients should be told that postoperative pain will be assessed with a conventional visual analog score (VAS), but more emphasis should be placed on recovery of function (bowel and bladder) and early ambulation. The perioperative management of pain for patients with a history of chronic pain or substance abuse adds challenges. Such patients tend to have a high tolerance for opioids and may experience severe postoperative pain. Those with a history of substance abuse can be at risk for relapse. The management of pain in patients with a history of substance abuse may require extra care, monitoring, documentation, or consultation with an expert.[4] In these situations, it is vital for patient assessment in the anesthesia perioperative medicine clinic or pain clinic to implement a clinical care pathway for pain management. Collaboration with a psychiatrist or addiction specialist may be necessary. For patients with a history of chronic pain who require opioid therapy, a multimodal approach and introduction of adjuvant therapy intraoperatively may improve postoperative pain control and reduce the risk for severe chronic pain. Collaborating with the surgeon and suggesting a minimally invasive procedure instead of a large open incision may assist in managing postoperative pain. The anesthesiologist, who plays a crucial role in the management of perioperative pain, should be an advocate for patients.

OPIOID TOLERANCE AND OIH

Chronic opioid exposure can lead to opioid tolerance or OIH. Clinical differentiation between them can be challenging. Opioid tolerance is a physiologic process in which a progressive lack of response to opioids requires an increase in dose to produce the same effect. There is a shift to the right of the dose-response curve. The lack of response is overcome by increasing the dose. During pharmacokinetic changes, upregulation of the metabolic process eliminates the drug. During pharmacodynamic changes, downregulation of the opioid receptor results in desensitization. The opioid receptor is linked to a G-protein, which, when activated, decreases cyclic adenosine 3,5-monophosphate (cAMP) and inhibits sodium and calcium influx. Over time, changes in G-protein function can lead to desensitization or opioid tolerance. OIH is a paradoxical response to opioids: patients with OIH experience a worsening of pain with administration of opioids.

RISK FACTORS AND MECHANISM OF ACTION FOR OIH

Why some patients develop OIH and others do not is not completely understood. In animal models, sex difference is one factor. After exposure to opioids, female rats develop OIH faster and for longer than male rats do.[5] Genetic predisposition may be a factor. Polymorphism in the catechol-*O*-methyltransferase (COMT) gene may predispose patients to OIH.[6] Patients with high levels of anxiety about postoperative pain may be more susceptible to OIH.[7]

Some of the proposed mechanisms of OIH involve the central glutaminergic system, spinal dynorphins, descending facilitation, genetic influence, and enhanced response to nociceptive neurotransmitters.[8] In the central glutaminergic system, the excitatory neurotransmitter glutamate and the *N*-methyl-D-aspartate (NMDA) receptor are activated. Prolonged exposure to morphine causes neurotoxicity by inducing NMDA receptor-mediated cell death in the dorsal horn.[9] Prolonged exposure to μ-receptor agonists increases levels of spinal dynorphins, which increases the release of excitatory neuropeptides.[10] Activation of descending facilitation from the rostral ventromedial medulla activates spinal nociceptive processing and increases excitatory neuropeptides.[11] Genetic variability of COMT affects central pain processing.[6]

MANAGEMENT OF OPIOID TOLERANCE AND OIH

OIH differs from opioid tolerance in that an increase in opioid dose worsens pain. Pain is lessened by lowering opioid dosage. Performing quantitative sensory testing (QST) before administration of opioids and at regular intervals may assist in the clinical diagnosis.[12]

OIH and opioid tolerance are two distinct phenomena that make postoperative pain difficult to control. Most practitioners may escalate an opioid dose. If no response is observed, OIH should be considered, and opioid dosing should be reduced or opioid rotation should be initiated. The mechanism of action and treatment options for OIH and opioid tolerance are summarized in Table 37.1.

When an anesthesiologist encounters patients with chronic pain and chronic opioid use, traditional intravenous opioids may not be efficient for pain relief. Multimodal therapy and adjuvant therapy (Table 37.2) may control postoperative pain and reduce the risk of developing OIH, opioid tolerance, or chronic postsurgical pain. Methadone has been used for treatment of chronic neuropathic and cancer pain. Its utilization for acute pain in the perioperative period has been minimal. PCA has been the foundation for the management of perioperative pain. Although PCA is superior to nurse-administered analgesia, PCA has its limitations. There are many misapprehensions regarding the onset, duration, and metabolism of methadone, making it less attractive for the acute pain setting. The myth that methadone has a slow onset of action, that duration of analgesia is shorter than elimination half-life, and that its highly variable clearance and interactions with other drugs make it unattractive for use in acute or perioperative settings have been disproven.[13] Methadone has several advantages over other narcotics for acute pain. It is a μ-receptor agonist that contains an NMDA antagonist property, which can counteract OIH.[14,15] It also inhibits reuptake of serotonin and norepinephrine (SSNRI), which has additional analgesic benefits. The initial studies on the use of methadone perioperatively were introduced by Gourlay et al.[16] In a double-blind, randomized trial comparing postoperative analgesia after perioperative loading doses of methadone or morphine, the difference in mean duration of pain relief between methadone (20.7 ± 2.2 hours) and morphine (6.3 ± 3.0 hours) was statistically significant.[17] In a prospective study of patients undergoing thoracolumbar spine surgery, patients were randomized to receive either methadone before surgical incision or a sufentanil loading dose followed by a sufentanil infusion. Perioperative treatment with a single intravenous bolus of methadone was superior and improved postoperative pain.[18] Methadone is rapidly growing as a first-line treatment for acute pain in patients with a history of chronic pain. The potential benefits include its duration of action and incomplete cross-tolerance with opioid rotation. It may, however, be associated with respiratory depression, sedation, and QTc interval prolongation. Doses range from 2.5 to 5 mg IV every 8 to 12 hours.

Buprenorphine is a partial μ-receptor agonist, opioid receptor like-1 (ORL-1) agonist, and κ-receptor antagonist. It may prevent OIH through its κ-receptor antagonist activity. Spinal dynorphin is a κ-receptor agonist that releases excitatory neurotransmitters.[8]

Cyclooxygenase inhibitors inhibit prostaglandin production, which facilitates the release of excitatory neurotransmitters and promotes peripheral and central sensitization.[19] Cyclooxygenase inhibitors can be used as adjuvant therapy in patients with a history of chronic pain. Adverse side effects include renal insufficiency, platelet inhibition, and gastrointestinal upset.

Ketamine is beneficial intraoperatively to reduce OIH and opioid tolerance.[20] It is an antagonist of the NMDA receptor. A bolus ranging range from 0.3 to 0.5 mg/kg is administered before incision, followed by a 2 to 5 μg/kg/min infusion. Adverse side effects include a sympathetic and psychotomimetic response.

Dexmedetomidine is an α_2-receptor agonist that may prevent OIH. Its agonistic property at the α_2-receptor in the spinal cord and locus ceruleus produces analgesia and sedation without respiratory depression. A bolus ranging from 0.5 to

Table 37.1. **MECHANISM OF ACTION AND TREATMENT OPTIONS FOR OPIOID-INDUCED HYPERALGESIA AND OPIOID TOLERANCE**

CAUSES OF OPIOID NONRESPONSIVENESS	MECHANISM OF ACTION	TREATMENT OPTIONS
Opioid tolerance	• Shift to the right of the dose-response curve. • Possible downregulation of receptors.	• Increase opioid dosage • Opioid rotation
Opioid-induced hyperalgesia	• Central glutaminergic system; NMDA receptor-mediated cell death in dorsal horn. • Enhanced response to nociceptive neurotransmitters. • Spinal dynorphin release. • Genetic polymorphism of COMT.	• Decrease opioid dosage • Discontinue opioid • Opioid rotation • NMDA receptor modulators

Abbreviations: COMT, catechol-*O*-methyltransferase; NMDA, *N*-methyl-D aspartate.

Table 37.2. ADJUNCT THERAPY

IV MEDICATION	DOSE	MECHANISM OF ACTION	POSSIBLE ADVERSE EFFECTS
Methadone	2.5–5 mg every 8–12 hr	μ-receptor agonist, NMDA receptor antagonist	Respiratory depression, sedation, prolonged QT interval
Buprenorphine	300 μg every 6–8 hr	Partial μ-receptor agonist, ORL-1 agonist, κ-receptor antagonist	Respiratory depression, sedation
Ibuprofen	400–800 mg every 6 hr	Inhibits cyclooxygenase	Renal insufficiency, platelet inhibition, GI upset
Acetaminophen	1 g every 6 hr	Unknown	Hepatic toxicity
Ketamine	0.3–0.5 mg/kg bolus before incision 2–5 μg/kg/min infusion	NMDA receptor antagonist	Psychotomimetic
Dexmedetomidine	0.5–2 μg/kg bolus before incision 0.2–0.7 μg/kg/hr infusion	Alpha 2 agonist	Hypotension, bradycardia, sedation

Abbreviations: GI, gastrointestinal; IV, intravenous; NMDA, *N*-methyl-D-aspartate; ORL-1, opioid receptor like-1.

2 μg/kg is administered before incision, followed by an infusion at 0.2 to 0.7 μg/kg/hr. The addition of dexmedetomidine to morphine PCA resulted in fewer morphine-induced adverse side effects and 29% less opioid consumption than in morphine PCA alone.[21] Adverse side effects were hypotension, bradycardia, and sedation.

Regional techniques (Table 37.3) can be considered a part of multimodal therapy in the treatment of postoperative pain. Thoracic epidural analgesia is a cornerstone for perioperative management after major thoracic and abdominal surgery. Advantages include analgesia, a decrease in perioperative cardiovascular events, and improved intestinal motility. Postoperative mortality was lower than with systemic opioid-based analgesia.[22] Contraindications to epidural analgesia are patient refusal or coagulopathy. The American Society of Regional Anesthesia (ASRA) has developed guidelines for the placement of single-shot or indwelling catheters and removal of indwelling catheters.[23] Controversy exists about the conservative nature of the recommendations. In a series of 4,365 patients undergoing hip and knee replacement surgery, removal of epidural catheters was uncomplicated despite INRs ranging from 1.5 to 5.9. Removal of the epidural catheters was timed to occur during initiation of warfarin therapy.[24] Warfarin inhibits protein C and factors II, VII, IX, and X. During initiation of warfarin therapy, the INR is initially dependent on levels of factor VII, as it has the shortest half-life. Vitamin K and factors II and X have a longer half-life and remain adequate, although an increase in INR is detected during the first 48 hours. For effective anticoagulation, these factors must be decreased.

The ASRA consensus guidelines recommend that the guidelines for neuraxial technique be followed for patients undergoing peripheral nerve and deep plexus block. Transversus abdominis plane (TAP) blocks and paravertebral blocks are peripheral nerve blocks that can be utilized for

Table 37.3. REGIONAL TECHNIQUES FOR ABDOMINAL SURGERY

REGIONAL TECHNIQUES	INDICATIONS	CONTRAINDICATIONS
Epidural analgesia	Provides analgesia to somatic and visceral organs.	Patient refusal, coagulopathy, infection at site
Transversus abdominis plane (TAP) block	Provides analgesia to skin and muscles of the anterior abdominal wall in lower abdomen Epidural contraindicated	Patient refusal, infection at site
Subcostal block	Provides analgesia to skin and muscles of the anterior abdominal wall in upper abdomen Epidural contraindicated	Patient refusal, infection at site
Paravertebral block	Provides analgesia to somatic and visceral organs	Patient refusal, coagulopathy, infection at site
PEC 1 and PEC 2 blocks	Provides analgesia to upper anterior chest wall and axilla (breast surgery)	Patient refusal, infection at site
Serratus anterior block	Provides analgesia to lateral chest wall (alternative to paravertebral block and thoracic epidural)	Patient refusal, infection at site

postoperative pain management. The TAP block was initially introduced in 2000 as a blind local anesthetic injection into Petit's lumbar triangle. Ultrasound-guided and surgically assisted methods have been described. The TAP is created by the fascial layer between the transverse abdominis muscle and the internal oblique muscle. The anterior rami of spinal nerves T7-L1 travel between these layers and innervate the anterior abdominal wall. The TAP block has been used for postoperative pain relief for several abdominal procedures.[25] It can be considered for patients undergoing abdominal surgery who are not candidates for epidural analgesia because of coagulopathies. TAP block is not technically challenging, but some complications, such as liver lacerations, have been reported.

Paravertebral blocks, which have been described for breast and thoracic surgery, are less frequently used for abdominal surgery. They can be incorporated in the multimodal treatment of postoperative abdominal pain.[26]

Because of concerns about pneumothorax and cord contusion and the lack of complete anesthesia coverage to the anterior chest wall via paravertebral blocks, the PEC 1 and PEC 2 block were introduced in 2012.[27] Later, the serratus anterior block was introduced for analgesia in the lateral chest wall as an alternative to paravertebral blocks and thoracic epidural analgesia.[28]

SPECIAL CONSIDERATIONS FOR PATIENTS WITH SUBSTANCE ABUSE

Acute and chronic pain are more difficult to treat in patients with a history of substance abuse. Patients with a history of substance abuse need opioids because adjuvant therapy alone is not sufficient. Although the potential for addiction is there, some suggest that pain may be protective against the rewarding effects of opiates. In animal studies using the conditioned place preference paradigm, morphine was less rewarding in the presence of pain.[29] Pain may lower, rather than increase, the risk of opiate addiction. Many physicians think that prescribing opioids to patients with a history of substance abuse and chronic pain feeds a habit and encourages dependence. A survey conducted by the Pain and Policy Group in Wisconsin among state medical board members compared responses from 1991, 1997, and 2004. On state medical boards, 75% of members are physicians, 20% are members of the public, and 5% are other health professionals. State board members are still skeptical about prescribing opioids for noncancer pain. A minority of board members considered it illegal to prescribe opioids to patients with a history of substance abuse,[30] although the DEA and the federation model policy permit their use. According to the model policy, the board considers the inappropriate treatment of pain a departure from standards of practice and will investigate such allegations.[4] In the survey, 18% of respondents reported addiction as being synonymous with physical dependence or tolerance. This misconception has potentially profound clinical implications because these views are held by members of a board that determines breach of professional conduct by physicians. Pain relief is a fundamental human right, even in patients with a history of substance abuse. The pain in patients with a history of chronic opioid or substance abuse can be challenging to manage, but incorporating multimodal treatment with pharmacologic and nonpharmacologic treatment options may improve outcome. Seeking consultation with experts in the field is highly recommended.

Table 37.4. **RISK FACTORS FOR CHRONIC POSTSURGICAL PAIN**

Surgical	Repeated surgical intervention Lengthy surgical time Surgery in previously traumatized area
Patient	Preexisting pain Female sex Young age Obesity Preoperative anxiety/catastrophizing
Anesthesia	General versus regional techniques

CHRONIC POSTSURGICAL PAIN SYNDROME

Chronic postsurgical pain syndrome (CPSP) was reported in 1998 in the United Kingdom. The etiology of pain in 40% of the chronic pain population was determined to be postsurgical in origin.[31] The International Association for the Study of Pain (IASP) defines CPSP as pain that persists for at least 2 months after a surgical intervention.[32] There is a strong positive correlation between the severity of acute postoperative pain and CPSP.[33] Risk factors have been identified for CPSP (Table 37.4).[34-38] Obesity is a risk factor, with the underlying mechanism associated with a pro-inflammatory state.[36] Anesthetic technique also has been implicated in CPSP. Retrospective data from hysterectomies and cesarean deliveries have shown a risk reduction of 50% with spinal anesthesia versus general anesthesia.[37,38]

CONCLUSION

- Perioperative pain management in patients with chronic pain and substance abuse requires special considerations and collaborative methods.
- OIH is a relatively new phenomenon that can encumber patient progress. Excessive opioid exposure worsens pain, rather than relieving it. Early recognition and management can improve outcomes.
- Opioid tolerance is common in patients who are on long-term opioid therapy for the management of a chronic pain syndrome. Opioid tolerance can lead to opioid nonresponsiveness and further hinder patient recovery.
- Attempts should be made to modify factors that increase the risk for chronic postsurgical pain. Certain patient factors and anesthetic and surgical techniques have been implicated.

- Incorporating multimodal methods for perioperative pain management using nonconventional opioids, such as methadone, cyclooxygenase inhibitors, NMDA antagonists, and regional techniques can improve outcomes and prevent OIH, opioid tolerance, and chronic postsurgical pain in patients on long-term opioid therapy.

REFERENCES

1. Apfelbaum JL, Chen C, Metha SS, et al. Postoperative pain experience. Results from a national survey suggest postoperative pain continues to be undermanaged. *Anesth Analg*. 2003;97:534–540.
2. International Narcotics Control Board. Narcotic drugs technical reports. Estimated world requirements for 2011. https://www.incb.org.
3. Janssen KJ, Kalkman CJ, Grobbee DE, et al. The risk of severe postoperative pain: modification and validation of clinical prediction rule. *Anesth Analg.* 2008;107:1330–1339.
4. Federation of State Medical Boards of the United States, Inc. *Model Policy for the Use of Controlled Substances for the Treatment of Pain.* 2004. Available from http://www.painpolicy.wisc.edu/sites/www.painpolicy.wisc.edu/files/model04.pdf.
5. Juni A, Cai M, Stankova M, et al. Sex-specific mediation of opioid-induced hyperalgesia by the melanocortin-1 receptor. *Anesthesiology*. 2010;112:181–188.
6. Jensen KB, Lonsdorf TB, Schalling M, et al. Increased sensitivity to thermal pain following a single opiate dose is influenced by the COMT Val (158) Met polymorphism. *PLoS ONE*. 2009;4:e6016.
7. Edward RR, Wasan A, Jamison R. Hyperalgesia in pain patients at elevated risk for opioid misuse. *J Pain*. 2010;11:S45.
8. Lee M, Silverman S, Hansen H, Patel V, Manchikanti L. A comprehensive review of opioid-induced hyperalgesia. *Pain Physician*. 2011;14:145–161.
9. Gardell LR, Wang R, Burgess SE, et al. Sustained morphine exposure induces a spinal dynorphin-dependent enhancement of excitatory transmitter release from primary afferent fibers. *J Neurosci.* 2002;22:6747–6755.
10. Morgan MM, Heinricher MM, Fields HL. Circuitry linking opioid-sensitive nociceptive modulatory systems in periaqueductal gray and spinal cord with rostral ventromedial medulla. *Neuroscience.* 1992;47:863–871.
11. Vanderah TW, Suenaga NM, Ossipov MH, Malan TP Jr, Lai J, Porreca F. Tonic descending facilitation from the rostral ventromedial medulla mediates opioid-induced abnormal pain and antinociceptive tolerance. *J Neurosci.* 2001;21:279–286.
12. Silverman S. Opioid induced hyperalgesia: Clinical implications for the pain practitioner. *Pain Physician*. 2009;12:679–684.
13. Kharasch ED. Intraoperative methadone: rediscovery, reappraisal and reinvigoration. *Anesth Analg*. 2011;112(1):15–16.
14. Manfredi PL, Houde RW. Prescribing methadone, a unique analgesic. *J Support Oncol.* 2003;1(3):2216–2220.
15. Toombs JD, Kral LA. Methadone treatment for pain states. *Am Fam Physician*. 2005;71(7):1353–1358.
16. Gourlay GK, Wilson PR, Glynn CJ. Pharmacodynamics and pharmacokinetics of methadone during perioperative period. *Anesthesiology.* 1982;57:458–467.
17. Chui PT, Gin T. A double-blind randomised trial comparing postoperative analgesia after perioperative loading doses of methadone and morphine. *Anaesth Intensive Care.* 1992;20(1):46–51.
18. Gotsschalk A, Durieux M, Nemergut E. Intraoperative methadone improves postoperative pain control in patients undergoing complex spine surgery. *Anesth Analg*. 2011;112:218–223.
19. Tröster A, Sittl R, Singler B, et al. Modulation of remifentanil-induced analgesia and postinfusion hyperalgesia by parecoxib in humans. *Anesthesiology*. 2006;105:1016–1023.
20. Koppert W, Sittl R, Scheuber K, et al. Differential modulation of remifentanil-induced analgesia and postinfusion hyperalgesia by S-ketamine and clonidine in humans. *Anesthesiology.* 2003;99:152–159.
21. Lin TF, Yeh YC, Lin FS, et al. Effect of combining dexmedetomidine and morphine for intravenous patient-controlled analgesia. *Br J Anaesth*. 2009;102:117–122.
22. Freise H, Van Aken H. Risk and benefits of thoracic epidural anaesthesia. *Br J Anaesth.* 2011;107(6):859–868.
23. Horlocker TT, Wedel DJ, Rowlingson JC, et al. Regional anesthesia in the patient receiving antithrombotic or thrombolytic therapy: American Society of Regional Anesthesia and Pain Medicine evidence-based guidelines (third edition). *Reg Anesth Pain Med.* 2010;35:64–101.
24. Liu S, Buvanendran A, Viscusi ER, et al. Uncomplicated removal of epidural catheters in 4365 patients with international normalized ratio greater than 1.4 during initiation of warfarin therapy. *Reg Anesth Pain Med.* 2011;36(3):231–235.
25. Siddiqui M, Sajid M, Uncles D, et al. A meta-analysis on the clinical effectiveness of transversus abdominis plane block. *J Clin Anesth.* 2011;23:7–14.
26. Finnerty O, Carney J, McDonnell JG. Truncal blocks for abdominal surgery. *Anaesthesia*. 2010;6(1):76–83.
27. Blanco R, Fajardo M, Parras Maldonado T, et al. Ultrasound description of PECS II (modified PECS I): a novel approach to breast surgery. *Rev Esp Anestesiol Reanim*. 2012;59(9):470–475.
28. Blanco R, Parras T, McDonnell JG, Prats-Galino A. Serratus plane block: a novel ultrasound-guided thoracic wall nerve block. *Anaesthesia.* 2013;68:1107–1113.
29. Betourne A, Familiades J, Lacassagne L, et al. Decreased motivation properties of morphine in mouse model of cancerous or inflammatory chronic pain: implication of supraspinal neuropeptide FF (2) receptors. *Neuroscience.* 2008;157(1):12–21.
30. Gilson A. State medical board members' attitudes about the legality of chronic prescribing to patients with noncancer pain: the influence of knowledge and beliefs about pain management, addiction, and opioid prescribing. *J Pain Symptom Manage.* 2010;40(4):599–612.
31. Crombie IK, Davies HT, Macrae WA. Cut and thrust: antecedent surgery and trauma among patients attending a chronic pain clinic. *Pain*. 1998;76:167–171.
32. Macrae WA, Davies HTO. Chronic postsurgical pain. In: Crombie IK, Linton S, Croft P, Von Korff M, LeResche L, eds. *Epidemiology of Pain.* Seattle, WA: IASP Press; 1999:125–142.
33. Yarnitsky D, Crispel Y, Eisenberg E, et al. Prediction of chronic postoperative pain: pre-operative DNIC testing identifies patients at risk. *Pain.* 2008;138:22–28.
34. Perkins FM, Kehlet H. Chronic pain as an outcome from surgery. A review of predictive factors. *Anesthesiology*. 2000;93:1123–1133.
35. Kehlet H, Jensen TS, Woolf CJ. Persistent postsurgical pain: risk factors and prevention. *Lancet*. 2006;367(9522):1618–1625.
36. Okifuji A, Donaldson GW, Barck L, Fine PG. Relationship between fibromyalgia and obesity in pain, function, mood, and sleep. *J Pain.* 2010;11:1329–1337.
37. Brandsborg B, Nikolajsen L, Hansen CT, et al. Risk factors for chronic pain after hysterectomy: a nationwide questionnaire and database study. *Anesthesiology*. 2007;106:1003–1012.
38. Nikolajsen L, Sorensen HC, Jensen TS, Kehlet H. Chronic pain following caesarean section. *Acta Anaesthesiol Scand.* 2004;48:111–116.

REVIEW QUESTIONS

1. A 32-year-old male with chronic back pain for which he takes hydrocodone/acetaminophen 10/325 mg every 4 hours undergoes a laparoscopic cholecystectomy. In the postoperative anesthesia care unit, he complains of sharp, excruciating pain at the incision site. He is tachypneic and unable to take deep breaths because of pain. He has received a total of 0.5 mg intravenous hydromorphone in the past hour.

Which of the following describes the cause for his opioid nonresponsiveness?

A. OIH
B. Opioid tolerance
C. Malingering
D. Physical dependence

2. Which of the following is not a mechanism for opioid tolerance?

A. Upregulation of the metabolic process that eliminates the drug
B. Downregulation of the opioid receptor
C. Shift to the right of the dose-response curve
D. Activation of the NMDA receptor

3. A 31-year-old Caucasian female with a body mass index of 60 is scheduled for an open appendectomy. She has had multiple abdominal surgeries and is very anxious about her upcoming surgery. Which of the following is not an indicator for an increased risk for chronic postsurgical pain?

A. Age
B. Gender
C. Race
D. Preoperative anxiety

ANSWERS

1. B. This patient's prior opioid exposure most likely causes a shift to the right of the dose-response curve. The patient needs large doses to produce the desired effect. Answer A is incorrect because the pain is consistent with the nociceptive nature typical of acute postoperative pain. In OIH, the pain tends to be neuropathic and located outside the surgical incision site.[8] Answer C is incorrect. The patient is distressed (tachypneic and unable to take deep breaths). Physical dependence means that the body relies on an external source of opioids to prevent withdrawal. This patient is not exhibiting symptoms or signs of withdrawal.

2. D. Activation of the NMDA receptor plays a role in developing OIH.[8] Answers A, B, and C are underlying mechanisms of opioid tolerance.

3. C. Race is not a risk factor for developing chronic postsurgical pain. Answers A, B, and D are risk factors for chronic postsurgical pain.[33] Patient, surgical, and anesthetic factors are positively correlated with developing chronic postsurgical pain. Young age, female sex, obesity, and preoperative anxiety are examples of patient factors. Surgery in a previously traumatized area (multiple abdominal surgeries before the open appendectomy) is a surgical factor that increases the risk for chronic postsurgical pain.

QUESTIONS AND ANSWERS

This chapter has accompanying questions and answers that are available to subscribers as part of the Oxford eLearning platform. To access the questions, follow the link below, or go to ✔ http://oxfordmedicine.com/painmanagementreview

38.

FIBROMYALGIA

Reem Jan and Dawen Zhang

STEM CASE AND KEY QUESTIONS

A 27-year-old Caucasian female is referred to your clinic with widespread pain. Her symptoms have been present since high school and she reports daily, migratory pain and stiffness in multiple joints, including her hands, wrists, shoulders, neck, and lower back that is present constantly without diurnal variation. She takes carisoprodol 250 mg at bedtime for her lower back pain and four to six tabs of hydrocodone-acetaminophen 7.5 mg/325 mg per day as needed for pain.

Despite pharmacotherapy, the patient has noted the severity of her pain has progressively increased over time. She tearfully admits that she recently ended a long-term relationship with her boyfriend. In the past couple of weeks, there were days where she was in "too much pain to function," had to take off work, and spent all day in bed. Despite sleeping 7 to 8 hours per day, she awakens unrefreshed and is fatigued. Her performance at work has been suffering because she has been unable to focus and to complete tasks on time. Recently, the patient experienced intermittent numbness and tingling in her face and hands. She previously underwent evaluation by gastroenterology for abdominal bloating and alternating diarrhea and constipation. Endoscopic studies were unremarkable.

WHAT PORTIONS OF HER HISTORY ARE CONSISTENT WITH FIBROMYALGIA?

Physical exam is notable for widespread pain to light touch, but a thorough joint examination reveals no focal areas of swelling or inflammation, nor does it show restricted range of motion in her joints.

ARE TENDER POINTS NECESSARY FOR A DIAGNOSIS OF FIBROMYALGIA?

Previous laboratory studies in the patient's chart include a chemistry panel, complete blood cell count, erythrocyte sedimentation rate (ESR), C-reactive protein (CRP), and thyroid-stimulating hormone (TSH); all were within normal limits.

SHOULD AN ANTINUCLEAR ANTIBODY (ANA), RHEUMATOID FACTOR (RF), OR ANTI-CITRULLINATED PROTEIN ANTIBODIES (ACPA) BE ORDERED AT THIS POINT TO RULE OUT AUTOIMMUNE AND RHEUMATIC PHENOMENA? WHAT OTHER LABORATORY TESTING SHOULD BE COMPLETED?

The patient brings up her back pain again and states that her back is often stiff as well. She saw a commercial that referred to ankylosing spondylitis and asks if she may have this condition. Her back pain is constant throughout the day and doesn't vary with activity. Her exam is not consistent with loss of range of motion in her axial skeleton, but she does note tenderness with even mild palpation at her sacroiliac joints.

WHAT FURTHER IMAGING IS WARRANTED AT THIS POINT?

You diagnose the patient with fibromyalgia, at which point she becomes defensive and accuses you of thinking that her symptoms are "all in my head." Tactfully, you explain that her symptoms and disease are indeed "real." You proceed to discuss the disease and counsel the patient in further detail.

An aerobic exercise regimen is encouraged and amitriptyline 10 mg 2 hours before bedtime is prescribed. A plan is put in place to slowly wean the patient off her narcotics. A week later, the patient calls your office saying that she has started jogging for 30 minutes every other day, but her pain and fatigue have worsened. You call her back saying that initial worsening of symptoms is not uncommon and it should subside with time. You encourage her to continue jogging.

She sees you in clinic for follow-up 3 months later and she is still complaining of fatigue and diffuse pain despite titrating amitriptyline to 25 mg at bedtime and continuing her jogging routine. Her lower back pain is the most troublesome today. The patient's friend has endorsed lumbar epidural steroid injections for his chronic back pain with significant improvement. She requests a trial of an epidural injection.

WHAT PROCEDURAL OR SURGICAL INTERVENTIONS HAVE A PLACE IN TREATING FIBROMYALGIA?

You explain that an epidural steroid injection is unlikely to help her and instead you start her on duloxetine 20 mg every morning, with plans to titrate slowly to 60 mg daily. Amitriptyline is discontinued. She returns in 3 months on 60 mg duloxetine; she is exercising daily and has had perceptible improvement in her pain and sleep.

DISCUSSION

Fibromyalgia is a chronic condition characterized by widespread musculoskeletal pain. For many years, clinicians had dismissed it as a psychosomatic or functional disorder, but a growing body of evidence shows consistent biochemical abnormalities in pain- processing pathways in patients with fibromyalgia. Although the life expectancy of patients with fibromyalgia is normal, there can be considerable morbidity and disability associated with the syndrome that in a significant subset of patients results in enormous personal and financial cost. A multidisciplinary approach to care that incorporates pharmacologic therapies, education, counseling, and exercise is required to lower pain levels and to restore function in this challenging disease.

Fibromyalgia occurs most commonly in perimenopausal women, but it can start in late childhood/adolescence with more localized pain issues, such as growing pains, irritable bowel syndrome, and recurrent headaches. The incidence in men has been historically underestimated as classic myofascial tenderness is less frequently seen in males; however, once new criteria are applied to diagnosis, the female to male ratio is found to be 3:1, rather than 9:1, as previously estimated.[1] There are equivalent rates of fibromyalgia across all socioeconomic and ethnic groups.[2]

PATHOPHYSIOLOGY

The principal mechanism of disease is deregulation of sensory pain pathways, leading to abnormally high levels of pain perception. For example, it has been demonstrated that serotonin levels are low and substance P levels are high in the CSF of patients who suffer from fibromyalgia compared to normal subjects.[3] The endogenous opioid receptors appear centrally attenuated, whereas glutamate activity is high in pain-processing regions of the brain, such as the insula.[4,5] Overall, these differential effects lead to both an increase in pain sensation and a decrease in the normal inhibitory mechanisms.

DIAGNOSTIC EVALUATION

History

Diffuse pain that cannot be explained fully by inflammation, degenerative disease, or trauma is the principal complaint in the presentation of fibromyalgia. Being central in nature, the pain is migratory, and it waxes and wanes. This contrasts with peripheral pain, which is more consistent in location and severity. Pain in fibromyalgia is musculoskeletal and is described as deep and aching, with intermittent sharp spasms. Some patients complain of tension in their muscles and being "tied in knots." Excessive tenderness is common and the slightest touch may cause severe pain.

Because all pain pathways are amplified, a range of other discomforting symptoms, such as chronic headaches, pelvic pain, chest pain, and irritable bowel syndrome, are frequently noted. Other common coexisting functional somatic disorders include chronic fatigue syndrome, temporomandibular joint syndrome, and interstitial cystitis.

Pain is frequently worsened by stressful physical or emotional events, but exacerbations can occur without any precipitating factors. Continuing the theme of central amplification, many patients have lower noxious thresholds for noises, odors, and other sensory stimuli.[6,7]

Fatigue affects almost all patients with fibromyalgia and is often debilitating, and 90% of patients complain of nonrestorative sleep (i.e., they are able to fall asleep, but they wake up tired and not refreshed).[8] The presence of disordered breathing, apnea, or snoring indicates a primary sleep disorder, such as obstructive sleep apnea, rather than fibromyalgia, which may in turn exacerbate pain perception. Cognitive difficulties occur frequently and are often described as "brain fog"; they are primarily difficulties with concentration and short-term memory.

Some fibromyalgia patients describe symptoms mimicking those of inflammatory arthritis, such as prolonged morning stiffness and swelling of extremities. However, in contrast to inflammatory disorders, fibromyalgia patients point to more diffuse swelling, rather than swelling around joint spaces, and there is no evidence of synovitis on physical examination.

Physical Exam/Laboratory Testing

A complete physical examination should be performed, with a focus on joint and neurologic testing. There are usually no abnormalities on exam, except for diffuse allodynia or hyperalgesia elicited on palpation and minor motor and sensory abnormalities.[9] The 1990 American College of Rheumatology (ACR) diagnostic criteria required the presence of 11 out of 18 tender points because fibromyalgia patients have pain thresholds at lower applied pressures. Assessment of tender points was important to ensure diagnostic homogeneity in clinical trials, but it was impractical in many routine clinical contexts. As a result, this provision was removed in the modified 2010 ACR criteria, which serve as an alternate method of diagnosis to the 1990 ACR criteria.[10]

Patients with fibromyalgia often present with certain dermatologic features that overlap with autoimmune disorders, including mild erythema of the digits and facial flushing that may mimic Raynaud's phenomenon and a malar rash to the untrained eye.

In terms of laboratory workup, a chemistry panel, complete cell count, ESR, CRP, and TSH are all that are necessary. There are no tests that are specific for fibromyalgia, so labs are useful only for ruling out alternative diagnoses. Particular care should be used to avoid expensive serologic testing, such as

Box 38.1. DIFFERENTIAL DIAGNOSIS OF FIBROMYALGIA

Polymyalgia rheumatica
Rheumatoid arthritis
Early autoimmune disease: Rheumatoid arthritis, systemic lupus erythematosus, Sjögren's syndrome
Myopathies
Hypothyroidism
Hepatitis C
Obstructive sleep apnea

ANA and RF, in the absence of specific symptoms or signs of an inflammatory or autoimmune disorder, as this may result in false-positive or weakly positive results.

It is important to distinguish fibromyalgia from conditions that may mimic or occur concurrently with the disease (see Box 38.1. This can in most cases be achieved with careful history and physical examination.

Diagnostic Criteria

The modified 2010 ACR fibromyalgia diagnostic criteria require widespread pain for at least 3 months that is not otherwise explained and that is found at 19 different, self-reported body locations (Widespread Pain Index [WPI]). Additionally, patients must have significant fatigue, nonrestorative sleep, cognitive symptoms, and certain somatic complaints (Summed Severity Score [SSS]). A sum of a WPI of ≥ 7 and a SSS ≥ 5, or a combination WPI between 3 and 6 and a SSS ≥ 9 supports a diagnosis of fibromialgia. These questions may be self-administered by the patient as a questionnaire.

The SSS adds the severity scores of four components: 1) fatigue, 2) unrefreshed upon waking, 3) cognitive symptoms, and 4) the extent of somatic symptoms. For the first three components, the scale ranges from 0 to 3. A component score of 0 signifies no problem while a score of 3 indicates a severe, pervasive and continuous problem.[10] The modified 2010 ACR criteria questionnaire had a sensitivity of 90.2% and specificity of 89.5% using clinical assessment by a rheumatologist as the gold standard.[11]

MANAGEMENT

Patients with fibromyalgia present with varying severity of pain responses, fatigue, sleep disturbances, and cognitive/psychologic burdens. Given the heterogeneity of the condition, it is important to tailor treatment to each individual, rather than following a strict algorithm. A combination of pharmacologic and nonpharmacologic treatment is often necessary to control symptoms.

PHARMACOLOGIC TREATMENT

Tricyclic Antidepressants (TCAs)

Amitriptyline and cyclobenzaprine have been widely studied and have been shown to be effective in fibromyalgia for improving pain, sleep, fatigue, and quality of life.[12,13] They inhibit serotonin and norepinephrine uptake at the synaptic cleft.[14] They also act as muscarinic and histamine receptor antagonists, and block sodium and calcium channel activity. Given their low cost and efficacy, TCAs are recommended as first-line treatment. TCAs improve symptoms by inhibition of norepinephrine and serotonin reuptake. Anticholinergic side effects are common and thus dosing should start low (10 mg of amitriptyline or 5 mg cyclobenzaprine 1 to 3 hours before bedtime). Amitriptyline should be titrated by 5 mg at 2-week intervals to a goal of 25 mg at bedtime. Higher dosing at 50 mg/day was no better than placebo.[12]

SEROTONIN-NOREPINEPHRINE REUPTAKE INHIBITORS (SNRIS OR DUAL REUPTAKE INHIBITORS)

Two SNRIs, duloxetine and milnacipran, have been shown to be effective in reducing pain and improving function in multicenter trials and are FDA approved for the treatment of fibromyalgia.[15,16] They have been shown to have efficacy similar to that of TCAs and are tolerated better than TCAs because they do not have anticholinergic side effects.[17] Duloxetine has 10 times the selectivity for serotonin over norepinephrine, but milnacipran is up to three times more selective toward norepinephrine reuptake.[14,18] Duloxetine is started at 30 mg every morning, then after a week it is increased to a maximum approved dose of 60 mg/day (although up to 120 mg/day was found to be safe during trials). Milnacipran should be started at 12.5 mg every morning, then titrated to a goal of 50 mg twice a day. Nausea and headaches are the most common side effects; other adverse symptoms are due to increased noradrenergic activation (dry mouth, hyperhidrosis, decreased appetite, constipation, agitation, and flushing).[16] Hypertension and tachycardia, while not common, should be carefully monitored for, especially with milnacipran. SNRIs are contraindicated with concurrent use of monamine oxidase inhibitors and in uncontrolled narrow-angle glaucoma. Venlafaxine is not recommended, given lack of study in trials.

Anticonvulsants (α_2-Ligands)

Pregabalin and gabapentin have been shown to improve pain, fatigue, physical function, and sleep quality. They are synthetic derivatives of GABA and bind to the alpha2/delta ($\alpha_2\delta$) subunit of the voltage-gated calcium channel in the CNS. They decrease nerve terminal calcium influx, which blocks release of glutamate, norepinephrine, and substance P.[19] Pregabalin is dosed at 25 to 50 mg at bedtime, then uptitrated weekly to 300 to 450 mg/day (either at night or in divided doses). Certain patients may respond well to lower doses (100 mg/day). With more limited evidence and less patient tolerability of uptitration to therapeutic doses, gabapentin may be considered if pregabalin is cost-prohibitive or not reimbursed.[20] The starting dose is 100 mg at bedtime, and the dose is titrated as tolerated to 1200 to 2400 mg/day in divided doses. Giving two-thirds or the entire daily dose of these anticonvulsants at bedtime may increase the tolerability of these drugs. Common side effects include weight gain, dizziness, somnolence, dry mouth, and peripheral edema.

In patients who do not respond to TCAs, or cannot tolerate TCAs because of side effects, the medication should be discontinued. If there is significant daytime fatigue, a SNRI, which will improve energy, may be initiated. If sleep disturbances predominate, an α_2-ligand may be started.

In patients with refractory disease on monotherapy, combination drug therapy should be explored. This has the benefit of targeting different symptoms in tandem. For example, an SNRI may be started in the morning in patients with poor energy levels and concentration, in combination with a TCA or α_2-ligand at night to alleviate insomnia. A combination of pregabalin with milnacipran has been shown to more effective than pregabalin alone.[21] Changing dosing times may improve tolerability as well; a patient may experience less daytime fatigue if dosing of pregabalin 75 mg twice a day is changed to 150 mg at bedtime.

Analgesia

Tramadol, alone or in combination with acetaminophen, may reduce pain, but does not improve function in fibromyalgia.[22,23] Tramadol is a weak mu opioid receptor agonist, but its analgesic effects in fibromyalgia are likely from its inhibition of serotonin and norepinephrine reuptake, as stronger opioids have been shown to be ineffective in treating pain in fibromyalgia. In fact, there is evidence that strong opioids lead to worsening long-term outcomes and therefore should be avoided.[24,25] Nonsteroidal anti-inflammatory drugs (NSAIDs) or other anti-inflammatories should not be considered for pain unless the patient has concurrent regional pain or inflammatory disorders.

OTHER THERAPIES

Exercise has consistently been shown to improve function and reduce the symptoms of fibromyalgia and it forms an integral part of the management of the disease.[26] In general, the advice is to start slowly with low-impact activity on a daily basis and gradually increase intensity and duration of exercise. Exercise can often be initiated a few weeks to months after a positive clinical response to medications. The evidence for homeopathic remedies and acupuncture is less robust and they should be recommended with caution.

It should be stressed to patients that fibromyalgia is indeed a real disease, rather than a psychosomatic condition. Realistic expectations should be provided; disease remission is not likely, but the illness is benign. Cognitive-behavioral therapy has been shown to reduce pain and function and may be initiated in patients who fail initial therapies.[27,28]

Selective serotonin reuptake inhibitors (SSRIs) have shown mixed results in small, randomized, controlled trials and should not be used solely for fibromyalgia symptoms until more proven medications have been tried. Older, less-selective SSRIs, such as fluoxetine or paroxetine, which have more noradrenergic activity, especially at higher doses, appear to be more efficacious than newer, more-selective SSRIs.[29]

It is important to recognize concurrent degenerative or connective tissue disease, but in the absence of these disorders, local therapies or procedures, such as steroid injections or joint replacement surgeries, will not impact the centralized pain of fibromyalgia and may lead to disappointing outcomes.[30]

EXPERIMENTAL THERAPIES

Small, single-center, randomized controlled trials have shown some medications to have early promising results. Naltrexone, pramipexole, and melatonin, with or without amitriptyline, were found to be superior to placebo at reducing pain.[31–33] Gamma-hydroxybutyrate (or sodium oxabate) has been shown to improve pain, sleep, and fatigue in high-quality studies, but the FDA did not approve the potent sedative for fibromyalgia given its abuse potential.[34,35]

Some early data have shown that nerve modulation techniques may be beneficial, but further study is needed before this is recommended. Transcranial stimulation, via either transcranial direct current stimulation (tDCS) or transcranial magnetic stimulation (TMS), with stimulation of the primary motor cortex or prefrontal cortex, has shown reduction in pain compared to sham procedure.[36,37] Transcutaneous electrical nerve stimulation (TENS) has shown some early promise, but so far has had mixed results in decreasing pain and improving function.[38–41]

CONCLUSIONS

Fibromyalgia is caused by amplification of central sensory and pain pathways and often manifests as chronic, widespread musculoskeletal pain, fatigue, sleep disturbances, and somatic complaints.

Physical examination elicits tenderness, but standardized tender point elicitation is not required based on the revised 2010 ACR criteria.

Lab testing should include only a chemistry panel, CBC, TSH, ESR, and CRP.

Treatment should be multidisciplinary and may include patient counseling and education, graded aerobic exercise, and pharmacologic therapy (with TCAs, SNRIs, and α_2-ligands).

REFERENCES

1. Vincent A, Lahr BD, Wolfe F, et al. Prevalence of fibromyalgia: a population-based study in Olmsted County, Minnesota, utilizing the Rochester Epidemiology Project. *Arthritis Care Res.* 2013;65(5):786–792. doi:10.1002/acr.21896.
2. Jones GT, Atzeni F, Beasley M, Fluss E, Sarzi-Puttini P, Macfarlane GJ. The prevalence of fibromyalgia in the general population: a comparison of the American College of Rheumatology 1990, 2010, and modified 2010 classification criteria. *Arthritis Rheumatol.* 2015;67(2):568–575. doi:10.1002/art.38905.
3. Russell IJ, Orr MD, Littman B, et al. Elevated cerebrospinal fluid levels of substance P in patients with the fibromyalgia syndrome. *Arthritis Rheum.* 1994;37(11):1593–1601.
4. Harris RE, Clauw DJ, Scott DJ, McLean SA, Gracely RH, Zubieta J-K. Decreased central mu-opioid receptor availability in

fibromyalgia. *J Neurosci.* 2007;27(37):10000–10006. doi:10.1523/JNEUROSCI.2849-07.2007.
5. Harris RE. Elevated excitatory neurotransmitter levels in the fibromyalgia brain. *Arthritis Res Ther.* 2010;12(5):141. doi:10.1186/ar3136.
6. McDermid AJ, Rollman GB, McCain GA. Generalized hypervigilance in fibromyalgia: evidence of perceptual amplification. *Pain.* 1996;66(2-3):133–144.
7. Gerster JC, Hadj-Djilani A. Hearing and vestibular abnormalities in primary fibrositis syndrome. *J Rheumatol.* 1984;11(5):678–680.
8. Bigatti SM, Hernandez AM, Cronan TA, Rand KL. Sleep disturbances in fibromyalgia syndrome: relationship to pain and depression. *Arthritis Rheum.* 2008;59(7):961–967. doi:10.1002/art.23828.
9. Watson NF, Buchwald D, Goldberg J, Noonan C, Ellenbogen RG. Neurologic signs and symptoms in fibromyalgia. *Arthritis Rheum.* 2009;60(9):2839–2844. doi:10.1002/art.24772.
10. Wolfe F, Clauw DJ, Fitzcharles M-A, et al. Fibromyalgia criteria and severity scales for clinical and epidemiological studies: a modification of the ACR preliminary diagnostic criteria for fibromyalgia. *J Rheumatol.* 2011;38(6):1113–1122. doi:10.3899/jrheum.100594.
11. Ferrari R, Russell AS. A questionnaire using the modified 2010 American College of Rheumatology criteria for fibromyalgia: specificity and sensitivity in clinical practice. *J Rheumatol.* 2013;40(9):1590–1595. doi:10.3899/jrheum.130367.
12. Nishishinya B, Urrutia G, Walitt B, et al. Amitriptyline in the treatment of fibromyalgia: a systematic review of its efficacy. *Rheumatology (Oxford).* 2008;47(12):1741–1746. doi:10.1093/rheumatology/ken317.
13. Tofferi JK, Jackson JL, O'Malley PG. Treatment of fibromyalgia with cyclobenzaprine: a meta-analysis. *Arthritis Rheum.* 2004;51(1):9–13. doi:10.1002/art.20076.
14. Sindrup SH, Otto M, Finnerup NB, Jensen TS. Antidepressants in the treatment of neuropathic pain. *Basic Clin Pharmacol Toxicol.* 2005;96(6):399–409. doi:10.1111/j.1742-7843.2005.pto_96696601.x.
15. Curran MP. Duloxetine: in patients with fibromyalgia. *Drugs.* 2009;69(9):1217–1227.
16. Clauw DJ, Mease P, Palmer RH, Gendreau RM, Wang Y. Milnacipran for the treatment of fibromyalgia in adults: a 15-week, multicenter, randomized, double-blind, placebo-controlled, multiple-dose clinical trial. *Clin Ther.* 2008;30(11):1988–2004. doi:10.1016/j.clinthera.2008.11.009.
17. Hauser W, Petzke F, Uceyler N, Sommer C. Comparative efficacy and acceptability of amitriptyline, duloxetine and milnacipran in fibromyalgia syndrome: a systematic review with meta-analysis. *Rheumatology (Oxford).* 2011;50(3):532–543. doi:10.1093/rheumatology/keq354.
18. Montgomery SA. Tolerability of serotonin norepinephrine reuptake inhibitor antidepressants. *CNS Spectr.* 2008;13(7)(suppl 11):27–33.
19. Wiffen PJ, Derry S, Moore RA, et al. Antiepileptic drugs for neuropathic pain and fibromyalgia—an overview of Cochrane reviews. *Cochrane Database Syst Rev.* 2013;11:CD010567. doi:10.1002/14651858.CD010567.pub2.
20. Arnold LM, Goldenberg DL, Stanford SB, et al. Gabapentin in the treatment of fibromyalgia: a randomized, double-blind, placebo-controlled, multicenter trial. *Arthritis Rheum.* 2007;56(4):1336–1344. doi:10.1002/art.22457.
21. Mease PJ, Farmer M V, Palmer RH, Gendreau RM, Trugman JM, Wang Y. Milnacipran combined with pregabalin in fibromyalgia: a randomized, open-label study evaluating the safety and efficacy of adding milnacipran in patients with incomplete response to pregabalin. *Ther Adv Musculoskelet Dis.* 2013;5(3):113–126. doi:10.1177/1759720X13483894.
22. Bennett RM, Kamin M, Karim R, Rosenthal N. Tramadol and acetaminophen combination tablets in the treatment of fibromyalgia pain: a double-blind, randomized, placebo-controlled study. *Am J Med.* 2003;114(7):537–545.
23. MacLean AJB, Schwartz TL. Tramadol for the treatment of fibromyalgia. *Expert Rev Neurother.* 2015;15(5):469–475. doi:10.1586/14737175.2015.1034693.
24. Ngian G-S, Guymer EK, Littlejohn GO. The use of opioids in fibromyalgia. *Int J Rheum Dis.* 2011;14(1):6–11. doi:10.1111/j.1756-185X.2010.01567.x.
25. Goldenberg DL, Clauw DJ, Palmer RE, Clair AG. Opioid use in fibromyalgia: a cautionary tale. *Mayo Clin Proc.* 2016;91(5):640–648.
26. Bidonde J, Busch AJ, Bath B, Milosavljevic S. Exercise for adults with fibromyalgia: an umbrella systematic review with synthesis of best evidence. *Curr Rheumatol Rev.* 2014;10(1):45–79.
27. Van Koulil S, van Lankveld W, Kraaimaat FW, et al. Tailored cognitive-behavioral therapy and exercise training for high-risk patients with fibromyalgia. *Arthritis Care Res.* 2010;62(10):1377–1385. doi:10.1002/acr.20268.
28. Glombiewski JA, Sawyer AT, Gutermann J, Koenig K, Rief W, Hofmann SG. Psychological treatments for fibromyalgia: a meta-analysis. *Pain.* 2010;151(2):280–295. doi:10.1016/j.pain.2010.06.011.
29. Walitt B, Urrutia G, Nishishinya MB, Cantrell SE, Hauser W. Selective serotonin reuptake inhibitors for fibromyalgia syndrome. *Cochrane Database Syst Rev.* 2015;6:CD011735. doi:10.1002/14651858.CD011735.
30. Brummett CM, Urquhart AG, Hassett AL, et al. Characteristics of fibromyalgia independently predict poorer long-term analgesic outcomes following total knee and hip arthroplasty. *Arthritis Rheumatol.* 2015;67(5):1386–1394. doi:10.1002/art.39051.
31. Younger J, Noor N, McCue R, Mackey S. Low-dose naltrexone for the treatment of fibromyalgia: findings of a small, randomized, double-blind, placebo-controlled, counterbalanced, crossover trial assessing daily pain levels. *Arthritis Rheum.* 2013;65(2):529–538. doi:10.1002/art.37734.
32. Holman AJ, Myers RR. A randomized, double-blind, placebo-controlled trial of pramipexole, a dopamine agonist, in patients with fibromyalgia receiving concomitant medications. *Arthritis Rheum.* 2005;52(8):2495–2505. doi:10.1002/art.21191.
33. De Zanette SA, Vercelino R, Laste G, et al. Melatonin analgesia is associated with improvement of the descending endogenous pain-modulating system in fibromyalgia: a phase II, randomized, double-dummy, controlled trial. *BMC Pharmacol Toxicol.* 2014;15:40. doi:10.1186/2050-6511-15-40.
34. Russell IJ, Holman AJ, Swick TJ, Alvarez-Horine S, Wang YG, Guinta D. Sodium oxybate reduces pain, fatigue, and sleep disturbance and improves functionality in fibromyalgia: results from a 14-week, randomized, double-blind, placebo-controlled study. *Pain.* 2011;152(5):1007–1017. doi:10.1016/j.pain.2010.12.022.
35. Spaeth M, Bennett RM, Benson BA, Wang YG, Lai C, Choy EH. Sodium oxybate therapy provides multidimensional improvement in fibromyalgia: results of an international phase 3 trial. *Ann Rheum Dis.* 2012;71(6):935–942. doi:10.1136/annrheumdis-2011-200418.
36. Fregni F, Gimenes R, Valle AC, et al. A randomized, sham-controlled, proof of principle study of transcranial direct current stimulation for the treatment of pain in fibromyalgia. *Arthritis Rheum.* 2006;54(12):3988–3998. doi:10.1002/art.22195.
37. Knijnik LM, Dussan-Sarria JA, Rozisky JR, et al. Repetitive transcranial magnetic stimulation for fibromyalgia: systematic review and meta-analysis. *Pain Pract.* 2016;16(3):294–304. doi:10.1111/papr.12276.
38. Noehren B, Dailey DL, Rakel BA, et al. Effect of transcutaneous electrical nerve stimulation on pain, function, and quality of life in fibromyalgia: a double-blind randomized clinical trial. *Phys Ther.* 2015;95(1):129–140. doi:10.2522/ptj.20140218.
39. Dailey DL, Rakel BA, Vance CGT, et al. Transcutaneous electrical nerve stimulation reduces pain, fatigue and hyperalgesia while restoring central inhibition in primary fibromyalgia. *Pain.* 2013;154(11):2554–2562. doi:10.1016/j.pain.2013.07.043.
40. Mutlu B, Paker N, Bugdayci D, Tekdos D, Kesiktas N. Efficacy of supervised exercise combined with transcutaneous electrical nerve stimulation in women with fibromyalgia: a prospective controlled study. *Rheumatol Int.* 2013;33(3):649–655. doi:10.1007/s00296-012-2390-8.

41. Lofgren M, Norrbrink C. Pain relief in women with fibromyalgia: a cross-over study of superficial warmth stimulation and transcutaneous electrical nerve stimulation. *J Rehabil Med*. 2009;41(7):557–562. doi:10.2340/16501977-0371.

REVIEW QUESTIONS

1. A 21-year-old male screams in pain during an uncomplicated peripheral IV insertion in the emergency department. What best describes this pain response?

   A. Hyperesthesia
   B. Allodynia
   C. Hyperalgesia
   D. Hyperpathia

2. A 39-year-old female is seen as a new patient in your clinic and fibromyalgia is the suspected cause of her complaints. She has muscle pain and joint pain, but no synovitis on exam. Which of the following laboratory testing is not indicated?

   A. Thyrotropin
   B. ANA
   C. CRP
   D. Complete blood count

3. Increased activity in which neurotransmitter pathways have been shown to improve symptoms in fibromyalgia?

   A. Substance P
   B. mu opioid receptor
   C. Glutamate
   D. Serotonin

ANSWERS

1. C. Hyperalgesia is the exaggerated response to normally painful stimuli, which is illustrated in this case. While starting peripheral intravenous access is often painful, the patient demonstrates a response out of proportion to the event. Hyperesthesia is the painful response to usually innocuous stimuli, such as light touch. Allodynia refers to pain caused by stimuli that are usually not noxious. Hyperesthesia, hyperalgesia, and allodynia are common in fibromyalgia. Hyperpathia usually denotes an increased pain response to repetitive pain stimuli, but in the context of a raised pain threshold.

2. B. ANA should not be ordered in this patient without symptoms or signs overtly pointing to a connective tissue disorder or autoimmune disease. A positive ANA in a patient with a low pretest probability of these diseases can be misleading and lead to both patient anxiety and increased utilization of expensive testing and specialist consultations. Thyrotropin (or TSH), CRP, complete blood count, chemistry panel, and ESR are often sufficient screening tests for alternate processes when the clinical suspicion for fibromyalgia is high.

3. D. Baseline mu opioid receptor is decreased in pain-processing areas of the brain and exogenous opioid use is not typically beneficial in this population. Norepinephrine (and its principal metabolite, 3-methoxy-4-hydroxyphenethylene [MPHG]) and serotonin (and its principal metabolite, 5-HIAA) are reduced in the CSF of patients with fibromyalgia. CSF levels of glutamate and substance P in patients with fibromyalgia are two to three higher than in controls and are thought to perhaps contribute to pathogenesis.

QUESTIONS AND ANSWERS

This chapter has accompanying questions and answers that are available to subscribers as part of the Oxford eLearning platform. To access the questions, follow the link below, or go to ✔ http://oxfordmedicine.com/painmanagementreview

39.

ANTICOAGULATION REGIMENS AND INTERVENTIONAL PAIN PROCEDURES

Christine Oryhan, Kevin Vorenkamp, and Daniel Warren

STEM CASE AND KEY QUESTIONS

A 71-year-old male with paroxysmal atrial fibrillation and depression presents to an interventional pain clinic with a 4-month history of left-sided low back pain that radiates down his left leg from his buttocks down the lateral aspect of his left thigh, crossing over to the medial aspect of his left lower leg and going down to his ankle. He has tried physical therapy without much benefit. He had a lumbar epidural steroid injection (LESI) for similar pain many years ago that relieved his pain. His medications include warfarin, which he had held for 5 days without a bridge, duloxetine, and naproxen as needed for pain.

WOULD YOU STILL CHECK AN INR IF THE PATIENT HAD HELD HIS WARFARIN FOR 5 DAYS? WOULD IT MAKE A DIFFERENCE IF HE HAD BEEN BRIDGED WITH HEPARIN OR ENOXAPARIN? IF HE WERE ALSO ON ASPIRIN 81 MG DAILY, WOULD YOU ASK HIM TO HOLD THE ASPIRIN OR CONTINUE IT? DULOXETINE IS AN ANTIDEPRESSANT; COULD IT HAVE ANY ANTICOAGULANT EFFECTS?

A recent lumbar MRI was reviewed and demonstrated a left paramedian disk bulge at L4-L5, multilevel degenerative disease with ligamentum flavum hypertrophy, and resultant mild to moderate central canal stenosis at L4-L5. The patient's INR was 1.4 upon arrival at the clinic. Because it was a Friday and he was planning to go out of town the next week, he was advised to restart his warfarin and to reschedule his procedure, but to hold his warfarin for 7 days prior to his next appointment. In the interim, the patient saw his primary care provider and was switched from warfarin to rivaroxaban, at the patient's request because he had seen it advertised on a commercial.

HOW LONG SHOULD THE PATIENT HOLD RIVAROXABAN? IS THERE A LABORATORY TEST TO CONFIRM SAFETY BEFORE PROCEEDING WITH A NEURAXIAL INTERVENTION?

The patient returns to the pain clinic after holding his rivaroxaban for 3 days. His last dose of naproxen was 2 days earlier. A LESI is performed under fluoroscopic guidance at L4-L5 using a parasagittal interlaminar approach. There were no immediate complications noted and the patient left the clinic in good spirits.

WHEN SHOULD THE PATIENT BE ADVISED TO RESTART HIS RIVAROXABAN? IF HE WAS STILL ON WARFARIN INSTEAD, WHEN SHOULD HE RESTART IT? DOES THE PATIENT NEED TO HOLD HIS NAPROXEN BEFORE A LESI? WHAT IF IT WERE A SPINAL CORD STIMULATOR (SCS) TRIAL?

The following day, the patient calls the pain clinic complaining of worsening pain in his back and some weakness in his legs that wasn't there before. He is advised to go to the emergency department (ED) as soon as possible. In the ED, he is found to have 4/5 strength in bilateral hip flexors but only 3/5 strength in bilateral knee flexion/extension and foot dorsal and plantar flexion. He has absent Achilles reflexes bilaterally, although they were present the day before. Given the high suspicion of spinal epidural hematoma, neurosurgery is consulted and a lumbar MRI is performed.

WHAT IF MRI WERE CONTRAINDICATED IN THIS PATIENT? IS THERE AN ALTERNATIVE IMAGING TEST THAT COULD BE PERFORMED?

The lumbar MRI demonstrated a spinal epidural hematoma extending from L3 to S1, with moderate to severe central canal stenosis, worst at the L4-L5 level. The patient was emergently brought to the operating room for hematoma evacuation, requiring L3-L5 laminectomies. Postoperatively, the patient noticed an immediate improvement in the pain but still had some mild residual lower extremity weakness, although he was able to ambulate. He did extensive physical therapy for 1 month and had a complete recovery of his neurologic deficits.

DISCUSSION

Interventional pain procedures carry a risk of bleeding, which can be minor if superficial or in a compressible area, but which can be potentially catastrophic if in a tight enclosed space, such as the epidural space. Spinal epidural hematomas can cause significant pressure on the spinal cord or nerve roots, resulting in irreversible paraplegia (or quadriplegia if in the cervical spine) if not treated emergently with hematoma evacuation, which often requires multilevel laminectomy.

While spinal hematomas after interventional pain procedures are rare, the few case reports were serious enough to prompt the American Society of Regional Anesthesia and Pain Medicine, in conjunction with other national and international societies, to develop guidelines specific for interventional pain procedures in patients on anticoagulant and antiplatelet therapy.[1] Prior to the development of these guidelines, pain medicine professionals were encouraged to apply the guidelines for regional anesthesia to interventional pain procedures. However, interventional pain procedures have varying levels of risk. While peripheral joint, nerve, and musculoskeletal injections are low-risk procedures for bleeding, SCS trials/implants, intrathecal catheter/pump implants, epiduroscopy, and vertebral augmentation are high-risk procedures. The majority of the remaining procedures fall into an intermediate-risk category (interlaminar/transforaminal epidural steroid injections, facet medial branch nerve blocks and thermal radiofrequency ablation, paravertebral blocks, sympathetic blocks, and peripheral nerve stimulator trial/implants). Stratifying the bleeding risk for the procedure must be balanced with the patient's bleeding risk when assessing the periprocedural management of anticoagulants/antiplatelets. Recently, additional cases of epidural hematoma following epidural steroid injections have been reported, both when the care had been discordant with the guidelines, and when care strictly adhered to the published recommendations.[2,3]

Advanced age, advanced liver or renal disease, female sex, history of bleeding diathesis, and concurrent or prolonged use of more than one anticoagulant/antiplatelet medication put patients at a higher risk of developing bleeding complications.[1,4] Difficult anatomy identified on radiographic imaging may also factor into risk of bleeding (i.e., nearby vascular structures, scar tissue from prior surgical intervention, degenerative osteophytes, severe central spinal canal stenosis). Chronic pain patients typically have altered anatomy and elderly patients with spinal stenosis tend to have less volume in the epidural space at baseline. Even a small volume of blood in this space can cause significant neurologic deficits.[5,6]

Knowledge of neuraxial vascular anatomy is important, particularly when considering risks associated with procedures like SCS implantation (Figure 39.1).

The anterior and lateral epidural venous plexuses are more prominent than the venous plexus in the posterior epidural space.[7] During a SCS trial or implantation, lead misplacement or migration into the anterior or lateral epidural space may increase the risk of bleeding in higher-risk patients. Anatomically difficult procedures can make vascular insult more likely as well.

ANTIPLATELET/ANTICOAGULANTS

Table 39.1 summarizes the recommended times for holding and restarting certain anticoagulant/antiplatelet medications for interventional pain procedures.[1] In general, the recommended time to hold antiplatelet and anticoagulant medications is based on time to return to normal platelet/coagulation function. For newer medications and those that have not been well studied, the recommendation is to hold for 5 half-lives, which means that about 3% of the drug remains in the plasma, assuming normal metabolism and elimination.

Historically, the most commonly used anticoagulants have been warfarin (oral), heparin (IV, subcutaneous), and enoxaparin (subcutaneous). Indications for use include prevention and treatment of venous thromboembolism, pulmonary embolism, and thromboembolic events associated with atrial fibrillation and heart valve replacements. Warfarin acts by inhibiting vitamin K-dependent clotting factors (factors II, VII, IX, and X). Warfarin has a narrow therapeutic window and must be monitored and adjusted to maintain a certain range of prothrombin time and international normalized ratio (PT/INR). Warfarin can be reversed with vitamin K or fresh frozen plasma (FFP) if emergent reversal is necessary. Heparin works by directly binding antithrombin (AT), thus enhancing its inhibitory effect on the coagulation cascade by inactivating thrombin and factors IXa and Xa.[8] Monitoring is done via activated partial thromboplastin time (aPTT) or anti-factor Xa activity level, and can be reversed with protamine. Enoxaparin, a low-molecular-weight heparin (LMWH), dose-dependently inhibits factor Xa and can also be monitored by anti-factor Xa activity. Another synthetic factor Xa inhibitor is fondaparinux, which is administered subcutaneously once daily and has the advantage of being less likely to cause heparin-induced thrombocytopenia (HIT) than heparin or LMWH.

Newer direct oral anticoagulants (DOACs) are now being used to treat thromboembolic diseases because they have a better safety profile and higher efficacy than warfarin and do not require monitoring. The DOACs include dabigatran (thrombin inhibitor), rivaroxaban, apixaban, and edoxaban (factor Xa inhibitors). While monitoring is not required, there are some laboratory measurements that indicate if the effect of the drug has diminished after cessation for a procedure. Normal thrombin time (TT) likely indicates no clinical levels of dabigatran, while normal anti-Xa levels likely indicate no clinically relevant levels of rivaroxaban, apixaban, and edoxaban.[9] See Table 39.1 for recommended holding time for DOACs prior to intervention. A 24-hour interval should be observed postprocedurally before restarting any of the DOACs.

Aspirin and other antiplatelet medications are primarily used for primary and secondary prevention of thrombotic cardiovascular and cerebrovascular events. Aspirin irreversibly inactivates COX-1 and blocks thromboxane production for the lifespan of platelets, which is about 7 to 10 days. Each day, about 10% of the existing platelets are replaced. Aspirin is therefore effective in inhibiting platelet activation, platelet aggregation, and thrombosis. While aspirin alone has traditionally been viewed as okay to continue for most neuraxial procedures, there have been several case reports of patients taking only aspirin, but who had other potential risk factors for bleeding, who developed spinal hematomas after interventional pain procedures, particularly high-risk procedures, such as SCS trials/lead removal.[10,11] It is also important to consider the cardiac and cerebrovascular risks associated with

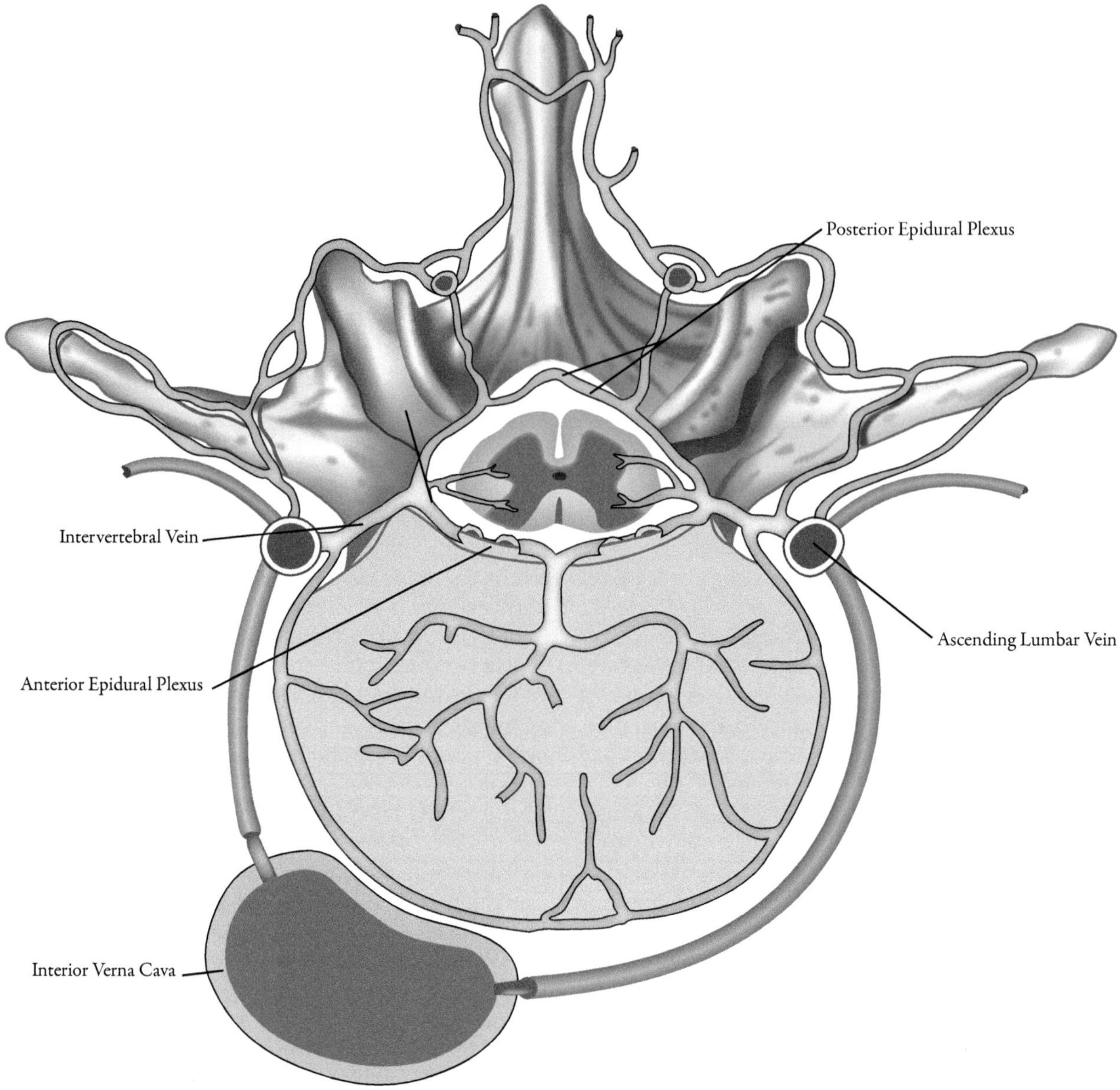

Figure 39.1. Axial view of neuraxial venous anatomy. Modified from Uflacker.[7]

discontinuing aspirin. While primary prophylaxis is used for preventing a primary occurrence of an event, secondary prophylaxis is used to prevent recurrence of an event, and discontinuation in the setting of preexisting disease is associated with significant risk of thromboembolic event.[1] After cessation of aspirin, a platelet rebound effect may occur that is characterized by a prothrombotic state.[12]

Phosphodiesterase (PDE) inhibitors, including cilostazol and dipyridamole, are also used as antiplatelet therapy, sometimes in combination with aspirin. Both of these medications have an elimination half-life close to 10 hours. While there are no recommendations for holding PDE inhibitors for low- and intermediate-risk procedures, five elimination half-lives or 2 days might be considered for high-risk procedures, especially in patients at higher risk for bleeding.[1]

P2Y12 inhibitors include clopidogrel, ticlopidine, prasurgel, and ticagrelor. Used in the treatment of cerebrovascular ischemic events, coronary syndrome, and peripheral vascular disease, they are often used concomitantly with aspirin as dual antiplatelet therapy after percutaneous coronary intervention (PCI). Guidelines for holding P2Y12 inhibitors are similar to those for regional anesthesia (see Table 39.1).

Other medications that may increase a patient's risk of bleeding complications include non-aspirin nonsteroidal anti-inflammatory drugs (NSAIDs) as well as antidepressants that inhibit serotonin reuptake, and herbal therapies that may affect coagulation status. While the anticoagulation effects of herbal therapies have not been well studied in the interventional pain population, providers should be aware of the herbal medications that may pose a risk, particularly when

Table 39.1. RECOMMENDED HOLDING TIMES FOR COMMON ANTICOAGULANTS BEFORE INTERVENTION

MEDICATION	RECOMMENDED HOLDING TIME			RECOMMENDED TIME TO RESTART
	HIGH-RISK PROCEDURE	INTERMEDIATE-RISK PROCEDURE	LOW-RISK PROCEDURE	
Aspirin	6 days for primary prophylaxis, ± based on risk factors for secondary prophylaxis	± based on other risk factors	No need to hold	24 hours
Phosphodiesterase inhibitors (cilostazol, dipyridamole)	2 days	No need to hold	No need to hold	24 hours
Coumadin	5 days, normal INR	5 days, normal INR	No need to hold	24 hours
Heparin (IV)	4 hours	4 hours	4 hours	2 hours, longer if bloody procedure
Heparin (subcutaneous)	8–10 hours	8–10 hours	8–10 hours	2 hours
LMWH (therapeutic)	24 hours	24 hours	24 hours	12–24 hours (4 hours after low- risk procedure)
LMWH (prophylactic)	12 hours	12 hours	12 hours	12–24 hours (4 hours after low-risk procedure)
Fondaparinux	4 days	4 days	± based on risk factors	24 hours
Dabigatran	4–5 days (6 days in renal dysfunction)	4–5 days (6 days in renal dysfunction)	± based on risk factors	24 hours
Rivaroxaban	3 days	3 days	± based on risk factors	24 hours
Apixaban	3–5 days	3–5 days	± based on risk factors	24 hours
P2Y12 inhibitors (clopidogrel, prasurgel, ticagrelor)	7 days	7 days	No need to hold	24 hours

Source: Modified from Narouze, et al.[1]

performing high-risk procedures in higher-risk patients. These include garlic, ginkgo biloba, ginseng, dong quai, and danshen.

Non-aspirin NSAIDs reversibly and competitively inhibit COX activity. The effect on platelets is related to the systemic plasma drug concentrations of the particular NSAID, and it is the degree of COX-1 inhibition that confers procedural bleeding risk. This can be affected by renal dysfunction (decreased NSAID binding to plasma proteins results in an increase in plasma concentration). Traditional NSAIDs, including indomethacin, naproxen, diclofenac, ibuprofen, and piroxicam, are nonselective and inhibit both COX-1 and COX-2. Some NSAIDs are more selective for COX-2 (meloxicam, etodolac, and nabumetone) and may be less likely to be associated with bleeding risk. Celecoxib is a selective COX-2 inhibitor and does not interfere with platelet function. There have been several case reports of spinal hematomas after interventional pain procedures in patients taking non-aspirin NSAIDs.[13] Given the variable half-lives of the NSAIDs and the fact that NSAIDs are not needed for management of thromboembolic disease, it is recommended to hold NSAIDs for 5 half-lives (Table 39.2).

Serotonin reuptake inhibitors (SRIs) include selective serotonin reuptake inhibitors (SSRIs), serotonin-norepinephrine reuptake inhibitors (SNRIs), and some tricyclic antidepressants (TCAs). Platelets require serotonin reuptake for serotonin-mediated platelet aggregation. While the risk of bleeding from SRIs is comparable to that with low-dose ibuprofen, the risk is increased in patients with advanced age, those with liver disease, and those taking concomitant antiplatelets or anticoagulants. Nonserotonergic antidepressants do not increase risk of bleeding. Common examples of SRIs and nonserotonergic antidepressants are listed in Table 39.3.[1] Cessation of SRIs prior to interventional pain procedures is not recommended on a routine basis. However, discontinuation of SRIs should be considered for 1 to 2 weeks (after gradual tapering) in patients with stable depression and at high risk of bleeding; SRIs can be restarted the day after surgery. Fluoxetine is unique in that it has an active metabolite with a long half-life and should be held for 5 weeks prior to a procedure (again after a gradual taper). Antidepressant management should be coordinated with the treating psychiatrist.

Table 39.2. **NONSTEROIDAL ANTI-INFLAMMATORIES (NSAIDS) AND THEIR RECOMMENDED HOLDING TIMES**

NSAID	HOLDING TIME FOR HIGH-RISK PROCEDURES (5 HALF-LIVES)
Diclofenac	1 day
Ketorolac	1 day
Ibuprofen	1 day
Etodolac	2 days
Indomethacin	2 days
Naproxen	4 days
Meloxicam	4 days
Piroxicam	10 days

Table 39.3. **SEROTONIN REUPTAKE INHIBITOR (SRI) AND NONSEROTONERGIC ANTIDEPRESSANTS**

SRI ANTIDEPRESSANTS	NONSEROTONERGIC ANTIDEPRESSANTS
Fluoxetine (SSRI)	Bupropion (misc)
Sertraline (SSRI)	Mirtazapine (α_2-antagonist)
Paroxetine (SSRI)	Nortriptyline (TCA)
Escitalopram (SSRI)	
Duloxetine (SNRI)	
Venlafaxine (SNRI)	

SIGNS AND SYMPTOMS OF SPINAL EPIDURAL HEMATOMA

Initial presentation of spinal epidural hematoma can vary, but it may include severe back pain and/or tenderness to palpation over the intervention site. Once the spinal cord is compressed, neurologic deficits may develop, including symptoms of cauda equina syndrome. This can include lower extremity weakness/paraplegia, lower extremity radicular pain, loss of reflexes (patellar, Achilles), saddle anesthesia, urinary retention, urinary overflow incontinence, and/or bowel incontinence. Onset of any of these "red flag" signs/symptoms in the hours to days after an interventional pain procedure should prompt immediate workup.

DIAGNOSIS OF SPINAL EPIDURAL HEMATOMA

In addition to history and physical exam, noncontrast MRI is the diagnostic imaging of choice for spinal epidural hematoma. Noncontrast CT may be performed if MRI cannot be used (Figure 39.2). Contraindications to MRI include having a pacemaker, metallic foreign body in the eye, or brain aneurysm clip. If there is any question about the presence of concerning symptoms of spinal epidural hematoma, the patient requires immediate assessment and there should be a low threshold for obtaining imaging.

TREATMENT OF SPINAL EPIDURAL HEMATOMA

Because a spinal epidural hematoma in the setting of neurologic deficits is a surgical emergency, expedited diagnosis and consultation with a neurosurgeon are essential. Spinal epidural hematomas require immediate evacuation of the hematoma

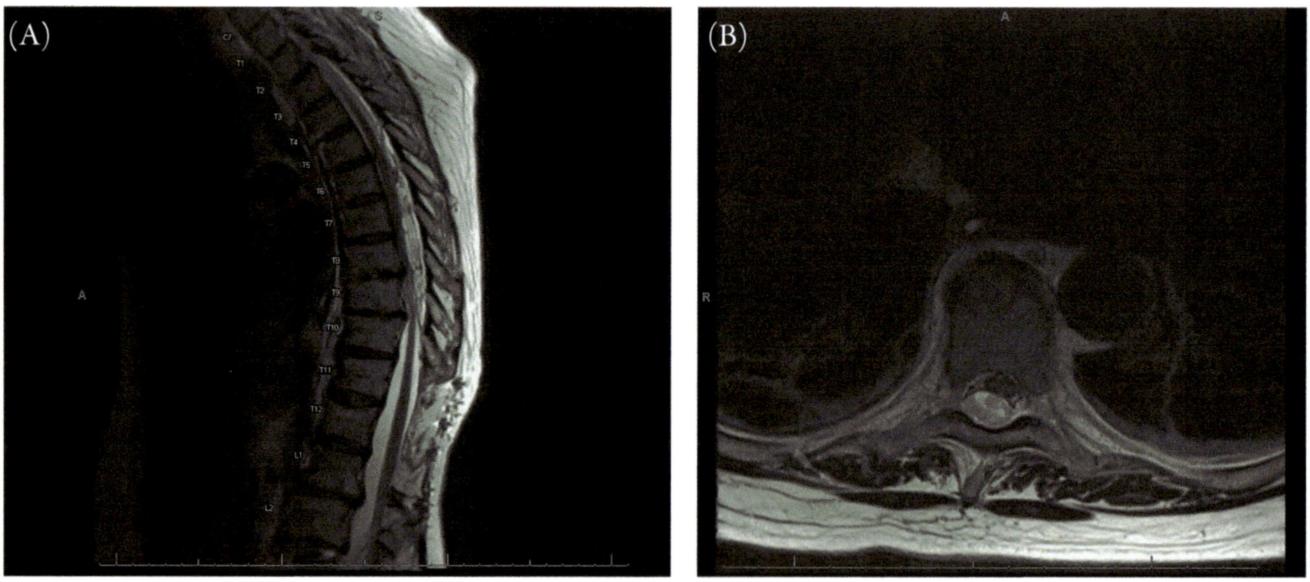

Figure 39.2. (A) Sagittal T2-weighted MRI of a patient with a thoracic epidural hematoma collection in the dorsal epidural space, resulting in anterior thecal sac displacement. (B) Axial T2-weighted MRI demonstrating the same epidural hematoma and anterior thecal sac displacement with cord compression.

and decompression of the spinal cord, which usually requires multilevel laminectomy. High-dose steroids may also be used, but they should not delay surgical treatment.

OUTCOMES AFTER SPINAL EPIDURAL HEMATOMA

Neurologic outcomes after development of a spinal epidural hematoma depend on several factors. The most important factor is prompt diagnosis and treatment. One study showed that patients taken to surgery within 12 hours of initial presentation had better neurologic outcomes than those who had delayed surgery.[14] A more severe degree of neurologic deficit before surgery also correlated with worse outcome.

CONCLUSIONS

As interventional pain physicians, we need to remain familiar with the continuously changing list of anticoagulant and antiplatelet medications. A systematic assessment of patient risk factors and current medications, including supplements, needs to be performed prior to neuraxial procedures. Advanced age, advanced liver or renal disease, female sex, history of bleeding diathesis and concurrent or prolonged use of more than one anticoagulant/antiplatelet medication put patients at a higher risk of developing bleeding complications.

Prompt diagnosis, imaging, and neurosurgical consultation are imperative if there is any concern about a spinal epidural hematoma.

REFERENCES

1. Narouze S, Benzon HT, Provenzano DA, et al. Interventional spine and pain procedures in patients on antiplatelet and anticoagulant medications: guidelines from the American Society of Regional Anesthesia and Pain Medicine, the European Society of Regional Anaesthesia and Pain Therapy, the American Academy of Pain Medicine, the International Neuromodulation Society, the North American Neuromodulation Society, and the World Institute of Pain. *Reg Anesth Pain Med.* 2015;40(3):182–212.
2. Benyamin RM, Vallejo R, Wang V, Kumar N, Cedeno DL, Tamrazi A. Acute epidural hematoma formation in cervical spine after interlaminar epidural steroid injection despite discontinuation of clopidogrel. *Reg Anesth Pain Med.* 2016;41(3):398–401.
3. Page J, Moisi M, Oskouian RJ. Lumbar epidural hematoma following interlaminar fluoroscopically guided epidural steroid injection. *Reg Anesth Pain Med.* 2016;41(3):402–404.
4. Horlocker TT, Wedel DJ, Rowlingson JC, et al. Regional anesthesia in the patient receiving antithrombotic or thrombolytic therapy: American Society of Regional Anesthesia and Pain Medicine evidence-based guidelines (third edition). *Reg Anesth Pain Med.* 2010;35(1):64–101.
5. Hebl JR, Horlocker TT, Kopp SL, Schroeder DR. Neuraxial blockade in patients with preexisting spinal stenosis, lumbar disk disease, or prior spine surgery: efficacy and neurologic complications. *Anesth Analg.* 2010;111(6):1511–1519.
6. Hooten WM, Hogan MS, Sanemann TC, Maus TJ. Acute spinal pain during an attempted lumbar epidural blood patch in congenital lumbar spinal stenosis and epidural lipomatosis. *Pain Physician.* 2008;11(1):87–90.
7. Uflacker R. *Atlas of Vascular Anatomy: An Angiographic Approach.* 2nd ed. Philadelphia, PA: Lippincott Williams & Wilkins; 2007.
8. Hirsh J, Anand SS, Halperin JL, Fuster V, American Heart Association. AHA Scientific Statement: Guide to anticoagulant therapy: heparin: a statement for healthcare professionals from the American Heart Association. *Arterioscler Thromb Vasc Biol.* 2001;21(7):E9-.
9. Burnett AE, Mahan CE, Vazquez SR, Oertel LB, Garcia DA, Ansell J. Guidance for the practical management of the direct oral anticoagulants (DOACs) in VTE treatment. *J Thromb Thrombolysis.* 2016;41(1):206–232.
10. Buvanendran A, Young AC. Spinal epidural hematoma after spinal cord stimulator trial lead placement in a patient taking aspirin. *Reg Anesth Pain Med.* 2014;39(1):70–72.
11. Giberson CE, Barbosa J, Brooks ES, et al. Epidural hematomas after removal of percutaneous spinal cord stimulator trial leads: two case reports. *Reg Anesth Pain Med.* 2014;39(1):73–77.
12. Gerstein NS, Schulman PM, Gerstein WH, Petersen TR, Tawil I. Should more patients continue aspirin therapy perioperatively? Clinical impact of aspirin withdrawal syndrome. *Ann Surg.* 2012;255(5):811–819.
13. Benzon HT, Huntoon MA. Do we need new guidelines for interventional pain procedures in patients on anticoagulants? *Reg Anesth Pain Med.* 2014;39(1):1–3.
14. Lawton MT, Porter RW, Heiserman JE, Jacobowitz R, Sonntag VK, Dickman CA. Surgical management of spinal epidural hematoma: relationship between surgical timing and neurological outcome. *J Neurosurg.* 1995;83(1):1–7.

REVIEW QUESTIONS

1. An 84-year-old woman with 7/10 right arm pain is scheduled for a cervical epidural steroid injection (CESI) for right cervical radiculopathy. She is taking clopidogrel for a history of transient ischemic attacks. What is the minimum length of time clopidogrel should be held prior to the CESI procedure?

A. 24 hours
B. 4 days
C. 7 days
D. 14 days

2. The same patient returns for her CESI after holding her clopidogrel for 10 days. A CESI is performed at C7-T1 without immediate complication. When is the earliest time the patient can resume taking her clopidogrel?

A. 6 hours
B. 24 hours
C. 4 days
D. 7 days

3. The same patient's husband calls the following morning reporting that the patient has new pain and weakness in her left arm. She denies fever, but is in 10/10 pain and is having difficulty lifting her left arm. What is the most appropriate next step in her care?

A. Instruct patient to take aspirin and call 9-1-1.
B. Prescribe gabapentin for the radicular pain.

C. Transfer to ED for urgent evaluation.
D. Instruct patient to increase her oxycodone and call back in 24 hours if not improved.

ANSWERS

1. C. Clopidogrel is a thienopyridine that blocks the ADP receptor, P2Y12 subtype. The maximum platelet inhibition is 50% to 60%, normalizing after 7 days. The ASRA guidelines recommend 7-day cessation for neuraxial procedures, but acknowledge that 5 days may be acceptable in higher-risk patients, in concordance with the American College of Cardiology recommendations. However, it is recommended that a platelet function test (P2Y12 assay) or thromboelastogram (TEG) be performed in the setting of 5-day discontinuation.[1]

2. B. Clopidogrel can be resumed 12 to 24 hours after the CESI.

3. C. The patient's symptoms are concerning for epidural hematoma and urgent evaluation is warranted. Aside from the prior clopidogrel use, the patient herself exhibits several other risks factors for epidural hematoma formation: female sex, increased age, and active or recent use of anticoagulant and/or antiplatelet medications.[4] Although clopidogrel was held for 10 days, exceeding the recommended minimum of 7 days, the patient may still be at increased risk.

QUESTIONS AND ANSWERS

This chapter has accompanying questions and answers that are available to subscribers as part of the Oxford eLearning platform. To access the questions, follow the link below, or go to ✔ http://oxfordmedicine.com/painmanagementreview

40.

PERIOPERATIVE EPIDURAL PAIN MANAGEMENT IN CHILDREN

Alina Lazar

STEM CASE AND KEY QUESTIONS

You are called to evaluate a 3-year-old, 15-kg male with stage IV neuroblastoma who is in the postanesthesia care unit (PACU) after undergoing exploratory laparotomy and resection of a retroperitoneal mass. He has no other medical problems or known allergies. Before surgical incision, a 20-G epidural catheter was inserted easily via a midline approach at T8-T9, following loss of resistance (LOR) to air at 1.8 cm, and was taped at 5 cm at the skin. Intravascular placement of the catheter was ruled out with a test dose of 1.5 mL of lidocaine 1.5% and 1:200,000 epinephrine. The catheter tip was visualized at T7 on an intraoperative chest X-ray. During surgery, which proceeded uneventfully, the patient received fentanyl 1 μg/kg/hr. When you arrive in the PACU, he is crying inconsolably and is trying to pull his dressings. His heart rate is 134 beats/min, blood pressure 107/68 mm Hg, respiratory rate 32 breaths/min, and oxygen saturation is 95%. The abdominal incision extends from the xiphoid process to 2 cm below the umbilicus.

HOW WOULD YOU DIFFERENTIATE INCISIONAL PAIN FROM OTHER SOURCES OF DISCOMFORT? HOW WOULD YOU EVALUATE THE FUNCTIONALITY OF THE EPIDURAL CATHETER? WOULD YOU TEST THE CATHETER AGAIN FOR INTRAVASCULAR PLACEMENT? HOW WOULD YOU ACTIVATE THE EPIDURAL CATHETER? WHAT TECHNIQUES CAN BE USED TO CHECK THE POSITION OF THE EPIDURAL CATHETER (INTRAOPERATIVELY AND POSTOPERATIVELY)?

After a negative test dose, a 3-mL bolus of 0.25% bupivacaine is given through the epidural catheter. The patient appears calm and his vital signs return to normal.

WHAT EPIDURAL INFUSION SOLUTION AND RATE WOULD YOU CHOOSE FOR POSTOPERATIVE PAIN CONTROL? WHAT ARE THE ADVANTAGES AND DISADVANTAGES OF VARIOUS LOCAL ANESTHETICS, OPIOIDS, AND ADJUVANTS IN PEDIATRIC PATIENTS?

Continuous epidural infusion of 2.5 mL/hr of bupivacaine 0.1% and hydromorphone 20 μg/mL is initiated. After spending 2 more hours in the PACU with good pain control, the patient is transferred to the floor. Soon after, the nurse calls you because the patient seems uncomfortable. She is also concerned that the epidural catheter may have dislodged, since she noticed fluid under the epidural dressings.

HOW DO YOU ADDRESS THE NURSE'S CONCERNS? WHAT WOULD BE A SAFE MAXIMUM INFUSION RATE FOR THE EPIDURAL SOLUTION FOR THIS PATIENT? WOULD THE RATE BE DIFFERENT IF THE EPIDURAL TIP WAS AT THE LUMBAR LEVEL?

The epidural infusion rate is increased to 3 mL/hr, but the patient continues to be intermittently fussy and grabbing at his intravenous (IV) and Foley catheters. A few hours later, after a dose of 15 μg of fentanyl is administered to facilitate the insertion of a nasogastric tube, the patient becomes unresponsive, with a respiratory rate of 4 breaths/min, and an oxygen saturation of 40%. Upon bag-mask ventilation and administration of naloxone, the patient becomes responsive and his vital signs return to normal. The epidural infusion is discontinued and the patient is transferred to the intensive care unit (ICU).

WHAT DO YOU THINK HAPPENED? DID THE EPIDURAL PLAY A ROLE IN THIS EVENT? COULD THE EVENT HAVE BEEN PREVENTED? SHOULD WE RESTART THE EPIDURAL INFUSION? AT WHAT RATE, AND WITH WHAT SOLUTION?

In the ICU, the patient becomes progressively agitated and restless, seemingly in pain. After a thorough discussion with the ICU and surgery teams, the epidural infusion is resumed, with a solution of bupivacaine 0.1% at 2.5 mL/hr, supplemented with IV morphine as needed, with good pain control overnight. On postoperative day 2, the tip of the epidural catheter is noted to be at T3. The patient is hemodynamically stable and seems comfortable. The apnea monitors have sounded a few times, but the alarms were short-lived.

WHAT CAN EXPLAIN THE CATHETER MIGRATION? ARE CERTAIN CATHETERS MORE LIKELY THAN OTHERS TO MIGRATE? WOULD YOU REMOVE THE CATHETER OR PULL IT BACK A FEW CENTIMETERS AND RETAPE IT?

The epidural is removed and pain control is maintained with a combination of opioids, ketorolac, and acetaminophen.

DISCUSSION

ORIGIN OF THE TECHNIQUE

The pediatric use of epidural analgesia was described in 1954 as an alternative to general anesthesia in high-risk neonates and children. Since its popularization in the 1980s with advances in technology to incorporate pediatric equipment sizes, this technique for intra- and postoperative pain relief has become standard. Demonstrating the feasibility of passing a catheter from the caudal to thoracic level in young children, Bösenberg and coworkers pioneered a new era of epidural use in pediatric patients.[1]

ADVANTAGES OF, AND INDICATIONS FOR, CONTINUOUS EPIDURAL ANALGESIA (CEA)

Medical literature on the advantages of epidural anesthesia in children is sparse. The proven benefits include decreased intraoperative requirements for anesthetics and their potential cardiodepressant and neurotoxic effects, better control of the surgical stress response than with opioids,[2] earlier tracheal extubation and return of gut function,[3] improved postoperative analgesia, and shorter ICU[4] and hospitalization stay.[5] In adults, pain control is improved and incidence of nausea and vomiting is decreased (Figure 40.1).[6]

The indications for use of CEA are open thoracic surgery, major intra-abdominal surgery with surgical dissection, extensive lower extremity surgery, and long-term pain management. Other surgeries are better managed with other techniques: paravertebral blockade, transabdominal plexus blocks, rectus sheath blocks, and lower limb blocks. CEA also has been successfully used for continuous sympathetic blockade in children with vascular insufficiency due to intense vasoconstriction (e.g., purpura fulminans) and in patients who have sickle cell trait with vaso-occlusive crisis.

ANATOMIC CONSIDERATIONS

In neonates and infants, the conus medullaris is located at the L3 vertebra, and it reaches the L1 level at approximately 1 year of age. In neonates, the intercristal line bisects the L5 vertebra. The sacral hiatus is located more cephalad than in adults, increasing the risk for dural puncture. Loosely packed epidural fat and lack of lumbar lordosis in nonwalking infants makes advancement of catheters from the caudal to the lumbar and thoracic levels relatively easy.[1] In infants up to the age of 6 months, the vertebral column remains cartilaginous, and epidural catheters can be visualized with ultrasonography. There is a more subtle "give" as the ligamentum flavum is pierced. As a general rule, the epidural space is found at 1 mm/kg of body weight; however, there is considerable individual variation (Table 40.1).[7]

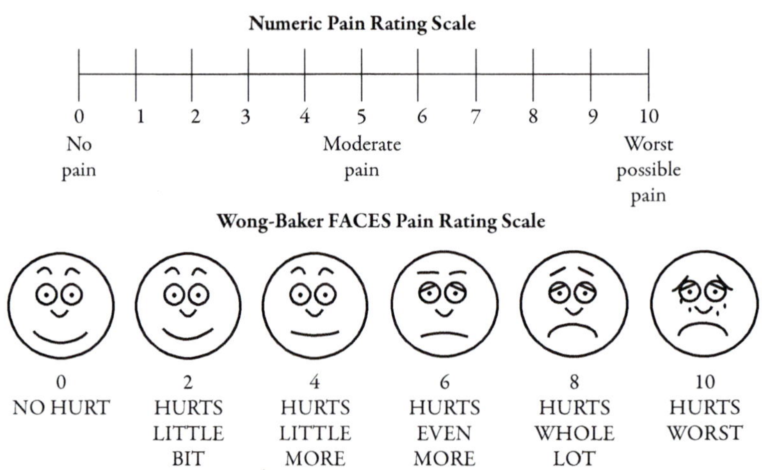

Figure 40.1. Numeric Pain Rating Scale.

Table 40.1. **DEPTH TO THE EPIDURAL SPACE IN CHILDREN**

Neonate	5–15 mm
Infants	~ 7.5 mm
Children 10–25 kg	~ 1 mm/kg
Children > 25 kg	0.8 + (0.05 × wt[kg]) = depth in cm

The wide variation in the depth of the epidural space means that a test for LOR should be performed as soon as the epidural needle has entered the supraspinous ligament.

A larger volume of local anesthetic for body weight is needed for epidural anesthesia in infants and children than in adults. The bolus and infusion doses are based on ideal body weight. The caudal space requires larger volumes for the same dermatome spread compared to the lumbar or thoracic region. Half of 5-year-old children have a probe-patent foramen ovale, with increased risk of massive air embolism through the epidural veins when LOR to air is used. Therefore, LOR to saline in the pediatric population is currently recommended.[8]

PHARMACOLOGIC CONSIDERATIONS

Because neonates have lower levels of plasma α_1-acid glycoprotein and albumin, binding of amide local anesthetics is reduced, and risk of local anesthetic toxicity is increased. Infants have rapid heart rates, which predisposes them to bupivacaine accumulation in the myocardium. The hepatic metabolism of amide local anesthetics does not mature until an infant is 6 months old. Pharmacokinetic studies in neonates show a significant increase in plasma bupivacaine levels after continuous epidural infusion. Thus, an infusion of bupivacaine at 0.2 mg/kg/hr in neonates should not be continued beyond 48 hr.[9,10] In contrast, ester local anesthetics, such as 2-chloroprocaine, are rapidly cleared, even in young infants.

PHYSIOLOGIC CONSIDERATIONS

The cardiovascular effects of a neuraxial block are less pronounced in children than in adults because of reduced sympathetic tone and less blood volume in the splanchnic circulation and lower limbs in children. In the absence of severe hypovolemia or high subarachnoid block, epidural analgesia in children less than 8 years old is associated with remarkable cardiovascular stability.[11]

ADVERSE EVENTS AND SIDE EFFECTS OF PEDIATRIC EPIDURAL ANESTHESIA

The rate of serious complications associated with pediatric epidural anesthesia is low. In the Pediatric Regional Anesthesia Network (PRAN) study, which evaluated the effects of 2,946 epidural catheters, there were no complications with long-term consequences lasting > 3 months. Catheter dislodgement or kinking, accidental dural puncture (0.9%), intravascular injection (2%), and local site inflammation or infection (11%) were the short-term adverse events.[12] In the U.K. pediatric epidural audit, the risk of serious complications was 1:2,000 and persistent complications were 1:10,000.[13] A retrospective analysis from Canada found that placement of caudothoracic epidurals is increasingly being used in neonates, despite a greater chance of complications in neonates than in older children.[14] In this series, five of seven complications in infants occurred in the postoperative period.

Neurologic Risks

In a U.K. audit of 10,633 pediatric epidurals, there were six events of neurologic injury, of which only one, cauda equina syndrome related to a drug infusion error, lasted more than 12 months.[13] Despite these generally reassuring data, catastrophic neurologic injury can occur, as shown in a recent report of four cases from institutions where pediatric epidurals are placed regularly.[15] Potential mechanisms of neurologic injury were high pressures created in the epidural place by the test and loading doses and infusions, and ischemic cord injury after systemic hypotension or epinephrine-induced vasoconstriction.[15] In animals, manipulation with large-bore styletted catheters in the epidural space caused detectible damage to the spinal cord.[16] In infants, depending on the anatomic level, clinical manifestations of neurologic injury may be persistent sensorimotor block, para- or tetraplegia, abnormal reflexes, continuous urine dribbling or urinary retention, rectal prolapse, or respiratory depression.

Infectious Risks

Catheter tip colonization occurs in 20% to 37% of caudal catheters and in only 4% of lumbar catheters. In a large series of 2,869 epidural catheters placed in infants, only two catheter-related infections were reported in the birth to 1-year-old age group; both catheters were inserted at a noncaudal level.[17] The U.K. prospective audit reported two epidural abscesses and a child with meningismus.[13] Several abscesses in this series were reported more than a day after catheter withdrawal. The risk of infection increases 2 to 3 days after catheter insertion. Subcutaneous tunneling of the catheter decreases the risk of infection with caudal placement of epidural catheters.[18]

Catheter Migration

Migration of epidural catheters may occur in approximately 40% of cases, and may result in perforation of dura, intravascular migration, high thoracic or cervical administration of epidural solution, or catheter dislodgement. Potential clinical manifestations are signs of a high neuraxial block, Horner's syndrome, bradycardia, local anesthetic toxicity, or loss of effective analgesia. The catheter may migrate cephalad after a change from prone or lateral position to supine position.[19] Compared to firm inelastic epidural catheters, the more stretchy and elastic Arrow Flex-Tip catheter may be predisposed to inward migration in active patients by a gripping motion of the ligamentum flavum[20] (Figure 40.2). In one

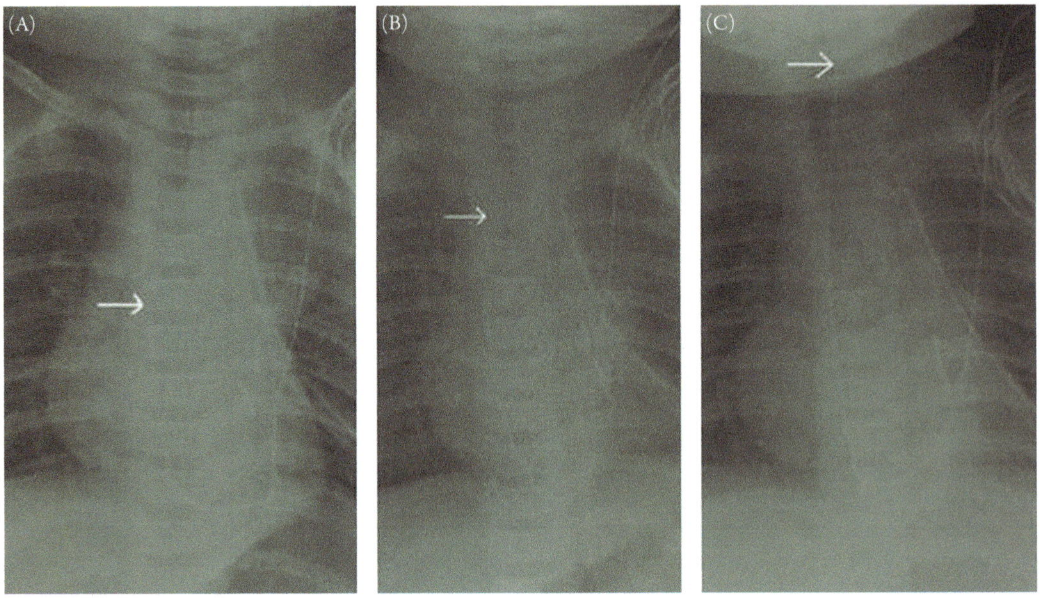

Figure 40.2. Migrating thoracic epidural catheter in an infant. Reproduced with permission from Thompson and Aasheim.[20]

series, the catheter migrated as many as 6.5 vertebral levels, and the migration tended to occur in smaller patients.[21] Leakage of infusion fluid around the catheter insertion site is a particular problem in small infants, because the epidural space may be only 7 to 10 mm deep, and the tissues through which the catheter passes are not dense. Application of a liquid topical adhesive, such as Dermabond, over the insertion site decreases problems with catheter leakage or migration. Other techniques of catheter fixation include Mastisol, Steri-strips (which may cause kinks in the catheter), commercial fixation devices (e.g., Simms Portex "lockit" device), and catheter tunneling.

Hemodynamic Effects and Total Spinal Anesthesia

Because the sympathetic system is immature in children up to 8 years old, cardiovascular stability is maintained even in high thoracic anesthesia, and in the presence of congenital heart disease.[11] Hypotension should prompt anesthesiologists to rule out total spinal anesthesia, intravascular injection, hypovolemia, decreased cardiac contractility, or excessive depth of anesthesia.

Dural Puncture

Given the variable and usually small distance from the skin to the epidural space, the risk of a dural puncture is high, with some series reporting rates up to 10%.[22] Post-dural-puncture headache (PDPH) is rare in the pediatric population. The low incidence may be explained by the shorter stature of infants and children.[23] Younger patients may not be able to clearly articulate symptoms related to dural puncture, and their behavior may be attributed to hunger, fatigue, illness, or medication side effects. The management of PDPH in children includes bed rest, hydration, analgesics, antiemetics, caffeine, and epidural blood patch. Caffeine is not frequently used in children, and the optimal dose is not known. Side effects—nausea, insomnia, and restlessness—are usually mild. The epidural blood patch (approximately 0.3 mL/kg) is performed in an awake or mildly sedated patient if possible, to detect the appearance of radicular symptoms.[24]

Epidural Hematoma

The reported incidence of epidural hematoma is 1 in 190,000 pediatric epidurals. The main risk factors are coagulopathy, thrombocytopenia, and full anticoagulation therapy.[11] In young, nonverbal or cognitively impaired children, epidural hematoma is suspected by acute-onset increase in motor block (not explained by changes in the epidural infusion), paraplegia, or urinary and fecal retention or incontinence. The diagnosis is confirmed by MRI.

COMPLICATIONS AND SIDE EFFECTS OF NEURAXIAL LOCAL ANESTHETIC ADMINISTRATION

Local Anesthetic Toxicity

Anesthetic toxicity can be caused by intravascular injection or by excessive bolus or infusion doses. In neonates and infants, cardiac dysrhythmia and apnea are more likely initial presentations than convulsions. Agitation, restlessness, and myoclonic movements may be incorrectly attributed to unrelieved pain. Dysrhythmia, bradycardia, and myocardial depression can be protracted if caused by bupivacaine. Intravenous intralipid (20% in a dose of 1.5 mL/kg every 3 to 5 min, followed by an infusion at a rate of 0.25 mL/kg/min) can be lifesaving in patients with malignant ventricular dysrhythmia.[25] The inadvertent intravascular administration of an epinephrine test dose (0.1 mL/kg solution containing epinephrine 1:200,000, maximum 3 mL) is signaled by an increase in the heart rate, hypertension or changes in T-wave appearance on the electrocardiogram. Since a negative test dose reduces, but does not eliminate, the possibility of intravascular injection, the utility of the test dose has been questioned. In one study, 27% of intravascular epinephrine injections in children were missed by heart rate criteria, and T- wave changes were unreliable in total IV anesthetics.[26]

Hypotension

Hypotension is rarely a problem in children less than 8 years old, but can occur in a high block or when the catheter migrates intrathecally.

Loss of Sensation

Lack of sensation in the postoperative period can mask undiagnosed compartment syndromes in children who have had surgery on a lower extremity. Heel blisters and pressure sores can also appear and may not be identified in a patient with an epidural.

COMPLICATION AND SIDE EFFECTS OF NEURAXIAL OPIOID ADMINISTRATION

The common side effects of neuraxial opioids are pruritus and nausea and vomiting.[27]

Pruritus may occur even when only epidural local anesthetics are used. Among the opioids, morphine is most likely to cause pruritus. To lessen the effect, decrease the rate of infusion, substitute an opioid less likely to induce pruritus, such as fentanyl, replace the epidural opioid with clonidine, and administer IV nalbuphine (50 to 75 μg/kg every 6 hours as needed), diphenhydramine (50 mg/kg every 6 hours as needed), or naloxone (0.25 to 1 μg/kg/hr).[28]

Nausea and vomiting are managed with ondansetron 0.1 mg/kg IV every 6 hours, metoclopramide 0.1 to 0.15 mg/kg IV every 6 to 8 hours, or naloxone 0.5 μg/kg IV every 4 hours as needed. A low-dose naloxone infusion effectively reduces nausea without reversing the analgesic effect of opioids.

The true incidence of urinary retention attributable to epidural analgesia is unknown, but it is higher in older children. Patients may require urinary catheter insertion, which is associated with a low but nonnegligible rate of complications. Some practitioners reserve the option of epidural catheterization for children who would usually undergo urinary catheterization for surgical indications.[11] Urinary retention is more frequently associated with morphine than with fentanyl.

Opioid-induced respiratory depression is more common with hydrosoluble opioids, whose rostral spread is more extensive, and in children at risk for apnea or hypoventilation (e.g., former preterm infants, or those with obstructive sleep apnea). Because of the synergistic depressant effect on respiration, neuraxial and IV or oral opioids should not be administered concurrently. The administration of an IV opioid in addition to a local anesthetic epidural infusion can treat pain from a patchy block or nonsurgical sites, and provides sedation.

Sedation in a child can be an early sign of toxic neuraxial opioids. Patients with epidural catheters should be frequently evaluated objectively with sedation scales.[28]

TECHNIQUES OF EPIDURAL CATHETER PLACEMENT

The midline approach is recommended for small children. LOR to saline is recommended to lessen the risk of embolism and neurologic injury with air injection.[29] Some experts still prefer LOR to air but try to avoid its injection.[30] For direct lumbar or thoracic level placement, the catheter is secured 1.5 to 2 cm into the epidural space. Alternatively, the needle insertion point may be selected a few levels below the desired dermatome and the catheter inserted 3 to 5 cm into the epidural space, to reduce the risk of dislodgement.

For caudal placement, the recommended needles are Crawford or a regular 18-G IV catheter. With the latter, there is concern about dural, vascular, rectal, or intraosseous puncture. (Tuohy needles are not used because getting the right alignment of the eye of the needle with the spinal canal is difficult.) The tip of the catheter is advanced easily up to the thoracic level (particularly in children weighing less than 5 kg). Although a high success rate has been claimed with blind insertion, numerous reports have shown that catheters threaded from the caudal space do not behave predictably, and that placement must be verified.

Lumbar-to-thoracic insertion is less successful than caudal-to-thoracic placement,[31] but the success rate improves at high lumbar levels of insertion. In one study, only 22% of catheters threaded from L4-L5 were advanced to predicted thoracic levels. Most catheters simply coiled within the epidural space close to their point of insertion.[32] There are reports of paraplegia from intraspinal hematoma during attempted lumbar block,[33] and this route is less preferred in neonates. When the catheter tip is far from the desired location, analgesia can be improved by increasing the volume of epidural infusion or administering hydrosoluble opioids epidurally.

Because risk is higher in neonates and small infants, direct thoracic insertion should be performed only by anesthesiologists highly experienced in this technique.

VERIFICATION OF CATHETER TIP POSITION

A radiopaque catheter facilitates the placement of the catheter tip at the desired dermatome. Injection of contrast through the catheter may help identify subdural or intravascular placement and predict analgesic coverage.[34] The disadvantages of this technique are cost and radiation and contrast exposure.

In the nerve stimulation (Tsui) technique, as the catheter is advanced, the operator is able to follow the muscular response.[35] A special kit is now commercially available (although it is quite expensive). With this technique, subarachnoid placement can be detected.

With ultrasound, the epidural puncture and catheter tip advancement can be visualized in real time.[36] Ultrasound-guided placement requires the help of an experienced assistant.

Table 40.2. **EPIDURAL INFUSION RATES PER SPINAL SEGMENT OF ANESTHESIA***

EPIDURAL LEVEL	INFUSION RATE (ML/KG/HR)
Lumbar lower thoracic (T10-S1)	0.06
Mid-thoracic (T6-T9)	0.03
Upper thoracic (T1-T5)	0.02

* The infusion rates are average starting doses for children less than 8 years old (30 kg). They may require adjustment based on the patient's response and the degree of proximity of the catheter tip to the spinal segments innervating the surgical area.

LOADING VOLUME

A good rule of thumb for calculating the loading volume is 0.05 mL/kg/dermatome. For midthoracic catheters, the loading volume should be reduced by 50%. Typical loading volumes are 0.3 mL/kg for thoracic epidurals and 0.5 mL/kg for lumbar epidurals. A dose equivalent with half of the initial bolus can be given 90 minutes after the initial dose.

An opioid may be co-administered with the local anesthetic in reduced doses in infants less than 6 months old: fentanyl (0.5 to 1 µg/kg), morphine (10 to 30 µg/kg), or hydromorphone (1 to 3 µg/kg). In neonates, and especially with the catheter tip at the thoracic level, respiratory depression may result.

CHOICE AND RATE OF INFUSIONS

Children often require anesthetic doses near the maximum acceptable. The first step in planning an epidural infusion is to determine the maximal amount of acceptable local anesthetic that may be infused per hour. Typical infusion rates per spinal segment of anesthesia and maximum safe rate for anesthetic are shown in Table 40.2 and Table 40.3, respectively. It may be necessary to reduce the planned concentration in order to keep the total dose to an acceptable amount.

Bupivacaine is the most commonly administered local anesthetic for routine postoperative analgesia in children. Administration of 0.2 mg/kg/hr of bupivacaine for longer than 48 hours could result in local anesthetic toxicity in neonates.[9] For adequate spread, an infusion of 0.05% bupivacaine and 1 µg/mL of fentanyl may be used at rates of 0.2 to 0.4 mL/kg/hr. Ropivacaine causes less motor block and less cardiac toxicity and neurotoxicity than equal concentrations of bupivacaine. It may be safer for postoperative epidural infusions because of more stable plasma concentrations than with bupivacaine.[37] Levobupivacaine causes less toxicity than bupivacaine and can be used in doses similar to racemic bupivacaine. The short half-life of 2-chloroprocaine (40 seconds in neonates), makes it particularly useful in small infants, patients requiring wide dermatomal coverage, and patients with decreased hepatic function (e.g., from prematurity, increased abdominal pressure, or liver resection). It can be used to test the functionality of an epidural catheter for which the proper positioning might be in question. Chloroprocaine 1.5% at 0.5 to 1 mL/kg/hr with or without fentanyl has been successfully used in neonates and infants.[38,39] Tachyphylaxis may limit the use of long-term infusions. Lidocaine is less cardiotoxic than bupivacaine and plasma levels can be monitored during infusion. Concerns regarding the rapid development of tolerance to lidocaine have limited its use. Plasma concentrations of lidocaine and its active metabolite, monoethylglycinexylidide, should be measured once a day in infants, and twice a day in neonates, because both compounds are epileptogenic.

Recommended administration of opioids for continuous epidural infusion in pediatric patients is shown in Table 40.4. The addition of an opioid to diluted anesthetics improves the quality of analgesia. In infants up to 6 months of age, epidural

Table 40.3. **RECOMMENDED RATES (UPPER END) OF LOCAL ANESTHETIC EPIDURAL INFUSION IN PEDIATRIC PATIENTS**

DRUG (COMMON CONCENTRATIONS)	RATE (µG/KG/HR)*		
	0–2 MONTHS	3–6 MONTHS	> 6 MONTHS
Bupivacaine (0.05%, 0.1%, 0.125%)	0.25	0.3	0.4
Levobupivacaine (0.1%, 0.125%)	0.25	0.3	0.4
Ropivacaine (0.1%)	0.3	0.4	0.4
Lidocaine (0.1%, 0.3%)	0.8	1	1.5 (Not commonly used)
Chloroprocaine (1.5%)	7.5 (mid-thoracic) 9–10.5 (lumbar and low thoracic)	7.5 (mid-thoracic) 9–10.5 (lumbar and low thoracic)	Rarely used

* Infusion rates should not exceed 15 mL/hr.

Table 40.4. **RECOMMENDED RATES OF ADJUVANTS FOR CONTINUOUS EPIDURAL INFUSION IN PEDIATRIC PATIENTS**

DRUG	DOSE* (μG/KG/HR)	TYPICAL CONCENTRATION (μG/ML)		
		NEONATES (0–2 MONTHS)	INFANTS	CHILDREN
Fentanyl	0.1–0.5	1–2	2 (2–5)	5 (2–5)
Hydromorphone	1.5–2.5	NR	NR	10–20**
Morphine	3–5	NR	NR	25–50**
Clonidine§	0.1–0.2	NR	0.4	0.4–1 (lumbar epidural tip) 0.4–0.6 (thoracic epidural tip)

NR, not recommended.

*Larger doses of opioids are indicated for opioid-tolerant patients.

**Administration of hydrophilic opioids through a thoracic epidural is not recommended.

§ When clonidine is added to an epidural solution, the epidural opioid dose should be reduced by 50%.

fentanyl (2 μg/mL) in combination with 0.1% bupivacaine improved postthoracotomy analgesia without an increase in side effects, compared with 0.1% bupivacaine alone.[40] Some experts avoid co-administration of opioid drugs in epidural catheters because of the risk of respiratory depression, urinary retention, or itching.[41] The higher cephalad spread of hydrosoluble opioids restricts their use to infants over 6 months old. Morphine has a higher rate of pruritus and nausea and vomiting than other epidural opioids.[42]

In very young infants, the use of clonidine has been associated with apnea, hypotension, and excessive sedation. An epidural clonidine infusion decreases the need for opioids, thus reducing the complications from nausea, pruritus, and respiratory depression. A continuous infusion of epidural clonidine at 0.08 to 0.12 μg/kg/hr produced dose-dependent analgesia when added to local anesthetic infusions,[43] and higher doses of clonidine alone (0.2 μg/kg/hr preceded by a bolus of 2 μg/kg) provided analgesia at rest after abdominal surgery.[44]

POSTOPERATIVE MONITORING OF PATIENTS WITH PEDIATRIC EPIDURAL INFUSIONS

Pain assessment may be quite difficult in children. Irritability or agitation, despite an apparently well-functioning epidural, may be caused by the presence of IV lines, a nasogastric tube, urinary catheter, or even the hospital environment. Self-report scales, such as Numeric Pain Rating Scale, and Wong Baker Faces Pain Rating Scale,[45] have been validated in patients 7 years old and older, and 3 years and older, respectively, (Figure 40.1). For patients who are unable or unwilling to report their pain, the pain assessment relies on observation of behavior. A commonly used scale recommended for patients 2 months to 7 years old is the Face, Legs, Activity, Cry, Consolability Scale (FLACC),[46] shown in Table 40.5. A revised FLACC scale for pain assessment in cognitively impaired patients incorporates additional descriptors associated with pain in this category of patients.[47] It is possible to assess dermatome levels in infants and nonverbal patients by carefully observing

Table 40.5. **THE FLACC BEHAVIORAL SCALE**[46]

CATEGORIES	SCORING 0	1	2
Face	No particular expression or smile	Occasional grimace or frown, withdrawn, not interested	Frequent to constant quivering chin, clenched jaw
Legs	Normal position or relaxed	Uneasy, restless, tense	Kicking, or legs drawn up
Activity	Lying quietly, normal position, moves easily	Squirming, shifting back and forth, tense	Arched, rigid, or jerking
Cry	No cry (awake or asleep)	Moans or whimpers, occasional complaint	Crying steadily, screams or sobs, frequent complaints
Consolability	Content, relaxed	Reassured by occasional touching, hugging, or being talked to, distractible	Difficult to console or comfort

Each of the five categories—(F) Face, (L) Legs, (A) Activity, (C) Cry, (C) Consolability—is scored from 0 to 2, which results in a total score between 0 and 10.

flinching and facial expression in response to ice on presumed blocked and unblocked dermatomes. Another method for determining the effectiveness of the regional blockade is to observe the patient's response to movement or to gentle palpation of the operative site.

A pain score of 3 or less is generally considered adequate pain control, requiring no intervention. Pain of 0/10 at rest and with activity at multiple hourly assessments suggests excessive medication and requires prompt reevaluation of the epidural infusion. Decrease or temporary discontinuation of the epidural infusion is indicated, especially if the pain score of 0/10 is correlated with excessive motor block or increased sedation.

A pain score of 4 or more with rest and activity might require adjustment of the epidural infusion by bolus and an increase of the continuous infusion rate. When in doubt regarding the source of distress, a trial of analgesic is both diagnostic and therapeutic. A test dose of lidocaine (0.5% to 1%, 3 to 5 mg/kg) may be used for this purpose, but caution should be exercised in infants receiving an amide local anesthetic infusion who could exceed maximum allowable doses for amide anesthetics. Alternatively, 3% chloroprocaine may be administered in incremental doses (total dose of 0.5 mL/kg, maximum 15 mL for patients > 50 kg) without the risk of toxicity. Chloroprocaine is metabolized by cholinesterase and has a short duration of action. Resolution of hypertension and tachycardia or lower extremity sensory or motor block (for a catheter tip at the lumbar level) after the administration of a lidocaine or chloroprocaine test dose supports correct catheter tip placement.

If analgesia is inadequate despite correct catheter tip position, consider increasing the local anesthetic concentration while maintaining the hourly dosing below the maximum safe rate. Alternatively, consider inclusion of an opioid, clonidine, or both, if the epidural solution does not include them already. If the catheter tip is in the lumbar region and remote from the segmental levels corresponding to the incisional area, a hydrophilic opioid may be added to the infusion. In young patients who are irritable despite adequate surgical-site analgesia, satisfactory sedation may be achieved by supplementing an anesthetic epidural infusion with IV opioids, or by adding clonidine to the epidural infusion.

Blood pressure, heart rate, respiratory rate, pulse oximetry, and EKG are measured hourly in the first 24 hours. Since blood pressure is relatively stable in children, assessment of respiratory rate, depth of respiration, and oxygen saturation may alert the physician to overmedication.

Motor block is assessed by the modified Bromage scale (Table 40.6).[48] A Bromage score of III or higher (lumbar epidural), or upper extremity weakness (thoracic epidural), and decreased or absent movement in response to touch suggest excessive epidural infusion rates, intrathecal migration of the catheter, or formation of an epidural abscess or hematoma. In younger or disabled children (who are unable to follow commands) movement and muscle tone are evaluated by tickling toes and gently flexing the knees or hips, respectively.

A sensory block above T3 may result in respiratory distress, bradycardia, numbness or tingling in the fingers or arms, loss of hand function, and Horner's sign. With excessive sedation, a patient is arousable only to deep stimuli, or unarousable. Contributing factors are excessive epidural clonidine or opioid administration, high block, oral or parenteral co-administration of sedatives and analgesics, or local anesthetic toxicity.

Table 40.6. **BROMAGE SCORE**

GRADE	CRITERIA	DEGREE OF BLOCK
I	Free movement of legs and knees	Nil (0%)
II	Just able to flex knees with free movement of feet	Partial (33%)
III	Unable to flex knees but with free movement of feet	Almost complete (66%)
IV	Unable to move legs or feet	Complete (100%)

The insertion site should be assessed frequently. Leakage of the epidural solution at the entry site is common in young children, and usually does not affect pain control. Leakage may be decreased by applying a pressure dressing over the catheter-occlusive dressing. Itching, nausea and vomiting, and urinary retention are common complications of epidurals and should be aggressively monitored in the postoperative period.

PATIENT-CONTROLLED EPIDURAL ANALGESIA (PCEA) IN THE PEDIATRIC POPULATION

Children as young as 5 years old have the cognitive ability to understand and the willingness to use PCEA.[49] In a group of 7- to 12-year-old children, the total amount of ropivacaine administered in the first 48 hours in the PCEA group was half that administered in the continuous epidural group, while pain scores were similar.[50] Follow-up studies showed the validity of PCEA in the pediatric population if a correct assessment of cognitive ability is made preoperatively by the anesthesiologist. A common PCEA regimen is described in Table 40.7.

CONCLUSIONS

- CEA in children is safe; however, neonates have a higher risk of complications than older children. The indications and choice of technique for CEA in children should be carefully weighed to optimize the risk–benefit ratio.

Table 40.7. **PCEA SETTINGS FOR PEDIATRIC PATIENTS USING BUPIVACAINE OR ROPIVACAINE INFUSIONS**

BASAL RATE	BOLUS	LOCKOUT INTERVAL	MAXIMUM HOURLY RATE
0.2 mg/kg/hr	0.1 mg/kg/hr	15 min	0.4 mg/kg/hr

- The most common problems with CEA are ineffectiveness, caused by incorrect dermatomal location; catheter problems (obstruction, leaking, or accidental displacement from the original position); inappropriate infusion rates or solutions; intravascular injection; and local site inflammation or infection.
- Infants and children have lower therapeutic indices for epidurally administered drugs. Therefore, the epidural catheter tip should be placed in close proximity to the dermatome to be blocked and its location confirmed via nerve stimulation, ultrasound, or radiography. Utmost care should be exercised in limiting the epidural infusion rate, concentration, and duration in this age group.
- Pain assessment is difficult in young or cognitively impaired children. Irritability and agitation are possible despite a working epidural. Patients may benefit from the sedative effects of epidural clonidine or IV opioids, in addition to a local anesthetic epidural infusion.
- For safe epidural management in children, calculate the maximum permissible local anesthetic infusion, determine the desired infusion rates, ensure that rates and concentration produce an acceptable dose of local anesthetic, determine the rate for the adjuvants, and calculate the required concentration of adjuvant in the epidural solution.

REFERENCES

1. Bösenberg AT, Bland BAR, Schulte-Steinberg O, et al. Thoracic epidural via the caudal route in infants. *Anesthesiology.* 1988;69;265–269.
2. Wolf AR, Eyres RL, Laussen PC, et al. Effect of extradural analgesia on stress response to abdominal surgery in infants. *Br J Anaesth.* 1993;70(6):654–660.
3. Bosenberg AT, Hadley GP, Wiersma R. Oesophageal atresia: caudo-thoracic epidural anesthesia reduces the need for postoperative ventilatory support. *Pediatr Surg Int.* 1992;7:289–291.
4. Di Pede A, Morini, F, Lombardi MH, et al. Comparison of regional vs systemic analgesia for post-thoracotomy care in infants. *Paediatr Anaesth.* 2014;24:569–573.
5. Wilson GA, Brown JL, Crabbe DG, Hinton W, McHugh PJ, Stringer MD. Is epidural analgesia associated with an improved outcome following open Nissen fundoplication? *Paediatr Anaesth.* 2001;11(1):65–70.
6. Nishimori M, Low JH, Zheng H, Ballantyne JC. Epidural pain relief versus systemic opioid-based pain relief for abdominal aortic surgery. *Cochrane Database Syst Rev.* 2012;11:7.
7. Bösenberg AT, Gouws E. Skin-epidural distance in children. *Anaesthesia.* 1995;50(10):895–897.
8. Brown TCK, Eyres RL, McDougall RJ. Local and regional anaesthesia in children. *Br J Anaesth.* 1999;83:65–77.
9. Larson BA, Lonnqvist PA, Olsson GL. Plasma concentrations of bupivacaine in neonates after continuous epidural infusion. *Anesth Analg.* 1997;84:501–505.
10. Berde C. Convulsions associated with pediatric regional anesthesia. *Anesth Analg.* 1992;75:164–166.
11. Rowney DA, Doyle E. Epidural and subarachnoid blockade in children. *Anaesthesia.* 1998;53:980–1001.
12. Polaner DM, Taebzer AH, Walker BJ, et al. Pediatric Regional Anesthesia Network (PRAN): a multi-institutional study of the use and incidence of complications of pediatric regional anesthesia. *Anesth Analg.* 2012;1156:1353–1364.
13. Llewellyn N, Moriarty A. National paediatric epidural audit. *Paediatr Anaesth.* 2007;17:520–532.
14. Wong GK, Arab AA, Chew SC, et al. Major complications related to epidural analgesia in children: a 15-year audit of 3,152 epidurals. *Can J Anaesth.* 2013;604:355–363.
15. Meyer MJ, Krane EJ, Goldschneider KR, et al. Case report: neurological complications associated with epidural analgesia in children: a report of 4 cases of ambiguous etiologies. *Anesth Analg.* 2012;115:1365–1370.
16. Gamble JJ, Ambros B, Seguin P, et al. Stimulating thoracic epidural placement via a lumbar approach causes significant spinal cord damage in a porcine model. *Can J Anaesth.* 2014;61:306–311.
17. Sethna NF, Clendenin D, Athiraman U, et al. Incidence of epidural catheter-associated infections after continuous epidural analgesia in children. *Anesthesiology.* 2010;113:224–232.
18. Bubeck J, Boos K, Krause H, et al. Subcutaneous tunneling of caudal catheters reduces the rate of bacterial colonization to that of lumbar epidural catheters. *Anesth Analg.* 2004;99(3):689–693.
19. Simpao AF, Gurnaney HG, Schwartz AJ, et al. Cephalad migration of pediatric caudal epidural catheters associated with change from prone to supine position. *Anesthesiology.* 2012;117:1353.
20. Thompson ME, Aasheim H. Migrating thoracic epidural catheter in an infant. *Paediatr Anaesth.* 2012;22:285–287.
21. Strandness T, Wiktor M, Varadajaran J, Weisman S. Migration of pediatric epidural catheters. *Paediatr Anaesth.* 2015;25:610–613.
22. Dalens B, Tanguy A, Haberer J-P. Lumbar epidural anesthesia for operative and postoperative pain relief in infants and young children. *Anesth Analg.* 1986;65:1069–1073.
23. Welch K. The intracranial pressure in infants. *J Neurosurg.* 1980;52:693–694.
24. López T, Sánchez FJ, Garzón JC, et al. Spinal anesthesia in pediatric patients. *Minerva Anestesiol.* 2012;78:78–87.
25. Neal JM, Bernards CM, Butterworth JF IV, et al. ASRA practice advisory on local anesthetic systemic toxicity. *Reg Anesth Pain Med.* 2010;35(2):152–161.
26. Polaner DM, Zuk J, Luong K, Pan Z. Positive intravascular test dose criteria in children during total intravenous anesthesia with propofol and remifentanil are different than during inhaled anesthesia. *Anesth Analg.* 2010;110:41–45.
27. Morton NS. Prevention and control of pain in children. *Br J Anaesth.* 1999;83:118–129.
28. Wood CE, Goresky GV, Klanssen KA, et al. Complications of continuous epidural infusion for postoperative analgesia in children. *Can J Anaesth.* 1994;41(7):613–620.
29. Flandin-Blety C, Barrier G. Accidents following analgesia in children. The results of a retrospective study. *Paediatr Anaesth.* 1995;5:41–46.
30. Johr M. Regional anaesthesia in neonates, infants and children. An educational review. *Eur J Anaesthesiol.* 2015;32:289–297.
31. Shenkeman Z, Hoppenstein D, Erez I, et al. Continuous lumbar/thoracic epidural analgesia in low-weight pediatric surgical patients: practical aspects and pitfalls. *Pediatr Surg Int.* 2009;25:623–634.
32. Blanco D, Llamazares J, Rincon R, et al. Thoracic epidural anesthesia via the lumbar approach in infants and children. *Anesthesiology.* 1996;84:1312–1316.
33. Breschan C, Krumholz R, Jost R, et al. Intraspinal haematoma following lumbar epidural anesthesia in a neonate. *Paediatr Anaesth.* 2001;11:105–108.
34. Taenzer AH, Cantwell CV, Kovarik WD. Experience with 724 epidurograms for epidural catheter placement in pediatric anesthesia. *Reg Anesth Pain Med.* 2010;35:432–435.
35. Tsui BC, Wagner A, Cave D, et al. Thoracic and lumbar epidural analgesia via the caudal approach using electrical stimulation guidance in pediatric patients: a review of 289 patients. *Anesthesiology,* 2004;100(3):683–689.
36. Willschke H, Bosenberg A, Marhofer P, et al. Epidural catheter placement in neonate: sonoanatomy and feasibility of

ultrasonographic guidance in term and preterm neonates. *Reg Anesth Pain Med,* 2007;32(1):34–40.
37. Bosenberg AT, Thomas J, Cronje L, et al. Pharmacokinetics and efficacy of ropivacaine for continuous epidural infusion in neonates and infants. *Paediatr Anaesth*. 2005;15:739–749.
38. Veneziano G, Iliev P, Tripi J, et al. Continuous chloroprocaine infusion for thoracic and caudal epidurals as a postoperative analgesia modality in neonates, infants and children. *Paediatr Anaesth.* 2016;26:84–91.
39. Muhly WT, Gurnaney HG, Kraemer FW, et al. A retrospective comparison of ropivacaine and 2-chloroprocaine continuous thoracic epidural analgesia for management of postthoracotomy pain in infants. *Paediatr Anaesth.* 2015;25:1162–1167.
40. Ganesh A, Adzick, NS, Foster T, et al. Efficacy of addition of fentanyl to epidural bupivacaine on postoperative analgesia after thoracotomy for lung resection in infants. *Anesthesiology.* 2008;109:890–894.
41. Marhofer P, Lonnqvist PA. The use of ultrasound-guided regional anaesthetic techniques in neonate and young infants. *Acta Anaesthesiol Scand*. 2014;58:1049–1060.
42. White MJ, Berghaussen EJ, Dumont SW, et al. Side effects during continuous epidural infusion of morphine and fentanyl. *Can J Anaesth*. 1996;51:1170–1172.
43. De Negri P, Ivani G, Visconti C, De Vivo P, Lonnqvist PA. The dose-response relationship for clonidine added to a postoperative continuous epidural infusion of ropivacaine in children. *Anesth Analg.* 2001;93:71–76.
44. Klamt JG, Garcia LV, Stocche RM, Meinberg AC. Epidural infusion of clonidine or clonidine plus ropivacaine for postoperative analgesia in children undergoing major abdominal surgery. *J Clin Anesth*. 2003;15:510–514.
45. Wong DL, Baker CM. Pain in children: comparison of assessment scales. *Pediatr Nurs*. 1988;14:9–17.
46. Merkel SI, Voepel-Lewis T, Shayevitz JR, Malviya S. The FLACC: a behavioral scale for scoring postoperative pain in young children. *Pediatr Nurs*. 1997;23(3):293–297.
47. Malviya S, Voepel-Lewis T, Burke C, Merkel S, Tait AR. The revised FLACC observational pain tool: improved reliability and validity for pain assessment in children with cognitive impairment. *Paediatr Anaesth*. 2006;16(3):258–265.
48. Bromage PR, ed. *Epidural Analgesia*. Philadelphia, PA: WB Saunders; 1978:144.
49. Birmingham PK, Wheeler M, Suresh S, et al. Patient-controlled epidural analgesia in children: can they do it? *Anesth Analg.* 2003;96:686–691.
50. Antok E, Bordet F, Duflo F, et al. Patient controlled epidural analgesia versus continuous epidural infusion with ropivacaine for postoperative analgesia in children. *Anesth Analg*. 2003;97:1608–1611.
51. Sethna NF, Berde CB. Venous air embolism during identification of the epidural space in children. *Anesth Analg*. 1993;76:925–927.
52. Byers K, Axelrod P, Michael S, Rosen S. Infections complicating tunneled intraspinal catheter systems used to treat chronic pain. *Clin Infect Dis*. 1995;21:403–408.
53. Sviggum HP, Jacob AK, Arendt KW, Mauermann ML, Horlocker TT, Hebl JR. Neurologic complications after chlorhexidine antisepsis for spinal anesthesia. *Reg Anesth Pain Med*. 2012;37(2):139–144.
54. Berde C. Convulsions associated with pediatric regional anesthesia. *Anesth Analg.* 1992;75:164–166.

REVIEW QUESTIONS

1. An epidural catheter is inserted in a 3-year-old patient undergoing femoral osteotomy under general anesthesia. The patient is intubated and her lungs are mechanically ventilated. Upon identification of the epidural space using the LOR to air technique, the SpO_2 decreases to 87% transiently, and the end-tidal CO_2 drops from 40 to 29 mm Hg. Which of the following clinical manifestations is not likely to accompany these findings?

   A. Pneumothorax
   B. Patchy analgesia
   C. Spinal cord ischemia
   D. Hemodynamic instability

2. A 5-month-old baby undergoes laparotomy for resection of a neuroblastoma. He is extubated and transferred to the pediatric ICU, where his pain is controlled with a thoracic epidural catheter with the tip placed at T7. On postoperative day 2, his breathing efforts are diminished, and his arterial oxygen saturation decreases to 93%. Which of the following could support the suspicion of epidural catheter erosion into the dural sac?

   A. Blood pressure 43/28 mm Hg
   B. Apnea
   C. Heart rate 189 beats/min
   D. Nausea

3. A neonate is undergoing thoracotomy for the management of congenital lobar emphysema. An epidural catheter is inserted in the caudal space and is advanced to T5-T6. Which of the following is recommended to reduce the risk of epidural catheter-related infection in this patient?

   A. Removing the catheter if the dressing is soiled.
   B. Disinfecting the skin with chlorhexidine before epidural placement.
   C. Tunneling of the catheter subcutaneously with the catheter exit point at the L4 level.
   D. Continuing IV antibiotic administration until the removal of the epidural catheter.

ANSWERS

1. A. LOR to air is associated with numerous complications, including nerve root compression, subcutaneous emphysema, pneumocephalus, incomplete analgesia (answer B), and paresthesia. In the pediatric population, venous air embolism represents a major concern because of the proportionally larger amount of air per body weight that could be inadvertently injected intravascularly. The up to 50% incidence of a patent foramen ovale in children younger than 5 years of age could lead to hemodynamic instability (answer D).[51] In a large retrospective study of pediatric epidural analgesia practice, LOR to air had been used in four of the five patients who developed severe neurologic deficits postoperatively (the fifth was unknown).[29] An air bubble trapped in an epidural vein may have caused local thrombosis and spinal ischemia (answer C). Considering the potential associated morbidity, testing by LOR to air is discouraged in children, particularly infants and neonates. Answer A is correct, because epidural needle insertion in the lumbar space is unlikely to cause a pneumothorax.

2. B. In young children with an immature sympathetic nervous system, accidental total spinal anesthesia manifests as apnea (answer B) or decreasing arterial oxygen saturation, rather than hypotension (answer A) or tachycardia (answer C). Hypotension is rarely associated with epidural anesthesia in children less than 8 years old. Although nausea can be a manifestation of complete spinal block in adults, infants and young children lack the ability to report this sensation; therefore, answer D is incorrect.

3. A. Fixing the catheter with occlusive dressing in a cephalad direction, removing the catheter when the dressing is soiled (answer A), and tunneling the catheter (typically for longer anticipated duration of CEA) reduce the risk of caudal catheter contamination by stool and urine. Answer C is incorrect because the exit point of the catheter at L4 (likely below the diaper line) is still exposed to stool. Answer D is incorrect because the benefit of prophylactic antibiotics before epidural catheterization is controversial. One study reported no association between the perioperative use of IV cefazolin and the risk of intraspinal catheter infection.[52] Given the low incidence of epidural infection and lack of a controlled trial, it is difficult to evaluate the efficacy of prophylactic antibiotics. Skin antisepsis is paramount in reducing catheter contamination. Alcohol-based chlorhexidine disinfectants are more effective than povidone iodine for reducing skin colonization. Although cases of severe arachnoiditis potentially associated with the use of chlorhexidine for skin disinfection have been reported, a recent large retrospective study of 12,465 patients showed no adverse effects after neuraxial anesthesia with chlorhexidine antisepsis.[53] Answer B is incorrect because chlorhexidine is not approved in children less than 2 months old.

QUESTIONS AND ANSWERS

This chapter has accompanying questions and answers that are available to subscribers as part of the Oxford eLearning platform. To access the questions, follow the link below, or go to ✔ http://oxfordmedicine.com/painmanagementreview

41.

NEURAXIAL ANESTHESIA IN COEXISTING NEUROLOGIC CONDITIONS

John Henry Harrison and Magdalena Anitescu

STEM CASE AND KEY QUESTIONS

A 71-year-old male, 82 kg, is scheduled for a rectal urethral fistula repair and ileal conduit. He reports uneventful surgeries under general anesthesia in the past. His medical history is significant for a cerebrovascular accident 10 years earlier with no sequelae. He was diagnosed 3 years earlier with Charcot-Marie-Tooth disease. He has leg fatigue and difficulty walking, so he often relies on a wheelchair for transportation. The cardiologist considers his cardiac risk for the scheduled surgery to be low.

WHAT WOULD YOUR ANESTHETIC PLAN BE? DO YOU NEED MORE INFORMATION BEFORE SURGERY? WOULD YOU PLACE AN EPIDURAL FOR POSTOPERATIVE PAIN CONTROL?

After discussion of the risks and benefits, an uneventful thoracic (T10-T11) epidural catheter is placed to alleviate postoperative pain. A bilateral T6 to L2 sensory, but not motor, block is achieved after 5 mL of the test dose (lidocaine 1.5% with 1:200,000 epinephrine). Vital signs are stable and no sympathectomy is observed.

WOULD YOU BOLUS THE EPIDURAL WITH THE INDUCTION OF ANESTHESIA? WOULD YOU USE THE EPIDURAL AS PART OF AN INTRAOPERATIVE ANESTHETIC OR WOULD YOU USE IT ONLY IN THE POSTOPERATIVE PERIOD?

After an uneventful induction of anesthesia with propofol and vecuronium, an endotracheal tube is placed without difficulty. Anesthesia is maintained for the 13-hour surgical procedure with 1.2 minimum alveolar concentration (MAC) isoflurane in 50% oxygen and 16 mg vecuronium. The patient also receives multiple blood products, albumin, and crystalloids for a 1500-mL estimated blood loss. The patient's vital signs are stable throughout the procedure. In the last hour, the patient is given an intravenous bolus of 500 μg fentanyl and 1.2 mg hydromorphone and no epidural medications.

WOULD YOU EXTUBATE THIS PATIENT? DOES THIS PATIENT HAVE OPTIMAL PAIN CONTROL? WOULD YOU CONSIDER ACTIVATING THE EPIDURAL?

The intubated patient is transported to the ICU after an epidural infusion of bupivacaine 0.125% at 6 mL/hr. Since the patient remains unresponsive for the next 16 hours, the epidural infusion is decreased to 4 mL/hr in the first 2 hours of his ICU stay.

WOULD YOU CONTINUE THE EPIDURAL INFUSION IN THIS INTUBATED PATIENT? WOULD THE UNDERLYING NEUROLOGIC DISEASE AFFECT YOUR DECISION FOR PERIOPERATIVE PAIN MANAGEMENT IN THIS CASE?

The patient is extubated when extubation criteria are met on postoperative day (POD) 1. He reports a pain score of 5/10 at the incision level. He currently has a T10-L2 sensory block bilaterally but no motor block. A 5-mL epidural bolus of 0.125% bupivacaine is administered. Patient-controlled epidural analgesia (PCEA) is implemented at an 8-mL/hr continuous rate and a 3-mL demand bolus every 20 minutes. The patient's pain score decreases to 0/10 at rest and with movement 1 hour after the changes.

IS THIS LEVEL OF PAIN RELIEF ACCEPTABLE? IS THE VISUAL ANALOG SCALE (VAS) THE ONLY MEASURE OF THE EFFICACY OF AN EPIDURAL?

On POD 2, approximately 20 hours after extubation and initiation of PCEA, the patient experiences motor block in both legs.

WHAT WOULD YOU DO? IS THIS EVENT AN EMERGENCY? WOULD YOU DISCONTINUE THE EPIDURAL?

The epidural infusion is discontinued. At 1-, 2-, and 4-hr neurologic evaluation of the patient, motor function does not improve. He feels no tenderness to palpation at the site of the epidural insertion and no additional discomfort. The epidural catheter is removed, and an MRI of the thoracolumbar spine is ordered, together with a neurology consult.

WOULD YOU REMOVE THE CATHETER AT THIS TIME? WHAT IS AN ALGORITHM TO REACH A POSITIVE DIAGNOSIS? WHAT IS THE DIFFERENTIAL DIAGNOSIS?

Neuroimaging shows no epidural hematoma. The patient's motor deficit lasts for the next 24 hours, after which motor function slowly returns to baseline. His pain is managed with a hydromorphone patient-controlled analgesia (PCA), and the VAS score is 1/10. Four days later, he is discharged from the hospital to a rehabilitation center.

DISCUSSION

In a 1956 review of regional techniques, neuraxial techniques were not recommended for patients with preexisting central and peripheral nervous system disorders.[1] For several decades, the risk of needle and catheter-induced mechanical trauma,[2] combined with a description of the double-crush phenomenon (preexisting neural compromise makes patients more susceptible to injury after an insult at another site), made regional techniques a rarity in neurologic patients undergoing various surgical procedures.[3] Many difficulties still remain in such patients. The perioperative analgesic plan must weigh the benefits of an epidural against the risks of aggravating an underlying neurologic abnormality.

In some conditions, such as brain tumors with severe intracranial hypertension or spinal tumors at the level of catheter insertion, neuraxial techniques are absolutely contraindicated.[4,5] In other neurologic disorders, such as multiple sclerosis (MS) or Guillain-Barré syndrome (GBS), the disease may be aggravated, and the decision to perform regional anesthesia must be weighed carefully.[6,7] Finally, in all cases of preexisting neuropathies, a neuraxial technique may confuse the clinical picture and possibly delay the diagnosis of an acute exacerbation of the disease in the immediate postoperative period.[5,6]

CHARCOT-MARIE-TOOTH DISEASE

The inherited neuropathy known as Charcot-Marie-Tooth disease (CMTD) was described in 1886 by Jean Martin Charcot and Pierre Marie in France and by Howard Henry Tooth in England.[8] It was called peroneal progressive muscular atrophy based on the observed clinical features of distal lower extremity muscle wasting, weakness, and sensory loss.[8] Hereditary sensory and motor peripheral neuropathy is the most common inherited neuromuscular disorder, affecting 150,000 people in the United States, with a worldwide incidence of 1:10,000 (1:2,500 in the United States).[8] CMTD is a genetically heterogeneous disorder with a common clinical phenotype: the distoproximal progression of muscle wasting.[9] Sensory loss also is common, and most phenotypes show a combined motor and sensory deficit.[9] Regardless of the original genetic defect (compaction of the myelin sheath or a defect in neuronal cytoskeleton, in axonal transport, or in mitochondrial metabolism) the common pathologic finding is axonal degeneration of large fibers[10] (Figure 41.1 and Figure 41.2).

The majority of cases manifest early, in the first to third decades of life.[9] In a few cases, patients are diagnosed in the sixth or seventh decade of life, when diagnostic tests are performed after another family member develops an unexplained weakness[11] (Table 41.1).

In patients with CMTD, the indication for a neuraxial technique depends upon the disease severity. Patients with onset of the disease during adolescence may develop musculoskeletal and respiratory comorbidities later in life.[12,13] When neuropathy debuts before the growth spurt, weakening of the

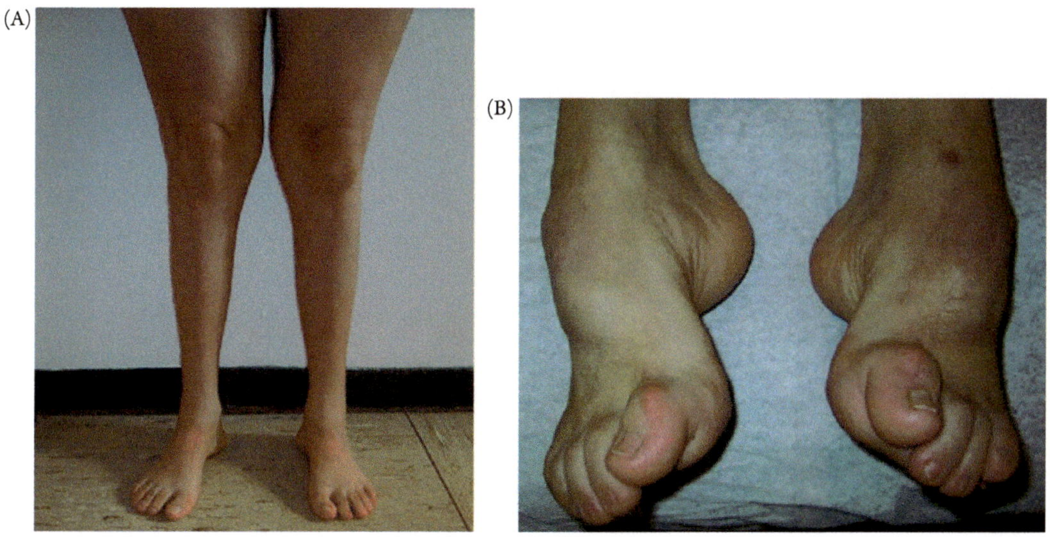

Figure 41.1. (A) Distoproximal progression of muscle wasting in Charcot-Marie-Tooth disease. (B) Foot deformities in Charcot-Marie-Tooth disease (high arch, hammertoes).[9]

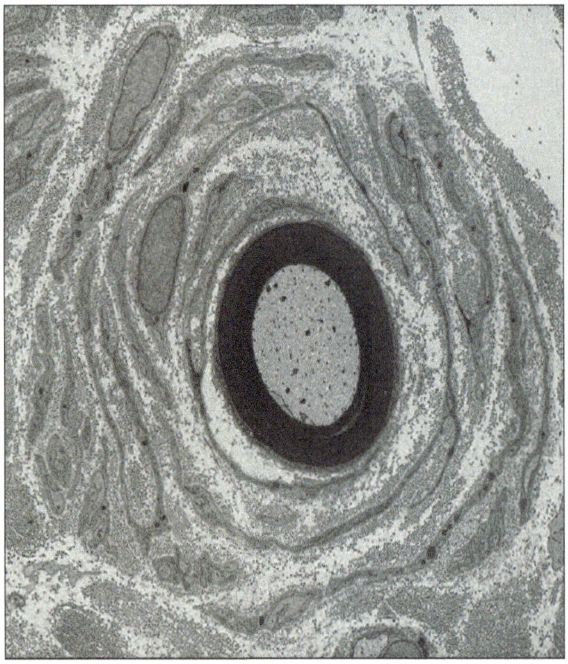

Figure 41.2. Electron micrograph of peripheral nerve biopsy in a patient with Charcot-Marie-Tooth disease showing onion-bulb (Schwann cell proliferation) surrounding an axon with decreased myelin.[15]

neuraxial skeleton predisposes patients to severe scoliosis and restrictive lung disease.[12,13] Pregnancy exacerbates neuromuscular manifestations,[14] and controversy exists about the use of a lumbar epidural as an analgesic technique in the laboring parturient. On the other hand, in patients with milder, late-onset clinical features, the disease is not exacerbated during pregnancy nor is the axial skeleton weakened. In these patients, neuraxial analgesia may be used for the same indications as in their healthy counterparts.[11] In severe cases, corrective spine fusion for scoliosis may be necessary,[12] making neuraxial block placement difficult. Coexisting restrictive pulmonary function and various cardiomyopathies complicate perioperative management.[13,15] In these situations, placement of the epidural for perioperative analgesia under direct vision in the fluoroscopic suite is suggested.

Recommendations for regional anesthesia for patients with CMTD are largely based on case reports and include use of ultrasound guidance, placing the block without a nerve stimulator, and low concentration of local anesthetic (LA).[7] Cytotoxicity is dose-dependent[16,17] and the use of ultrasound guides the administration of LA and minimizes needle manipulation and needle trauma.[18] Demyelination and decreased nerve excitability make nerve stimulation unreliable; thus, an ultrasound technique is favored.[19,20]

GBS

Because the incidence of GBS is 1.2 cases per 100,000 in developed countries, patients with the syndrome present for surgery.[21] GBS is an acute demyelinating polyradiculoneuropathy characterized by areflexia and diffuse ascending neuromuscular paralysis.[22] In this autoimmune inflammatory state, patchy segmental demyelination occurs along peripheral nerves and nerve roots.[21] The inflammatory infiltrates are lymphocytes, monocytes, and plasma cells.[21] The autoimmune inflammation is thought to be spurred by an infection or other insult to the immune system; triggers may include pregnancy, vaccinations, immunosuppression, systemic illnesses, infection, and transfusion[23] (Figure 41.3).

Regional anesthesia in patients with GBS is generally avoided and GBS is considered by some to be a relative contraindication to neuraxial anesthesia.[24,25] Evidence in support is largely limited to case reports of neuraxial techniques in obstetric patients.[22] Concerns include recrudescence or worsening of disease or severe autonomic responses during neuraxial anesthetic placement because of autonomic instability.[26] Needle trauma to nerve roots may initiate or exacerbate a cascade of immunologic events leading to demyelinating neuropathy.[27] Interaction of LA with myelin is a contributing factor.[27]

Table 41.1. **CLASSIFICATION OF HEREDITARY SENSORY AND MOTOR PERIPHERAL NEUROPATHIES OF CHARCOT-MARIE-TOOTH DISEASE (CMTD)**

TYPE	PATHOLOGY	INHERITANCE	ONSET	CLINICAL FEATURES
CMTD I	Demyelination (hypertrophic, onion bulb appearance of myelin)	AD	Adolescence	Commonest are weakness, atrophy, sensory loss in legs
CMTD II	Neuronal disorder (axonal degradation)	AD	Later age	Mild, distal weakness
CMTD III (Déjérine-Sottas)	Severe demyelination (thinning of myelin sheath)	AD and AR	Infancy	Rare, delayed developmental milestones and motor skills
CMTD IV	Demyelination (hypertrophic, onion bulb appearance of myelin)	AR	Early childhood	Rare, leg weakness
CMTD X	Defect in communication between Schwann cells and axons	X-linked	Late childhood, adolescence	Rare, male > female, moderate to severe motor and sensory neuropathy

Original table based on Pareyson and Marchesi.[9]

Abbreviations: AD, autosomal dominant; AR, autosomal recessive.

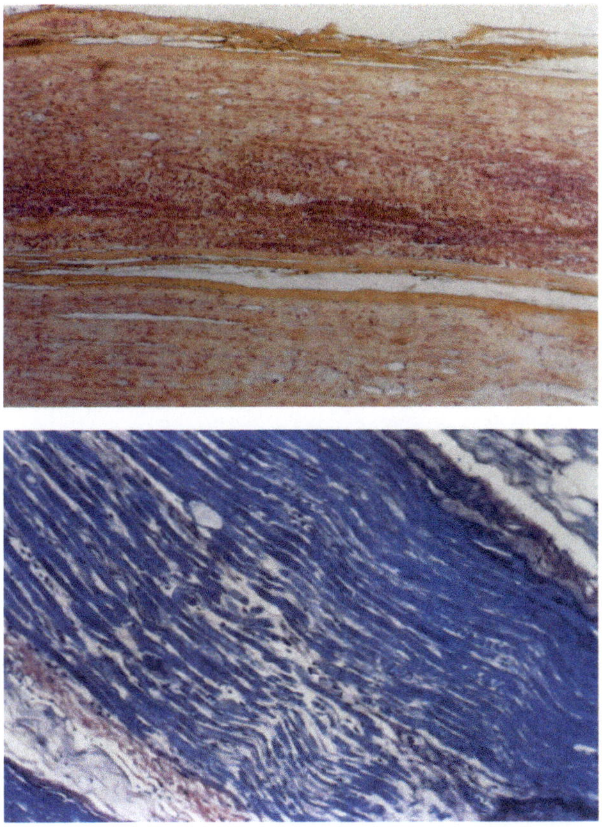

Figure 41.3. Photomicrographs of tissue from patients with Guillain-Barré syndrome. (A) Sural nerve tissue with lymphocyte and macrophage infiltration and severe demyelination. (B) Tibial nerve tissue showing demyelination without lymphocyte infiltration.[24]

Quantifying the contribution of neuraxial anesthesia to disease recrudescence or exacerbation is difficult. The stress of surgery itself exacerbates the disease.[28,29] Ultimately, the decision to perform regional anesthesia in patients with GBS should be made on a case-by-case basis after a thorough conversation about risks and benefits.[22]

MS

MS, another autoimmune disease, is characterized by inflammation, demyelination, and axonal damage to the CNS. Global median prevalence for MS is 30 per 100,000 people.[30] However, in the United States, its overall prevalence varies from 50 to 140 per 100,000 persons. Choosing an optimal anesthetic technique depends largely on respiratory function and drug interactions with medications the patient may be taking. Weakness of the respiratory muscles is possible later in the course of the disease.[6] In cases of limited respiratory reserve, mild residual effects of muscle relaxants may lead to respiratory compromise postoperatively.[31] Response to nondepolarizing neuromuscular blockers may be altered by baseline weakness or from interactions with medications, such as carbamazepine.[6] The minimum alveolar concentration of inhalational agents should be reduced, and there is a potential for delayed emergence.[32] Relying on regional or neuraxial techniques instead of general anesthesia may be of benefit in certain cases.

AMYOTROPHIC LATERAL SCLEROSIS

Amyotrophic lateral sclerosis, a progressive disease, results in the death of upper and lower motor neurons throughout the CNS. Weakness of the respiratory muscles occurs earlier than with MS. The overall prevalence rate is 3.9 per 100,000 persons in the United States.[6] Bulbar involvement increases the risk of aspiration, and neuromuscular blockade is prolonged, making postoperative respiratory complications a concern when general anesthesia is used.[30]

Neuraxial anesthesia may exacerbate CNS diseases by the double-crush phenomenon, when neurons are exposed to mechanical injury, LA cytotoxicity, or ischemia, thus increasing susceptibility to disease progression.[22] Surgery itself contributes to disease exacerbation and quantification of anesthetic risk in these patients is difficult. Certain risk factors increase the likelihood of exacerbation during surgery include extremes of age, body habitus, surgical trauma, stress of surgery, and patient positioning.[22] Yet in a retrospective cohort study of 136 surgical patients with CNS disease, all received some form of neuraxial anesthesia for surgery (epidural, spinal, combined spinal epidural, continuous spinal) and no new or worsened postoperative neurologic deficits were found in any.[2]

Although there is no strong evidence, an epidural may be preferable to a spinal technique in patients with preexisting CNS disease.[6] Epidural anesthesia is associated with lower intrathecal concentrations of LA, thus decreasing exposure of the spinal cord to LA cytotoxic effect and mitigating direct neuronal damage.[6]

MUSCULAR DYSTROPHY

Duchenne muscular dystrophy, an X-linked autosomal recessive disease, causes progressive muscle degeneration and muscle weakness.[33] Cardiac muscle may also be involved.[33] Myocardial dysfunction and conduction abnormalities increase the risk of cardiac complications from the effects of anesthetic drugs or from rhabdomyolysis and hyperkalemia.[6] Respiratory muscle weakness and sensitivity to neuromuscular blockers increase the risk for postoperative respiratory complications.[6,33]

Myotonic dystrophy is characterized by both myotonia and muscular dystrophy. It is an autosomal dominant disorder.[34] Cardiac and respiratory muscles are involved, and myotonia and chronic contractures are usually present.[6] Contractures are not treated by neuraxial blockade and may be provoked by shivering from sympathectomy and loss of body heat.[6] Normothermia should be maintained, and placement of neuraxial blockade can be challenging if scoliosis has resulted from chronic contractures.[6] There have been case reports of success with the neuraxial technique.[34]

MYASTHENIA GRAVIS

Myasthenia gravis (MG) is an autoimmune disorder in which autoantibodies destroy postsynaptic acetylcholine nicotinic receptors in the neuromuscular junction.[35] The destruction results in muscle weakness, and a major anesthetic consideration is respiratory failure after surgery.[35] Leventhal et al. created

Table 41.2. **LEVENTHAL CRITERIA FOR PREDICTING NEED FOR POSTOPERATIVE MECHANICAL VENTILATION IN PATIENTS WITH MYASTHENIA GRAVIS***

PREDICTING FACTORS	WEIGHTED SCORE
Duration of disease > 6 years	12 points
Other comorbid pulmonary disease	10 points
Dose of pyridostigmine > 750 mg/day	8 points
Preoperative vital capacity < 2.9 L	4 points

Original table based on Leventhal et al.[36] and Cardone et al.[37]

* Four criteria are weighted based on predictive value. A score of 10 or greater is said to identify patients who will require postoperative mechanical ventilation.[36,37]

a scoring system to predict the need for postoperative mechanical ventilation in such patients after surgery. Metrics used for scoring appear in Table 41.2.[36] When scoring, each measure is weighted based on predictive value.[37] A score of 10 or greater identifies patients who will need postoperative mechanical ventilation.[37] The criteria lack sensitivity (22.2%) and have a low positive predictive value (25%).[37] The specificity of the test is 77.8% and the negative predictive value is 75%.[37]

Patients with MG are less sensitive to depolarizing neuromuscular blockade and more sensitive to nondepolarizing neuromuscular blockers. Respiratory failure from residual neuromuscular blockade is a potential complication of general anesthesia. A large single-shot intrathecal dose of LA may be less predictable and cause respiratory weakness more than would a continuous epidural. Using the lowest amount of LA and supplementing with opioids may prevent respiratory weakness.[6]

INDICATIONS FOR NEURAXIAL ANESTHESIA

Optimal dynamic pain relief for early recovery of organ function is the key for quick postoperative rehabilitation. A multimodal (balanced) method combines techniques and medications for synergistic effects on pain control and functional rehabilitation.[38] A continuous epidural infusion is a superior analgesic technique for patients with severe postoperative pain. It is one of the multimodal analgesic tools often used for efficient perioperative pain control.[39,40]

The consequences of surgical procedures (orthopedic, abdominal, thoracic) require procedure-specific techniques for pain relief (Table 41.3).[38–44]

The anesthesiologist individualizes a comprehensive analgesic regimen, with pain procedures directed toward expedited functional convalescence.[45]

CONTRAINDICATIONS TO NEURAXIAL ANESTHESIA

Neuraxial anesthesia should be viewed in the context of its risks and benefits. The absolute contraindications to neuraxial anesthesia are listed in Table 41.4.[46] Relative contraindications include preexisting neurologic conditions, but evidence for this recommendation is lacking.[47]

Table 41.3. **CURRENT RECOMMENDATIONS FOR COMMON PROCEDURE-SPECIFIC NEURAXIAL AND REGIONAL ANALGESIC REGIMENS IN THE PERIOPERATIVE PERIOD**

SURGERY	NEURAXIAL TECHNIQUES	REGIONAL TECHNIQUES
Laparoscopic cholecystectomy	Not recommended (low risk/benefit ratio)	TAP block
Cesarean section	Recommended	TAP block
Open colonic resection	Recommended	TAP block
Thoracotomy	Recommended	Paravertebral block
Total knee replacement	Recommended	Adductor canal block versus femoral nerve block

Original table based on Chou et al.,[41] Saliminia et al.,[42] Srivastava et al.,[43] and Gao et al.[44]

Abbreviation: TAP, Transversus abdominis plane.

NERVE INJURY IN REGIONAL AND NEURAXIAL ANESTHESIA

When axoplasmic flow is impaired, as in neurologic disorders, a new injury by needle or catheter placement, by epinephrine-induced vasoconstriction, or by LA neurotoxicity may create damage synergistic with the initial injury and complete an irreversible denervation.[26]

The perineurium normally protects the nerve from cytotoxic effects of LA.[48] After intrafascicular injection, axonal degradation disrupts the blood–nerve barrier.[16,17] The degree

Table 41.4. **ABSOLUTE AND RELATIVE CONTRAINDICATIONS TO NEURAXIAL ANESTHESIA**

ABSOLUTE CONTRAINDICATIONS	RELATIVE CONTRAINDICATIONS
Infection at site of insertion	Bacteremia
Severe malformations of spine/spinal cord, increased intracranial pressure	Preexisting neurologic disorders (MS, myelopathy, spina bifida)*
Patient refusal or inability to remain still during neuraxial procedure	Aortic stenosis*
Bleeding diathesis	

Original table based on Miller and Manuel.[47]

*Theoretical concerns for major morbidity associated with neuraxial anesthesia; however, evidence is lacking. Therefore, it is recommended to proceed on a case-by-case basis with caution and after weighing risks/benefits.

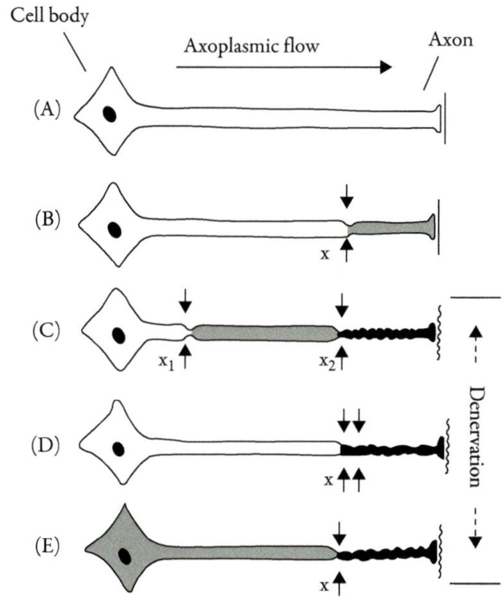

Figure 41.4. Double-crush phenomenon. (A) Normal axoplasmic flow. (B) One minor injury to the neuron not affecting axoplasmic flow. (C) Two minor neuronal injuries causing denervation. (D) Severe neuronal injury at one site, causing denervation. (E) One minor injury in a diseased neuron causing denervation.[52]

of nerve injury is proportional to concentration of LA and duration of exposure.[16,17] Mechanisms for cell injury are numerous, and elevations in intracellular calcium play a central role.[48] High calcium levels alter energy metabolism and activate kinases, leading to apoptosis.[48] Lidocaine has been shown to activate the proapoptotic p38 MAP kinase in primary sensory neurons.[26] Susceptibility to injury is increased, lending credit to the double-crush phenomenon (Figure 41.4).

Transient neurologic symptoms are the result of temporary nerve impairment from LA.[49] They are characterized by slight to severe pain in the buttocks and legs. Symptoms usually develop within a few to 24 hours after spinal anesthesia and last up to 5 days.[49] Lidocaine is linked to the highest incidence of transient neurologic symptoms when administered intrathecally; however, in vitro models have shown bupivacaine to be the most cytotoxic.[49,50]

Vasoconstriction by LA decreases blood flow to neurons. Ischemia alters metabolic supply/demand and after reperfusion, oxygen free radicals may form.[48]

Mechanical trauma interrupts the blood–nerve barrier, leading to nerve injury.[48] Intrafascicular injection of LA and the cytotoxic effects of subsequent injections of LA through the misplaced needle are likely the main source of nerve injury.[48] For example, fascicular penetration without injection of LA did not affect nerve function.[51,52] Similarly, intrafascicular injection of normal saline does not alter microscopic anatomy or the blood–nerve barrier.[17] Other sources of nerve trauma are tourniquets or patient positioning.

DAILY EPIDURAL MANAGEMENT

Monitoring the efficacy of an epidural is aggressive in the immediate postoperative period in order to achieve pain control and to limit side effects. The pain is measured by the VAS, a 100-mm line whose ends are labeled "no pain" and "the worst pain imaginable." This method has been shown to be accurate, valid, reliable, and reproducible.[53] Pain is assessed at rest and with activity. A numerical rating scale (NRS) is another way to assess patients' pain. A NRS value of 3 or below is generally considered adequate pain control, requiring no intervention. A score of 4 or above with rest and activity requires adjustment of the epidural infusion.

Pain of 0/10 at rest and with activity at multiple hourly assessments suggests excessive medication and requires prompt reevaluation of the epidural infusion. A decrease or temporary discontinuation of the epidural infusion is indicated, especially if the pain score of 0/10 is correlated with excessive motor block from the LA or sedation from the accumulation of neuraxial opioid.

Vital signs (blood pressure, heart rate, respiratory rate, pulse oximetry, ECG) are measured hourly in the first 24 hours to alert the physician to patient overmedication. Hypotension, depressed respiratory rate, or decreased pulse oximetry values may be early signs of excessive neuraxial anesthetics or opioids. With such signs, the rate of the epidural infusion is promptly reduced or discontinued.

LAs differentially block autonomic, sensory, and motor neurons. Increasing nerve diameter is proportional to increasing resistance to LA blockade. The true cause for varying resistance to blockade among nerve fiber types includes factors such as nerve fiber length, distribution of Na^+,K^+ channels, effects on other ion channels, and nerve fiber anatomic distribution. Myelination increases susceptibility to LA blockade.[46]

Small myelinated autonomic neurons need the lowest concentration of LA for blockade, and the blockade is typically the most extensive. Neuraxial spread is approximately two to four levels above and below the site of injection, with incremental increases in LA concentration. Neuraxial opioids do not result in autonomic or motor blockade (Table 41.5).[54]

The Bromage scale measures the degree of motor block (Table 41.6).[55]

Sedation in a patient with an epidural is assessed by the Ramsay Sedation Scale.[56] Excessive sedation correlates with excessive neuraxial opioids, especially in the elderly (Table 41.7).

Evaluation of a sensory block by light touch, ice, or pinprick validates congruency between type of surgery and epidural effectiveness. One study found light touch to be most accurate.[57] Light touch sensation is tested with a tapered wisp of cotton stroked once across an area not to exceed 1 cm of skin with the patient's vision blocked.[58] Pinprick sensation may be tested with a disposable safety pin. Cold sensation is tested with ice inside a disposable glove or with ethyl chloride spray.[57] Testing begins several dermatomes either caudad or cephalad to the suspected border of sensation loss, and moves toward the border in 2- to 3-cm increments.[57] Table 41.8 shows recommended vertebral levels for epidural catheter placement based on the corresponding surgery.[59–62] When possible, the lumbar levels are not blocked, in anticipation of mobility postoperatively.[62]

Table 41.5. **SUSCEPTIBILITY OF NERVE FIBERS TO LA BLOCKADE**

TYPE (*SUBTYPE*)	MYELINATED	DIAMETER (μM)*	FUNCTION	CONDUCTION VELOCITY	NEURAXIAL BLOCK SUSCEPTIBILITY	NEURAXIAL SPREAD OF BLOCKADE
A (*Aα*)	Yes	12–20	Large motor nerve impulses, proprioception	Fast	Low	Least spread
A (*Aβ*)	Yes	5–15	Small motor nerve impulses, touch, pressure	Fast	Low	
A (*Aγ*)	Yes	3–8	Muscle tone	Fast	Low	
A (*Aδ*)	Yes	2–5	Sharp fast pain, temperature	Fast	Low	
B	Yes	3	Preganglionic autonomics	Slow	High	Two to four levels above/below motor
C	No	0.3–1.5	Dull slow pain, temperature, postganglionic autonomics	Slow	Moderate	Two to three levels above/below motor

Original table based on Brull et al.[46]

* Increasing diameter decreases susceptibility to LA blockade, and myelination increases susceptibility to LA blockade. Concentration of LA decreases at neuraxial sites progressively higher and lower than the injection site. The decreasing concentration results in differential blockade of autonomic (two to four levels beyond motor) and sensory fibers (two to three levels beyond motor).

Table 41.6. **BROMAGE MOTOR BLOCKADE SCALE**

GRADE	CRITERIA	DEGREE OF BLOCK
I	Free movement of legs and knees	0%
II	Flex knees, free movement of feet	33%
III	Unable to flex knees, free movement of feet	66%
IV	Unable to move legs or feet*	100%

Original table based on Bromage.[55]

*The inability to move the lower extremities suggests an excessive infusion or intrathecal migration of the catheter.

Table 41.7. **RAMSEY SEDATION SCALE**[56]

SCORE	RESPONSE
1	Anxious, restless
2	Cooperative, oriented, tranquil
3	Responding to commands
4	Brisk response to stimulus
5	Sluggish response to stimulus
6	No response to stimulus

ADVERSE EVENTS

The site of an epidural catheter insertion is assessed two to three times per day for the duration of the epidural infusion. Infection is promptly treated, and the epidural catheter is discontinued. Tenderness over the epidural site represents an early sign of a hematoma, especially if associated with mild neurologic deficits. An epidural hematoma can progress within 6 to 8 hours to permanent paralysis if unrecognized and untreated.

Table 41.8. **RECOMMENDED VERTEBRAL LEVEL FOR EPIDURAL CATHETER PLACEMENT BY SURGERY TYPE**

SURGICAL SITE	LEVEL OF EPIDURAL CATHETER INSERTION
Thoracic	T4-T6
Upper abdominal (esophagus, stomach, pancreas, liver, spleen)	T4-T6
Mid abdominal surgery (small bowel, colon)	T8-T9
Lower abdominal surgery (sigmoid colon, rectum)	T10-T11
Urologic (radical cystectomy)	T9-T11
Gynecologic	T8-T10
Orthopedic	L3-L5

Original table based on References 56 to 62.

In a study of 704,000 central neuraxial blocks in the United Kingdom, the incidence of permanent injury was 4.2:100,000 and of paraplegia or death, 1.8:100,000.[63] The analysis was conducted on 704,000 central neuraxial blocks performed in 1 year. Most side effects resolved in the first 6 months.[63]

With the advent of fast track surgery, better surgical techniques, shorter operating times, and newer general anesthetic techniques, the risks of serious complications associated with general anesthesia are reduced.[64] The large systematic reviews demonstrating decreased risk of pulmonary and thromboembolic complications associated with neuraxial anesthesia are decades old.[65] Newer studies suggest less of a difference in serious complications between neuraxial and general anesthesia.[64] When the POISE trial investigated the risk of cardiac morbidity and mortality in high-risk cardiac patients undergoing general or neuraxial anesthesia for surgery, patients undergoing neuraxial anesthesia were at increased risk of cardiovascular death, nonfatal MI, and nonfatal cardiac arrest.[66]

Dural Puncture

Coexisting degenerative disorders of the spine add to the challenge of epidural catheter placement. Elderly patients with calcified ligamentum flavum and spinal stenosis may be prone to a dural puncture even in the absence of free needle backflow. Unrecognized, an epidural catheter placed intrathecally can have a significant adverse outcome, given the ratio of 1:10 of spinal:epidural medication dose.

Intravascular Injection

Negative blood aspiration from the epidural catheter does not preclude intravascular placement. Partial intravascular injection of a test dose might not be evident in a patient taking beta-blockers because the heart rate may not increase. The intravascular injection of bupivacaine can be dangerous, especially in elderly patients in whom accumulation of this drug can lead to seizures and arrhythmias.

Epidural Abscess

Epidural abscess is rare; its incidence is difficult to estimate, and the overall incidence of epidural abscess ranges from 1:1,000 to 1:50,000 epidural catheterizations.[67,68] An abscess may develop 5 days after the initial placement. The gold standard for diagnosing an abscess is an MRI.[69]

Epidural Hematoma

Epidural hematoma is another potential, but rare, complication. Its appearance is usually associated with the concomitant presence of a coagulopathy. More recent evidence points toward an increase in incidence of epidural hematomas worldwide with newer anticoagulants or in patients with comorbidities undergoing extensive and complex surgeries.[70]

Analysis of case reports suggest varying rates of epidural hematoma depending on the patient population. At the lowest risk for epidural hematoma are obstetric patients, with an incidence in one case report of 1:200,000.[70] In another large study involving neuraxial blockade in 79,837 parturients, no epidural hematomas occurred.[71] HELLP syndrome (hemolysis, elevated liver enzymes, and low platelet count) increases risk for epidural hematoma.[67]

Among nonobstetric patients, the incidence of epidural hematoma has been shown to range between 1:1,000 and 1:9,000.[70,71] Risk factors include thromboprophylaxis and coagulation disorders. Thrombocytopenia (platelets < 150,000/mm^3) and INR > 1.4 are also risk factors. Anatomic deformities, such as ankylosing spondylitis, increase the risk for epidural hematoma, as does osteoporosis.[67] Older age also appears to increase risk.[70]

New guidelines on perioperative use of anticoagulants and the placement or removal of neuraxial peripheral nerve catheters have been recently developed to help the clinician identify the best candidates for regional anesthesia and analgesia (Table 41.9).[72]

In the absence of a preoperative neurologic baseline and with lack of recovery from neuraxial block despite discontinuation of anesthetic infusions, anesthesiologists should rely on neuroimaging for establishing a positive diagnosis.

Lack of sensation in response to LA during the postoperative period can mask undiagnosed compartment syndromes in surgery on lower extremities or the abdomen. Pressure sores or an acute abdomen may not be identified in a patient with an epidural. A LA can mask progression of an underlying neurologic disorder, such as MS.

Pruritus, Nausea, and Vomiting

Common dose-dependent side effects of neuraxial opioids are pruritus, nausea, and vomiting, which are easily treated.[73] Morphine and fentanyl, mu agonists, cause more pruritus than the partial agonists buprenorphine and butorphanol.[74] Butorphanol added to fentanyl and administered epidurally resulted in less pruritus than fentanyl alone. It is believed that kappa receptor stimulation mitigates opioid-induced pruritus.[74] A single epidural injection of buprenorphine or butorphanol alone does not provide adequate postoperative analgesia.

Pruritus is unreliably treated with antihistamines. Low-dose naloxone or butorphanol more reliably relieves pruritus but increasing doses come at the cost of analgesia. Ondansetron is more effective at relieving pruritus than diphenhydramine.[74]

Nausea and vomiting associated with neuraxial opioid administration depend on the type of opioid used.[74] Neuraxial morphine causes nausea and vomiting more than the lipophilic opioids, such as fentanyl and sufentanil.[74] Ondansetron, dexamethasone, droperidol, and metoclopramide decrease the incidence of nausea and vomiting associated with neuraxial opioid administration.[74]

Urinary Retention

Urinary retention is associated more with the use of neuraxial morphine than with fentanyl.[75] Because urinary retention is dose-dependent, using the lowest long-acting opioid dose possible for effective pain control is recommended.

Table 41.9. **INTERVENTIONAL SPINE AND PAIN PROCEDURES IN PATIENTS ON ANTIPLATELET AND ANTICOAGULANT MEDICATIONS***

THERAPEUTIC CLASS	DRUG	WHEN TO STOP	WHEN TO RESTART
Aspirin	Aspirin, primary prophylaxis	6 days	24 hr
	Aspirin, secondary prophylaxis	Shared assessment	Shared assessment
NSAIDs	Diclofenac	1 day	24 hr
	Ketorolac	1 day	24 hr
	Ibuprofen	1 day	24 hr
	Etodolac	2 days	24 hr
	Indomethacin	2 days	24 hr
	Naproxen	4 days	24 hr
	Meloxicam	4 days	24 hr
	Nabumetone	6 days	24 hr
	Oxaprozin	10 days	24 hr
	Piroxicam	10 days	24 hr
Phosphodiesterase inhibitors	Cilostazol	2 days	24 hr
	Dipyridamole	2 days	N/A
	Aspirin combinations	See Aspirin	See Aspirin
Thromboprophylaxis	Enoxaparin (≤ 40 mg/day)	12 hr	4 hr
	Enoxaparin (30 mg twice a day or 40 mg twice a day)	12 hr	4 hr
	Fondaparinux (≤ 2.5 mg/day)	4 days	24 hr
	Unfractionated heparin (5,000 units twice a day)	8–10 hr	2 hr
	Unfractionated heparin (5,000 units three times a day)	8–10 hours	2 hr
	Rivaroxaban (10 mg daily)	No recommendations	No recommendations
Therapeutic anticoagulants	Enoxaparin (1 mg/kg every 12 hr)	24 hr	4 hr
	Enoxaparin (1.5 mg/kg every 24 hr)	N/A	N/A
	Fondaparinux (5–10 mg/day)	4 days	24 hr
	Unfractionated heparin, intravenous	4 hr	2 hr
	Rivaroxaban (20–30 mg/day)	3 days	24 hr
	Dabigatran	4–5 days	24 hr
	Apixaban	3-5 days	24 hr
	Edoxaban	N/A	N/A
	Argatroban	N/A	N/A
	Warfarin	5 days, normal INR	24 hr
P2Y12 inhibitors	Clopidogrel	7 days	12 hr
	Prasugrel	7–10 days	24 hr
	Ticagrelor	5 days	24 hr

* 2015 guidelines from the American Society of Regional Anesthesia and Pain Medicine. From Narouze et al.[72]

Respiratory Depression

Opioid-induced respiratory depression can be diagnosed easily by continuous pulse oximetry in the immediate postoperative period. The risk of respiratory depression is increased with morphine.[73] Morphine remains in the cerebrospinal fluid (CSF) for a longer period of time than other more lipophilic opioids.[73] The higher concentration in the CSF is thought to result in a rostral spread of hydrophilic opioids, with penetration into the brainstem.[73] Patients with preexisting neurologic disease and respiratory compromise have less respiratory reserve and are at increased risk for respiratory depression.[76]

Sedation

Sedation can be an early sign of toxic neuraxial opioids. The patient with an epidural catheter should be evaluated frequently by sedation scales.

CONCLUSIONS

- Neuraxial anesthesia is not contraindicated in patients with neurologic disease.
- After neuraxial anesthesia in patients with preexisting neurologic conditions, prolonged LA effect on injured nerves may result in slow recovery from sensory, autonomic, and motor blocks.
- Prolonged sensory and motor blockade after neuraxial analgesia and anesthesia in patients with preexisting neurologic disease raises concern about rare neuraxial complications, such as epidural hematoma and abscess.
- In the setting of preexisting neurologic disease, a lower concentration of LA might be of benefit.

REFERENCES

1. Dripps RD, Vandam LD. Exacerbation of pre-existing neurologic disease after spinal anesthesia. *N Engl J Med.* 1956;255:843–849.
2. Hebl JR, Horlocker TT, Schroeder DR. Neuraxial anesthesia and analgesia in patients with pre-existing central nervous system disorder. *Anesth Analg.* 2006;103:223–228.
3. Upton AR, McComas AJ. The double crush in nerve entrapment syndromes. *Lancet.* 1973;2(7825):359–362.
4. Allen DJ, Chae-Kim SH, Trousdale DM. Risks and complications of neuraxial anesthesia and the use of anticoagulation in the surgical patient. *Baylor Univ Med Cent Proc.* 2002;15(4):369–373.
5. Klingler W, Lehmann-Horn F, Jurkat-Rott K. Complications of anesthesia in neuromuscular disorders. *Neuromusc Disord.* 2005;15:195–206.
6. Vercauteren M, Heytens L. Anaesthetic considerations for patients with a pre-existing neurological deficit: are neuraxial techniques safe? *Acta Anaesthesiol Scand.* 2007;51:831–838.
7. McSwain J, Doty J, Wesley W, Sylvia H. Regional anesthesia in patients with pre-existing neurologic disease. *Curr Opin Anaesthesiol.* 2014;27(5):538–543.
8. Ionasescu VV. Charcot-Marie-Tooth neuropathies: from clinical description to molecular genetics. *Muscle Nerve.* 1995;18:267–275.
9. Pareyson D, Marchesi C. Diagnosis, natural history and management of Charcot-Marie-Tooth disease. *Lancet Neurol.* 2009;8:654–667.
10. Bösenberg A, Larkin K. Anaesthesia and Charcot-Marie-Tooth disease. *S Afr J Anaesth Analg.* 2006;12(4):131–133.
11. Greenwood JJ, Scott WE. Charcot-Marie-Tooth disease: peripartum management of two contrasting clinical cases. *Int J Obstet Anesth.* 2007;16:149–154.
12. Karol L, Elerson E. Scoliosis in patients with Charcot-Marie-Tooth disease. *J Bone Joint Surg Am.* 2007;89(7):1504–1510.
13. Marques W, Alcantara M, Nogueira-Barbosa M, et al. Respiratory dysfunction in Charcot-Marie-Tooth disease type 1A. *J Neurol.* 2015;262:1164–1171.
14. Awater C, Zerres K, Rudnik-Schoneborn S. Pregnancy course and outcome in women with hereditary neuromuscular disorders: comparison of obstetric risks in 178 patients. *Eur J Obstet Gynecol Reprod Biol.* 2012;162:153–159.
15. Reily M. Classification and diagnosis of the inherited neuropathies. *Ann Indian Acad Neurol.* 2009;12(2):80–88.
16. Selander D, Brattsand R, Lundborg G, Nordborg C, Olsson Y. Local anesthetics: importance of mode of application, concentration and adrenaline for the appearance of nerve lesions. An experimental study of axonal degeneration and barrier damage after infrafascicular injection or topical application of bupivacaine (Marcain). *Acta Anaesthesiol Scand.* 1979;23(2):127–136.
17. Gentili F, Hudson AR, Hunter D, Kline DG. Nerve injection injury with local anesthetic agents: a light and electron microscopic, fluorescent microscopic, and horseradish peroxidase study. *Neurosurgery.* 1980;6:263–272.
18. Neal JM, Bernards CM, Hadzic A, et al. ASRA practice advisory on neurologic complications in regional anesthesia and pain medicine. *Reg Anesth Pain Med.* 2008;33:404–415.
19. Dhir S, Balasubramanian S, Ross D. Ultrasound-guided peripheral regional blockade in patients with Charcot-Marie-Tooth disease: a review of three cases. *Can J Anaesth.* 2008;55(8):515–520.
20. Eltawansy SA, Bakos A, Checton J. Noncompaction cardiomyopathy with Charcot-Marie-Tooth disease. *Case Rep Cardiol.* 2015;2015:646890.
21. Pascuzzi R, Fleck J. Acute peripheral neuropathy in adults: Guillain-Barre syndrome and related disorders. *Neurol Clin.* 1997;15(3):529–547.
22. Kopp S, Jacob A, Hebl J. Regional anesthesia in patients with preexisting neurologic disease. *Reg Anesth Pain Med.* 2015;40(5):467–478.
23. Pithadia AB, Kakadia N. Guillain-Barré syndrome (GBS). *Pharmacol Rep.* 2010;62:220–232.
24. Ropper A. The Guillain-Barre syndrome. *N Engl J Med.* 1992;326:1130–1136.
25. Kattula A, Angelini G, Arndt G. Regional anesthesia in the presence of neurologic disease. In: Finucane BT, ed. *Complications of Regional Anesthesia.* 2nd ed. New York, NY: Springer; 2007:373–385.
26. Lirk P, Birmingham B, Quinn H. Regional anesthesia in patients with preexisting neuropathy. *Int Anesth Clin.* 2011;49(4):144–165.
27. Steiner I, Argov Z, Cahan C, et al. Guillain-Barre syndrome after epidural anesthesia: direct nerve root damage may trigger disease. *Neurology.* 1985;35:1473–1475.
28. Kuok C, Tsai P, Hsu Y, Ko Y, Huang C, Chen C. Postoperative delayed respiratory failure caused by Guillain-Barre syndrome—a case report. *Acta Anaesthesiol Taiwan.* 2007;45(1):43–46.
29. Hekmat M, Ghaderi H, Foroughi M, Mirjafari S. Guillain-Barre syndrome after coronary artery bypass graft surgery: a case report. *Acta Med Iran.* 2016;54(1):76–78.
30. Pasternak JJ, Lanier WL Jr. Spinal cord disorders. In: Hines RL, Marschall KE, eds. *Stoelting's Anesthesia and Co-Existing Diseases.* 6th ed. Philadelphia, PA: Elsevier Saunders; 2012.
31. Dorotta I, Schubert A. Multiple sclerosis and anesthetic implications. *Curr Opin Anaesthesiol.* 2002;15(3):365–370.
32. Sladen RN, Playford H. Multiple sclerosis. In: Sladen RN, Coursin DB, Ketzler JT, Playford H, eds. *Anesthesia and Co-Existing Disease* (Cambridge Pocket Clinicians). 1st ed. Cambridge, United Kingdom: Cambridge University Press; 2007:329.

33. Bang SU, Kim YS, Kwon WJ, Lee SM, Kim SH. Peripheral nerve blocks as the sole anesthetic technique in a patient with severe Duchenne muscular dystrophy. *J Anesth.* 2016;30:320–323.
34. Aquilina A, Groves J. A combined technique utilising regional anaesthesia and target-controlled sedation in a patient with myotonic dystrophy. *Anaesthesia.* 2002;57:385–386.
35. Blichfeldt-Lauridsen L, Hansen B. Anesthesia and myasthenia gravis. *Acta Anaesthesiol Scand.* 2012;56:17–22.
36. Leventhal S, Orkin F, Hirsh R. Prediction of the need for postoperative mechanical ventilation in myasthenia gravis. *Anesthesiology.* 1980;53:26–30.
37. Cardone A, Congedo E, Aceto P, et al. Perioperative evaluation of myasthenia gravis. *Ann Ital Chir.* 2007;78:359–365.
38. White PF, Kehlet H. Improving postoperative pain management: what are the unresolved issues? *Anesthesiology.* 2010;112:220–225.
39. Ballantyne JC, McKenna JM, Ryder E. Epidural analgesia—experience of 5628 patients in a large teaching hospital derived through audit. *Acute Pain.* 2003;4:89–97.
40. Moraca RJ, Sheldon DG, Thirlby RC. The role of epidural analgesia and anesthesia in surgical practice. *Ann Surg.* 2003;238:663–673.
41. Chou R, Gordon D, Leon-Casasola O, et al. Management of postoperative pain: a clinical practice guideline from the American Pain Society, the American Society of Regional Anesthesia and Pain Medicine, and the American Society of Anesthesiologists' Committee on Regional Anesthesia, Executive Committee, and Administrative Council. *J Pain.* 2016;17(2):131–157.
42. Saliminia A, Azimaraghi O, Babayipour S, Ardavan K, Movafegh A. Efficacy of transverse abdominis plane block in reduction of postoperative pain in laparoscopic cholecystectomy. *Acta Anaesthesiol Taiwan.* 2015;53(4):119–122.
43. Srivastava U, Verma S, Singh T, et al. Efficacy of trans abdominis block for post cesarean delivery analgesia: a double-blind, randomized trial. *Saudi J Anaesth.* 2015;9(3):298–302.
44. Gao F, Ma J, Sun W, Guo W, Li Z, Wang W. Adductor canal block versus femoral nerve block for analgesia after total knee arthroplasty: a systematic review and meta-analysis. *Clin J Pain.* 2017;33(4):356–368.
45. Caumo W, Schmidt AP, Schneider CN, et al. Preoperative predictors of moderate to intense acute postoperative pain in patients undergoing abdominal surgery. *Acta Anaesthesiol Scand.* 2002;46:1265–1271.
46. Brull R, Macfarlane AJ, Chan V. Spinal, epidural, and caudal anesthesia. Miller's Anesthesia, 8th ed. Philadelphia, PA: Elsevier Saunders; 2014:1691–1693.
47. Miller R, Manuel P. Basics of Anesthesia. 6th ed. Philadelphia, PA: Elsevier Saunders; 2011:262–263.
48. Hogan Q. Pathophysiology of peripheral nerve injury during regional anesthesia. *Reg Anesth Pain Med.* 2008;33(5):435–441.
49. Zaric D, Christiansen C, Pace N, Punjasawadwong Y. Transient neurologic symptoms (TNS) following spinal anaesthesia with lidocaine versus other local anaesthetics. *Cochrane DB Syst Rev.* 2003;(2):CD003006.
50. Perez-Castro R, Patel S, Garavito-Aguilar Z, et al. Cytotoxicity of local anesthetics in human neuronal cells. *Anesth Analg.* 2009;108(3):997–1007.
51. Lofstrom B, Wennberg A, Wien L. Late disturbances in nerve function after block with local anaesthetic agents. *Acta Anaesthesiol Scand.* 1966;10:111–122.
52. Hebl J, Horlocker T, Pritchard D. Diffuse brachial plexopathy after interscalene blockade in a patient receiving cisplatin chemotherapy: the pharmacological double crush syndrome. *Anesth Analg.* 2001;92(1):249–251.
53. Scott J, Huskisson E. Graphic representation of pain. *Pain.* 1976;2(2):175–184.
54. Wheatley R, Schug S, Watson D. Safety and efficacy of postoperative epidural analgesia. *Br J Anaesth.* 2001;87:47–61.
55. Bromage PR. *Epidural Analgesia.* Philadelphia, PA: WB Saunders; 1978:144.
56. Ramsay M, Savege T, Simpson B, Goodwin R. Controlled sedation with alphaxolone-alphadalone. *BMJ.* 1974;2:656–659.
57. Russell I. A comparison of cold, pinprick and touch for assessing the level of spinal block at caesarean section. *Int Obstet Anesth.* 2004;13:146–152.
58. Kirshblum S, Burns S, Biering-Sorensen F, et al. International standards for neurological classification of spinal cord injury (revised 2011). *J Spinal Cord Med.* 2011;34(6):535–546.
59. Brodner G, Van Aken H, Hertle L, et al. Multimodal perioperative management— combining thoracic epidural analgesia, forced mobilization, and oral nutrition reduces hormonal and metabolic stress and improves convalescence after major urologic surgery. *Anesth Analg.* 2001;92(6):1594–1600.
60. Ahmed A, Latif N, Khan R. Post-operative analgesia for major abdominal surgery and its effectiveness in a tertiary care hospital. *J Anaesthesiol Clin Pharmacol.* 2013;29(4):472–477.
61. Yun M, Kwon M, Kim D, Lee J. Combined spinal-epidural anesthesia using a reduced-dose of spinal bupivacaine and epidural top up leads to faster motor recovery after lower extremity surgeries. *Korean J Anesthesiol.* 2014;66(1):28–33.
62. Agenjo F, Carli F. Neural blockade for abdominal and thoracic (non-vascular) surgery. In: Cousins MJ, Horlocker TT, Carr DB, Bridenbaugh PD, eds. Cousins and Bridenbaugh's Neural Blockade in Clinical Anesthesia and Pain Medicine. 4th ed. Philadelphia, PA: Lippincott Williams & Wilkins; 2009:522.
63. Cook TM, Counsell D, Wildsmith JA, et al. Major complications of central neuraxial block: report on the Third National Audit Project of the Royal College of Anesthetists. *Br J Anaesth.* 2009;102:170–190.
64. Harsten A, Kehlet H, Ljung P, Toksvig-Larsen S. Total intravenous general anaesthesia vs. spinal anaesthesia for total hip arthroplasty: a randomised, controlled trial. *Acta Anaesthesiol Scand.* 2015;59:298–309.
65. Rodgers A, Walker N, Schug S, et al. Reduction of postoperative mortality and morbidity with epidural or spinal anaesthesia: results from overview of randomised trials. *BMJ.* 2000;321:1493.
66. Leslie K, Myles P, Devereaux P, et al. Neuraxial block, death and serious cardiovascular morbidity in the POISE trial. *Br J Anaesth.* 2013;111(3):382–390.
67. Moen V, Dahlgren N, Irestedt L. Severe neurological complications after central neuraxial block in Sweden 1990–99. *Anesthesiology.* 2004;101:950–959.
68. Christie IW, McCabe S. Major complications of epidural analgesia after surgery: results of a six-year survey. *Anaesthesia.* 2007;62:335–341.
69. Wilmink J. MR imaging of the spine: trauma and degenerative disease. *Eur Radiology.* 1999;9:1259–1266.
70. Popping D, Zahn P, Van Aken H, Boche R, Pogatzki-Zahn E. Effectiveness and safety of postoperative pain management: a survey of 18,925 consecutive patients between 1998 and 2006 (2nd version): a database analysis of prospectively raised data. *Br J Anaesth.* 2008;101(6):832–840.
71. Bateman B, Mhyre J, Ehrenfeld J, et al. The risk and outcomes of epidural hematomas after perioperative and obstetric epidural catheterization: a report from the Multicenter Perioperative Outcomes Group Research Consortium. *Anesth Analg.* 2013;116(6):1380–1385.
72. Narouze S, Benzon H, Provenzano D, et al. Interventional spine and pain procedures in patients on antiplatelet and anticoagulant medications: guidelines from the American Society of Regional Anesthesia and Pain Medicine, the European Society of Regional Anaesthesia and Pain Therapy, the American Academy of Pain Medicine, the International Neuromodulation Society, the North American Neuromodulation Society, and the World Institute of Pain. *Reg Anesth Pain Med.* 2015;40(3):182–212.
73. Armstrong S, Fernando R. Side effects and efficacy of neuraxial opioids in pregnant patients at delivery: a comprehensive review. *Drug Safety.* 2016;39(5):381–399.

74. Ackerman W, Juneja M, Kaczorowski D, Colclough G. A comparison of the incidence of pruritus following epidural opioid administration in the parturient. *Can J Anaesth.* 1989;36(4):388–391.
75. Liang C, Chang S, Wong S, Chang Y, Cheng P. Effects of postoperative analgesia on postpartum urinary retention in women undergoing cesarean delivery. *J Obstet Gynaecol Res.* 2010;36(5):991–995.
76. Carvalho B. Respiratory depression after neuraxial opioids in the obstetric setting. *Anesth Analg.* 2008;107(3):956–961.

REVIEW QUESTIONS

Box 41.1. **PATIENT INFORMATION**

A 35-year-old pregnant female at 39 weeks 5 days presents in active labor. Her past medical history is only significant for MS. Her BMI is 58 and her airway is Class IV. The fetus is in breech position and several attempts at external cephalic version have failed. The obstetrician would like to proceed with cesarean delivery. A combined spinal epidural neuraxial technique is used.

After a successful cesarean delivery, the patient requests a tubal ligation. The epidural catheter is left in place overnight and a tubal ligation is performed the next morning. Lidocaine is dosed through the epidural catheter for surgical anesthesia. Several hours later, the patient complains of severe pain in her buttocks and legs.

1. Refer to the patient information in Box 41.1. When neuraxial anesthesia is performed in patients with MS, which of the following is true?

   A. Add epinephrine to LA to help increase duration of blockade.
   B. Use lowest possible dose of LA.
   C. Chronic contractures may cause scoliosis and difficult placement of the block.
   D. MS is a contraindication to neuraxial anesthesia.

2. Refer to the patient information in Box 41.1. Transient neurologic symptoms (TNS) typically resolve within:

   A. 24 hours
   B. 5 days
   C. 2 weeks
   D. 1 month

3. Refer to the patient information in Box 41.1. Which of the following is most often associated with transient neurologic symptoms:

   A. Lidocaine
   B. Bupivacaine
   C. Tetracaine
   D. Chloroprocaine

ANSWERS

1. B. In patients with MS, lower intrathecal concentrations of LA decrease exposure of the spinal cord to the detrimental effects of LA and help mitigate direct neurotoxic effects, therefore answer B is correct. Also, prolonging spinal cord exposure to LA with epinephrine should be avoided, therefore answer A is incorrect.[6] Chronic contractures are not a hallmark of MS, but rather myotonic dystrophy, so answer C is incorrect. MS is not a contraindication to neuraxial anesthesia, and in this case the risk of exacerbation of MS disease maybe less significant when compared to the risk of manipulating a potentially difficult airway in a pregnant patient with critical consequences on the life of mother and baby.[6]

2. B. TNS are characterized by slight to severe pain in the buttocks and legs, with symptoms usually developing within a few hours to 24 hours after spinal anesthesia. TNS last in most cases up to 5 days.[49]

3. A. Direct toxic effects on nerve fibers have been reported as complications of LA.[48] Lidocaine is linked to the highest incidence of transient neurologic symptoms; however, in vitro models have shown bupivacaine to be the most cytotoxic.[50]

QUESTIONS AND ANSWERS

This chapter has accompanying questions and answers that are available to subscribers as part of the Oxford eLearning platform. To access the questions, follow the link below, or go to
✔ http://oxfordmedicine.com/painmanagementreview

42.

THE VASOVAGAL REFLEX AND NEURAXIAL TECHNIQUES

Magdalena Anitescu and Chirag Shah

STEM CASE AND KEY QUESTIONS

A 52-year-old female with a medical history of ovarian cancer is scheduled for a total abdominal hysterectomy, bilateral salpingo-oophorectomy, and retroperitoneal lymph node dissection. Anxious, she reports a "fainting" episode at her varicose vein surgery 1 month ago. She has a fear of doctors and both her sons faint at the sight of needles. She requests placement of an indwelling epidural catheter for postoperative pain relief because of low tolerance for pain. An indwelling catheter is planned as part of a multimodal approach to relieve pain after surgery.

WOULD YOU PLACE AN EPIDURAL CATHETER FOR POSTOPERATIVE PAIN RELIEF OR WOULD YOU DECLINE TO PLACE A CATHETER BECAUSE OF HER HISTORY OF A VASOVAGAL EPISODE? WOULD YOU INQUIRE ABOUT ANYTHING ELSE?

After standard monitors are applied, the patient is placed in a sitting position and 2 mg IV midazolam is administered in preparation for epidural catheter placement. The patient remains calm and converses throughout positioning. With sterile preparation and after identification of the interlaminar space between T10 and T11, 2 mL of 1% lidocaine is injected through a 25-G, 1¾-inch needle. The patient reports slight discomfort, does not change position, and has stable vital signs.

WOULD YOU ANESTHETIZE THE SKIN MORE OR ADMINISTER MORE ANXIOLYTICS? WOULD YOU GIVE IV OPIOIDS? WOULD YOU WAIT 1 OR 2 MINUTES FOR THE LOCAL ANESTHETIC TO TAKE EFFECT OR PLACE THE NEEDLE IMMEDIATELY?

One minute after the skin wheal is placed, a 17-G epidural needle is placed 1 inch deep into the skin and subcutaneous tissues. The patient is observed slouching forward. Her heart rate (HR) decreases to 40 beats per minute (bpm) and her blood pressure is 70/40 mm Hg. The patient moans incoherently.

WHAT IS THE NEXT STEP? KEEP GOING? ABORT THE EPIDURAL PLACEMENT?

The needle is withdrawn from the patient's skin, and she is positioned supine with her head down. She is unresponsive. Her blood pressure is 50/30 mm Hg, and her HR is 25 bpm. Resuscitation measures are started immediately with fluids (normal saline 1 L bolus), a vasopressor (ephedrine), and an anticholinergic (atropine). Within 30 seconds, the patient regains consciousness. Vital signs stabilize in the next 5 minutes. Arterial blood pressure is measured and two large-bore IVs are placed.

WOULD YOU PROCEED WITH SURGERY? WOULD YOU PLACE AN EPIDURAL AFTER THE PATIENT RECOVERS FROM THIS EPISODE? WOULD YOU CONSIDER PLACING THE EPIDURAL POSTOPERATIVELY OR WHILE THE PATIENT IS ASLEEP?

The team decides against placing an epidural catheter. During recovery from the suspected vasovagal episode, ST depression is seen in leads II and V5. A 12-lead electrocardiogram (ECG) confirms the finding with a 3-mm ST depression in leads II, aVF, V5, and V6. The team is worried about lateral and inferior wall ischemia, although the patient does not complain of chest pain or discomfort. She reports symptoms similar to those after previous "fainting" spells, such as nausea, dizziness, and diaphoresis. The case is cancelled and a cardiology consult is requested. The cardiologist recommends the patient undergo serial cardiac enzyme testing and a nuclear stress test.

IS THAT THE COURSE OF ACTION YOU WOULD CONSIDER? IS THERE ANYTHING ELSE THAT MAY CONTRIBUTE TO ESTABLISHING A DIAGNOSIS? WOULD THE ECG CHANGES SUGGEST AUTOMATIC INVASIVE TESTING? WHAT ARE THE WORKING AND DIFFERENTIAL DIAGNOSES FOR THIS CASE? WOULD A DETAILED PERSONAL AND FAMILY HISTORY HAVE HELPED?

The second series of cardiac enzymes shows a tenfold increase of troponin levels and normal creatine kinase. The patient continues to be asymptomatic, with no chest discomfort. The symptoms from the episode resolve, and the ST depressions decrease slightly, to 2 mm in the same leads.

IS A NUCLEAR STRESS TEST THE BEST WAY TO EVALUATE AN ACUTE CARDIAC EVENT? DO OTHER NONINVASIVE TESTS HAVE A ROLE? COULD THE PATIENT HAVE UNDERLYING PATHOLOGY UNRELATED TO THE EVENT, SUCH AS SILENT CORONARY ARTERY DISEASE, UNDIAGNOSED SICK SINUS SYNDROME, OR VALVULOPATHY?

Minutes after increased troponin values are identified, the cardiologist cancels the stress test in favor of emergent cardiac catheterization. Results show no evidence of coronary artery disease, with all vessels patent and no appreciable vessel obstruction. Vital signs have been stable since the syncopal episode. The patient remains asymptomatic. In view of a normal coronary angiogram, the cardiologist thinks that the transient troponin elevation was likely caused by demand ischemia during a hypotensive/bradycardic syncopal episode. The patient is taken to the floor from the PACU 14 hours after her syncope episode.

SHOULD THIS EPISODE BE INVESTIGATED BEFORE PROCEEDING TO SURGERY? WOULD YOU CANCEL OR POSTPONE THE SURGERY? IS A TILT-TABLE TEST OR AN ECHOCARDIOGRAM NEEDED TO IDENTIFY THE CAUSE OF SYNCOPE? SHOULD SURGERY PROCEED THE NEXT DAY WITHOUT ADDITIONAL TESTING?

The patient is admitted overnight to the intensive care unit. The arterial line is discontinued. The first 3-mm ST depression returns to normal by the morning of surgery. She undergoes abdominal surgery but no epidural catheter is placed. Cardiac enzymes, including troponin levels, are normal by the third set. The patient tolerates the surgery well, with normal vital signs. Her pain is well controlled with hydromorphone via patient-controlled anesthesia. The hospital course is uneventful, with no other syncopal episodes or ECG changes. No other tests are initiated during the hospitalization.

IS CARDIAC FOLLOW-UP NECESSARY FOR THIS PATIENT?

Upon discharge from the hospital, the patient is advised to arrange for an appointment for evaluation of the causes of her neurally mediated syncope. Although the working diagnosis is vasovagal reflex, the underlying causes may be vasovagal disease, sick sinus syndrome, or postural syncope.

HOW WOULD YOU POSITIVELY DIAGNOSE A PATIENT'S SYNCOPE? WHAT TESTS CAN BE HELPFUL IN THE DIFFERENTIAL DIAGNOSIS OF A NEURALLY MEDIATED SYNCOPE? HOW IMPORTANT IS HISTORY-TAKING IN SUCH CASES? HOW WOULD YOU ANESTHETIZE A PATIENT WITH VASOVAGAL SYNCOPE? WOULD YOU MODIFY THE ANESTHETIC TECHNIQUE IF A PATIENT SUFFERS FROM ANXIETY?

During outpatient evaluation by an electrophysiologist, the patient's medical, syncopal, and family histories are obtained. She undergoes tilt-table testing and continuous Holter monitoring. Findings are nonspecific. The electrophysiologist determines that the vasovagal episode was caused by anxiety and preoperative dehydration. The patient is advised to continue anxiety treatment and to maintain normovolemia by fluid intake. She is also instructed to undergo thorough preoperative evaluation before any future surgery and to present the electrophysiologist's findings to the anesthesiologist. If normovolemia and anxiolysis are maintained perioperatively, vasovagal syncope may be prevented.

DISCUSSION

Sudden, transient loss of consciousness with inability to maintain postural tone and position characterize syncope. Syncope accounts for approximately 1% to 3% of emergency department visits and is the sixth leading cause of hospitalization for people more than 65 years old.[1,2] The four pathophysiologic mechanisms leading to syncope are listed in Table 42.1.[3]

Neurally mediated syncopal syndromes may be vasovagal or situational. An abnormal neural reflex leads to a syncopal episode. In orthostatic syncope, the sympathetic nervous system fails to respond to a change in position from supine to upright. Cardiac syncope is caused by arrhythmias, cardiomyopathy, or structural heart diseases. Cerebrovascular syncope results from migraines, steal syndromes, or transient ischemic attacks.

Table 42.1. **CLASSIFICATION AND CAUSES OF SYNCOPE**

CLASSIFICATION AND PRINCIPAL CAUSES OF SYNCOPE			
NEURAL, REFLEX	ORTHOSTATIC	CARDIAC ARRHYTHMIA	STRUCTURAL CARDIOVASCULAR
• Vasovagal syncope • Carotid sinus syndrome • Situational: cough, postmicturition	• Drug-induced • Atrial node syndrome (primary or secondary)	• Bradyarrhythmia (e.g., sick sinus syndrome, atrioventricular block) • Tachycardia (ventricular tachycardia, supraventricular tachycardia) • Channelopathies	• Aortic stenosis • Ischemic cardiomyopathy, nonischemic cardiomyopathy • Pericardial dysfunction/tamponade • Pulmonary hypertension • Aortic dissection • Subclavian steal
60%	15%	10%	5%
Unknown cause = 10%			

Modified from Benditt and Nguyen.[1]

The clinical manifestations of syncope are summarized in Table 42.2. Our focus is on neurally mediated vasovagal syncope, which may occur during a procedural intervention perioperatively or in the pain clinic. The momentary loss of control of circulation in neurally mediated syncope is a reflex. It accounts for approximately 66% of all syncope[4] and has various triggers.[5] Of the types of neurally mediated syncope, the one most often encountered in the general population is the vasovagal reflex. Approximately 37% of the population experience fainting from a vasovagal episode at least once.[6] The most common triggers of a vasovagal episode are listed in Table 42.3.[2]

In vasovagal syncope, a decrease in cerebral perfusion pressure initiates loss of consciousness. The abnormal myoclonic jerks present in 12% to 90% of patients are frequently misdiagnosed as seizures.[7] The prevalence of anxiety and mood disorders in patients with vasovagal syncope might be as high as 26%.[8] Patients with panic disorders may have exaggerated declines in cerebral blood flow; vagal hyperactivity has been observed in patients with blood phobia. Treatment of minor psychiatric disorders resulted in a significant decrease in syncope recurrence. Vasovagal syncope also appears to be a familial disease. Although the exact gene for transmission is unknown, several familial studies suggest an autosomal recessive condition with a common frequency of the recessive allele (the first locus identified, on chromosome 15q26, belonged to a family with autosomal dominant vasovagal syncope; Figure 42.1).[9,10]

Table 42.2. **COMMON SYMPTOMS AND PROGNOSTIC IMPLICATIONS OF SYNCOPAL EPISODES**

CAUSE OF SYNCOPE	SYMPTOMS AND SIGNS	PROGNOSTIC IMPLICATIONS
Cardiopulmonary disease (structural changes)	Related to underlying disease	Moderate to Severe
Neurally mediated Vasovagal syncope Carotid sinus syndrome Volume depletion	Warmth Nausea Diaphoresis	Benign
Orthostatic	Warmth Nausea Diaphoresis	Benign
Vascular steal (neurologic)	Seizure Transient ischemic attack Focal neurologic deficit	Moderate
Psychiatric	No injury	Benign

Modified from Rosanio et al.[3]

CAUSES OF VASOVAGAL SYNCOPE

The cause of vasovagal syncope is controversial.[10] A distinction should be made between an isolated episode and vasovagal disease (Table 42.4).[11] Fainting in a syncopal episode may contribute to preserving vital functions while blood pools in dependent structures (Figure 42.2).[12] Several factors and reflexes affecting the heart have been implicated as causes.

Sinoatrial Node

Stretching of the sinoatrial node contributes directly to HR variations; increase in blood volume increases HR through a mechanism devoid of outside neural control.

Veno-Atrial Junction Receptors

Atrial stretch with volume increase initiates afferent transmission through the vagus nerve to the vasomotor centers in the medulla oblongata. Myelinated fibers arising from these centers are coupled with efferent paths through cardio-accelerator fibers to increase the HR. Sympathetic outflow is limited to the sinoatrial node, with no extension to the ventricles or increase in inotropic state. Nonmyelinated fibers are less sensitive

Table 42.3. **TRIGGERS FOR SYNCOPE IN ADULTS OF VARIOUS AGES**

TRIGGER	GANZENBOOM ET AL. (2013)	PROVIDENCIA ET AL. (2011)	O'DWYER ET AL. (2012)	GRAHAM ET AL. (2001)
Number with syncope	154/394	598/2011	219/219	62/62
Mean age (years)	21	22	36	50
Warm environment (%)	31	22	23	37
Prolonged standing (%)	27	12	55	27
Pain (%)	25	12	2.7	
Illness (%)	18	4.5	1.4	
Alcohol (%)	13	8	10	10
Emotion (%)	11	13	21	21
Venipuncture (%)	10	13	15	11
Multiple triggers (%)	55	33	48	

Other triggers: fasting, fatigue, drugs, menstruation, epileptic features, accident, meals, sitting, and during and after physical exercise.

Modified from Kenny et al.[2]

and need greater atrial distension to be stimulated. They can be stimulated by rapid stretches. Their efferent paths stimulate receptors responsible for bradycardia and vasodilatation.

Bezold-Jarisch Reflex

Initially described in 1867 by von Bezold, the reflex was confirmed by Jarisch in 1937. The reflex originates in the lungs and heart (stretching of receptors in the inferoposterior wall of the left ventricle) and then travels to the medullary centers via the vagus nerve. Efferent fibers, in response to chemical or mechanical stretches, are responsible for bradycardia and hypotension.

Baroreceptor Reflex

The baroreceptor reflex originates in the baroreceptors of the carotid sinus and aortic arch. Afferent input, triggered by an

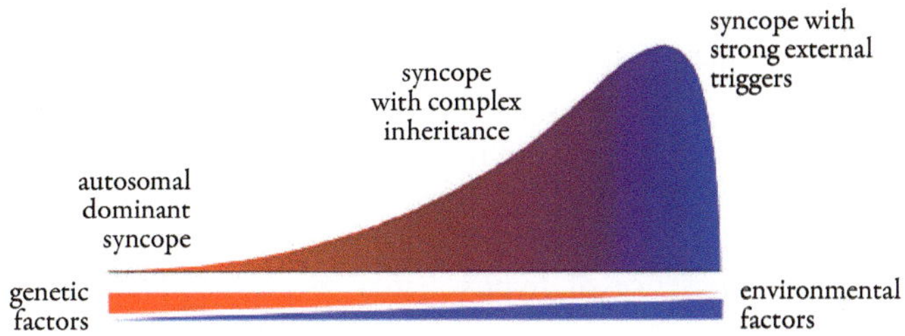

Figure 42.1. Conceptualization of the genetic architecture of syncope. The x-axis shows the spectrum of syncope, with predominant genetic factors on the left and predominant external factors on the right. The y-axis shows the assumed frequency of the different forms. Syncope due to strong environmental triggers, where genetic factors are less relevant, is assumed to be the most frequent. Autosomal dominant vasovagal syncope is least common. Reproduced with permission from Klein KM, Berkovic SF. Genetics of vasovagal syncope. *Auton Neurosci.* 2014; pii: S1566-0702(14)00056-3.

Table 42.4. **DIFFERENCE BETWEEN VASOVAGAL SYNCOPE AND VASOVAGAL DISEASE**

ISOLATED VASOVAGAL SYNCOPE	VASOVAGAL DISEASE
Onset: Younger age	Onset: Older age
Otherwise healthy patients	Comorbidities: Cardiovascular and neurologic diseases
Typical vasovagal prodrome/ triggers	No prodrome/triggers
Affects 50% of all individuals	Diagnosed after positive head-up tilt test
70% of population predisposed	Overlap with carotid sinus syndrome
Frequent spontaneous disappearance with age	Sometimes progressively worsening over time

Modified from Brignole.[11]

increase in arterial pressure, travels with the vagus in the nucleus tractus solitarius in the medulla. Efferent interneurons inhibit sympathetic outflow, which decreases blood pressure. Excitatory efferents toward the nucleus ambiguus, a vagal nucleus, increase the vagal tone and diminish the HR.

Chemoreceptor Reflex

Chemoreceptors in the carotid sinus and the aortic arch respond to variations in oxygen, carbon dioxide, and hydrogen ion concentrations. Acidosis and hypoxemia stimulate respiration, usually accompanied by vagal inhibition. In vasovagal syncope, sympathetic tone increases with fear or anxiety to affect heart inotropy.[13] Subsequent vagal action slows the HR,

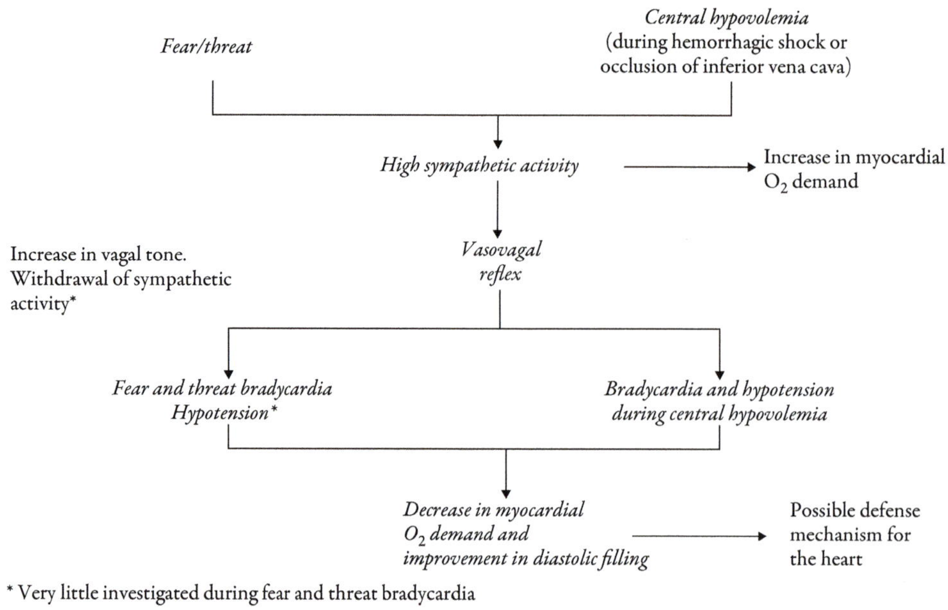

Figure 42.2. Fainting after the vasovagal reflex promotes restoration of blood volume. Based on this explanation, vasovagal syncope is compared to the "playing dead" reaction seen in some animals under extreme stress. Reproduced with permission from Alboni P, Alboni M, Bertolelle G. The origin of vasovagal syncope: to protect the heart or to escape predation? *Clin Auton Res*. 2008; 18: 170–178.

while sympathetic inhibition and peripheral vasodilatation lower blood pressure.

Neural Pathways

Two neural mechanisms are activated in the vasovagal response. The corticohypothalamo-medullary path carries neural information from the superior structures to the medullary cardiovascular centers. Receptors in the sinoatrial node of the heart perceive the sudden decrease in venous return as hypovolemia, and HR slows. Heart inotropy, which precedes the Bezold-Jarisch reflex, triggers the receptors in the inferoposterior wall of the left ventricle. The sudden decrease in venous return empties the heart quickly, and bradycardia and hypotension result via a reflex completed in the medulla oblongata. After sympathetic stimulation with emptying in the atria, the atrial receptors are activated. A false signal of overfilling travels through the myelinated or nonmyelinated vagal fibers to the medullary centers. A signal of reduced venous return activates two opposing reflex mechanisms. The baroreceptor reflex restores blood pressure by increasing the sympathetic outflow and vagal inhibition. The depressor reflex slows HR to restore cardiac filling and decrease oxygen demand.

DIFFERENTIAL DIAGNOSIS OF VASOVAGAL SYNCOPE

Placement of a neuraxial local anesthetic affects the heart and circulation. In true vasovagal syncope, loss of consciousness is accompanied by bradycardia, hypotension, diaphoresis, and feelings of weakness and nausea. It appears with infiltration of a local anesthetic, with prepping of the back, or with insertion of a catheter in highly anxious individuals who have a history of similar episodes or familial occurrence. Seizure-like movements are common and patients can lose consciousness or be semiresponsive. If the triggering action is eliminated and the episode is aggressively treated with fluids and pressors, the condition is self-limited and benign. Vasovagal syncope may occur in pain clinics during cervical epidural steroid injections, in excessively anxious, unsedated patients, or during placement of an epidural catheter perioperatively. A test dose through an epidural catheter can result in hypotension and tachycardia or bradycardia if the catheter has migrated intrathecally. An intravascular injection may be associated with transient tachycardia and hypertension. In outpatient pain clinics, the administration of a test dose has become common before administration of therapeutic medication to alert a physician to vascular uptake. During neuraxial injections of local anesthetics, an accidental intrathecal test dose, unrecognized intrathecal migration of an epidural catheter, or excessive administration of local anesthetic via an epidural catheter, blocks the sympathetic chain and leads to hypotension and bradycardia. With complex spine pathology, intrathecal migration of the needle tip is possible. Failure to recognize an intrathecal injection by fluoroscopic image has devastating consequences in cervical spine injections. High spinals should also be suspected after lumbar or thoracic epidural steroid injections if low volume of local anesthetic renders a patient severely hypotensive and bradycardic.

In the presence of hypovolemia in an anxious patient, a vasovagal reflex can be exaggerated by the sympathectomy induced from a neuraxially delivered local anesthetic. Cardiocirculatory collapse can be profound, refractory to treatment, and accompanied by respiratory collapse requiring airway support. Every attempt should be made to prevent a potential vasovagal episode by relieving anxiety with benzodiazepines. Yet patients should maintain consciousness during neuraxial procedures to prevent potential nerve injury. Thus, during epidural placement preoperatively or epidural steroid injections administered in outpatient pain clinics, sedation should be administered with the goal of a relaxed, conversant, but immobile patient. Standard monitors are required to capture an early event.

Postural Tachycardia Syndrome (POTS)

POTS is defined by orthostatic intolerance. Patients have tachycardia and complaints of palpitations, fatigue, and syncope or near syncope that arise when standing and resolve when sitting down.[14] HR increases at least 30 bpm or exceeds 120 bpm within 10 minutes of standing. Blood pressure is not necessarily decreased. Severe autonomic nervous system disorders or vascular unresponsiveness is responsible for the condition.[15] Peripheral neuropathy leads to an inability of the vasculature to maintain tone during gravitational stress, and blood pools in the lower extremities.[16] Some patients will have symptoms of adrenergic stimulation, including tachycardia, tremor, and anxiety. Patients may also have elevated norepinephrine levels.[17]

Sick Sinus Syndrome

In sick sinus syndrome, patients suffer from deteriorating end-organ perfusion. They faint or have episodes of light-headedness, fatigue, confusion, oliguria, and heart failure.[18] Cardiac impulse formation is abnormal, and propagation from the sinoatrial node deteriorates pacemaker function. Tachycardia or bradycardia may manifest, as well as sinus pauses or arrest and sinoatrial exit block.[19] HR response to exercise or sympathetic stimulation is inadequate, not meeting the body's physiologic requirements for cardiac output. The intrinsic causes of sick sinus syndrome are changes to the sinoatrial node itself: degenerative fibrosis, ion channel dysfunction, and remodeling.[20] Intrinsic causes are age-related and increase in the elderly. Approximately 1 in 600 cardiac patients more than 65 years old is affected by the syndrome. Extrinsic causes of the syndrome are autonomic dysfunction, electrolyte abnormalities, and certain drugs, which are listed in Table 42.5.[20]

Table 42.5. CAUSES OF SICK SINUS SYNDROME

INTRINSIC CAUSES	EXTRINSIC CAUSES THAT MIMIC OR EXACERBATE SICK SINUS SYNDROME
Degenerative fibrosis	Autonomic dysfunction Carotid sinus hypersensitivity Neurocardiogenic syncope Vasovagal syncope
Infiltrative disease process Amyloidosis Connective tissue disease Hemochromatosis Sarcoidosis	Increased vagal tone (occurs in athletes and during sleep)
Ion channel dysfunction	Metabolic disturbances Hyper- and hypokalemia Hypocalcemia Hypothermia Hypothyroidism Hypoxia
Remodeling of the sinoatrial node	Obstructive sleep apnea
	Pharmacologic agents Antiarrhythmic medications (Class I and III) Beta-blockers Calcium channel blockers (nondihydropyridine) Digoxin Lithium Sympatholytic medications
	Toxins

Modified from Semelka M, Gera J, Usman S. Sick sinus syndrome: a review. *Am Fam Physician.* 2013;87:691–696.

NEURAXIAL PROCEDURES AND THE VASOVAGAL REFLEX

Preprocedure Factors

During skin infiltration and superficial placement of an epidural or spinal needle, vasovagal syncope may cause bradycardia, hypotension, diaphoresis, fainting, or loss of posture. During placement of an epidural or spinal needle deep in a ligament, vasovagal syncope may result if the structures are not well anesthetized by local infiltration or if preparation for the procedure takes long in an extremely anxious patient. With sudden accidental injection of air intrathecally during the process of loss of resistance to air, a patient may become unresponsive. Seizurelike activity or severe headache from pneumocephalus may result, even though vital signs are maintained. During placement of an epidural catheter or injection of medication into the epidural space, the injectate can trigger the reflex. In cardiac compromised patients, epinephrine in an intravascular test dose can contribute to cardiac injury. Signs of ventricular ischemia will appear on the ECG. Sudden loss of consciousness is considered cardiac syncope and is less likely to be a benign reflex. Depending on the level of epidural insertion, loss of consciousness can be accompanied by hypotension and tachycardia (below T4) or hypotension and bradycardia (above T4).

Intraoperative Factors

In the presence of excessive neuraxial delivery of local anesthetic in an anesthetized patient with undiagnosed high sensory and sympathetic levels, certain surgical procedures (bowel manipulation, catheter placement for peritoneal dialysis, retroperitoneal exploration) can stimulate vagal tone. Severe, refractory bradycardia or asystole with profound hypotension may be the result.

Postoperative Factors

Pain contributes to the reflex, especially when an epidural catheter is not yet activated. When it is activated, sudden sympathectomy and brief loss of consciousness may occur in

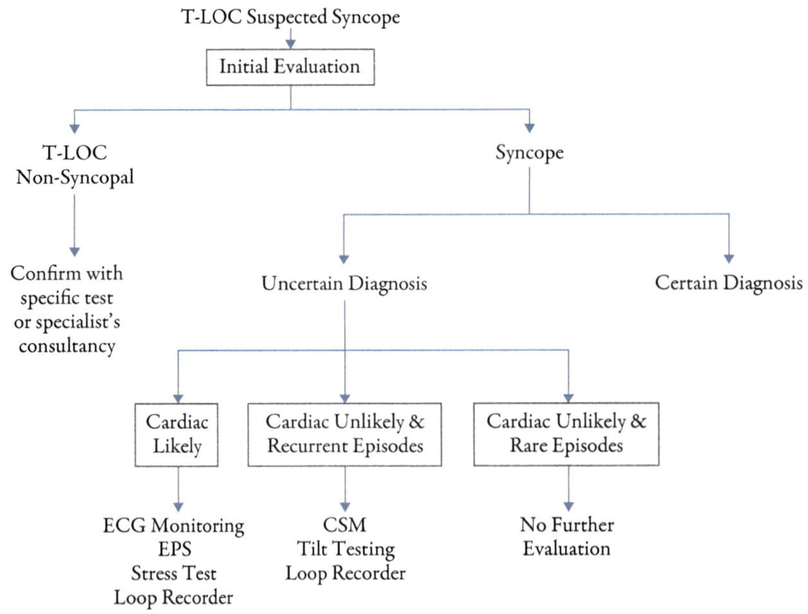

Figure 42.3. The general strategy for evaluation of syncope as recommended in the European Society of Cardiology's *Syncope Practice Guidelines*. Abbreviations: CSM, carotid sinus massage; EPS, electrophysiology studies; T-LOC, transient loss of consciousness. Reproduced with permission from Benditt DG, Nguyen JT. Syncope, therapeutic approaches. *J Am Coll Cardiol.* 2009; 53(19): 1741–1751.

a hypovolemic patient who suffered intraoperative blood loss severe enough for hemorrhagic anemia.

Outpatient Peripheral Nerve Blocks or Joint Injections

Nerve blocks in the upper extremities of anxious patients can contribute to vasovagal reflexes. When a local anesthetic is accidentally injected intravascularly, sudden loss of consciousness is accompanied by seizures and cardiac compromise that requires cardiocirculatory intervention to maintain vital signs.

DIAGNOSING VASOVAGAL SYNCOPE

A general strategy for identifying the pathophysiologic mechanism of syncope and for diagnosing a vasovagal episode can be found in the practice guidelines proposed by the European Society of Cardiology (Figure 42.3).

Patient History

Thorough medical and family histories are essential. During detailed interviews, triggering events and their frequency can be identified.

Electrocardiography

After an acute episode, a 12-lead ECG may direct attention to a concomitant cardiac event. The event, triggered by hypotension or bradycardia associated with syncope, may uncover a previously undiagnosed cardiac abnormality.

Blood Pressure Monitoring

Some patients have consistent and persistent low blood pressure for as long as 24 hours. Low blood pressure may aggravate a syncopal episode.

Holter Monitoring

If syncope is severe and frequent, long-term cardiac monitoring may show arrhythmias; however, the sensitivity of a positive test by Holter monitoring is only 10% in unexplained syncope.

Echocardiography

Not routinely used for diagnosis of vasovagal reflex, an echocardiogram can eliminate coexisting cardiac disease from the differential diagnosis, especially when ECG changes can be attributed to bradycardia and hypotension during syncope.

Electrophysiologic Tests

An electrophysiologic test is offered to patients with suspected structural disease, such as sick sinus syndrome. In structural disease, hypotension and bradycardia after a vasovagal episode are refractory to treatment and are accompanied by changes in the ECG.

Tilt-Table Test

A tilt-table test is the only modality available to diagnose neurocardiogenic syncope. Lying supine on a table, a patient is monitored with an ECG. HR and blood pressure are evaluated when the table changes the patient's position from reclining to standing. A positive test is one that provokes hypotension, triggering the patient's symptoms. The reproducibility of the test is 80% to 95% for a negative test but only 30% to 90% for a positive test. The hemodynamic effects are milder than in spontaneous vasovagal episodes.

Implantable Loop Recorders

Small recorders, placed subcutaneously, store 45 minutes of ECG waves. This method is reserved for patients with

Table 42.6. EFFICACY OF TREATMENT FOR VASOVAGAL SYNCOPE

TREATMENT	TREATMENT EFFECT	EVIDENCE*
Educational and lifestyle changes		
a. Increase salt and fluid	Probably helpful	Moderate
b. Physical exercise	Debatable effect	Weak
c. Physical counterpressure	Probably helpful	Good
d. Tilt training	Debatable effect	Moderate, Good
Pharmacologic therapy		
a. Beta-blockers	Probably unhelpful	Good
b. Selective serotonin reuptake inhibitor	Debatable effect	Moderate
c. Midodrine	Probably helpful	Good
d. Fludrocortisone	Debatable effect	Weak
Cardiac pacemaker		
a. Routine use	Probable unhelpful	Good
b. Refractory cases	Debatable effect	Weak

* Good evidence from randomized studies and meta-analysis, moderate evidence from nonrandomized trials, and weak evidence from consensus opinions.

recurrent syncope and uncertain diagnosis. The diagnostic yield is approximately 40% when the device is used for 8 to 10 months.[21,22]

TREATMENT OF VASOVAGAL SYNCOPE

When a regional or neuraxial technique is anticipated, aggressive treatment is initiated. Otherwise, supportive measures are used during vasovagal episodes. When supportive measures are exhausted, pharmacologic therapy or surgical intervention is suggested (Table 42.6).

Among supportive measures are the following:

Correction of existing hypovolemia. Central neuraxial blockade in a hypovolemic patient can become life-threatening hypotension and bradycardia. Fluid boluses restore normovolemia.

Limiting the maximum level of sensory blockade. With incremental small doses of local anesthetic through an epidural catheter, sensory blockade can be controlled and the effect on blood pressure and HR is limited.

Reconsidering preload. Maintaining normovolemia is superior to force loading with crystalloids and colloids, especially in cardiac-disabled individuals.

Relying on gravity. During neurocardiogenic syncope, when neuraxial blockade with local anesthetics results in acute sympathectomy, venous return decreases. Thus, neuraxial procedures, such as spinals and epidurals, may be performed with patients prone or in the lateral decubitus position.

Treatment of bradycardia. For mild or gradual bradycardia, atropine or glycopyrrolate is administered. For sudden severe bradycardia, venous return is restored with epinephrine or intravenous fluids. The patient is placed in the Trendelenburg position, head down with legs elevated.

Treatment of hypotension. Ephedrine acts directly on alpha- and beta-receptors and indirectly on postganglionic presynaptic adrenergic nerve endings. Phenylephrine acts on alpha-receptors to constrict resistance and capacitance vessels. During vasovagal syncope, phenylephrine may aggravate bradycardia.

Recommended lifestyle changes. Patients with recurrent episodes benefit from fluid intake of 2 L/day and salt intake of 6 to 9 g/day. Regarding physical exercise, patients are advised to follow a balanced schedule. Isometric contraction of the legs (by crossing the legs) or the arms and hands (by pulling apart gripped hands) are movements best performed during presyncopal periods. The maneuvers are suggested for patients who experience long prodromal episodes. Leg-crossing increases cardiac output up to 10% and arterial blood pressure up to 8%. Passive tilt training daily with the goal of gradually increasing symptom-free stand-up time is not encouraged in symptomatic patients.

Pharmacologic therapy. A trial using beta-blocker therapy showed identical outcome rates with placebo or metoprolol. Other studies have shown that beta-blockers reduce the recurrence of syncope. Clinical evidence is mixed about the manipulation of central serotonin levels for the treatment of vasovagal syncope. Selective serotonin reuptake inhibitors are not the first line of treatment. Midodrine, a peripherally active alpha-agonist that crosses the blood–brain barrier, is used to treat reduced sympathetic outflow responsible for venous pooling. In several randomized, controlled studies of patients treated with midodrine, vasovagal episodes decreased fourfold compared to the number in the placebo group. Midodrine is used in symptomatic patients whose quality of life is affected because of frequent syncopal episodes. Fludrocortisone, a corticosteroid with mineralocorticoid activity, induces water and sodium retention and potassium excretion. No data exist on fludrocortisone in adult patients and studies in the pediatric population had conflicting results.

Surgical interventions. Routine, benign, incidental vasovagal episodes require no treatment. Frequent documented syncopal episodes with severe bradycardia not responsive to a conservative regimen may require invasive treatment, such as pacemaker placement. Older unblinded studies show the efficacy of pacemakers in the treatment of recurrent vasovagal episodes. Newer randomized trials show no difference between the placebo and study groups. A recently published double-blind, randomized, placebo-controlled trial showed that permanent pacing is effective in reducing recurrence of syncope in patients ≥ 40 years old who suffered from severe, asystolic, neurally mediated syncope.[23]

CONCLUSIONS

- Neurocardiogenic syncope appears in susceptible individuals as a result of excessive peripheral venous pooling with sudden decline in peripheral venous return to the right ventricle.

- A cardiac "hypercontractile" state activates mechanoreceptors (otherwise responding only to stretch). Increased neural afferent traffic to the brain provokes an apparent paradoxical bradycardia and a decline in peripheral vascular resistance.
- In regional or neuraxial techniques, the superimposed sympathectomy in response to administration of a local anesthetic can result in excessive, refractory, life-threatening bradycardia and hypotension.
- Prevention by maintaining normovolemia while administering small incremental doses of neuraxial local anesthetic and prompt treatment with anticholinergics and pressors may limit complications as well as cardiac, circulatory, and neurologic sequelae.

REFERENCES

1. Benditt DG, Nguyen JT. Syncope, therapeutic approaches. *J Am Coll Cardiol.* 2009;53(19):1741–1751.
2. Kenny RA, Bhangu J, King-Kallimanis BL. Epidemiology of syncope/collapse in younger and older Western patient populations. *Prog Cardiovasc Dis.* 2013;55:357–363.
3. Rosanio S, Schwarz ER, Ware D L, Vitarelli A. Syncope in adults: systematic review and proposal of a diagnostic and therapeutic algorithm. *Int J Cardiol.* 2013;162:149–157.
4. Brignole M. Diagnosis and treatment of syncope. *Heart.* 2007;93:130–136.
5. Chen-Scarabelli C, Scarabelli TM. Neurocardiogenic syncope. *BMJ.* 2004;329:336–341.
6. Kuriachan V, Sheldon RS, Platonov M. Evidence-based treatment of vasovagal syncope. *Heart Rhythm.* 2008;5:1609–1614.
7. Josephson CB, Rahey S, Sadler RM. Neurocardiogenic syncope: frequency and consequences of its misdiagnosis as epilepsy. *Can J Neurol Sci.* 2007;34:221–224.
8. Leftheriotis D, Michopoulos I, Flevari P, et al. Minor psychiatric disorders and syncope: the role of psychopathology in the expression of vasovagal reflex. *Psychother Psychosom.* 2008;77(6):372–376.
9. Newton JL, Kerr S, Pairman J, et al. Familial neurocardiogenic (vasovagal) syncope. *Am J Med Genet A.* 2005;133A:176–179.
10. Klein KM, Berkovic SF. Genetics of vasovagal syncope. *Auton Neurosci.* 2014;184:60–65.
11. Brignole M. Vasovagal syncope and vasovagal disease. *Hellenic J Cardiol.* 2008;49:61–64.
12. Grubb BP. Neurocardiogenic syncope. *N Engl J Med.* 2005;352:1004–1010.
13. Stienstra R. Mechanisms behind and treatment of sudden, unexpected circulatory collapse during central neuraxis blockade. *Acta Anesthesiol Scand.* 2000;44:965–971.
14. Grubb BP. Postural tachycardia syndrome. *Circulation.* 2008;117:2814–2817.
15. Thieben MJ, Sandroni P, Sletten DM, et al. Postural tachycardia syndrome: the Mayo Clinic experience. *Mayo Clin Proc.* 2007;82:308–313.
16. Grubb BP, Kanjwal Y, Kosinski D. The postural tachycardia syndrome: a concise guide to diagnosis and management. *J Cardiovasc Electrophysiol.* 2006;14:108–112.
17. Shannon JR, Flattem NL, Jordan J, et al. Orthostatic intolerance and tachycardia associated with norepinephrine-transporter deficiency. *N Engl J Med.* 2000;342:541–549.
18. Adán V, Crown LA. Diagnosis and treatment of sick sinus syndrome. *Am Fam Physician.* 2003;67(8):1725–1732.
19. Dobrzynski H, Boyett MR, Anderson RH. New insights into pacemaker activity: promoting understanding of sick sinus syndrome. *Circulation.* 2007;115(14):1921–1932.
20. Semelka M, Gera J, Usman S. Sick sinus syndrome: a review. *Am Fam Physician.* 2013;87:691–696.
21. Vaddadi G, Lambert E Corcoran SJ, Esler MD. Postural syncope: mechanisms and management. *Med J Aust.* 2007;187: 299–304.
22. Jhanjee R, van Dijk JG, Sakaguchi S, Benditt DG. Syncope in adults: terminology, classification and diagnostic strategy. *Pacing Clin Electrophysiol.* 2006;29:1160–1169.
23. Fu Q, Levine BD. Pathophysiology of neurally mediated syncope: role of cardiac output and total peripheral resistance. *Autonom Neurosci.* 2014;184:24–26.

REVIEW QUESTIONS

1. An 81-year-old healthy female presents to the operating room for a right knee arthroplasty. You decide to provide anesthesia for the case with a combined spinal epidural. Upon inserting the epidural needle, the patient becomes hypotensive, with a MAP of 30 and bradycardic at 40 bpm. What is the first step you would take?

   A. Administration of fluid
   B. Removal of the epidural needle
   C. Administration of atropine
   D. Administration of epinephrine

2. A 75-year-old patient with a history of localized endometrial cancer is scheduled to undergo a curative surgical procedure under general anesthesia. During the preoperative epidural placement, she develops 4-mm ST depressions in leads V5 and V6 during a benign and mild vasovagal episode. Which myocardial wall is suspected to be exposed to ischemia in this asymptomatic patient?

   A. Lateral wall
   B. Inferior wall
   C. Septal wall
   D. Anterior wall

3. In a follow-up consultation regarding her recent uncomplicated syncopal episode during an aborted cervical epidural steroid injection in the sitting position, a highly educated 60-year-old patient inquires about the cause of the episode. While explaining the possible pathophysiology implicated, you mention that afferent transmission to the vasomotor center in the medulla oblongata from the veno-atrial junction is carried by which cranial nerve?

   A. VII
   B. VIII
   C. IX
   D. X

ANSWERS

1. B. From the listed possibilities, remove of the epidural needle and positioning the patient in an optimal manner for resuscitation maneuvers is the best initial maneuver. Answers A, C, and D are all options in the resuscitation algorithm, but not the first step. Medical management should come after supportive measures are exhausted. After medical management is optimized, investigation related to the cause of the syncopal episode may direct further diagnostic and treatment possibilities.

2. A. Myocardial ischemia is associated with ST depression. The greater the depression, the more significant the ischemia (ST depression of 1 mm is less severe than a 4-mm depression). Other causes of ST segment depression, such as hypokalemia and left ventricular hypertrophy, should be considered in the differential diagnosis of a completely asymptomatic patient with ST depression. Lateral wall ischemia occurs as an insufficiency of the left circumflex coronary artery and most ECG signs are best shown by leads I, aVL (high lateral left ventricle wall), V5, and V6 (lateral left ventricle wall). Inferior wall ischemia is best shown by leads II, III, and aVF. Septal wall ischemia is best shown by leads V1 and V2. Anterior wall ischemia is best shown by leads V3 and V4. ST depression is consistent with subendocardial injury and imbalance of oxygen supply and demand, as seen in ischemia; ST elevation injury is associated with acute coronary myocardial infarction (Table 42.7).

3. D. The vagus nerve (X) provides afferent transmission for parasympathetic control from the heart and digestive tract.

Table 42.7. **ECG CHANGES WITH CORONARY ISCHEMIA**

ECG CHANGES	VENTRICLE	ARTERIAL SUPPLY
V1, V2	Septal wall	Left anterior descending coronary artery
V2-V5	Anterior wall	
V5, V6	Lateral wall	Left circumflex coronary artery
I, aVL	High lateral wall	Left circumflex coronary artery
II, III, aVF	Inferior wall	Right coronary artery
rV3, rV4	Right ventricle	

CN VII, the facial nerve, is important for facial expression. CN IX is the vestibulocochlear nerve and plays an important role in hearing and balance. CN IX is the glossopharyngeal nerve and is relevant for sensation, taste, and salivation.

QUESTIONS AND ANSWERS

This chapter has accompanying questions and answers that are available to subscribers as part of the Oxford eLearning platform. To access the questions, follow the link below, or go to ✔ http://oxfordmedicine.com/painmanagementreview

43.

LOCAL ANESTHETIC SYSTEMIC TOXICITY: DIAGNOSIS, PREVENTION, AND MANAGEMENT

Alexandra Dubikovsky Golden and David Dickerson

STEM CASE AND KEY QUESTIONS

A 57-year-old male with a history of end-stage renal disease (ESRD), chronic hepatitis, diabetes, and systolic heart failure with ejection fraction (EF) of 40% presents for open reduction internal fixation (ORIF) of the ankle. During the preoperative interview, it becomes apparent that his daily medication regimen includes 15 different medications for his various comorbidities. Regional anesthesia is planned for the case, along with light sedation with propofol and midazolam.

WHAT ARE THE RISK FACTORS THAT COULD LEAD TO LOCAL ANESTHETIC SYSTEMIC TOXICITY (LAST) IN PATIENTS WITH COMORBID CONDITIONS UNDERGOING SURGERY UNDER REGIONAL ANESTHESIA? WHICH ARE PRESENT IN THIS PATIENT?

Generally, patients' comorbid conditions that should be considered in regional anesthesia and risk for LAST are: extremes of age, high-cardiac-output states that increase absorption of local anesthetics, low-cardiac-output states that lead to reduced clearance of local anesthetics, reduced plasma proteins that increase free fraction of local anesthetics, pregnancy (with both increased cardiac output and lower proportional plasma proteins), and the concomitant use of beta blockers, digoxin, calcium channel blockers, and cytochrome P450 inhibitors.

This patient has likely low cardiac output and decreased plasma proteins, as well as a history of polypharmacy. His diabetes is probably associated with peripheral neuropathy, which should be carefully considered when a regional anesthetic technique is planned.[1]

YOU DECIDE TO PERFORM AN ADDUCTOR CANAL BLOCK AS WELL AS A POPLITEAL NERVE BLOCK. WHAT LOCAL ANESTHETIC WOULD YOU USE (DRUG, CONCENTRATION, TOTAL VOLUME AT EACH SITE)?

The surgery is planned for approximately 3 hours; therefore, a longer-acting local anesthetic, such as bupivacaine, should be considered. Because the planned anesthetic is regional, an anesthetic concentration is indicated. Therefore, the blocks are performed with bupivacaine 0.5% with epinephrine, 15 mL at each site.

WHAT TECHNIQUES WOULD YOU USE TO REDUCE THE RISK OF LAST DURING THE PROCEDURE?

To avoid accidental intravascular injection of the local anesthetic, direct visualization of needle and injection is indicated. Both blocks are therefore performed under direct ultrasound visualization, with aspiration after every 3 to 5 mL incremental injection.[1–4]

YOU DECIDE TO PROCEED WITH THE BLOCKS AND ADMINISTER SEDATION. GIVEN THE PATIENT'S COMORBID CONDITIONS, YOU INCREMENTALLY GIVE 15 ML OF 0.375% BUPIVACAINE WITH 1:200,000 EPINEPHRINE TO THE ADDUCTOR CANAL. THE PATIENT REPORTS PRODROMAL SYMPTOMS, SEDATION, AND SLIGHT TWITCHING OF THE EYELIDS, BUT EXHIBITS NO CHANGE IN HEART RATE. DOES THIS CONCERN YOU? WOULD YOU PROCEED WITH THE POPLITEAL BLOCK?

The symptoms described are consistent with central nervous system (CNS) effects and therefore you immediately suspect LAST from likely local anesthetic uptake into the neighboring blood vessels. Even in the absence of cardiac symptoms, this presentation should alert the physician to LAST, because this condition's symptoms can be incredibly varied in presentation, and it should prompt the physician to stop further injections and to assess the patient.[5,6]

AFTER YOU WAIT 5 MINUTES AND THE PATIENT IS AGAIN RESPONSIVE AND FULLY AWAKE, YOU DECIDE TO CONTINUE WITH THE POPLITEAL BLOCK. UPON INJECTION OF AN ADDITIONAL 15 ML OF BUPIVACAINE 0.375% WITH EPINEPHRINE, THE PATIENT DEVELOPS ADDITIONAL PRODROMAL SYMPTOMS AND BECOMES ANXIOUS BUT IS STILL INTERACTIVE. WOULD YOU ADMINISTER EMULSION THERAPY? WHAT WOULD DETERMINE YOUR NEXT STEPS IN TREATMENT?

Upon complaints form the patient of feeling anxious you look at the monitors and see significant tachycardia; you suspect that further local anesthetic vascular uptake has taken place and you call for backup, consider placing an arterial line, and begin steps to immediately administer lipid emulsion therapy, as early initiation is crucial to the success of the treatment.[7–9]

THE PATIENT LOSES CONSCIOUSNESS. WHAT WOULD YOU DO NEXT?

As LAST is quickly developing, you activate a code, start chest compressions, administer epinephrine, continue lipid emulsion therapy, and notify the cardiac surgery team for cardiopulmonary support.[7–9]

WOULD YOU USE A COGNITIVE TOOL, SUCH AS A CHECKLIST? WHY OR WHY NOT?

Because this is an emergency, to ensure that all elements of LAST treatment are properly done, during the resuscitation efforts, you ask your helper to pull out the LAST protocol checklist secured to the regional anesthesia cart. This step is essential for optimal recovery of the patient and to ensure that no aspects of the emergency protocol are missed.[5,10]

WOULD YOU INTUBATE THE PATIENT? WHY OR WHY NOT?

Because the patient is unresponsive, placement of an endotracheal tube is important for airway protection. Additionally, prevention of respiratory acidosis is important for cardiac stability in a patient with LAST.[7–9,11,12]

WHEN WOULD YOU GIVE LIPID EMULSION THERAPY? WHAT DOSE?

When the patient lost consciousness, together with the call for help, you started 20% lipid emulsion therapy, with a bolus of 1.5 mL/kg and then infusion at 0.25 to 0.5 mL/kg (while continuing chest compressions), and continue the therapy until 10 minutes after return of spontaneous circulation (ROSC). Bolus can be repeated two to three times every 5 minutes.[10]

AFTER RECEIVING A 500-ML BAG OF 20% LIPID EMULSION, THE PATIENT DEVELOPS SINUS RHYTHM AND RETURN OF PULSE. WOULD YOU CONTINUE TO ADMINISTER LIPID EMULSION THERAPY?

Lipid emulsion therapy should be continued for a minimum of 10 minutes after ROSC.[10] Five minutes after the intralipid is administered, the patient suddenly develops supraventricular tachycardia, with very frequent ventricular extrasystole, a rhythm that at times switches to ventricular tachycardia.

YOU CALL FOR ANOTHER BAG OF LIPID EMULSION THERAPY AND ARE TOLD IT IS THE ONLY ONE THAT WAS AVAILABLE FOR USE AND THAT THERE ARE NO OTHER BAGS OF LIPID EMULSION THERAPY. WHAT ELSE CAN BE CONSIDERED FOR RESUSCITATING THIS PATIENT?

You call the vascular and cardiac surgeons and consider placing the patient on ECMO until stabilized, with continued use of amiodarone and epinephrine. Propofol can be considered, but it is a poor alternative, given its hemodynamic effects.[13,14]

THE PATIENT GOES TO THE ICU, INTUBATED AND ON AN AMIODARONE DRIP. HIS ANKLE SURGERY IS RESCHEDULED. IN RETROSPECT, WHAT WOULD YOU HAVE DONE DIFFERENTLY?

You could consider using lower doses of local anesthetic, with incremental dosing and aspiration under the guidance of ultrasound. If a practitioner is not comfortable with the blocks required for a case, general anesthesia with a good postoperative analgesic plan is a viable alternative.[15]

DISCUSSION

HISTORY AND MEDICAL PERTINENCE

Local anesthetics have been used for surgical and medical pain management since 1884.[16] While the benefits of local anesthetics in pain reduction are well known, the widespread use of these drugs has uncovered a multitude of adverse effects,[17–20] primarily due to the vascular uptake of local anesthetics, with subsequent development of toxicity. The toxic states, all part of LAST, include, but are not limited to, respiratory failure, seizures, palpitations, and irregular cardiac function leading to cardiovascular collapse.[19–22] These occurrences are relatively rare, currently estimated to have an incidence ranging from 2.5 to 10 events in every 10,000 blocks. The low incidence is thought to be due to improvements in administration safety.[23,24] Increased awareness by proceduralists of safety steps, the advent of lipid emulsion therapy, and the development of checklists for

Table 43.1. CHARACTERISTICS OF LOCAL ANESTHETICS

DRUG	PKA	PERCENT NONIONIZED AT PHYSIOLOGIC PH	POTENCY*	MAXIMUM DOSE (MG)	DURATION AFTER INFILTATION (MIN)
Procaine	8.9	3	1	500	45–60
Chlorprocaine	8.7	5	2	600	30–60
Tetracaine	8.5	7	8	75	180–600
Lidocaine	7.9	24	2	300	60–120
Mepivacaine	7.6	39	2	300	90–180
Prilocaine	7.9	24	2	400	60–120
Bupivacaine	8.1	17	8	150	240–480
Ropivacaine	8.1	17	6	200	240–480

Original table based on Miller.[59]

* Relative potencies vary based on experimental model or route of administration. Doses are for a 75 kg person and without addition of epinephrine.

treatment should the toxic events occur, all aid in making LAST a rare event and, when it occurs, an event with reduced morbidity and mortality.[24,25]

The mechanism of action of local anesthetics is straightforward: binding of the agent to sodium channels leads to blocking of the excitation threshold in nociceptive afferent neurons.[26,27] Other mechanisms of action of local anesthetics are their effects on decreasing inflammatory mediators and reducing hyperexcitability at the level of the dorsal horn of the spinal cord and brain.[27–29]

Because of the differences in their chemical structures, which dictate solubility, protein binding, and charge status at physiologic pH, each local anesthetic has properties that determine its suitability for various clinical situations[27,30] (Table 43.1).

An understanding of these properties guides the appropriate selection of drug and dose best suited to the patient, procedure, or practice setting, with the ultimate goal of better pain control and good outcomes for patients.

THE ROLE OF LOCAL ANESTHETICS IN ANESTHESIA PRACTICE

As evidenced by current literature and the ongoing prevalence of use, local anesthetics have a prominent role in anesthesia care.

As part of a multimodal perioperative analgesic approach, local anesthetics have a variety of benefits, including improved quality of recovery, decreased risk of chronic postsurgical pain, decreased incidence of postoperative nausea and vomiting, and a decrease in the use of opioids and in their corresponding side effects, as well as a shorter length of hospital stay, potentially leading to decreased overall medical costs.[31,32]

In the field of chronic pain management, local anesthetics frequently provide diagnostic information for ruling in or out various pain generators when applied in discrete volumes.

Additionally, local anesthetics can be delivered through a variety of routes. Commonly used routes of administration include systemic infusions, perineural injections, peri-incisional delivery, intracompartmental and intra-articular injections, localized intravenous (Bier) blocks, and transdermal delivery. The delivery route impacts an anesthetic's risks and benefits; appropriately tailored delivery can be matched to patient needs, with the hope of decreasing the risk of LAST. On the contrary, haphazard administration can lead to failure of pain control, reversible or permanent nerve injury, and toxic systemic effects that cause catastrophic injury, including death.[33]

LAST is the primary limiting factor in the use of local anesthetics.[6,33] Their administration should be optimized by careful evaluation of anatomic site-specific dosing while considering the patient's size, weight, and medical condition. Choosing and understanding the pharmacokinetic profile of each local anesthetic, as well as addition of adjuvants (epinephrine), is essential in reducing the risk of LAST during local anesthetic administration.[5]

Relatively recently, liposomal bupivacaine has been approved for single-dose wound infiltration and administration as a depot local anesthetic. The liposomal form of bupivacaine was developed to provide sustained analgesic concentrations for better control of patients' pain without causing the rapid rise in serum concentration seen with nonliposomal local anesthetics.[34] However, a clear benefit of depot local anesthetics in terms of cost-effectiveness and safety profile, especially when used in conjunction with nonliposomal local anesthetics, has yet to be fully elucidated. Further studies, including the investigation of bupivacaine-impregnated collagen, are currently underway and provide hope for the development of techniques that lead to improved postoperative pain control without the increased risk of LAST.

SIGNS AND SYMPTOMS OF LOCAL ANESTHETIC TOXICITY

The clinician using local anesthetics must understand the pathophysiology of LAST in order to successfully manage a toxicity event. Cardiac collapse is the most profound cause of morbidity and mortality.[5,6,32,33,35] In the majority of cases, it is preceded by CNS toxicity, including a prodrome of anxiety, circumoral numbness, seizures, and loss of consciousness. Although not in the majority of cases, cardiovascular symptoms, such as arrhythmia and cardiac arrest, can occur without prodromal or CNS symptoms.[6,33] Each local anesthetic has its own ratio of cardiovascular to CNS toxicity.[6]

Cardiac toxicity is the primary cause of injury and/or death. There are two proposed mechanisms of cardiac toxicity with local anesthetics: impaired electrophysiologic function of the heart and the loss of cardiac energy at the mitochondrial level. In order to create impaired signal transmission in the heart, local anesthetics bind the voltage-gated sodium channels that the cardiac myocytes rely on to produce the rhythmic depolarization in the cardiac cycle. Blocking this physiologic process can lead to conduction and contractility abnormalities that produce unstable ventricular arrhythmias. Local anesthetics decrease fatty acid transport into the inner mitochondrial membrane, thereby inhibiting energy production by oxidative phosphorylation and functionally starving cardiac myocytes of energy.[6,28,32,33]

CNS toxicity is also a considerable concern with local anesthetic administration. Suggested mechanisms include local anesthetic inhibition of gamma-aminobutyric acid (GABA) and potassium (TASK—Twik-related acid-sensitive K^+ channel) channels, causing neuronal hyperexcitability and instability, leading to the altered sensorium and, ultimately, the induction of seizures.[5,11,12,26,28,32]

In order to effectively treat LAST, timely and proper recognition of its occurrence is crucial. Classically, systemic toxicity begins with prodromal symptoms, such as perioral numbness, tinnitus, and dysgeusia; subsequently, there is progression to CNS hyperexcitabilty and cardiovascular instability (although it is important to note that the findings differ based on the local anesthetic used). In one study, however, it was found that only 60% of cases presented in the classic pattern and that up to 18% of cases presented with only cardiovascular symptoms.[6,32] While the findings arguably could be confounded by the presence of heavy sedation or even general anesthesia, the atypical presentations are important points for clinicians to consider.[35–37]

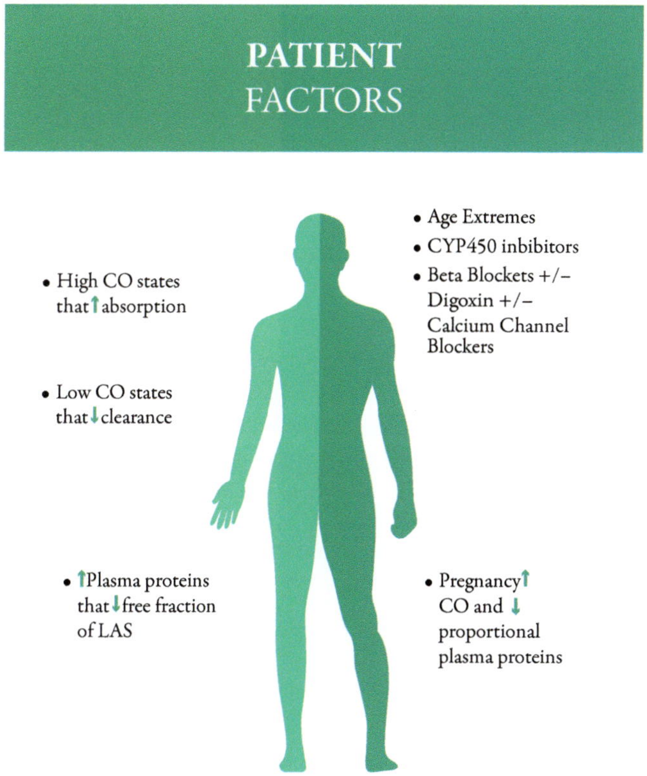

Figure 43.1. Patient characteristics that increase incidence of LAST. Original art based on Neal et al.[1]

PREVENTING LAST

A variety of patient characteristics increase the incidence of LAST. These include, but are not limited to, extremes of age, high-cardiac-output states that increase absorption, low-cardiac-output states that lead to reduced clearance, reduced plasma proteins that increase the free fraction of local anesthetics, pregnancy (with both increased cardiac output and lower proportional plasma proteins), and the concomitant use of beta blockers, digoxin, calcium channel blockers, and cytochrome P450 inhibitors[1] (Figure 43.1).

Besides being able to recognize the onset of LAST, it is also of utmost importance that the anesthesiologist be aware of how technique can reduce its incidence. Technical factors include: limiting the cumulative dose, as dictated by patient factors and drug pharmacokinetics; using ultrasound for catheter and single-shot block placement; test dosing; utilizing incremental injections of local anesthetics; confirmation and interval reconfirmation of negative catheter/needle aspiration; and close adherence to published guidelines regarding LAST prevention and treatment.[1,2,5,38–40] While each of these steps can be helpful in decreasing toxicity, the combined use of several or all of these techniques leads to improved patient safety.

In the outpatient setting, it is equally important to recognize symptoms and presentation of local anesthetic toxicity associated with various commonly performed procedures in chronic pain management. For example, stellate ganglion block can be complicated by vertebral artery injection, which may present as loss of consciousness before the onset of seizures. In addition to being aware of such presentations, the clinician must also be aware of patient and clinical factors that can increase the incidence of these complications. This includes being aware of altered anatomy after surgical procedures, radiation, and trauma (Figure 43.2).

In order to fully explore the safety implications of each of the steps in prevention, it is important to consider each precautionary measure individually.

First, limiting the cumulative dose of local anesthetic drugs reduces the chances of systemic toxicity.[38,39] Because multiple local anesthetics and modes of delivery can be used in a single patient within a procedure, it is crucial to account for additive effects. For example, all incisional injections of local anesthetics by the surgical team need to be discussed with the

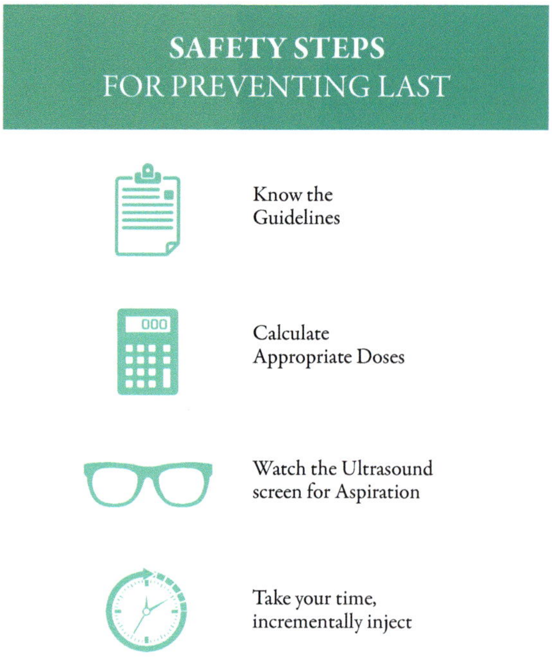

Figure 43.2. Steps for the prevention of LAST. Original art based on References 17, 22, 24, 25, 28, and 29.

Table 43.2. **TEST DOSE AGENTS, AMOUNT, AND EXPECTED RESPONSE AFTER ADMINISTRATION**

TEST DOSE AGENTS	TOTAL DOSE ADMINISTERED/ TEST DOSE ATTEMPT	DIAGNOSTIC PARAMETERS OF INTRAVASCULAR TEST DOSE INJECTION
Epinephrine	15 μg	• HR increase > 10 beats/min • SBP increase > 15 mm Hg • T-wave increase by > 25%
Local anesthetics	• Chlorprocaine/ lidocaine 100 mg • Bupivacaine 25 mg • Ropivacaine 60 mg	• Circumoral numbness • Metallic taste • Auditory changes
Air	2 mL	Audible response of precordial Doppler
Opioids	Fentanyl 100 μg	• Sedation • Decreased respiratory drive
Isoproterenol	3 μg	HR increase > 20 beats/min

Original table based on Wolfe and Butterworth,[29] Du, Chen, and Todorovic,[30] and Pu.[31]

anesthesiologists taking care of the patient, so that overdosing does not occur. Additionally, weight-based dosing has a poor correlation with ultimate serum concentrations and toxicity can occur at lower than expected dosing levels.[3,4,28] Therefore, current ASRA guidelines suggest that the lowest concentration and dose necessary for neuraxial anesthesia be used in each setting, a concept that can readily be applied to other applications of local anesthetics, such as peripheral nerve blocks and catheters.[1] Topical application and tumescent injection of local anesthetics during cosmetic and plastic surgery procedures, such as liposuction, provide a unique challenge to the anesthesiologist, given that these modes of delivery typically require higher weight-based doses of local anesthetics, although historically they have a relatively low incidence of toxicity.[4] Nonetheless, LAST can occur with any administration route and should be considered in every case where these drugs are used.

Despite a paucity of data regarding incremental injection—typically 3 to 5 mL—and catheter aspiration during local anesthetic administration with peripheral nerve blocks and placement of infusion catheters, consensus-based guidelines recommend both of these precautionary measures. Incremental injection and negative catheter aspiration aim to limit the amount of inadvertent intravascular injection that can occur. With frequent aspiration and wait time between incremental injections, the proceduralist allows an appropriate amount of circulatory time between each incremental injection, thus allowing quick identification of LAST symptoms. This is the recommended practice for limiting LAST.[1]

Test dosing for intravascular injection is a common practice for assessing proper placement of local anesthetics in both neuraxial and peripheral nerve block anesthesia.[40] Despite the fact that few studies have identified evidence-based techniques for catheter test dosing, there are various experience-based techniques that are commonly employed. Test dose agents that are co-administered with local anesthetics include epinephrine, air, opioids, and isoproterenol.[40–42] Of these, epinephrine is used most commonly, as its intravascular injection will change the patient's vital signs, namely heart rate and blood pressure, which can alert the clinician to systemic effects of both co-administered drugs (Table 43.2).

The use of ultrasound has become widely accepted as a safety measure for the administration of local anesthetics. Although the use of ultrasound does not preclude the possibility of intravascular injection, the lack of spread of medication on the ultrasound image can alert the anesthesiologists to accidental intravascular injection and can be the impetus for preparing for the consequences of LAST at an earlier time point.[15,43–46] In a similar manner, the use of dye to prevent intravascular injection in fluoro-guided procedures in outpatient pain centers can act as a visual feedback mechanism for spread and action of injected medications.

TREATMENT OF LAST

Despite the safety measures and guidelines used to limit the possibility of LAST, it still occurs. Increased awareness of LAST and its treatment is crucial for the practicing anesthesiologist.[47,48] It is especially important because the treatment of cardiovascular compromise caused by local anesthetic varies significantly from the conventional cardiac arrest algorithm. Specifically, ventilatory support and optimization of oxygenation are of the utmost importance in LAST, because prevention of low oxygen tension and subsequent acidosis from tissue ischemia may attenuate some of the negative consequences of systemic toxicity, such as cardiovascular collapse and seizures.[11,12] When seizures are present, the administration of benzodiazepines or neuromuscular blocking drugs can minimize the acidosis stemming from sustained muscle contraction.[48,49]

When cardiac arrest is present, chest compressions continue to be the mainstay of treatment initiation. However, the dose of epinephrine administered in LAST with cardiovascular compromise is significantly lower than the conventional dosing parameters, < 1 µg/kg, due to the increased incidence of persistent arrhythmias at higher doses. When persistent ventricular arrhythmias do occur, amiodarone is the agent of choice. Other drugs used in conventional cardiac protocols, such as beta blockers and calcium channel blockers, are not recommended in LAST due to their negative inotropic effect. Without appropriate patient improvement with these established measures, cardiopulmonary bypass should be considered, and it is prudent to alert the members of the cardiac team when the first signs of LAST are recognized.[7–9,49,50]

Most importantly, the rapid initiation of lipid emulsion therapy has been shown in multiple studies to prevent or slow the progression of cardiovascular collapse and worsening acidosis.[7,8] Because of this, there is an increased need for clinicians to be well versed in the administration and use of lipid emulsion therapy when using local anesthetics in their clinical practices, including both inpatient and outpatient settings.

Because of the efficacy of lipid emulsion therapy in LAST treatment, it has rapidly been added to resuscitation guidelines internationally. While the exact mechanism of action of lipid emulsion therapy has not been fully established, there are several promising proposed mechanisms. It has been suggested that lipid emulsion therapy acts as a "lipid sink" for the dissociation of local anesthetics from cardiac sodium channels.[51,52] By binding free drug within the circulation, lipid emulsion therapy can promote metabolism and clearance of local anesthetics without allowing them to interfere with important physiologic functions. Additionally, it has been proposed that lipid emulsion therapy can act as a direct source of energy to the inhibited myocardium through the production of mitochondrial adenosine triphosphate. Increased ATP production and triglyceride levels can positively impact myocardial contractility, leading to increased cardiac output and maintenance of systemic cardiovascular tone.[52–55]

While further studies are still underway, the optimal administration of lipid emulsion therapy has been formulated through clinical experience. Current guidelines recommend an initial bolus of lipid emulsion therapy at 1.5 mL/kg, followed by an infusion at 0.25 mL/kg/min. Furthermore, the therapy should be continued for a minimum of 10 minutes after ROSC. It has been shown in several case studies that cardiovascular compromise can recur after the cessation of lipid emulsion therapy.[13] For this reason, it is important to continue to monitor the patient after spontaneous circulation has been reinstated and to have an adequate supply of lipid emulsion therapy at any location where local anesthetics are being administered.[14,56] This is especially important to consider in the outpatient pain clinic setting, where resources are often more limited than in the hospital setting.[10]

While lipid emulsion therapy has rapidly become a mainstay of LAST treatment and has considerable benefits for patients, it nonetheless carries risks associated with administration. Allergic reactions, especially to egg, soy, and peanut cross-reactivity, have been seen with lipid emulsion therapy. Additionally, hyperthermia, pancreatitis, hypercoagulability, antineutrophil reactions, and elevated liver aminotransferases have occurred after lipid emulsion therapy was used.[56,57]

Pertinent to this discussion is the realization that the ability to appropriately recognize patients and situations at risk of LAST is critical for the prevention, recognition, and timely treatment of this emergency. Once these factors are recognized, additional safety measures for increased vigilance and preparedness can be initiated. This includes closer monitoring of patients with exposure to local anesthetics in every part of the perioperative setting or pain clinic, presence of trained personnel and readily available ASRA checklists wherever local anesthetics are being administered, and effective follow-up upon discharge.[1,10,14,58] Because LAST is a rare event, training of anesthesiologists through simulations to provide familiarity with the LAST checklist and through practiced encounters can create safer environments for patients. While no one part of the guidelines is most important, the comprehensive availability of continued awareness, resuscitative equipment, standard monitors, lipid emulsion therapy, and skilled practitioners is integral to safe patient outcomes with local anesthetic use.

CONCLUSION

The underlying mechanism of action of local anesthetics is straightforward: binding of sodium channels leads to blocking of the excitation threshold in nociceptive afferent neurons.

As part of a multimodal analgesic approach, local anesthetics have a variety of benefits, including improved quality of recovery, decreased risk of chronic postsurgical pain, decreased incidence of postoperative nausea and vomiting, a decrease in the use of opioids and their corresponding side effects, and a shorter length of hospital stay, potentially leading to decreased overall medical costs.

Increased awareness by proceduralists of safety steps, the advent of lipid emulsion therapy, and the development of checklists for treatment all aid in making LAST a rare event and, when it occurs, an event with reduced morbidity and mortality.

Cardiac collapse is the most profound cause of morbidity and mortality with LAST. In 60% of cases, hemodynamic instability is preceded by CNS toxicity, including a prodrome of anxiety, circumoral numbness, seizures, and loss of consciousness.

Table 43.3. **LAST TREATMENT SUMMARY**

1. Recognize LAST and call for help

2. Ventilate with 100% oxygen

- mask ventilation followed by intubation

- ACLS with low-dose epinephrine (10–100 μg)

- call for cardiopulmonary bypass back-up

3. Infuse 20% lipid emulsion

- bolus 1.5 mL/kg over 1 minute

- follow with continuous infusion of 0.25 mL/kg/min

- if patient is still unstable, double continuous dose

- continue ACLS, monitor ABGs for acidosis and hypoxia

4. Continued support

- if patient is still unstable, consider initiating cardiopulmonary bypass

- if patient is stabilizing, infuse lipid emulsion for additional 10 minutes and monitor for recurrence

The two proposed mechanisms of cardiac toxicity with local anesthetics are impaired electrophysiologic function of the heart and the loss of cardiac energy at the mitochondrial level.

Suggested mechanisms for neuronal hyperexcitability and instability leading to altered sensorium and seizures include local anesthetic inhibition of GABA and TASK channels.

A variety of patient characteristics increase the incidence of LAST. These include extremes of age, high-cardiac-output states that increase absorption, low-cardiac-output states that lead to reduced clearance, reduced plasma proteins that increase free fraction of local anesthetics, pregnancy, and the concomitant use of beta blockers, digoxin, calcium channel blockers, and cytochrome P450 inhibitors.

Prevention of LAST includes limiting the cumulative dose, using ultrasound for catheter and single-shot block placement, test dosing, utilizing incremental injections of local anesthetics, confirmation and interval reconfirmation of negative catheter aspiration, and close adherence to published guidelines.

A summary of the LAST treatment algorithm is shown in Table 43.3.

REFERENCES

1. Neal JM, Bernards CM, Butterworth JF, et al. ASRA practice advisory on local anesthetic systemic toxicity. *Reg Anesth Pain Med.* 2010;35:152–161.
2. Mulroy MF, Norris MC, Liu SS. Safety steps for epidural injection of local anesthetics: review of the literature and recommendations. *Anesth Analg.* 1997;85:1346–1356.
3. Schoenmakers KP, Vree TB, Nigel TJ, et al. Pharmacokinetics of 450 mg ropivacaine with and without epinephrine for combined femoral and sciatic nerve block in lower extremity surgery: a pilot study. *Br J Clin Pharmacol.* 2012;75(5):1321–1327.
4. Ostad A, Kageyama N, Moy RL. Tumescent anesthesia with a lidocaine dose of 55 mg/kg is safe for liposuction. *Dermatol Surg.* 1996;22:921–927.
5. Neal JM, Barrington MJ, Brull R, et al. The second ASRA practice advisory on neurologic complications associated with regional anesthesia and pain medicine: executive summary 2015. *Reg Anesth Pain Med.* 2015;40(5):401–430. doi:10.1097/AAP.0000000000000286.
6. Di Gregorio G, Neal JM, Rosenquist RW, et al. Clinical presentation of local anesthetic systemic toxicity: a review of published cases, 1979 to 2009. *Reg Anesth Pain Med.* 2010;35(2):181–187.
7. Weinberg G, Vadeboncouer T, Ramaraju GA, Garcia-Amaro MF, Cwik MJ. Pretreatment or resuscitation with a lipid infusion shifts the dose-response to bupivacaine-induced asystole in rats. *Anesthesiology.* 1998;88:1071–1075.
8. Weinberg G, Ripper R, Feinstein DL, Hoffman W. Lipid emulsion infusion rescues dogs from bupivacaine-induced cardiac toxicity. *Reg Anesth Pain Med.* 2003;28:198–202.
9. Rosenblatt MA, Abel M, Fischer GW, Itzkovich CJ, Eisenkraft JB. Successful use of a 20% lipid emulsion to resuscitate a patient after a presumed bupivacaine-related cardiac arrest. *Anesthesiology.* 2006;105:217–218.
10. Neal JM, Mulroy MG, Weinberg GL. American Society of Regional Anesthesia and Pain Medicine checklist for managing local anesthetic systemic toxicity: 2012 version. *Reg Anesth Pain Med.* 2012;37(1):16–18.
11. Moore DC, Crawford RD, Scurlock RD. Severe hypoxia and acidosis following local anesthetic-induced convulsions. *Anesthesiology.* 1980;53(3):259–260.
12. Moore DC, Thompson GE, Crawford RD. Long-acting local anesthetic drugs and convulsions with hypoxia and acidosis. *Anesthesiology.* 1982;56(3)230–232.
13. Marwick PC, Levin AI, Coetzee AR. Recurrence of cardiotoxicity after lipid rescue from bupivacaine-induced cardiac arrest. *Anesth Analg.* 2009;108(4):1344–1346.
14. Association of Anesthetists of Great Britain and Ireland. Intralipid in the management of LA toxicity: guidance from the Association of Anesthetists of Great Britain and Ireland (AAGBI), 2007. http://www.aagbi.org/publications/guide-lines/docs/latoxicity07.pdf.
15. Orebaugh SL, Kentor ML, Williams BA. Adverse outcomes associated with nerve stimulator-guided and ultrasound-guided peripheral nerve blocks by supervised trainees: update of a single-site database. *Reg Anesth Pain Med.* 2012;37:577–582.
16. Bier AKG. Experiments in cocainization of the spinal cord, 1899. In: Faulconer A, Keys TE, trans. *Foundations of Anesthesiology.* Springfield, IL: Charles C Thomas; 1963:854.
17. Adverse reactions with bupivacaine. *FDA Drug Bull.* 1983;13:23.
18. Albright GA. Cardiac arrest following regional anesthesia with etidocaine or bupivacaine. *Anesthesiology.* 1979;51:285–287.
19. Auroy Y, Narchu P, Messiah A, et al. Serious complications related to regional anesthesia: results of a prospective survey in France. *Anesthesiology.* 1997;87:479–486.
20. Auroy Y, Benhamou D, Laurent B, et al. Major complications of regional anesthesia in France. *Anesthesiology.* 2002;97(5):1274–1280.
21. Brown DL, Ransom DM, Hall JA, et al. Regional anesthesia and local anesthetic-induced systemic toxicity: seizure frequency and accompanying cardiovascular changes. *Anesth Analg.* 1995;81:321–328.
22. Barrington MJ, Watts SA, Gledhill SR, et al. Preliminary results of the Australasian regional anaesthesia collaboration. *Reg Anesth Pain Med.* 2009;34(6):534–541.
23. Sites BD, Taenzer AH, Herrick MD, et al. Incidence of local anesthetic systemic toxicity and postoperative neurologic symptoms associated with 12,668 ultrasound-guided nerve blocks: an analysis from a prospective clinical registry. *Reg Anesth Pain Med.* 2012;37:478–412.
24. Zetlaoui PJ, Labbe JP, Benhamou D. Ultrasound guidance for axillary plexus block does not prevent intravascular injection. *Anesthesiology.* 2008;108:761–762.
25. Whiteman DM, Kushins SI. Case report: successful resuscitation with intralipid after marcaine overdose. *Aesthetic Surg J.* 2014;34:738–740.

26. Fukuda K, Nakajima T, Viswanathan PC, Balsar JR. Compound-specific Na+ channel pore conformational changes induced by local anesthetics. *J Physiol.* 2005;564(pt 1):21–31.
27. Ritchie JM, Ritchie B, Greengard P. The active structure of local anesthetics. *Pharmacol Exp Ther.* 1965;150(1):152–159.
28. Butterworth J. Models and mechanisms of local anesthetic cardiac toxicity: a review. *Reg Anesth Pain Med.* 2010;35:167–176.
29. Wolfe JW, Butterworth JF. Local anesthetic systemic toxicity: update on mechanisms and treatment. *Curr Opin Anaesthesiol.* 2011;24:561–566.
30. Du G, Chen X, Todorovic MS, et al. TASK channel deletion reduces sensitivity to local anesthetic-induced seizures. *Anesthesiology.* 2011;115(5):1003–1011.
31. Pu LLQ. The use of a pain pump for optimal postoperative pain management. *Plast Reconstr Surg.* 2006;117:2066–2069.
32. Andreae MH, Andreae DA. Local anaesthetics and regional anaesthesia for preventing chronic pain after surgery. *Cochrane Database Syst Rev.* 2012;10:CD007105.
33. Liu S, Ortolan S, Vizarreta Sandoval M, et al. Cardiac arrest and seizures caused by local anesthetic systemic toxicity after peripheral nerve blocks: should we still fear the reaper? *Reg Anesth Pain Med.* 2015;41.
34. Weller WJ, Azzam MG, Smith RA, Azar FM, Throckmorton TW. Liposomal bupivacaine mixture has similar pain relief and significantly fewer complications at less cost compared to indwelling interscalene catheter in total shoulder arthroplasty. *J Arthroplasty.* 2017;32(11): 3557–3562. doi:10.1016/j.arth.2017.03.017.
35. Copeland SE, Ladd LA, Gu X, Mather LE. The effects of general anesthesia on whole body regional pharmacokinetics of local anesthetics at toxic doses. *Anesth Analg.* 2008;106(5):1440–1449.
36. Tanaka M, Sato M, Kimura T, Nishikawa T. The efficacy of simulated intravascular test dose in sedated patients. *Anesth Analg.* 2001;93:1612–1617.
37. Takahashi S, Tanaka M, Toyooka H. The efficacy of hemodynamic and T-wave criteria for detecting intravascular injection of epinephrine test dose in propofol- anesthetized adults. *Anesth Analg.* 2002;94:717–722.
38. Petrar S, Montemurro T. Total local anesthetic administered is integral to the syndrome of local anesthetic systemic toxicity. *Anesthesiology.* 2014;121(5):1130–1131. doi:10.1097/ALN.0000000000000425.
39. Rosenberg PH, Veering BT, Urmey WF. Maximum recommended doses of local anesthetics: a multifactorial concept. *Reg Anesth Pain Med.* 2004;29:564–575.
40. Norris MC, Ferrenbach D, Dalman H, et al. Does epinephrine improve the diagnostic accuracy of aspiration during labor epidural analgesia? *Anesth Analg.* 1999;88:1073–1076.
41. McCartney CJ, Murphy DB, Iagounova A, Chan VW. Intravenous ropivacaine bolus is a reliable marker of intravascular injection in premedicated healthy volunteers. *Can J Anaesth.* 2003;50:795–800.
42. Leighton BL, Gross JB. Air: an effective indicator of intravenously located epidural catheters. *Anesthesiology.* 1989;71:848–851.
43. Neal JM, Brull R, Horn JL, et al. The second American Society of Regional Anesthesia and Pain Medicine evidence-based medicine assessment of ultrasound-guided regional anesthesia: executive summary. *Reg Anesth Pain Med.* 2016;41(2):181–194.
44. Salinas FV, Hanson NA. Evidence-based medicine for ultrasound-guided regional anesthesia. *Anesthesiol Clin.* 2014;32(4):771–787. doi:10.1016/j.anclin.2014.08.001.
45. Barrington MJ, Kluger R. Ultrasound guidance reduces the risk of local anesthetic systemic toxicity following peripheral nerve block. *Reg Anesth Pain Med.* 2013;38:289–297.
46. Abrahams MS, Axix ME, Fu RF, Horns JL. Ultrasound guidance compared with electrical neurostimulation for peripheral nerve block: a systematic review and metaanalysis of randomized controlled trials. *Br J Anesth.* 2009;102:408–417.
47. Fettiplace MR, Weinberg G. Past, present, and future of lipid resuscitation therapy. *JPEN.* 2015;39(suppl 1):72S–83S. doi:10.1177/0148607115595979.
48. Neal JM. Local anesthetic systemic toxicity: improving patient safety one step at a time. *Reg Anesth Pain Med.* 2013;38(4):259–261.
49. Weinberg GL. Treatment of local anesthetic systemic toxicity (LAST). *Reg Anesth Pain Med.* 2010;35(2):188–193.
50. *Support.* Schaumburg, IL: Committee on Critical Care Medicine, Society of Critical Care Anesthesiologists, and American Society of Anesthesiologists; 2008.
51. Kuo I, Akpa BS. Validity of the lipid sink as a mechanism for the reversal of local anesthetic systemic toxicity: a physiologically based pharmacokinetic model study. *Anesthesiology.* 2013;118(6):1350–1361.
52. Nouette-Gaulain K, Capdevila X, Robin F, Beloeil H. Intravenous lipid emulsion and local anesthetic-induced systemic toxicity: mechanisms and limits. *Ann Fr Anesth Reanim.* 2014;33(6):411–417. doi:10.1016/j.annfar.2014.03.012.
53. Shi K, Zia Y, Wang Q, et al. The effect of lipid emulsion on pharmacokinetics and tissue distribution of bupivacaine in rats. *Anesth Analg.* 2013;116(4):804–809.
54. Coat M, Pennec JP, Guillouet M, Arvieux CC, Gueret G. Haemodynamic effects of intralipid after local anaesthetic intoxication may be due to a direct effect of fatty acids on myocardial voltage-dependent calcium channels. *Ann Fr Anesth Reanim.* 2010;29(9):661.
55. Cave G, Harvey M. Intravenous lipid emulsion as antidote beyond local anesthetic toxicity: a systematic review. *Acad Emerg Med.* 2009;16(9):815–824.
56. Driscoll DF. Lipid injectable emulsions: pharmacopeial and safety issues. *Pharm Res.* 2006;23(9):1959–1969.
57. Cave G, Harvey M, Willers J, et al. LIPAEMIC report: results of clinical use of intravenous lipid emulsion in drug toxicity reported to an online lipid registry. *J Med Toxicol.* 2014;10(2):133–142. doi:10.1007/s13181-013-0375-y.
58. Fencl JL. Local anesthetic systemic toxicity: perioperative implications. *AORN J.* 2015;101(6):697–700. doi:10.1016/j.aorn.2015.03.002.
59. Miller RD. *Miller's Anesthesia.* 7th ed. Philadelphia, PA: Churchill Livingstone/Elsevier; 2010.

REVIEW QUESTIONS

1. Which of the following is the mechanism of action of local anesthetics?

   A. Binding of sodium channels, leading to blocking of the excitation threshold in nociceptive afferent neurons
   B. Increase in inflammatory modulators
   C. Increase in hyperexcitability at the level of the dorsal horn
   D. Increase in excitability at the level of the ventral horn

2. The use of local anesthetics in the multimodal pain control approach leads to:

   A. A potential decrease in the use of opioids
   B. Increased postsurgical chronic pain
   C. Longer hospital stays
   D. Delayed extubation

3. What is the most common cause of morbidity and mortality with LAST?

   A. Uncontrolled seizures
   B. Cardiovascular collapse
   C. Respiratory compromise
   D. Renal failure

ANSWERS

1. A. Local anesthetics work by binding sodium channels, which leads to blocking of the excitation threshold in nociceptive afferent neurons.[26,27] This leads to decreased pain signal transmission to the intracranial and spinal pain-processing centers. Local anesthetics have also been shown to decrease systemic and CNS inflammatory modulators, as well as to decrease hyperexcitability at the level of the dorsal horn.[27–29] Local anesthetics do not act at the level of the ventral horn; instead, the ventral horn governs motor nerve conduction and transmission.

2. A. As part of a multimodal analgesic approach, local anesthetics have a variety of benefits, including improved quality of recovery, decreased risk of chronic postsurgical pain, decreased incidence of postoperative nausea and vomiting, a decrease in the use of opioids and their corresponding side effects, and a shorter length of hospital stay, potentially leading to decreased overall medical costs.[31,32] Through these mechanisms, local anesthetics help mitigate the risk of prolonged intubation due to uncontrolled pain.

3. B. Cardiac collapse is the most profound cause of morbidity and mortality with LAST.[5,6,32,33,35] Uncontrolled seizures due to neuronal hyperexcitability via GABA and TASK channelopathies also occur commonly with LAST.[5,11,12,26,28,30,32] While respiratory compromise can occur with inadequate oxygenation and ventilation, requiring high inspired oxygen levels during LAST, respiratory compromise itself is not a direct presentation of toxicity.[11,12] Renal failure is also not a direct consequence of local anesthetic toxicity, although acute renal injury can occur secondary to prolonged ischemic time from cardiovascular collapse of any etiology.

QUESTIONS AND ANSWERS

This chapter has accompanying questions and answers that are available to subscribers as part of the Oxford eLearning platform. To access the questions, follow the link below, or go to ✔ http://oxfordmedicine.com/painmanagementreview

44.

INTERSCALENE CATHETERS: COMPLICATIONS AND MANAGEMENT

Hassan Aboumerhi and Tariq M. Malik

STEM CASE AND KEY QUESTIONS

A 55-year-old male with chronic obstructive pulmonary disease (COPD) and chronic back pain, for which he takes oxycodone 5 mg three times a day, suffers from right shoulder pain from a rotator cuff tear after playing baseball in the park with his son. His sports medicine orthopedist has scheduled him for an arthroscopic rotator cuff repair in an ambulatory care center. The patient is obese, but has no history of problems with anesthesia during previous surgeries. Pain control after previous surgeries was poor, however, and the patient is concerned about the postsurgical pain.

WHAT TYPE OF PAIN CONTROL WOULD YOU RECOMMEND FOR THIS PATIENT? WHY?

The patient's COPD is well controlled. His lumbar degenerative disk disease causes chronic back pain, managed with oxycodone daily. After discussing various options with the patient, you suggest an interscalene block with catheter placement. You plan to use minimal sedation intraoperatively and to keep the catheter in place for 3 days or more for postprocedure pain relief. The patient agrees to your plan.

WHAT IS THE OPTIMAL TECHNIQUE FOR PLACING AN INTERSCALENE CATHETER IN THIS PATIENT?

The patient is taken to a designated block room, where emergency equipment and drugs are readily available. Standard monitors recommended by the American Society of Anesthesiologists are applied. A catheter is placed under ultrasound guidance using an in-plane needle method. Hydrodissection confirms the needle tip location. Minimal sedation is used for catheter insertion, with 2% lidocaine incrementally until a surgical block is achieved in the C5-C6 distribution. The patient needs 15 mL of 2% lidocaine. After the patient is observed for 15 minutes with no change in cardiopulmonary status, he is transferred to the operating room and is placed in the beach-chair position for surgery. He suddenly feels anxious and tachypneic. His oxygen saturation drops to 93% from 100% on nasal cannula.

HOW DO YOU ASSESS THE PATIENT'S BREATHING COMPLAINT? WHAT IS THE DIFFERENTIAL DIAGNOSIS?

The oxygen rate from the nasal cannula is increased from 2 L/min to 6 L/min. The patient is in no acute distress and his lungs are clear to auscultation bilaterally. Ultrasound examination of the chest rules out pneumothorax. His saturation is stable at 95%. You suspect phrenic nerve dysfunction that does not appear to compromise his respiratory status. You proceed with the surgery, which is uneventful.

THE SURGEON IS CONCERNED ABOUT THE PATIENT AND DECIDES TO KEEP HIM IN THE HOSPITAL OVERNIGHT. HE WANTS TO KNOW IF KEEPING THE CATHETER IN PLACE IS SAFE. WHAT WOULD YOU ADVISE?

The patient is doing well in the recovery area. His surgical dressing is intact and there is no swelling or discoloration at the catheter insertion site. Its marking at the skin is unchanged. Aspiration of the catheter is negative for blood. You keep the catheter in place and set the catheter infusion to 0.125% bupivacaine at 5 mL per hour to avoid phrenic nerve dysfunction.

THE PACU NURSE CALLS YOU CLAIMING THE BLOCK MAY NOT BE WORKING BECAUSE THE PATIENT IS HAVING PAIN ON THE INSIDE OF HIS ARM. HOW DO YOU PROCEED?

In the PACU, the patient's vital signs are stable. He can move his fingers and wrist. His shoulder and the base of his thumb feel numb. You explain to the patient and nurse that the C5 and C6 dermatomes are covered. Movement of fingers is not a sign of block failure. You administer a 5 mL bolus of bupivacaine and increase the infusion rate. You prescribe oral ibuprofen 600 mg for pain. The patient is observed for 30 minutes, after which his pain decreases and he is discharged to the floor.

THE FLOOR NURSE CALLS THE ON-CALL PAIN TEAM RESIDENT BECAUSE THE CATHETER HAS DISCONNECTED FROM THE INFUSION PUMP AND THE PATIENT IS NOW IN PAIN. SHE WANTS YOU TO EVALUATE THE PATIENT BECAUSE SHE DOES NOT KNOW HOW TO RECONNECT THE CATHETER.

You instruct the resident to change the tubing and catheter connector and then reconnect the two. You also instruct the resident to give the patient a 5 mL bolus with 1% lidocaine to activate the catheter before starting the infusion. The patient feels better within 10 minutes. The resident observes the patient for another 5 minutes, and the patient feels comfortable enough to sleep.

THE NURSE CALLS THE RESIDENT EMERGENTLY BECAUSE THE PATIENT IS UNRESPONSIVE.

The patient is unresponsive, hypotensive, bradycardic, and breathing poorly. The infusion is stopped. He is emergently intubated for airway protection and vasopressors are started to support circulation. He is taken to the ICU, where he recovers after 3 hours of care. After a negative cardiac workup, he is extubated without issue and returned to the floor. You instruct the resident to remove the catheter, but it is now stuck. The catheter is left in place.

HOW DO YOU HANDLE A STUCK CATHETER?

The patient is seen in the morning. He has no residual block in the arm. Tugging on the catheter causes shooting pain down his arm. The wire-reinforced catheter is incompatible with MRI. A CT scan of the neck reveals that the catheter tip is close to the neural foramen, but it is not embedded in neuronal tissue. The tip is bent and hooked around a nerve root. You explain the situation to the patient and recommend removing the catheter under fluoroscopic guidance.

THE PATIENT IS TAKEN TO A FLUOROSCOPY SUITE. THE AREA AROUND THE CATHETER IS PREPPED AND DRAPED WITH STERILE TOWELS. ANY SPECIAL CONCERN WHEN REMOVING THE CATHETER?

One more pull on the catheter still causes paresthesias down the arm and you stop manipulation. You anesthetize the skin and soft tissue surrounding the catheter insertion site with local anesthetic. A 2-inch plastic angiocatheter without a needle is threaded over the stuck catheter to loosen up the tissue around the catheter. The angiocatheter is threaded carefully all the way up to the tip of the stuck catheter under fluoroscopic guidance. The catheter is then gently tugged until it slowly slips out with constant gentle traction. After inspection, the catheter tip is found to be intact. Physical examination of the patient reveals no sensory or motor deficit.

DISCUSSION

Orthopedic surgeries are among the most painful postoperatively. Regional anesthesia is superior to other options for pain control perioperatively, and continuous brachial plexus blocks are better than single-shot blocks for pain relief after shoulder surgery. Interscalene catheters are most commonly used to mitigate pain after rotator cuff repair or total shoulder arthroplasty.

For interscalene block and catheter placement, the roots or trunks of the brachial plexus are accessed between the anterior and middle scalene muscles. The catheter is placed just outside the epineurium. Because the space communicates freely with the epidural and prevertebral proximal spaces, many side effects are possible with a block.

Absolute contraindications are infection or malignant tumor at the surgical site, allergy to local anesthetic, or patient refusal. Complications after catheter placement come from anatomic disturbance after needle placement or from the pharmacologic effects of the local anesthetic as it blocks various nerves when it spreads. The sympathetic and phrenic nerves are affected by the block, and if local anesthetic spreads to the epidural space, extensive blockage can be life-threatening. The pharmacologic effects are compounded if the patient has poor functional reserve.

Before an interscalene block and catheter placement are undertaken, the cardiovascular and respiratory reserve of the patient must be assessed. A history of pneumonectomy or preexisting phrenic nerve palsy will tax the pulmonary reserve too much, even if the block is perfectly placed, because the phrenic nerve is paralyzed with every interscalene block.

Diaphragmatic paralysis results in dyspnea and anxiety when the phrenic nerve is paralyzed via direct block or local anesthetic spread. The phrenic nerve originates at C3-C5, with nerves that run through the interscalene groove. The incidence of iatrogenic palsy is 100% after block under fluoroscopic guidance,[1] and 10% of patients experience clinically significant palsy and became dyspneic.[2] Patients with COPD usually do not have the pulmonary reserve to compensate for palsy. The treatment is supportive respiratory care in anticipation of respiratory decompensation. The incidence of phrenic nerve dysfunction can be reduced by diluting the local anesthetic solution, decreasing injection volume, or lowering the site of injection.[3]

Nerve injury results in numbness, paresthesia, or weakness in the ipsilateral arm of the block. There is a 5% to 10% incidence of short-term paresthesias lasting weeks to months.[4] The incidence of continued nerve deficits lasting longer than 6 months is 0.02% to 0.2%.[5] It is unclear whether reported postblock paresthesias are caused by needle trauma, local anesthetic, perioperative positioning, or the surgery itself. If postoperative paresthesia is persistent, follow-up with neurology for electromyogram is recommended.

The early symptoms of local anesthetic systemic toxicity (LAST) are tinnitus and a metallic taste in the mouth. Patients may then develop a sense of impending doom, become unconscious, or experience seizures. Death is possible in extreme cases. LAST may be caused by direct vascular injection into the ipsilateral carotid, vertebral artery, or external jugular, or slow tissue absorption of local anesthetic. The incidence is 0.08%.[6] Standard monitoring and administration of oxygen before beginning the procedure are recommended. Emergency induction medications and airway intubation material should be readily available. Intralipid is administered in the event of a LAST-induced code.

Hoarseness is possible after interscalene block or catheter administration of local anesthetic despite no physical manipulation of the posterior oropharynx or larynx; it occurs due to vasodilation in the laryngeal blood supply or from recurrent laryngeal nerve palsy. The incidence of this complication is 30%.[7] Airway stability must be monitored, because recurrent laryngeal nerve palsy can cause airway obstruction. As with paresthesias, reassure the patient that recovery is likely and schedule follow-up. Most cases of hoarseness after interscalene block resolve spontaneously.

If a patient suffers ipsilateral miosis, ptosis, or anhidrosis after interscalene catheter placement, it may be caused by Horner's syndrome from local anesthetic sympathectomy. The incidence is 50% to 75%.[8] As with hoarseness and paresthesias, the mainstay of treatment is reassurance and observation.

Pneumothorax from pleural trauma is a serious complication, with dyspnea, loss of ipsilateral breath sounds, and hypoxia. Tracheal deviation develops, along with hemodynamic instability. Although the incidence is rare, the consequences can be dire.[9] Ultrasound can rule out pneumothorax intraoperatively. The sensitivity and specificity of ultrasound are better than those of chest X-ray. Proper ultrasound examination requires imaging of the chest at the highest intercostal space, looking for lung movement, which is often described as a "sliding sign" or "comet tail" appearance. On M-mode, a normal lung gives the appearance of a "seashore." Absence of this sign requires immediate chest X-ray to quantify the size of the pneumothorax. Mainstem intubation results in absence of the sliding sign on the contralateral side, even though there is no pneumothorax. Phrenic nerve block can eliminate lung movement, although accessory muscles should mobilize the lungs sufficiently to create the sliding sign. If the sliding sign is absent on ultrasound lung examination, pneumothorax must be ruled out even after an interscalene block.

Epidural or intrathecal injection is another rare, yet serious, complication after interscalene catheter placement. It happens when a needle is inserted toward the spinal cord or when the dural sleeve is punctured.[12] Then the local anesthetic tracks the brachial plexus roots to the epidural space. At the time of placement, it can be recognized immediately or may be found later after catheter migration. Intrathecal injection of a large amount of local anesthetic causes immediate cardiovascular collapse, dyspnea, and bilateral upper extremity weakness. Symptoms may progress to apnea and hemodynamic instability. Treatment is respiratory support or intubation and vasopressors to treat cardiovascular compromise.

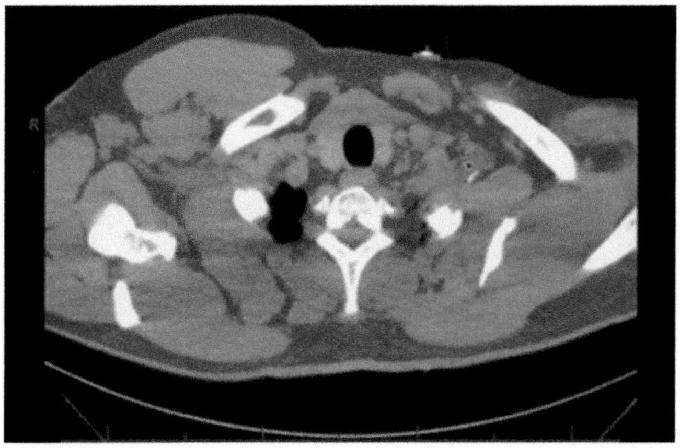

Figure 44.1. Arrow pointing to retained interscalene catheter on CT scan.

Depending on the degree of the block, treatment may range from supportive care and resuscitation to acute critical care of hemodynamic collapse.

A stuck catheter is an uncommon, but real, problem. Published reports of catheters for postsurgical pain control discuss a malpositioned or stuck catheter, but the reports are not comprehensive and complications may be underreported (Figure 44.1).

A catheter should be removed only when the anesthetic effect has worn off. Should catheter removal tug on a nerve, the patient will feel pain. If the patient is in pain, all efforts to pull the catheter are stopped. With MRI-compatible catheters, an MRI rules out abnormal kinking or knotting of the catheter around a nerve. A radiopaque catheter can be removed in a procedure suite under fluoroscopic guidance. The removal requires a sterile technique, numbing of the area around the catheter, and blunt dissection around the catheter using a regular intravenous, angiocath cannula, which is threaded over the catheter. The catheter is mobilized from the surrounding soft tissue for easy removal. If an MRI or CT scan shows that the catheter is knotted around a nerve or plexus, a surgical consult may be warranted (Figure 44.2).

A catheter may get stuck if its tip is bent into a hook shape. This happens when the catheter is threaded against resistance. The metal tip of a nerve-stimulating catheter, for example, can bend during threading to become a hook. If a stylet can be successfully inserted, the tip may be straightened for removal without open exploration. If stylet insertion fails to straighten the tip, a plastic angiocatheter or a dilator from a central line kit can be threaded over the catheter up to the bent tip to help remove it. The most difficult removal is of a catheter that has been placed intraneurally. Tugging on these catheters may cause severe paresthesias. An MRI of the brachial plexus and symptoms of paresthesias confirm intraneural catheter placement. Shearing of a nerve upon tugging can be disastrous and avulsion of the nerve has been reported.[13] If only a minimal part of the catheter is intraneural, its removal can be attempted with careful monitoring. In the procedure suite, the catheter insertion site is prepped and draped. The area around the catheter is numbed using 1% lidocaine. Then using blunt dissection, an 18-G or 16-G intravenous angiocatheter

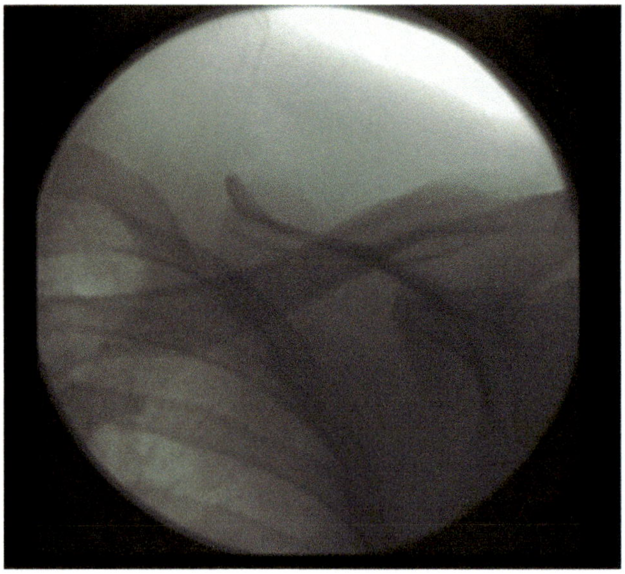

Figure 44.2. Retained interscalene catheter on fluoroscopy.

is threaded over the catheter up to the plexus using ultrasound guidance. The angiocatheter frees the regional catheter from adhesions and stabilizes the plexus, minimizing any stretch of the nerves during tugging while the angiocatheter is held in a fixed position. Gentle persistent traction may help the regional catheter slip out. The key in this maneuver is an awake patient who can complain of pain or paresthesia. No excessive force should be applied. If these maneuvers are unsuccessful, a surgical consult is needed (Figure 44.3).

CONCLUSIONS

Interscalene block is a useful technique for quality perioperative and postoperative pain control with shoulder surgery. As with any procedure, there are multiple risks that must be discussed with the patient before administering the block. A good anesthesia care provider is adaptable and is always prepared. Apply standard monitors and oxygen before beginning the procedure. Have emergency drugs and an airway kit on hand. After the block, as long as local anesthetic is flowing through the catheter, the patient is still subject to complications. Have a low threshold to assess for catheter migration.

In the event of a complication, assess the patient closely for risk of cardiorespiratory decompensation. Be prepared to admit the patient for supportive or acute critical care if needed.

A stuck peripheral nerve catheter is an uncommon, but not a rare, complication. The catheter can be removed without surgical exploration most of the time, but surgical removal should never be discounted.

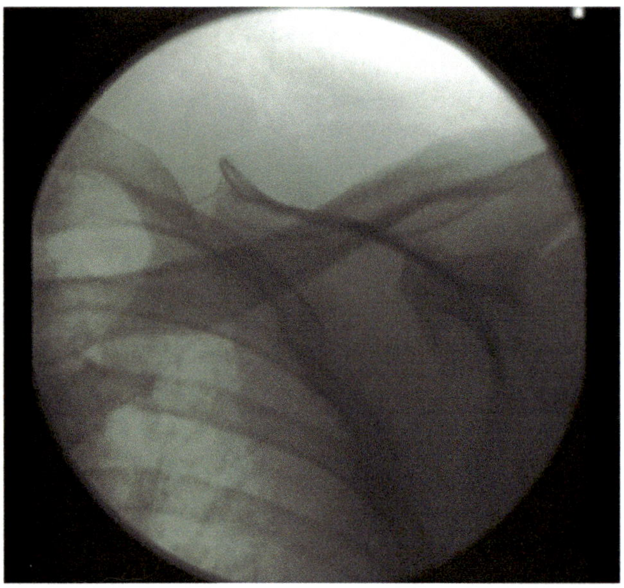

Figure 44.3. Fluoroscopy revealing successful removal of interscalene catheter.

REFERENCES

1. Urmey WF, Talts KH, Sharrock NE. One hundred percent incidence of hemidiaphragmatic paresis associated with interscalene brachial plexus anesthesia as diagnosed by ultrasonography. *Anesth Analg.* 1991;72(4):498–503.
2. Liu SS, Gordon MA, Shaw PM, Wilfred S, Shetty T, Yadeau JT. A prospective clinical registry of ultrasound-guided regional anesthesia for ambulatory shoulder surgery. *Anesth Analg.* 2010;111(3):617–623.
3. Verelst P, van Zundert A. Respiratory impact of analgesic strategies for shoulder surgery. *Reg Anesth Pain Med.* 2013;38(1):50–53.
4. Borgeat A, Ekatodramis G, Kalberer F, Benz C. Acute and nonacute complications associated with interscalene block and shoulder surgery: a prospective study. *Anesthesiology.* 2001;95(4):875–880.
5. Auroy Y, Benhamou D, Bargues L, Ecoffey C, Falissard B, Mercier FJ. Major complications of regional anesthesia in France: the SOS Regional Anesthesia Hotline Service. *Anesthesiology.* 2002;97(5):1274–1280.
6. Sites BD, Taenzer AH, Herrick MD, et al. Incidence of local anesthetic systemic toxicity and postoperative neurologic symptoms associated with 12,668 ultrasound-guided nerve blocks: an analysis from a prospective clinical registry. *Reg Anesth Pain Med.* 2012;37(5):478–482.
7. Liu SS, Gordon MA, Shaw PM, Wilfred S, Shetty T, Yadeau JT. A prospective clinical registry of ultrasound-guided regional anesthesia for ambulatory shoulder surgery. *Anesth Analg.* 2010;111(3):617–623.
8. Vester-Andersen T, Christiansen C, Hansen A, Sørensen M, Meisler C. Interscalene brachial plexus block: area of analgesia, complications and blood concentrations of local anesthetics. *Acta Anaesthesiol Scand.* 1981;25(2):81–84.
9. Graber R, Raghavendra M. Interscalene nerve block. *Medscape.* Available at http://emedicine.medscape.com/article/2000151-overview#showall.

REVIEW QUESTIONS

1. Interscalene blocks are most suitable for which of the following surgeries?

   A. Neck dissection
   B. Shoulder arthroscopy
   C. Brachial arteriovenous fistula placement
   D. Hand surgery

2. You perform an interscalene block on a young, healthy patient in the ambulatory surgical center. She becomes worried

because she feels like she cannot take a deep breath, although her hemodynamics are stable. What is the risk of this event?

A. 10%
B. 25%
C. 50%
D. 100%

3. Given no other respiratory conditions in the patient from the question above except mild intermittent asthma, how would you treat this patient?

A. Emergent intubation
B. Continuous positive airway pressure
C. Bilevel positive airway pressure
D. Reassurance and monitoring

ANSWERS

1. B. Interscalene blocks are suitable for shoulder arthroscopy and total shoulder arthroplasty. The block targets the nerve roots and trunks of C5-C6, which carry the sensory supply from the shoulder joint. The block is placed high in the interscalene region to numb the suprascapular nerve, which comes off the superior trunk of the brachial plexus. An interscalene block is not adequate analgesia for surgery outside the C5-C6 distribution, including surgical manipulation below the mid arm.

2. E. The patient is exhibiting signs of iatrogenic phrenic nerve palsy, which occurs in 100% of interscalene blocks with injection volumes more than 20 mL. The incidence is 20% if the volume of local anesthetic is kept at 5 mL or less and is deposited outside the plexus sheath.

3. D. Given no compromising respiratory issues and stable hemodynamics, a patient with interscalene block phrenic nerve palsy can be reassured and monitored until recovery. The block affects ventilatory capacity by increasing the PCO_2 level, rather than by causing hypoxia, unless the patient has severe lung disease. Respiratory acidosis can affect pulmonary vasculature and precipitate right heart failure. Barring such dramatic compromise, reassurance is all that is needed. Bilevel positive airway pressure and intubation are forms of support used only to treat decompensated hypercapnia.

QUESTIONS AND ANSWERS

This chapter has accompanying questions and answers that are available to subscribers as part of the Oxford eLearning platform. To access the questions, follow the link below, or go to ✔ http://oxfordmedicine.com/painmanagementreview

45.

ACUTE PAIN IN THE OPIOID-TOLERANT PATIENT

Ignacio Badiola, Tulsi Singh, Jiabin Liu, and Nabil Elkassabany

STEM CASE AND KEY QUESTIONS

A 32-year-old male with a history of heroin abuse presents to the emergency department (ED) with a proximal humerus fracture. He has abstained from heroin use for 7 years and is in a methadone maintenance program. He is unsure of his methadone dosage and states his last dose was yesterday morning. He has been evaluated by orthopedics and is scheduled for an open reduction and internal fixation later today. In the ED, he receives 2 mg of IV hydromorphone along with ketorolac 30 mg, but he continues to report 10/10 pain on the numeric rating scale. The ED physicians consult the acute pain service for guidance on how to best manage his pain.

WHAT IS A METHADONE MAINTENANCE PROGRAM (MMP)?

MMPs have been used to treat opioid dependence and addiction since the 1930s. Methadone is a substitute given to treat opioid addiction (due to medical or illicit use) in those who have failed detoxification. Dosing varies greatly and can range from 20 mg to 150 mg (or more) a day. In the acute pain management of a patient enrolled in an MMP, it is important to ascertain the exact dose that is used daily. This may involve contacting the MMP. Knowledge of the exact dose allows the acute pain management clinician to ensure that the patient receives his maintenance methadone (or an equianalgesic opioid) during his acute pain episode. Failure to continue methadone or an equianalgesic opioid may lead to withdrawal and futility in the acute management of the patient's current pain.

ASIDE FROM PHARMACOLOGIC AGENTS TO HELP TREAT HIS ACUTE PAIN, WHAT OTHER OPTION CAN BE INSTITUTED TO HELP MANAGE HIS ACUTE/PERIOPERATIVE PAIN?

Regional anesthesia is an excellent technique that can help with opioid sparing, as well as avoid the adverse effects of higher opioid doses and other adjunct medications. A patient with a proximal humerus fracture may be a good candidate for an interscalene brachial plexus block with placement of a perineural catheter for more prolonged perioperative analgesia.

WHAT IS THE BEST WAY TO MANAGE THIS PATIENT'S OPIOID THERAPY TO TREAT HIS ACUTE PAIN ISSUES?

There are no evidence-based clinical trials of how to best manage acute pain problems in patients who are opioid dependent/tolerant. Providers must obtain a thorough history with exact doses of chronic opioids, as maintaining these opioids (or an equianalgesic opioid) is important. Additionally, higher doses of opioids may be required due to opioid tolerance. Adjuncts, such as nonsteroidal anti-inflammatory drugs (NSAIDs), gabapentanoids, and regional anesthesia techniques, should be used if possible.

BEFORE SURGERY, THE ANESTHESIOLOGIST DECIDES TO PERFORM A FENTANYL CHALLENGE. WHAT IS A FENTANYL CHALLENGE?

A fentanyl challenge is an analgesic modality that can help anesthesiologists with intraoperative and postoperative dosing of opioids in opioid-dependent/tolerant patients. In one study evaluating this modality, chronic opioid-consuming patients received a fentanyl infusion at 2 µg/kg/min until their respiratory rates were < 5 breaths per minute. Once respiratory depression ensued, pharmacokinetic simulation software was used to estimate the effect-site concentration of fentanyl. This information was used to predict the patient-controlled analgesia (PCA) settings that would deliver an effect-site concentration of fentanyl equivalent to 30% of that observed with respiratory depression. This infusion rate was continued intraoperatively and in the postanesthesia care unit (PACU). Postoperatively, the PCA basal infusion was set to 50% of the predicted hourly requirement and the remaining 50% of the hourly analgesic requirement was divided in demand doses every 15 min (up to 4 doses/hr). The basal rate was adjusted according to the patient's demand-dosing requirements. At less than one demand dose an hour, the basal rate was decreased by 20%. If there were more than three demand doses an hour, it was increased by 20%. Out of 18 patients, seven required no PCA adjustments, eight required a single adjustment, and three required more than one adjustment.[1]

DISCUSSION

Opioids are commonly prescribed for both acute and chronic pain. In fact, they are so prevalent that every adult in the United States could own an entire bottle of pills.[2] Twenty percent of patients presenting to a physician's office with noncancer pain will receive a prescription for opioids.[3] In light of these statistics, it is important that those involved in the care of patients with acute pain (almost all medical specialties) be aware of methods to manage this patient population.

While many patients will benefit from opioids, there has also been a significant increase in opioid abuse, misuse, and opioid-related morbidity and mortality.[4] Although this is a major national crisis, less is discussed about the difficulty of managing patients in acute pain who are using opioids for chronic pain conditions or misusing/abusing opioids. Currently, there are no randomized controlled studies available to guide management, and clinicians rely mostly on case reports, institutional practice guidelines, or recommendations from other clinicians who have cared for opioid-tolerant patients.

Methadone is a commonly prescribed opioid agonist with high affinity for mu and delta opioid receptors. It also has activity on serotonergic and *N*-methyl-D-aspartate (NMDA) receptors. In the past, it has been used mostly as maintenance therapy for patients addicted to opiates; however, its use as an agent in chronic opioid therapy (COT) for chronic pain has increased.[5] It is highly lipophilic, is stored in fat, and is slowly released into plasma. Elimination is biphasic, with an alpha phase (8 to 12 hours) and a beta phase (30 to 60 hours), with the alpha phase corresponding to analgesia. The long beta phase prevents withdrawal symptoms. The slow clearance allows for once daily dosing for maintenance.[6] More frequent dosing (i.e., every 6 hours) is typically used for analgesia. Like all opioids, methadone may lead to tolerance, opioid-induced hyperalgesia (OIH), and addiction.

Opioid tolerance occurs in patients who are prescribed opioids for chronic pain (cancer or noncancer) as well as in those who misuse/abuse opioids. Tolerance results in a reduction in drug effect after repeated administration. It can be overcome by increasing the dose.[7] This differs from OIH, which is a state of enhanced sensitization to pain as a result of COT.[8] OIH is unlike opioid tolerance in that increasing the opioid dose does not improve analgesia, and may paradoxically worsen pain. The mechanism of OIH involves NMDA and the central glutaminergic system. NMDA receptors, when inhibited, may prevent OIH. Several studies looking at perioperative use of ketamine (an NMDA antagonist) in patients using long-term opioids for chronic pain have been published. The results have been mixed, with some showing benefit[9,10] and others not.[11] It is difficult to make generalizations on the use of ketamine in these patients because ketamine dose, length of treatment, and timing (i.e., only intraoperative or also postoperative) are unknown.

Managing acute pain in opioid-tolerant patients includes providing adequate analgesia, preventing drug withdrawal, and assisting with social, psychiatric, or behavioral issues.[7] Those unfamiliar with the management of these patients must be aware that patients may have an opioid requirement beyond what the staff is accustomed to prescribing and administering. "Persistently high pain scores as well as misplaced assumptions about 'pain patients' and 'addicts' can hinder assessment and diagnosis."[7]

Whenever possible, non-opioid (i.e., NSAIDs) and nonpharmacologic (i.e., regional anesthesia) modalities should be implemented. The patient's chronic opioid drug, dose, and schedule should be verified by the patient's provider/pharmacy. This dose should be continued throughout the acute pain event, and it should not be assumed to adequately manage the patient's acute pain symptoms, regardless of dosage. During surgery, opioid-tolerant patients have a higher intraoperative opioid need than providers expect, but it is difficult to quantify exactly how much. One suggestion is to wait until the patient is breathing spontaneously, and then up-titrate opioids with a goal respiratory rate of 10 breaths per minute.[7]

Continuous monitoring for opioid-related side effects, including decreased respiratory rate and sedation, is required as much in opioid-tolerant patients as in opioid-naïve patients. Although tolerance to many of these side effects can develop quickly, rapid escalation of doses and boluses for breakthrough pain can still lead to adverse effects and morbidity.

PCA may be useful in this patient population because it gives patients a sense of control and may minimize the risk of underdosing. Staff must continue to review needs frequently, because opioid-tolerant patients will usually require more opioids than what is considered "standard." A retrospective review of 202 patients undergoing various surgical procedures noted that chronic pain patients used a mean of 135.8 mg of morphine equivalents over 24 hours, whereas control patients used 42.8 mg.[12] As noted previously, the patient's baseline opioid should be continued through the acute pain event. PCA can facilitate this by using a basal infusion of the patient's baseline opioid and dose (or if not available, an equivalent dose of a different opioid with a reduction for incomplete cross-tolerance). For example, a patient on 30 mg of sustained-release morphine three times a day is using a total daily morphine dose of 90 mg. One milligram of morphine IV equals 3 mg of morphine orally, and accordingly, this patient will require 30 mg of morphine IV as a baseline. When divided over 24 hours, this equals 1.25 mg/hour as a basal infusion. Bolus dose estimation is more challenging, and most patients will require frequent dose adjustments until a proper bolus dose and time interval are determined. Various models to predict opioid dosing have been proposed, including the fentanyl challenge[1]; however, frequent monitoring of patients and pain assessments are the best guides to therapy.

In conclusion, managing acute pain in opioid-tolerant patients presents a significant challenge because there is a profound lack of research to help guide therapy. Staff caring for these patients must obtain a detailed history of the patient's prior opioid use and employ a multimodal therapy regimen, with the use of adjunct medications (i.e., NSAIDs, gabapentanoids), as well as regional anesthetic techniques when appropriate.

CONCLUSIONS

- Acute pain management in opioid-tolerant/dependent patients is a growing concern in the United States due to increasing numbers of patients utilizing opioids for legitimate medical reasons and illicit reasons.
- No clinical trials are available on how to best manage patients with acute pain issues who are opioid-dependent/tolerant.
- It is imperative that clinicians caring for these patients note the exact type and dose of opioid being utilized by the patient prior to the inciting event.
- The patient's baseline opioid (or equianalgesic opioid) and opioid dose should be continued through the acute pain episode and should not be assumed to provide sufficient analgesia, regardless of dose.
- A multimodal approach to pain management should be instituted, including adjunct medications (i.e., NSAIDs, gabapentanoids) and regional anesthesia when appropriate

REFERENCES

1. Davis JJ, Swenson JD, Hall RH, et al. Preoperative "fentanyl challenge" as a tool to estimate postoperative opioid dosing in chronic opioid-consuming patients. *Anesth Analg*. 2005;101:389–395.
2. Paulozzi LJ, Mack KA, Hockenberry JM, Centers for Disease Control and Prevention, National Center for Injury Prevention, Division of Unintentional Injury Prevention. Vital signs: variation among states in prescribing of opioid pain relievers and benzodiazepines—United States, 2012. *MMWR*. 2014;63:563–568.
3. Daubresse M, Chang HY, Yu Y, et al. Ambulatory diagnosis and treatment of nonmalignant pain in the United States, 2000–2010. *Med Care*. 2013;51:870–878.
4. Cheatle MD. Prescription opioid misuse, abuse, morbidity, and mortality: balancing effective pain management and safety. *Pain Med*. 2015;16(suppl 1):S3–S8.
5. Kuehn BM. Methadone overdose deaths rise with increased prescribing for pain. *JAMA*. 2012;308:749–750.
6. Singh N FS, Tokarz K. Methadone for chronic pain. In: Deer TR, Leong MS, Buvanendran A, Gordin V, Kim PS, Panchal SJ, Ray AL, eds. *Comprehensive Treatment of Chronic Pain by Medical, Interventional and Integrative Approaches*. New York, NY: Springer; 2013:145–150.
7. Huxtable CA, Roberts LJ, Somogyi AA, MacIntyre PE. Acute pain management in opioid-tolerant patients: a growing challenge. *Anaesth Intensive Care*. 2011;39:804–823.
8. Yi P, Pryzbylkowski P. Opioid induced hyperalgesia. *Pain Med*. 2015;16(suppl 1):S32–S36.
9. Urban MK, Ya Deau JT, Wukovits B, Lipnitsky JY. Ketamine as an adjunct to postoperative pain management in opioid tolerant patients after spinal fusions: a prospective randomized trial. *HSS J*. 2008;4:62–65.
10. Loftus RW, Yeager MP, Clark JA, et al. Intraoperative ketamine reduces perioperative opiate consumption in opiate-dependent patients with chronic back pain undergoing back surgery. *Anesthesiology*. 2010;113:639–646.
11. Subramaniam K, Akhouri V, Glazer PA, et al. Intra- and postoperative very low dose intravenous ketamine infusion does not increase pain relief after major spine surgery in patients with preoperative narcotic analgesic intake. *Pain Med*. 2011;12:1276–1283.
12. Rapp SE, Ready LB, Nessly ML. Acute pain management in patients with prior opioid consumption: a case-controlled retrospective review. *Pain*. 1995;61:195–201.
13. Mahathanaruk M, Hitt J, de Leon Casasola OA. Perioperative management of the opioid tolerant patient for orthopedic surgery. *Anesthesiol Clin*. 2014;32:923–932.
14. Alford DP, Compton P, Samet JH. Acute pain management for patients receiving maintenance methadone or buprenorphine therapy. *Ann Intern Med*. 2006;144:127–134.

REVIEW QUESTIONS

1. A 32-year-old female with a history of fibromyalgia presents to the emergency department complaining of pain uncontrolled on her current opioid regimen. You suspect this patient has opioid dependence. Which of the following is a sign of dependence?

   A. Development of withdrawal symptoms with dose reductions, irritability, and weakness
   B. An obsession with taking psychotropic substances, sacrificing hobbies for further drug consumption, as well as irritability
   C. Sacrificing hobbies for further drug consumption, weakness, and development of withdrawal symptoms with dose reduction
   D. Development of withdrawal symptoms with dose reductions, an obsession with taking psychotropic substances, and sacrificing hobbies for further drug consumption

2. A 57-year-old male with a history of L4-L5 radiculopathy on COT has just undergone left hip replacement, and he is now complaining of increased pain unrelieved with oxycodone on postoperative day 2. Which of the following is not an effective treatment for OIH?

   A. Transdermal fentanyl
   B. Ketamine
   C. Clonidine
   D. COX inhibitors

3. What is the mechanism responsible for OIH?

   A. Upregulation of NMDA receptors leading to increased release of excitatory neurotransmitters
   B. Downregulation of NMDA receptors leading to increased release of excitatory neurotransmitters
   C. Upregulation of NMDA receptors leading to increased release of inhibitory neurotransmitters
   D. Downregulation of NMDA receptors leading to increased release of inhibitory neurotransmitters

ANSWERS

1. D. According to the 10th revision of the *International Statistical Classification of Diseases and Related Health Problems* (ICD-10), dependence is defined by the presence of three or more of the following criteria simultaneously within the last year: Inability to control the amount of drug taking (including initiation and quitting), signs of tolerance, continued drug consumption in spite of unwanted consequences, development of withdrawal symptoms with dose reductions, an obsession with taking psychotropic substances, and sacrificing hobbies for further drug consumption. Answer D encompasses the last three signs; therefore, it is correct.

2. A. All opioids cause a dose-dependent reduction in the pain threshold. Ketamine reduces this effect when given simultaneously with opioids. Clonidine reduces noradrenaline release presynaptically. COX inhibitors decrease spinal excitatory neurotransmitter release while acting synergistically with NMDA receptor antagonists. Pain is paradoxically worsened by opioids in OIH.

3. A. Hyperalgesia occurs due to activation of the NMDA system and increased release of excitatory neurotransmitters. NMDA receptors are increased, leading to a decrease in opioid receptors, decreasing the effect of opioid medications.

QUESTIONS AND ANSWERS

This chapter has accompanying questions and answers that are available to subscribers as part of the Oxford eLearning platform. To access the questions, follow the link below, or go to
✔ http://oxfordmedicine.com/painmanagementreview

46.

ANTICOAGULATION IN REGIONAL ANESTHESIA

Issam A. Mardini, Jiabin Liu, and Nabil Elkassabany

STEM CASE AND KEY QUESTIONS

A 57-year-old man presents to the surgical suite for elective bilateral total knee arthroplasty (TKA). The patient has a history of atrial fibrillation and has been maintained on dabigatran (Pradaxa) for 3 months. The patient had coronary angioplasty with placement of a drug-eluting stent (DES) about 9 months ago and was maintained on clopidogrel (Plavix) and aspirin after the procedure. Clopidogrel was discontinued after 6 months of dual antiplatelet therapy (DAPT), when dabigatran was initiated due to the onset of atrial fibrillation. Aspirin has been continued at 81 mg orally daily.

In preparation for his planned bilateral knee surgeries, dabigatran was stopped 5 days before the scheduled surgery and the patient has been maintained on subcutaneous enoxaparin (Lovenox) 40 mg once daily instead. The last dose was administered at 6 pm the night before the surgery. The consensus among your anesthesia group is to offer spinal anesthesia for primary unilateral TKA and combined spinal epidural (CSE) techniques for bilateral cases. Either femoral nerve or adductor canal block is routinely offered as part of the postoperative analgesia regimen.

WHAT ARE THE RISKS ASSOCIATED WITH DABIGATRAN USE FOR PATIENTS SCHEDULED TO RECEIVE REGIONAL ANESTHESIA? DOES DISCONTINUATION OF DABIGATRAN 5 DAYS BEFORE SURGERY SUFFICE TO ELIMINATE THE RISKS?

Dabigatran (Pradaxa) is a direct inhibitor of thrombin that is available as an oral prodrug dabigatran etexilate mesylate, which is rapidly converted to dabigatran in the body, with a peak onset of action of 2 hours. The half-life is 12 to 14 hours, with a predictable anticoagulant response that does not require routine coagulation monitoring. The drug has been approved by the Food and Drug Administration (FDA) since 2010 for prevention of stroke[1] and systemic blood clots in patients with atrial fibrillation, as well as for treatment and prevention of deep venous thrombosis (DVT) and pulmonary embolism. Dabigatran is associated with a significantly increased risk of bleeding and the drug had no antidote for emergency situations until October 2015 when the FDA approved idarucizumab (Praxbind). The reversal is achieved 4 hours after administration of Praxbind intravenously.[2,3] Prior to the availability of the specific reversal agent, the interval recommended by ASRA for discontinuation of dabigatran was 5 days before routine neuraxial and other regional anesthesia procedures. The use of antidote or withholding dabigatran for 5 days may be associated with significantly increased risk of clot formation and therefore higher risk of stroke in atrial fibrillation patients.

The ASRA guidelines published as a draft in 2015 recommended 5 days of discontinuation of dabigatran prior to neuraxial procedures. The recommendation was based on exceeding five times the half-life of dabigatran, which is in the range of 12 to 14 hours, and the same principle was adopted for the European and Scandinavian guidelines.[4,5] According to the Scandinavian guidelines, dabigatran may be resumed about 8 hours after removal of an epidural catheter.[4]

ASPIRIN HAS NOT BEEN STOPPED UNTIL THE NIGHT BEFORE SURGERY. WHAT ARE THE RISKS ASSOCIATED WITH NONSTEROIDAL ANTI-INFLAMMATORY DRUGS (NSAIDS) AND ASPIRIN IN PARTICULAR FOR A PATIENT UNDERGOING REGIONAL ANESTHESIA?

ASRA guidelines have consistently indicated no evidence of increased risk of spinal hematoma with the use of NSAIDs, including aspirin. Aspirin irreversibly inactivates cyclooxygenase (COX) in platelets, which blocks their thromboxane pathway and results in inhibition of platelet aggregation. Aspirin has higher affinity for cyclooxygenase-1 (COX-1), which is the constitutive enzyme in multiple cellular functions in the body, including in platelets. The affected platelets will continue to have blockade of their COX pathway for their life cycle, which averages 7 to 10 days. COX blockade by all other NSAIDs is mediated via competitive binding.[6,7] The half-life of the different commonly used NSAIDs is variable and ranges from 1 to 2 hours to 1 to 2 days.[6,7]

Aspirin has been in wide use for primary or secondary prevention of cardiovascular events. The risk of cardiac complications or stroke when a patient is ordered to discontinue aspirin prior to a procedure may be high, so the decision has to be made very carefully.

The risk of spinal hematoma is almost impossible to define when multiple agents are used that interfere with hemostasis through different mechanisms (e.g., platelet aggregation, thrombin inhibition, or LMWH). ASRA guidelines suggest taking extra caution when multiple agents that disturb hemostasis are used in a patient. The decision to proceed with a regional technique should be taken on a case-by-case basis, assessing risks and benefit for each individual patient.

CLOPIDOGREL MAY NEED TO BE RESTARTED (PATIENT DEVELOPED NEW ANGINA 3 DAYS POSTOPERATIVELY THAT REQUIRES A NEW STENT). WHAT ARE THE RISKS OF CLOPIDOGREL FOR A PATIENT UNDERGOING REGIONAL ANESTHESIA?

Clopidogrel is a direct platelet inhibitor (P2Y12 receptor inhibitor) that is frequently used among cardiac patients. The current cardiology recommendation[8,9] is to continue DAPT (i.e., clopidogrel and aspirin) for at least 6 months after placement of a DES. The DES in the coronaries may pose a significant reclotting risk with potential myocardial infarction if platelet inhibition is interrupted.[8,9]

ASRA guidelines recommend 5 to 7 days of discontinuation of clopidogrel prior to a neuraxial procedure.[10] ASRA recommends avoiding restarting clopidogrel after procedures involving placement of catheters in general. If a single-shot spinal or nerve block is done, it is recommended that clopidogrel be delayed for 2 to 6 hours after the procedure.[10] The same delay is recommended after removal of an epidural catheter.

The same guidelines from ASRA pertaining to neuraxial anesthesia are recommended for peripheral nerve blocks (PNBs). Nevertheless, the risks of bleeding in PNBs may be outweighed by the benefit achieved from a more effective regional analgesia versus the use of systemic opioid therapy. The balance of risks and benefits has to be evaluated on an individual basis.

ENOXAPARIN WAS ADMINISTERED 12 HOURS BEFORE SURGERY. IS THIS A SAFE INTERVAL BEFORE PERFORMANCE OF A REGIONAL ANESTHESIA TECHNIQUE? WHAT ARE THE RISKS FOR EPIDURAL ANESTHESIA OR SPINAL ANESTHESIA VERSUS BILATERAL FEMORAL NERVE BLOCKS?

Enoxaparin is a low-molecular-weight heparin (LMWH) that became available in the 1990s. Enoxaparin binds to and accelerates the activity of antithrombin III.[11] The advantage of this drug includes sustained benefit by subcutaneous injection that can provide prophylactic or therapeutic anticoagulation without the need for an infusion or regular laboratory blood work.[11] The introduction of this medication in the 1990s was associated with an increased incidence of spinal hematomas, which prompted the FDA to add a black box warning to Lovenox[12] warning practitioners of the increased risk of spinal hematoma in patients receiving enoxaparin or other LMWH drugs.

The current ASRA guidelines recommend delaying neuraxial needle placement at least 12 hours after the last LMWH dose if the patient is on a prophylactic once-daily regimen.[10] The recommended interval when using higher doses of enoxaparin or with dalteparin (Fragmin) is 24 hours before any neuraxial needle placement.[10] It is also recommended that at least 24 hours' delay be observed before any subsequent dosing of LMWH postoperatively.[10]

If an epidural catheter or peripheral nerve catheter is inserted, no LMWH should be given while the catheter is in place.[10] The interval between removal of the catheter and subsequent dosing of LMWH has been updated recently by the FDA[12] to 4 hours, based on information provided to the FDA by the manufacturer of Lovenox, Sanofi-Aventis. Subsequently, ASRA has adopted the same interval recommendation of 4 hours after catheter removal.[10]

DISCUSSION

TKA lends itself to multiple options for anesthesia and postoperative analgesia. The surgery may be performed under spinal anesthesia, epidural anesthesia, CSE, or general anesthesia. Epidural analgesia and bilateral femoral or adductor canal blocks are some of the options that may be utilized in the postoperative pain management protocol. Recent literature suggests that regional anesthesia may offer some advantages over general anesthesia.[13,14] PNBs have also been shown to be more effective and to reduce opioid use and its associated side effects in the immediate postoperative period.[15]

A complex anticoagulation history provides a unique opportunity to discuss the risks and limitations of regional techniques with patients. The discussion should include consideration of available recommendations from the FDA as well as guidelines formulated by ASRA and other professional societies regarding use of anticoagulants in relationship to regional anesthesia and analgesia.

It has to be noted that the risk of spinal hematoma has to be weighed against the presumed benefits of regional anesthesia in each individual patient. Clinical judgment has to be exercised and should guide clinical decision-making. Strictly adhering to the guidelines decreases the risk of bleeding complications but does not eliminate this risk. The guidelines seem to be a little unclear about bleeding risks in patients using anticoagulants and undergoing PNBs. Perceived benefits of the given block, its location (superficial versus deep), and consequences of bleeding in the given block location should be considered. The guidelines are similar for deeper blocks and neuraxial techniques; however, they allow more room for clinical judgment if the block is in a more compressible location.

Some authors challenged the recommendation to consider an INR (international normalized ratio) of >1.4

unsafe for removal of an epidural catheter based on correlation with the level of factor VII and its activity in patients receiving warfarin therapy.[16] Similarly, Chelly et al. have also challenged recommendations against removal of lumbar plexus catheters in patients with an INR > 1.4.[17] Other studies have demonstrated the safety of PNBs in patients receiving thrombophylaxis in different settings.[18,19] In summary, ASRA guidelines are considered by some groups to err on the side of caution, especially pertaining to PNBs, without taking into account their potential benefits over alternative therapies.[20] In 2015, ASRA published guidelines that were geared specifically toward interventional pain and spine procedures.[21] The European Society of Anesthesiology also published its recommendation to guide the practice of regional anesthesia in patients receiving antithrombotic agents.[5] In collaboration with Vanderbilt University, ASRA created a smart phone application (app) to be a decision support tool for the published guidelines. The app provides a mechanism for rapidly disseminating guidelines and facilitates distribution of frequent updates.[22]

CONCLUSIONS

- The ASRA guidelines represent the best available evidence and the collective experience of experts in the field of regional anesthesia and anticoagulation. Adherence to the guidelines does not guarantee safety against bleeding complications. Risks and benefits of regional anesthesia have to be assessed individually.
- Dabigatran and other new oral anticoagulants provide an attractive option for patients with atrial fibrillation for prevention of stroke and cardiovascular events. The recommended interval of discontinuation of these drugs is five times the known half-life of the agents. This interval is approximately 5 days for dabigatran.
- Use of aspirin and other NSAIDs has not been shown to be associated with increased risk of spinal hematomas in patients undergoing neuraxial blocks. Although NSAIDs other than aspirin that are usually used for arthritis symptoms may be discontinued preoperatively, aspirin may need to be continued in many patients in the perioperative period due to its important role for secondary prevention of cardiovascular events. The risk from using multiple agents that might interfere with hemostasis cannot be defined.
- Direct platelet inhibitors, such as clopidogrel, pose a significant risk for bleeding in the perioperative period and should be discontinued at least 7 days prior to placement of neuraxial blocks.
- LMWH provides anticoagulation in many patients, especially as a bridge to other agents before surgery. Waiting 12 hours after the last prophylactic dose of enoxaparin, or 24 hours after higher doses of enoxaparin, is considered safe for performance of neuraxial or other regional anesthesia blocks. If a catheter is placed epidurally or perineurally, the use of LMWH is not recommended while the catheter is in place. After removal of an epidural catheter, subsequent dosing of enoxaparin should be delayed for 4 hours.

REFERENCES

1. Connolly SJ, Ezekowitz MD, Yusuf S, et al. Dabigatran versus warfarin in patients with atrial fibrillation. *N Engl J Med*. 2009;361(12):1139–1151. doi:10.1056/NEJMoa0905561.
2. Pollack CV Jr, Reilly PA, Bernstein R, et al. Design and rationale for RE-VERSE AD: a phase 3 study of idarucizumab, a specific reversal agent for dabigatran. *Thromb Haemost*. 2015;114(1):198–205. doi:10.1160/TH15-03-0192.
3. Pollack CV Jr, Reilly PA, Eikelboom J, et al. Idarucizumab for dabigatran reversal. *N Engl J Med*. 2015;373(6):511–520. doi:10.1056/NEJMoa1502000.
4. Breivik H, Bang U, Jalonen J, Vigfusson G, Alahuhta S, Lagerkranser M. Nordic guidelines for neuraxial blocks in disturbed haemostasis from the Scandinavian Society of Anaesthesiology and Intensive Care Medicine. *Acta Anaesthesiol Scand*. 2010;54(1):16–41. doi:10.1111/j.1399-6576.2009.02089.x.
5. Gogarten W, Vandermeulen E, Van Aken H, et al. Regional anaesthesia and antithrombotic agents: recommendations of the European Society of Anaesthesiology. *Eur J Anaesthesiol*. 2010;27(12):999–1015. doi:10.1097/EJA.0b013e32833f6f6f.
6. Brune K. Persistence of NSAIDs at effect sites and rapid disappearance from side-effect compartments contributes to tolerability. *Curr Med Res Opin*. 2007;23(12):2985–2995. doi:10.1185/030079907X242584.
7. Brune K, Furst DE. Combining enzyme specificity and tissue selectivity of cyclooxygenase inhibitors: towards better tolerability? *Rheumatology (Oxford)*. 2007;46(6):911–919. doi:10.1093/rheumatology/kem070.
8. Levine GN, Jeong YH, Goto S, et al. World Heart Federation expert consensus statement on antiplatelet therapy in East Asian patients with ACS or undergoing PCI. *Glob Heart*. 2014;9(4):457–467. doi:10.1016/j.gheart.2014.08.001.
9. Levine GN, Jeong YH, Goto S, et al. Expert consensus document: World Heart Federation expert consensus statement on antiplatelet therapy in East Asian patients with ACS or undergoing PCI. *Nat Rev Cardiol*. 2014;11(10):597–606. doi:10.1038/nrcardio.2014.104.
10. Horlocker TT, Wedel DJ, Rowlingson JC, et al. Regional anesthesia in the patient receiving antithrombotic or thrombolytic therapy: American Society of Regional Anesthesia and Pain Medicine evidence-based guidelines (third edition). *Reg Anesth Pain Med*. 2010;35(1):64–101.
11. Turpie AG, Levine MN, Hirsh J, et al. A randomized controlled trial of a low-molecular-weight heparin (enoxaparin) to prevent deep-vein thrombosis in patients undergoing elective hip surgery. *N Engl J Med*. 1986;315(15):925–929. doi:10.1056/NEJM198610093151503.
12. Food and Drug Administration. *Updated recommendations to decrease risk of spinal column bleeding and paralysis in patients on low molecular weight heparins*. Available from https://www.fda.gov/downloads/Drugs/DrugSafety/UCM373735.pdf.
13. Memtsoudis SG, Sun X, Chiu YL, et al. Perioperative comparative effectiveness of anesthetic technique in orthopedic patients. *Anesthesiology*. 2013;118(5):1046–1058. doi:10.1097/ALN.0b013e318286061d.

14. Liu J, Ma C, Elkassabany N, Fleisher LA, Neuman MD. Neuraxial anesthesia decreases postoperative systemic infection risk compared with general anesthesia in knee arthroplasty. *Anesth Analg.* 2013;117(4):1010–1016. doi:10.1213/ANE.0b013e3182a1bf1c.
15. Memtsoudis SG, Poeran J, Cozowicz C, Zubizarreta N, Ozbek U, Mazumdar M. The impact of peripheral nerve blocks on perioperative outcome in hip and knee arthroplasty—a population-based study. *Pain.* 2016;157(10):2341–2349. doi:10.1097/j.pain.0000000000000654.
16. Benzon HT, Avram MJ, Benzon HA, Kirby-Nolan M, Nader A. Factor VII levels and international normalized ratios in the early phase of warfarin therapy. *Anesthesiology.* 2010;112(2):298–304. doi:10.1097/ALN.0b013e3181ca6cfc.
17. Chelly JE, Szczodry DM, Neumann KJ. International normalized ratio and prothrombin time values before the removal of a lumbar plexus catheter in patients receiving warfarin after total hip replacement. *Br J Anaesth.* 2008;101(2):250–254. doi:10.1093/bja/aen132.
18. Chelly JE, Schilling D. Thromboprophylaxis and peripheral nerve blocks in patients undergoing joint arthroplasty. *J Arthroplasty.* 2008;23(3):350–354. doi:10.1016/j.arth.2007.05.045.
19. Buckenmaier CC III, Shields CH, Auton AA, et al. Continuous peripheral nerve block in combat casualties receiving low-molecular weight heparin. *Br J Anaesth.* 2006;97(6):874–877. doi:10.1093/bja/ael269.
20. Chelly JE. The most recent recommendations for "deep blocks" and thromboprophylaxis: evidence not supporting a "thromboprophylaxis therapeutic window." *Reg Anesth Pain Med.* 2010;35(4):402, author reply 403. doi:10.1097/AAP.0b013e3181e861a6.
21. Narouze S, Benzon HT, Provenzano DA, et al. Interventional spine and pain procedures in patients on antiplatelet and anticoagulant medications: guidelines from the American Society of Regional Anesthesia and Pain Medicine, the European Society of Regional Anaesthesia and Pain Therapy, the American Academy of Pain Medicine, the International Neuromodulation Society, the North American Neuromodulation Society, and the World Institute of Pain. *Reg Anesth Pain Med.* 2015;40(3):182–212. doi:10.1097/AAP.0000000000000223.
22. Gupta RK, McEvoy MD. Initial experience of the American Society of Regional Anesthesia and Pain Medicine Coags regional smartphone application: a novel report of global distribution and clinical usage of an electronic decision support tool to enhance guideline use. *Reg Anesth Pain Med.* 2016;41(3):334–338. doi:10.1097/AAP.0000000000000391.

REVIEW QUESTIONS

1. What is the current recommendation on discontinuing dabigatran before placing a PNB?

   A. hours before surgery
   B. 3 days before surgery
   C. 5 days before surgery
   D. There is no need to withhold dabigatran for superficial PNB.

2. What is the current recommendation on withholding clopidogrel before elective surgery in a patient with a DES placement who is scheduled for neuraxial anesthesia?

   A. to 7 days, 3 months after DES placement
   B. to 7 days, 6 months after DES placement
   C. 7 days, 9 months after DES placement
   D. 7 days, 12 months after DES placement

3. Which of the following statements is/are correct?

   A. Prophylactic dose of enoxaparin should be withheld 8 hours before regional anesthesia.
   B. Therapeutic twice-daily dose of enoxaparin should be withheld 24 hours before regional anesthesia.
   C. Enoxaparin can be administered with an existing epidural catheter.
   D. Enoxaparin should be administered no less than 2 hours after epidural catheter removal.

ANSWERS

1. C. The current ASRA guideline recommends withholding dabigatran 5 days, based on the reported half-life of 12 to 14 hours.

2. B. Clopidogrel is a direct platelet inhibitor (P2Y12 receptor inhibitor) that is frequently used among cardiac patients. The ASRA guideline recommends withholding clopidogrel 5 to 7 days before performing neuraxial anesthesia. The 2016 updated cardiology recommendation was revised to state that elective surgery could be considered after 6 months of DAPT.

3. B. Enoxaparin is a LMWH. Per ASRA guidelines, it is held 12 hours (prophylactic) and 24 hours (therapeutic) before neuraxial needle placement. It should not be administered with a catheter in place and should be restarted 4 hours (per FDA recommendations) after catheter removal.

QUESTIONS AND ANSWERS

This chapter has accompanying questions and answers that are available to subscribers as part of the Oxford eLearning platform. To access the questions, follow the link below, or go to ✔ http://oxfordmedicine.com/painmanagementreview

INDEX

Note: Page numbers followed by *b*, *f*, and *t* indicate a box, figure, and table.